Metabolites as Signals in Immunity and Inflammation

Developments in Immunology Series

Metabolites as Signals in Immunity and Inflammation

Edited by

Tristram A.J. Ryan
Harvard Medical School, and Division of Immunology, Division of Gastroenterology, Boston Children's Hospital, Boston, MA, United States

Luke A.J. O'Neill
Trinity College Dublin, School of Biochemistry and Immunology, Dublin, Ireland

Zbigniew Zasłona
Molecure SA, Warsaw, Poland

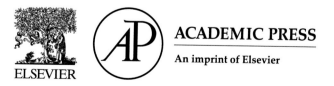

Academic Press is an imprint of Elsevier
125 London Wall, London EC2Y 5AS, United Kingdom
525 B Street, Suite 1650, San Diego, CA 92101, United States
50 Hampshire Street, 5th Floor, Cambridge, MA 02139, United States

Copyright © 2025 Elsevier Inc. All rights are reserved, including those for text and data mining, AI training, and similar technologies.

For accessibility purposes, images in electronic versions of this book are accompanied by alt text descriptions provided by Elsevier. For more information, see https://www.elsevier.com/about/accessibility.

Publisher's note: Elsevier takes a neutral position with respect to territorial disputes or jurisdictional claims in its published content, including in maps and institutional affiliations.

No part of this publication may be reproduced or transmitted in any form or by any means, electronic or mechanical, including photocopying, recording, or any information storage and retrieval system, without permission in writing from the publisher. Details on how to seek permission, further information about the Publisher's permissions policies and our arrangements with organizations such as the Copyright Clearance Center and the Copyright Licensing Agency, can be found at our website: www.elsevier.com/permissions.

This book and the individual contributions contained in it are protected under copyright by the Publisher (other than as may be noted herein).

Notices
Knowledge and best practice in this field are constantly changing. As new research and experience broaden our understanding, changes in research methods, professional practices, or medical treatment may become necessary.

Practitioners and researchers must always rely on their own experience and knowledge in evaluating and using any information, methods, compounds, or experiments described herein. In using such information or methods they should be mindful of their own safety and the safety of others, including parties for whom they have a professional responsibility.

To the fullest extent of the law, neither the Publisher nor the authors, contributors, or editors, assume any liability for any injury and/or damage to persons or property as a matter of products liability, negligence or otherwise, or from any use or operation of any methods, products, instructions, or ideas contained in the material herein.

ISBN: 978-0-443-15447-8

For Information on all Academic Press publications
visit our website at https://www.elsevier.com/books-and-journals

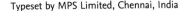

Publisher: Stacy Masucci
Acquisitions Editor: Wendi Baker
Editorial Project Manager: Deepak Vohra
Production Project Manager: Punithavathy Govindaradjane
Cover Designer: Mark Rogers

Typeset by MPS Limited, Chennai, India

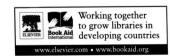

Contents

List of contributors xi

Chapter 1: The metabolism revolution: you need energy to fight and to live 1
Tristram A.J. Ryan, Luke A.J. O'Neill and Zbigniew Zasłona
References 5

Chapter 2: Host–microbe interactions in the lung and the role of immunometabolism 7
Sebastián A. Riquelme, Ayesha Zainab Beg, Tania Wong Fok Lung and Alice Prince

Introduction 7
Immunometabolites in the infected airway 8
Pulmonary immunometabolites and the pathogenesis of bacterial infection 9
Succinate 9
Pseudomonas aeruginosa infection is fueled by succinate in the lung 10
Itaconate 12
Pseudomonas aeruginosa forms biofilms in response to itaconate 12
The *Pseudomonas aeruginosa* transcription factor RpoN responds to immunometabolites 13
Staphylococcus aureus adapts to airway immunometabolites 14
Glucose utilization, proline, and glycolysis by *Staphylococcus aureus* in vivo 15
Itaconate and *Staphylococcus aureus* clearance by neutrophils 16
Itaconate and *Staphylococcus aureus* biofilm production 16
Klebsiella pneumoniae pathotypes direct the immunometabolic response in the lung 18
Production of host antiinflammatory metabolites is stimulated by *Klebsiella pneumoniae* 19
Klebsiella pneumoniae responds to immunometabolic pressure through the type 6 secretion system 20

Conclusions 21
Acknowledgments 22
Disclosures 22
References 22

Chapter 3: Crosstalk between metabolites and myeloid cell biology 27
Brian P. Goldspiel, Mikel D. Haggadone, Sunny Shin and Will Bailis

Chapter introduction—metabolites: friend or foe? 27
Metabolic and innate immune signaling 30
    mTORC1 30
    MAPK 33
    SREBP 35
Stress responses in myeloid cells 37
Crosstalk between tissue microenvironment and tissue-resident macrophage metabolism 39
Metabolic and functional specialization of macrophages during homeostasis 39
    Tissue fuels as drivers of inflammation 42
Concluding thoughts 44
References 45

Chapter 4: Immunometabolism in macrophage cell death 63
Sara Cahill, Laurel Stine and Fiachra Humphries

Introduction 63
Macrophage programmed cell death 64
Ferroptosis 67
The Warburg effect primes macrophage activation 69
Metabolic regulation of cell death 70
Regulation of pyroptosis by fumarate 70
Itaconation in cell death and tolerance 71
Mitochondrial reactive oxygen species prime pyroptosis 73
Summary and future directions 75
References 76

Chapter 5: Computational modeling of metabolism in oncology 81
Linda Fong, Meng Jin, Samir Kharbanda, Marc Creixell, Xiumin Wu, David Zhang, Juan Dubrot, Kathleen Yates, Robert Manguso, Benjamin Kauffman-Malaga, Sean Hackett and Jonathan Powell

Introduction 81
    Metabolism as a therapeutic avenue in oncology 81

Uncovering potential targets: altered metabolic programs in cancer cells 82
　　　Emerging importance of metabolites as signals for immune cells and
　　　stromal cells 83
　　　Computational models help provide a comprehensive and unifying picture 89
　Development of genome-scale metabolic models and applications of
　constraint-based modeling in oncology 90
　　　Constraint-based modeling utilizes genome-scale metabolic models 90
　　　Validating constraint-based metabolic models for tumor cells in
　　　preclinical settings 92
　　　Adapting constraint-based models for single-cell RNA sequencing
　　　(scRNA-seq) data 94
　Utilization of single-cell transcriptomic data for model customization 95
　　　Single-cell metabolic modeling in immune cells 95
　　　Applying metabolic models to clinical data 98
　Perspectives on the implementation of metabolic models in target discovery
　and clinical development 99
　References 101

Chapter 6: Immunometabolic contributions to the pathogenesis of cardiovascular disease 109

Emily Anne Day

Introduction 109
　　　Immune cells in cardiovascular disease 109
　　　Atherosclerotic plaque structure and environment 110
　　　Immune cell metabolism 111
Metabolites in the pathogenesis of cardiovascular disease 111
　　　Cholesterol and lipid metabolites 111
　　　Glucose metabolism and metabolites 113
　　　Amino acid metabolites 115
　　　Tricarboxylic acid cycle intermediates 118
　　　Short-chain fatty acids 120
Conclusion 120
AI disclosure 121
References 121

Chapter 7: Damage-associated molecular patterns as metabolic regulators of innate immunity 129

Tristram A.J. Ryan, Ivan Zanoni and Marco Di Gioia

Introduction 129

Intracellular metabolites function as damage-associated molecular patterns intrinsically modulating pathogen-associated molecular patterns-induced responses 130
    Succinate...132
    Fumarate...135
    Itaconate 136
    Metabolites and their derivatives: contrasting results in the context of type I interferons 139
    An ever-expanding array of immunomodulatory metabolites.......................140
Extracellular damage-associated molecular patterns as extrinsic regulators of pathogen-associated molecular pattern-initiated immunometabolism: the case of oxidized phospholipids.. 141
    oxPLs modulate early metabolic reprogramming and block antiinflammatory responses...142
    oxPLs modulate long-term metabolic processes and boost inflammatory responses..144
    oxPLs induce hyperinflammation...145
Conclusion 147
References 147

Chapter 8: Adaptive immunity and metabolism 157
Katherine C. Verbist, Piyush Sharma, Helen Beere and Douglas R. Green

Introduction... 157
Metabolism of the antigen-presenting cells 158
Metabolism of $CD8^+$ T cells 158
    Naïve T cell metabolism 158
    T cell activation 159
    Mitochondrial metabolism dynamics in T cell activation 160
    Fatty-acid metabolism in activated T cells 161
    Amino acid metabolism in activated T cells 161
    Effector and memory $CD8^+$ T cells..162
    T cell exhaustion...163
Metabolism of $CD4^+$ T cells 164
    Metabolism of $CD4^+$ Treg cells..164
    Targeting Treg metabolism 166
    Metabolism of $CD4^+$ Th1 T cells..167
    Targeting Th1 metabolism 168
    Metabolism of $CD4^+$ Th2 cells...168
    Targeting Th2 metabolism 169
    Metabolism of $CD4^+$ Th9 T cells..169

  Metabolism of CD4⁺ Th17 T cells 170
  Targeting Th17 metabolism 171
  Metabolism of CD4⁺ Tfh cells 172
  Targeting Tfh metabolism 173
 Metabolism of humoral immunity 173
  B cell development 174
  B cell activation 175
  Germinal center reaction 176
 References 178

Chapter 9: Regulation of cytokine secretion by immunometabolites 191
Alexander Hooftman

IL-1β 191
TNF-α and IL-6 195
Type I interferons 196
T cell cytokines 199
 T cell–derived metabolites 199
 Tumor cell–derived metabolites 200
 Myeloid cell–derived metabolites 201
Concluding remarks 202
References 202

Chapter 10: Omics metabolism tools in antiaging drug discovery 209
Rafael Tiburcio, Jay Rappaport and Clovis Palmer

Introduction 209
Genomics in disease prognosis and personalized medicine 210
Transcriptomics and repurposing of drugs for antiaging effects 211
 Overlapping mechanisms between viral infection and aging 213
Proteomics for senolytic biomarkers and drug discovery 214
 Senotherapeutics and aging 214
 Characterization of senescence-associated secretory phenotype
 and senescence-associated proteins 215
 High-throughput proteomic technologies for novel SASP and
 senescence-associated proteins 215
Metabolomics and metabolite profiling 216
 Metabolites in aging diseases 217
 Targeting the sphingomyelin pathway in AD 219
Bioinformatics: integrating omics data 219
Challenges and future directions 221

Conclusion 221
Acknowledgment 222
References 222

Chapter 11: Neuroimmunometabolism as a regulator of obesity 227
Charles A.P. Sweeney and Ana I. Domingos

Introduction..227
Body weight homeostasis and thermogenesis...228
    Central modulation..228
    Neuroanatomy of the sympathetic nervous system............................229
    Physiology of white, brown and beige adipocytes..............................231
    The neuro-adipose synapse and browning...233
Immunometabolism..235
    Macrophages role in insulin resistance in white adipose tissue and brown adipose tissue...236
    Aging effect on lipolysis..239
    Eosinophils...239
Bridging the neuroendocrine-immunometabolomic gap 240
    Sympathetic perineurial cells critical immunomodulatory signaling in adipose tissue...241
    "Sailing under false colors": $LepR^+$ SPCs secrete IL-33 to mask the redox immunogenic niche they ensheathe 244
    Is the sympathetic perineurial cell barrier a mediator of immune privilege?...........249
References 252

Chapter 12: Clinical stage drugs utilizing cellular metabolism pathways 263
Tristram A.J. Ryan, Luke A.J. O'Neill and Zbigniew Zasłona

Introduction..263
Metabolites as clinical biomarkers...263
Targeting—and manipulating—immunometabolism for clinical therapies 264
Drugs modulating glycolysis..266
Targeting mitochondrial biology..269
Targeting the tricarboxylic acid cycle 270
Metabolism as a portal to new therapeutics...271
Acknowledgments..272
References 272

Index..**275**

List of contributors

Will Bailis   Department of Pathology and Laboratory Medicine, Children's Hospital of Philadelphia, Philadelphia, PA, United States; Department of Pathology and Laboratory Medicine, Perelman School of Medicine, University of Pennsylvania, Philadelphia, PA, United States

Helen Beere   Department of Immunology, St. Jude Children's Research Hospital, Memphis, TN, United States

Ayesha Zainab Beg   Department of Pediatrics, Division of Infectious Diseases, Columbia University Irving Medical Center, New York, NY, United States

Sara Cahill   Division of Innate Immunity, Department of Medicine, UMass Chan Medical School, Worcester, MA, United States

Marc Creixell   Calico Life Sciences, LLC, South San Francisco, CA, United States

Emily Anne Day   Department of Physiology and Pharmacology, Schulich School of Medicine and Dentistry, The University of Western Ontario, London, ON, Canada

Marco Di Gioia   Harvard Medical School, and Division of Immunology, Division of Gastroenterology, Boston Children's Hospital, Boston, MA, United States

Ana I. Domingos   Department of Physiology, Anatomy and Genetics, University of Oxford, Oxford, United Kingdom

Juan Dubrot   Clinica Universidad do Navarra, Madrid, Spain

Linda Fong   Calico Life Sciences, LLC, South San Francisco, CA, United States

Brian P. Goldspiel   Medical Scientist Training Program, Perelman School of Medicine, University of Pennsylvania, Philadelphia, PA, United States; Department of Pathology and Laboratory Medicine, Children's Hospital of Philadelphia, Philadelphia, PA, United States

Douglas R. Green   Department of Immunology, St. Jude Children's Research Hospital, Memphis, TN, United States

Sean Hackett   Calico Life Sciences, LLC, South San Francisco, CA, United States

Mikel D. Haggadone   Department of Microbiology, Perelman School of Medicine, University of Pennsylvania, Philadelphia, PA, United States

Alexander Hooftman   Swiss Federal Institute of Technology Lausanne (EPFL), Global Health Institute, Lausanne, Switzerland

Fiachra Humphries   Division of Innate Immunity, Department of Medicine, UMass Chan Medical School, Worcester, MA, United States

Meng Jin   Calico Life Sciences, LLC, South San Francisco, CA, United States

Benjamin Kauffman-Malaga   CA, United States

Samir Kharbanda Calico Life Sciences, LLC, South San Francisco, CA, United States

Tania Wong Fok Lung Department of Microbiology, Biochemistry & Molecular Genetics, Rutgers NJ Medical School, Center for Immunity and Inflammation, Newark, NJ, United States

Robert Manguso Broad Institute of MIT & Harvard, Cambridge, MA, United States

Luke A.J. O'Neill Trinity College Dublin, School of Biochemistry and Immunology, Dublin, Ireland

Clovis Palmer Tulane National Primate Research Center, Covington, LA, United States; Department of Microbiology and Immunology, Tulane University School of Medicine, New Orleans, LA, United States

Jonathan Powell Calico Life Sciences, LLC, South San Francisco, CA, United States

Alice Prince Pediatrics, Division of Infectious Diseases, Columbia University, John M. and Yvonne T. Driscoll, New York, NY, United States

Jay Rappaport Tulane National Primate Research Center, Covington, LA, United States; Department of Microbiology and Immunology, Tulane University School of Medicine, New Orleans, LA, United States

Sebastián A. Riquelme Immunology, Department of Pediatrics, Division of Infectious Diseases, Columbia University Irving Medical Center, New York, NY, United States

Tristram A.J. Ryan Harvard Medical School, and Division of Immunology, Division of Gastroenterology, Boston Children's Hospital, Boston, MA, United States

Piyush Sharma Department of Immunology, St. Jude Children's Research Hospital, Memphis, TN, United States

Sunny Shin Department of Microbiology, Perelman School of Medicine, University of Pennsylvania, Philadelphia, PA, United States

Laurel Stine Division of Innate Immunity, Department of Medicine, UMass Chan Medical School, Worcester, MA, United States

Charles A.P. Sweeney Department of Physiology, Anatomy and Genetics, University of Oxford, Oxford, United Kingdom

Rafael Tiburcio Division of Experimental Medicine, Department of Medicine, University of California, San Francisco, CA, United States

Katherine C. Verbist Department of Immunology, St. Jude Children's Research Hospital, Memphis, TN, United States

Xiumin Wu CA, United States

Kathleen Yates Broad Institute of MIT & Harvard, Cambridge, MA, United States

Ivan Zanoni Harvard Medical School, and Division of Immunology, Division of Gastroenterology, Boston Children's Hospital, Boston, MA, United States

Zbigniew Zasłona Molecure SA, Warsaw, Poland

David Zhang Yale University, New Haven, CT, United States

CHAPTER 1

The metabolism revolution: you need energy to fight and to live

Tristram A.J. Ryan[1], Luke A.J. O'Neill[2] and Zbigniew Zasłona[3]

[1]*Harvard Medical School, and Division of Immunology, Division of Gastroenterology, Boston Children's Hospital, Boston, MA, United States,* [2]*Trinity College Dublin, School of Biochemistry and Immunology, Dublin, Ireland,* [3]*Molecure SA, Warsaw, Poland*

In times when only single-cell organisms populated the earth, some evolved to use energy from oxygen. Then, one of these aerobic bacteria formed an endosymbiotic alliance with larger anaerobic bacteria. The smaller cell continued to use oxygen as a source of energy but continued to do so from the safety of a new home. As a means to pay rent, it started to share its energy with the host. In evolutionary terms, this deal offered the platform to dominate other forms of simple organisms, eventually forming eukaryotic cells as we know them today. The small ingested cell became the mitochondrion, increasing mutual dependence with the bigger cell, but retaining its main task of harnessing energy from oxygen consumption. This helped to build other specialized organelles within the bigger cell in time leading to multicellular organisms, including human beings. This deal made a long time ago determined the world as we know it and is responsible for all of the diversity around us. In this book, while we will not cover topics as broad as the foundation and evolution of our species, we will focus specifically on how regulation of cellular energy affects immune cell functions, enabling host defense during infection or injury. Employing multiple examples, we will illustrate how studying cellular energy of the immune system can be exploited to fight diseases.

From the beginning of our existence, we had to fight. When we were not frightened by big predators, we were most vulnerable to viral and bacterial infections. This has changed very recently in human evolution—with the invention of antibiotics and vaccinations, infectious diseases are no longer in first place in the ranking of human killers (the idea for this book came before COVID-19). Nowadays, autoimmune disorders, cancers, and other so called occupational diseases have become our biggest threat. The immune system, however, has not adapted so fast and is still designed to be primarily ready to rapidly respond to infections. This feature of our defense system comes with a substantial energy cost. Our immune cells, by default, are equipped with metabolic regulation which can facilitate mechanisms that require massive boosts of energy in a timely manner.

It is crucial for the immune system to fulfill functions rapidly, as following infection, it is a matter of life and death for the host. Every day our body produces over 100 billion leukocytes [1]. B cells can produce as much as 18 mg of free λ type light chain per 10^6 cells per day or 6000 λ chain molecules per cell per second [2]. This type of response has to match, for instance, viral replication. Macrophages can eat—nonstop—up to 70 dead cells per day and at a time can ingest particles 1.44 times their diameter, or 3 times their volume [3]. Collectively, this requires a major metabolic output. This is necessary during infection but also during homeostasis and resolution of inflammation, where phagocytosis is a natural process necessary to keep our bodies healthy. Neutrophils, innate cousins of macrophages, can ingest up to 100 *Staphylococcus aureus* or *Escherichia coli* in 30 minutes [4]. Compared with macrophages, they are short-lived since body safety rules require that this kind of killing spree should be controlled in a timely fashion. A single natural killer (NK) cell, a trained killer from the adaptive immunity family of cells, can kill multiple target cells—this can extend up to 10 target cells over a 6-hour period [5]. This activity is crucial in controlling the growth of any cancer in our bodies. The lifespan of dendritic cells is approximately one week, but they are a very dynamic cell type, continuously migrating throughout all of the body's tissues in order to recognize foreign or cancer motifs, before capturing, processing, and presenting them to T cells. That is quite a different lifestyle compared with macrophages, who prefer a stationary lifestyle by finding a local tissue and residing for years at a time. Thanks to macrophage phenotype plasticity, their long lifespan, and their ability to shape the microenvironment, they have become an interesting therapeutic target. Specifically, macrophages have the capacity to restore homeostasis after their initial inflammatory response—a process that can be regulated by modulation of cellular energy.

Interest in immunometabolism is ever-growing, reflected by the advent of new journals and conferences that suck in old-school immunologists, but also researchers from different scientific fields. Traditional metabolism research dates to the awarding of the 1902 Nobel Prize in Chemistry to Hermann Emil Fischer "for his work on sugar and purine syntheses" [6], decades before Otto Heinrich Warburg was awarded the 1931 Nobel Prize in Physiology or Medicine "for his discovery of the nature and mode of action of the respiratory enzyme" [7,8]. Warburg, whose name to this day is innately interwoven with "the Warburg effect"—a process whereby cancer cells switch their metabolism toward aerobic glycolysis for energy production, much like immune cells during inflammation—was a critical catalyst in the rapid expansion of metabolic research.

The 1930s witnessed the publication of two fundamental discoveries in metabolism from Sir Hans Adolf Krebs, who had trained with Warburg in Berlin. In collaboration with his student Kurt Henseleit, Krebs first described the urea cycle—also termed the ornithine cycle—in 1932 which outlines the processes by which ammonia and carbon dioxide—breakdown products of amino acid catabolism which are toxic if accumulated—are excreted by the liver and kidneys [9]. Five years later, in 1937, in collaboration with another of his students, William Johnson, Krebs, using a model of pigeon breast muscle, demonstrated that the metabolite citrate could be oxidized sequentially into a series of different metabolites with each reaction being catalyzed by specific enzymes [10,11]. Importantly, Krebs found that the final metabolite described, oxaloacetic acid, could be re-converted to citrate in the presence of an unknown molecule (later defined as acetyl coenzyme A). Thus Krebs simultaneously confirmed previous findings by Albert Imre Szent-Györgyi, a Hungarian biochemist who had discovered that cellular respiration occurs as a consequence of oxidation of triose (acetyl-CoA) by oxaloacetate and also that conversion of oxaloacetate back into citrate was the result of a cyclical process [12]. This became known as the Krebs cycle or tricarboxylic acid (TCA) cycle, and it is the primary pathway used by aerobic organisms for energy generation from nutrients and food via oxidation of water and carbon dioxide. Krebs was jointly awarded the 1953 Nobel Prize in Physiology or Medicine with Fritz Albert Lipmann "for his discovery of the citric acid cycle."

In 1961 Peter Mitchell proffered a new theory for the molecular mechanisms by which living organisms breakdown fuel to generate energy. Mitchell theorized that the electron transport chain in the mitochondrial inner membrane generates a proton and voltage gradient via a "proton motive force," which is coupled to ATP production in a process termed oxidative phosphorylation, the final step of cellular respiration [13]. Although met with skepticism and resistance within the field at first, this discovery led to the study of bioenergetics and Mitchell's awarding of the 1978 Nobel Prize in Chemistry "for his contribution to the understanding of biological energy transfer through the formulation of the chemiosmotic theory."

Building on these seminal breakthroughs in metabolism research, scientists began to study the crosstalk between metabolism and the immune system, with immunometabolism studies coming to the fore as a field of research in its own right. To highlight this explosion in immunometabolism research, a search for "immunometabolism" in the National Center for Biotechnology Information's (NCBI) PubMed tool returns 19 publications before 2011. Since then, 4177 manuscripts (as of January 2025) have been published containing the term "immunometabolism." Recent advances can partially be explained by the rapid development of research tools. Metabolomics analyses, facilitated by dedicated mass spectrometry and isotope-assisted tracing, have identified key metabolites involved in cellular functions relevant for fundamental immune responses. Seahorse technology has allowed for real-time measurements in live cells of mitochondrial respiration and glycolysis and their relative contribution to energy production. As has happened previously in the history of science, we can expect that technology will catch up if researchers realize that it can open doors to nature's secrets. In the near future, the importance of metabolites as signaling molecules will increase in comparison to proteins. The degree to which we understand proteins is somewhat due to our better understanding of the processes of transcription and translation. With the ever-growing arsenal of new research tools at our disposal, we will be able to comprehensively delineate complex metabolic processes.

Another reason for the recent surge in interest in immunometabolism is the collective, global, and highly collaborative response to the COVID-19 pandemic. This led to the rapid development of effective and safe vaccines—a perfect and encouraging example of industry and academia working together to bring new technology into medical practice. Pandemic times were also the triumph of immunology as a whole field—vaccine-driven boosting of our immune system saved many lives. Importantly, pandemic times increased humanity's awareness of a conventional definition of metabolism. Lifestyle, diet, and exercise suddenly became more relevant when listed as factors which can determine the final outcome of COVID-19 infection. All these factors reminded societies in different countries of the pressing need to find novel ways of treatment for the increasingly aging global population.

This book, "*Metabolites as signals in immunity and inflammation,*" serves to offer a resource to the wider scientific community by detailing the crosstalk of immunity, pathophysiological states, and cellular metabolism, collectively termed immunometabolism. The aim of this book is to encapsulate the critical role of immunometabolism in the regulation of inflammation in health and disease. Each chapter, contributed by global research leaders in their respective fields, captures the core background, research, and future potential of immunometabolism in different contexts of immune responses and provides suggestions for future research directions. The field has rapidly expanded as a new frontier in human health leading to expectations that the study of immunometabolism will identify new therapies. Greater understanding of immunometabolic pathways will help to achieve this goal. In this book, we cover how the immune system manipulates metabolism—and vice versa—to regulate its interactions with both nonimmune cells and invading pathogens that can lead to pathophysiological states [14,15], with particular focus on the latest immunometabolism discoveries in the context of cellular processes integral to pathological states such as cell death [16], cancer [17], obesity [18], and the regulation of the cardiovascular system [19]. We also address the crosstalk between metabolism and innate and adaptive immunity [20,21], and how metabolites themselves can trigger immune activation via cytokine secretion [22]. Finally, we examine recently developed research tools which have revolutionized drug discovery in the field of immunometabolism [23] and present novel therapeutic opportunities [24]. We hope that this book will provide a bedrock of fundamental principles as an introduction to immunometabolism and act as a guide to open future directions of research. In addition, we hope to make immunometabolism more accessible to readers, especially those who are still hesitant to enter the field.

References

[1] Britannica: The Editors of Encyclopaedia Britannica. White Blood Cell [Internet]. Britannica; 2024 [cited 2024 Sep 6]. Available from: https://www.britannica.com/science/white-blood-cell.

[2] Kruse Jr P, Patterson Jr M. Tissue culture: methods and applications, Vol. 1. Academic Press; 1973. p. 868.

[3] Wang Y, Subramanian M, Yurdagul A, Barbosa-Lorenzi VC, Cai B, de Juan-Sanz J, et al. Mitochondrial fission promotes the continued clearance of apoptotic cells by macrophages. Cell 2017;171(2):331–45 e22.

[4] Gordon DL, Rice JL, McDonald PJ. Regulation of human neutrophil type 3 complement receptor (iC3b receptor) expression during phagocytosis of Staphylococcus aureus and Escherichia coli. Immunology 1989;67(4):460–5.

[5] Choi PJ, Mitchison TJ. Imaging burst kinetics and spatial coordination during serial killing by single natural killer cells. Proc Natl Acad Sci U S A 2013;110(16):6488–93.

[6] Fischer E. Synthese des Traubenzuckers. Berichte der Deutschen Chemischen Ges 1890;23:799–805.

[7] Warburg O, Wind F, Negelein E. The metabolism of tumors in the body. J Gen Physiol 1927;8(6):519–30.

[8] Warburg O. On the origin of cancer cells. Science 1956;123(3191):309–14.

[9] Henseleit K, Krebs HA. Untersuchungen über die Harnstoffbildung im tierkorper. Z Physiol Chem 1932;210:33–66.

[10] Krebs HA, Johnson WA. Metabolism of ketonic acids in animal tissues. Biochem J 1937;31(4):645–60.

[11] Krebs HA, Johnson WA. The role of citric acid in intermediate metabolism in animal tissues. FEBS Lett 1980;117(Suppl):K1–10.

[12] Annau E, Banga I, Gözsy B, Huszák B, Laki K, Straub B, et al. Über die Bedeutung der Fumarsäure für die tierische Gewebsatmung. Biol Chem 1935.

[13] Mitchell P. Coupling of phosphorylation to electron and hydrogen transfer by a chemi-osmotic type of mechanism. Nature 1961;191:144–8.

[14] Riquelme SA, Beg AZ, Wong Fok Lung T, Prince A. Host–microbe interactions in the lung and the role of immunometabolism. Metabolites Signals Immun Inflammation. 2025. Chapter 2, pp. 7–26.

[15] Goldspiel BP, Haggadone MD, Shin S, Bailis W. Crosstalk between metabolites and myeloid cell biology. Metabolites Signals Immun Inflammation. 2025. Chapter 3, pp. 27–61.

[16] Cahill S, Stine L, Humphries F. Immunometabolism in macrophage cell death. Metabolites Signals Immun Inflammation. 2025. Chapter 4, pp. 63–80.

[17] Linda F, Meng J, Samir K, Marc C, Xiumin W, David Z, et al. Computational modeling of metabolism in oncology. Metabolites Signals Immun Inflammation. 2025. Chapter 5, pp. 81–107.

[18] Sweeney CAP, Domingos AI. Neuroimmunometabolism as a regulator of obesity. Metabolites Signals Immun Inflammation. 2025. Chapter 11, pp. 227–62.

[19] Day EA. Immunometabolic contributions to the pathogenesis of cardiovascular disease. Metabolites Signals Immun Inflammation. 2025. Chapter 6, pp. 109–28.

[20] Ryan TAJ, Zanoni I, Di Gioia M. Damage-associated molecular patterns as metabolic regulators of innate immunity. Metabolites Signals Immun Inflammation. 2025. Chapter 7, pp. 129–55.

[21] Verbist KC, Sharma P, Beere H, Green DR. Adaptive immunity and metabolism. Metabolites Signals Immun Inflammation. 2025. Chapter 8, pp. 157–90.

[22] Hooftman A. Regulation of cytokine secretion by immunometabolites. Metabolites Signals Immun Inflammation. 2025. Chapter 9, pp. 191–208.

[23] Tiburcio R, Rappaport J, Palmer C. Omics metabolism tools in antiaging drug discovery. Metabolites Signals Immun Inflammation. 2025. Chapter 10, pp. 209–25.

[24] Ryan TAJ, O'Neill LAJ, Zasłona Z. Clinical stage drugs utilizing cellular metabolism pathways. Metabolites Signals Immun Inflammation. 2025. Chapter 12, pp. 263–74.

CHAPTER 2

Host—microbe interactions in the lung and the role of immunometabolism

Sebastián A. Riquelme[1], Ayesha Zainab Beg[2], Tania Wong Fok Lung[3] and Alice Prince[4]

[1]Immunology, Department of Pediatrics, Division of Infectious Diseases, Columbia University Irving Medical Center, New York, NY, United States, [2]Department of Pediatrics, Division of Infectious Diseases, Columbia University Irving Medical Center, New York, NY, United States, [3]Department of Microbiology, Biochemistry & Molecular Genetics, Rutgers NJ Medical School, Center for Immunity and Inflammation, Newark, NJ, United States, [4]Pediatrics, Division of Infectious Diseases, Columbia University, John M. and Yvonne T. Driscoll, New York, NY, United States

Introduction

The pathogenesis of pulmonary infection is initiated by inhaled pathogens that are able to rapidly adapt to the conditions in the airway, including the diverse metabolites generated by both host and pathogen. Among the many different microbes that can access the respiratory tract, a relatively small number are routinely associated with human infection. Opportunistic bacteria, such as the ESKAPE pathogens, have tremendous metabolic and genetic flexibility that enable adaptation to the human airway and coordinated gene expression to optimize their persistence in the lung [1,2]. Such is the case of *Staphylococcus aureus* and *Pseudomonas aeruginosa*, bacteria commonly associated with colonization in patients with cystic fibrosis (CF), and *Klebsiella*, *Acinetobacter* and a few other opportunists that successfully infect individuals with damaged airways, as occurs in ventilator-associated pneumonias (VAP), chronic obstructive pulmonary disease (COPD), and bronchiectasis. Pathogens must immediately identify and metabolize new carbon sources, as well as compete for essential nutrients such as carboxylates, amino acids, fatty acids, carbohydrates and key metals that support their bioenergetic integrity, including iron, copper, and zinc. The presence of bacteria in the airway and lung triggers a robust immune response that successful pathogens must counter. A variety of bacterial virulence factors participate in establishing and maintaining infection: toxins that destroy host immune cells, proteases that target epithelial and endothelial tight junctions to promote invasion, secreted factors that inactivate immunoglobulins and thwart phagocytosis, or indiscriminately alter T cell effector fate. Basic bacterial functions, such as flagella and pilin-associated motility function in pathogenesis, as do the extracellular polysaccharides that form the biofilms that interfere with phagocytosis. The abundance of these bacterial gene products is regulated by microbial metabolism, which in turn is dictated by the constraints of the local microenvironment. Not only do the bacteria alter their basal metabolic configuration to optimize their ability to proliferate in the lung, but the host also responds to the bacterial mass with major changes in its metabolic program, especially through the production of immunometabolites.

The airway provides an array of potential substrates for bacterial proliferation. These include the constituents of airway fluid, secreted mucins, and the debris from cell turnover. In the setting of inflammation, there is the recruitment of immune cells and their products, immunometabolites that help to direct immune clearance and counter the effects of damaging inflammation. In contrast to the fastidious upper airway pathogens, such as *Hemophilus influenzae*, opportunists like *S. aureus*, *P. aeruginosa*, and *Klebsiella pneumoniae* have substantially greater metabolic flexibility, as well as greater resistance to immune clearance mechanisms. In this chapter, we will focus on a few opportunistic pathogens that are associated with persistent and potentially fatal pneumonia and explore the mechanisms through which they are able to adapt to and exploit the abundant immunometabolites generated over the course of pulmonary infection.

Immunometabolites in the infected airway

Exactly what immunometabolites are available in the airway? Do they serve as carbon sources for specific microorganisms or activate bacterial gene expression? It has been difficult to obtain accurate data to detail the composition of human airway fluid. Data sets from the SARS-CoV-2 epidemic [2] and from ongoing studies of patients with CF and diseased controls [3] document the composition of the airway fluid obtained via bronchoscopy in bronchoalveolar lavage (BAL) fluid. However, many of the compounds important in immunometabolism, such as the TCA cycle components, succinate, fumarate, and itaconate, are not specifically quantified in many studies. In adults, glucose in BAL, a preferred substrate for *S. aureus*, was only 10% of the serum levels, suggesting that even in diabetics with elevated blood sugars that are a substrate for bacterial growth, this is not an exceptionally increased amount [4]. Data from clinical studies using primarily infected CF and non-CF subjects who are undergoing BAL (bronchoalveolar lavage) is the source of much information regarding the immunometabolites that predominate during infection. From these studies, we find that both succinate and itaconate are especially abundant [5,6], observations that are replicated in mouse models of infection. Each of these dicarboxylates has major effects on bacterial physiology, as well as shaping the host immune response (Fig. 2.1).

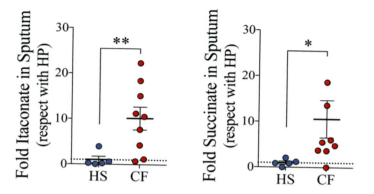

Figure 2.1
Metabolite profiling of sputum from healthy subjects (HS) versus CF patients. *CF*, Cystic fibrosis.

Pulmonary immunometabolites and the pathogenesis of bacterial infection

The airway mucosa is continually exposed to the environment, to particulate matter, allergens, and to potential pathogens. The mucociliary escalator helps to maintain unobstructed airways, especially in the setting of mucosal injury. During infection, resident and recruited phagocytes accumulate around the pathogen niche, producing and releasing mitochondrial metabolites with major immunomodulatory properties, such as succinate and itaconate. Here, we will discuss the role of each of these factors in pulmonary homeostasis, particularly during acute and chronic infection by ESKAPE opportunists.

Succinate

Succinate is a crucial mitochondrial metabolite involved in energy generation, epigenetic regulation, and cell-to-cell communication [7]. In airway cells, succinate is produced by succinyl-CoA ligase, which couples succinyl-CoA with ADP to generate succinate, CoA, and ATP. Succinate is further oxidized by succinate dehydrogenase (Complex II), reducing FAD^+ to $FADH_2$ [7]. $FADH_2$ then donates electrons to ubiquinone, which transports these electrons within the inner membrane of the mitochondria to Complex III [8,9]. Complex III transfers these electrons to Complex IV, where oxygen (O_2) is reduced to water (H_2O) [8,9]. As a result of this process, many protons are pumped out from the mitochondrial matrix into the intermembrane space, creating a proton gradient across the inner mitochondrial membrane. When these protons flow back into the matrix through Complex V (ATP synthase), they drive the condensation of ADP and Pi, which generates ATP [8]. Thus succinate plays an essential role in the bioenergetic integrity of pulmonary cells.

During respiratory injury affecting the architecture of the tissue (acute lung injury, following intubation, sepsis), airway cells experience hypoxia, which activates hypoxia-induced factor 1a (HIF1a) [10–14]. In type II airway epithelial cells, HIF1a promotes the internalization of glucose, replenishing the acetyl-CoA pool and fueling the TCA cycle [14–16]. This stimulation of the TCA cycle leads to an accumulation of succinate, which is then released and interacts with its surface receptor SUCNR1 [14]. By stimulating SUCNR1, succinate promotes signaling through the inflammatory cytokine IL-1b, aggravating tissue damage [14]. Thus exogenous succinate plays a key role in aggravating respiratory pathology.

Recent studies have linked the accumulation of succinate in peripheral tissues to the progression of idiopathic pulmonary fibrosis (IPF) [17–19]. Patients with IPF exhibit elevated succinate levels in both circulation and airway fluids, alongside augmented expression of the succinate receptor SUCNR1 [17]. These findings have been observed in both humans and animal models of IPF, such as those induced by bleomycin [17,18]. Mechanistically, succinate augmented fibrosis in the respiratory tract, leading to augmented deposition of fibronectin and scar tissue. The administration of succinate dehydrogenase inhibitors, such as dimethyl malonate (DMM) and IR-780, limited IPF by bleomycin, suggesting that the mechanism by which succinate promotes respiratory fibrosis is through oxidative metabolism [18].

Pseudomonas aeruginosa *infection is fueled by succinate in the lung*

One of the earliest methods of bacterial classification was by the metabolic activity of specific cocci or rods, characterized as Gram (+)or Gram (-) by the presence or absence of lipopolysaccharide (LPS). *P. aeruginosa* is a motile nonlactose fermenter, which preferentially consumes succinate to generate energy in the TCA cycle [20,21]. Carbon source utilization is regulated by the carbon catabolite repressor system (CCR), consisting of small RNAs that force *P. aeruginosa* to prioritize succinate consumption over other available nutrients until the supply is exhausted [20]. CCR provides a hierarchical distribution of substrate consumption which dictates the bacterial nutritional program in environments rich in succinate, such as the inflamed lung [22]. Upon infection, respiratory phagocytes, such as alveolar macrophages, accumulate and release succinate [22,23]. Succinate not only promotes the activation of the inflammasome and the release of IL-1b [24] but also serves as a major nutritional source for *P. aeruginosa*, enhancing its growth and proliferation [22]. Consequently, the local inflammatory response triggered by this pathogen is directly linked to its capacity to thrive by consuming locally available substrates [20,22] (Fig. 2.2).

Alveolar macrophages release succinate in response to LPS during *P. aeruginosa* and other Gram-negative infection [22,25,26]. The display of LPS on the bacterial surface is regulated by the transporter LptD [27,28]. Of note, this LptD-mediated mobilization of LPS can be

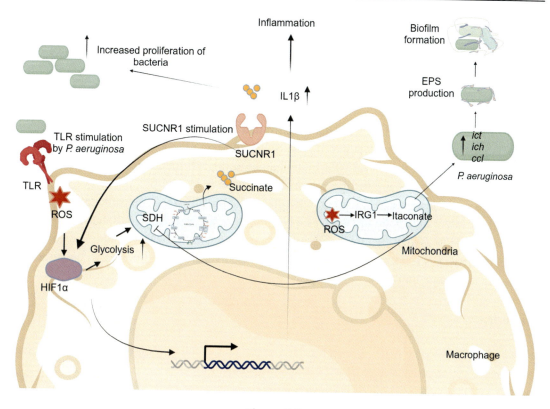

Figure 2.2
Schematic overview of interplay between host immunometabolites and *Pseudomonas aeruginosa* adaptation.

limited during chronic infection decreasing the immunogenicity of the organisms [29]. Upon activation of toll-like receptor 4 (TLR4), LPS not only activates NF-kB proinflammatory signaling but also compromises host mitochondrial stability, prompting an array of adaptations that lead to the generation of succinate [24,30]. This succinate leaks into the cytoplasm of LPS-activated cells, is excreted into the extracellular milieu, and is assimilated by *P. aeruginosa* [22].

In *P. aeruginosa*, succinate is oxidized by succinate dehydrogenase in the TCA cycle [20–22]. By extracting electrons from succinate, this enzyme stimulates the formation of $FADH_2$, which further promotes the generation of bacterial energy through oxidative phosphorylation (OXPHOS). This bioenergetic program enables *P. aeruginosa* to produce sufficient ATP to grow, generating rapidly proliferating communities that outcompete host immune defenses [20–22]. The impact of succinate on *P. aeruginosa* pathogenesis is clearly illustrated in the airways of patients with cystic fibrosis (CF) who exhibit increased susceptibility to *P. aeruginosa* pulmonary infection [22,31]. CF is produced by mutations in the CF transmembrane conductance regulator (CFTR), which limit the translocation of this molecule to the cell membrane and/or impair its function [32]. Lack of CFTR in the membrane compromises its interaction with the phosphatase PTEN, a mitochondria-associated metabolic checkpoint that regulates succinate biology [5]. Lack of the CFTR-PTEN complex promotes the release of high levels of succinate from airway cells of individuals with CF, enriching the respiratory lumen with this factor, which is a preferred substrate for *P. aeruginosa* consumption [22]. *P. aeruginosa* assimilates this succinate to both thrive and elicit inflammasome signaling, leading to more succinate excretion and inflammatory tissue damage [22]. Drugs that improve CFTR mobilization to the cell membrane increase CFTR-PTEN interaction and decrease the generation of succinate [22]. The predilection of *P. aeruginosa* for succinate helps to explain why this metabolically versatile pathogen, and not others with different metabolic preferences, predominates in CF. Based upon in vitro data, it seems reasonable to predict that the CFTR modulators currently in widespread use would increase CFTR-PTEN association and result in decreased succinate and possibly decreased proinflammatory signaling [33].

Itaconate

Itaconate is a carboxylate derived from the TCA cycle, specifically produced in phagocytes like macrophages but not bacteria, and one of the most abundant metabolites in the infected airway fluid [34,35]. It is synthesized by the enzyme immune-responsive gene 1 (IRG1), also known as aconitate decarboxylase 1 (ACOD1), from cis-aconitate, an intermediate of the TCA cycle [36,37]. Itaconate plays a significant role in immunoregulation by modulating inflammatory responses, particularly those associated with destructive inflammation, such as the inflammasome [36,38–40]. It acts as a potent immunosuppressive agent, interfering with the activity of succinate dehydrogenase and thereby reducing the production of proinflammatory cytokines such as IL-1β [41]. Itaconate can modify the function of nuclear factor erythroid 2–related factor 2 (NRF2), a key regulator of antioxidant responses, enhancing the expression of genes that protect against oxidative stress, such as heme oxygenase 1 (*Hmox1*), although the importance of this effect in human macrophages may be more limited [42,43]. However, itaconate acts not only as a major immunomodulatory metabolite but also as a strong bactericidal agent [44–47]. Many pathogens are susceptible to itaconate, both intracellularly and extracellularly. Through these mechanisms, itaconate helps to control pathogen burden and excessive inflammation and maintain immune homeostasis, making it a crucial component in maintaining the body's response to infection and tissue damage.

Pseudomonas aeruginosa *forms biofilms in response to itaconate*

A hallmark of *P. aeruginosa* chronic infection is the emergence of bacterial communities that produce biofilm [48,49]. These pathogens proliferate less, allocating most of their energy into the synthesis of complex exopolysaccharides (EPS) [48,50–52]. These EPS facilitate not only the attachment of *P. aeruginosa* to the respiratory mucosa but also function as a barrier that protects the community from phagocytes, from the oxidants released as well as interfering with uptake and killing [52]. Accumulating evidence suggests that itaconate stress may be a factor in driving the metabolic switch as *P. aeruginosa* convert from planktonic growth to biofilm formation in the human lung [29].

As one of the most abundant metabolites in the infected airway, itaconate induces acute membrane stress in *P. aeruginosa*, prompting a series of adaptive changes in the pathogen, leading to the synthesis of EPS that form biofilm [6]. By producing biofilms in response to itaconate, *P. aeruginosa* coopts the immunometabolic response orchestrated by effector phagocytes against the infection, enabling persistence and proliferation in the lung. This is a major cause of the pulmonary pathology caused by *P. aeruginosa* in people with CF [6]. These subjects, lacking function of the CFTR-PTEN complex, release elevated levels of itaconate as well as succinate into airway fluids [5,22]. In this environment, *P. aeruginosa* forms specialized bacterial communities programmed to generate biofilms, thus establishing a direct link between host immunometabolites and bacterial persistence.

In addition to rewiring its metabolic activity in response to itaconate, *P. aeruginosa* can also deplete this metabolite by consuming it as a carbon source [6,53]. *P. aeruginosa* has a dedicated TRAP family transporter that is regulated by the presence of itaconate, along with the *ict-ich-ccl* locus that mediates its assimilation [54]. *P. aeruginosa* can break down itaconate into acetyl-CoA and pyruvate, replenishing the bacterial TCA cycle and generating the energy needed for the maintenance of critical biomass [55]. Although succinate and itaconate are similar dicarboxylates, *P. aeruginosa* uses an RpoN-dependent transport system to acquire succinate, whereas itaconate uptake is through a different mechanism [55,56]. Thus *P. aeruginosa* is a metabolically sophisticated opportunist that can leverage the advantages provided by both itaconate and succinate in the human lung that is heavily populated by effector phagocytes which produce both of these carboxylates (Fig. 2.2).

The Pseudomonas aeruginosa *transcription factor RpoN responds to immunometabolites*

P. aeruginosa is equipped to sense environmental signals and adapts to establish a bacterial community in the lung. The availability of dicarboxylates such as itaconate and succinate act as signals that are integrated to optimize bacterial bioenergetics to fuel ongoing metabolism and pathoadaptive strategies. The activation of specific transcription factors provides an efficient mechanism to coordinate gene expression in response to such environmental cues. In *P. aeruginosa*, PAO1 cellular regulation is dependent on a combination of 550 transcriptional regulators and 24 sigma factors [57]. Among these sigma factors, 19 were identified as extracytoplasmic function (ECF) sigma factors that respond to environmental stimuli, such as immunometabolites [58]. The alternative sigma factor *rpoN* is widely conserved among many different Gram-negative bacteria and in *P. aeruginosa* senses succinate, as well as other C-4 and C-5 dicarboxylates, including itaconate, that accumulate in the infected airway. In response to succinate, RpoN directs the expression of a specific succinate transporter, providing the bacteria with a favored carbon source [59]. The C-5 dicarboxylate itaconate provides an alternative carbon source as the organisms adapt to the milieu within the infected airway. In *P. aeruginosa* isolates from chronic infection in CF, there are often mutations in *rpoN* limiting succinate uptake, but not the metabolism of itaconate [60].

RpoN further coordinates much of the metabolic response to these immunometabolites that fuel infection. The glyoxylate shunt, directed by RpoN and *aceA* activity, drives the production of gluconeogenic precursors for biofilm biomass, the predominant bacterial growth modality in the infected lung. RpoN has multiple effects on genes involved in quorum sensing and ultimately in biofilm formation; thus it has a major role in directing the adaptation of the bacteria to the conditions in the infected lung. For example, during evolution of CF isolates in the infected airway, mutations in *rpoN* result in low succinate assimilation and higher *aceA* activity, rewiring bacterial metabolism to support the biofilm lifestyle [61].

Many bacterial signaling networks are activated or suppressed by RpoN activity [62]. The metabolic networks involved in nitrogen sensing and metabolism, the response to oxidants and pyochelin production, as well as those important in motility and scavenging carbon sources, are all under the positive or negative regulation of RpoN. Thus the ability of carboxylate immunometabolites to trigger RpoN responses is a major factor in driving the adaptation and success of *P. aeruginosa*.

Staphylococcus aureus *adapts to airway immunometabolites*

S. aureus is a Gram-positive pathogen that is a frequent cause of pulmonary infection, especially in individuals with damaged airways. As an opportunist with substantial metabolic flexibility, *S. aureus* can readily adapt to many different tissues, including skin, bone, and especially the lung. *S. aureus* shares many of the same ecological niches as *P. aeruginosa*, especially the damaged lung as seen in patients with CF, in which it is the most common pathogen early in the disease process. From longitudinal studies of CF clinical isolates, the ongoing metabolic adaptation of *S. aureus* to airway metabolites can be followed over decades of infection [63,64]. The success of *S. aureus* as a pathogen is often attributed to its formidable array of toxins and proteins that specifically thwart the activity of the immune system, T cells, B cells, and phagocytes [65]. It expresses several virulence determinants that interfere with opsonization and phagocytosis by neutrophils [66]. *S. aureus* also responds to the metabolic activity of neutrophils, their robust production of itaconate and are able to evade efficient killing by these phagocytes through their own metabolic adaptation. The ability of *S. aureus* to modify their own metabolic activity in response to host production of immunometabolites is a major factor in their success as pulmonary pathogens.

Glucose utilization, proline, and glycolysis by Staphylococcus aureus *in vivo*

S. aureus prefers to use glycolysis and glucose as a carbon source, as well documented in numerous metabolic studies [67]. However, in vivo there is competition for the relatively limited supplies of glucose in the airway. Studies of BAL fluids composition from infected patients indicated levels of glucose approximately 10% of the glucose found in serum [4]. *S. aureus* must compete with neutrophils which also prefer to utilize glucose for their metabolic needs and are the major phagocyte recruited to the site of *S. aureus* infection [66]. Sensing limited glucose in the setting of chronic infection, the carbon catabolite repression system directs *S. aureus* metabolism and directs the utilization of proline [68]. Over the course of persistent infection, *S. aureus* upregulate the expression of proline transporters. Proline, a major constituent of collagen, is a product of activated airway fibroblasts involved in the maintenance of airway integrity, via collagen deposition [64]. With ongoing collagen deposition as a component of airway repair, *S. aureus* residing in the airway are provided with an abundant carbon source. Moreover, proline as a component of the citrulline super pathway provides the building blocks for the production of extracellular polysaccharides and biofilm.

Within the lung, *S. aureus* assumes a biofilm mode of growth to maintain persistent infection. Energy is diverted into the production and maintenance of biofilm components using amino acid metabolism and the TCA cycle. In addition, small colony variants (SCV) of *S. aureus* are often recovered from biofilms in CF pulmonary infections. These mutants can use glycolysis and generate mitochondrial ROS and inflammation, despite slow growth rates [69]. However, consistent with the abundance of succinate in the chronically inflamed CF lung, *S. aureus* SCV strains often have upregulated Sdh expression and excrete succinate [70]. While they may prefer to utilize glycolysis, they rely upon an intact TCA cycle to adapt to the constraints of biofilm growth in vivo. The recovery of SCVs from clinical infections is common and problematic as these organisms persist intracellularly and are antibiotic resistant due to both slow growth and their metabolic inability to accumulate antibiotics intracellularly.

Itaconate and Staphylococcus aureus *clearance by neutrophils*

Immunometabolites provide strong selective pressure for *S. aureus* adaptation to the lung. *S. aureus*, despite its lack of LPS, is a potent stimulator of *Irg1* (*Acod1*) expression and itaconate production, especially by neutrophils, the major phagocyte responsible for staphylococcal clearance [71]. *S. aureus* glycolysis, its preferred mechanism to generate energy, stimulates host itaconate production. While initially considered to have antimicrobial activity [44–47], itaconate does not have potent anti-*S. aureus* activity. $Irg1^{-/-}$ mice that are unable to produce itaconate clear *S. aureus* more readily than WT C57Bl mouse controls at 24 hours of infection [71]. However, itaconate inhibits glycolysis in the host, especially in neutrophils [71]. Diminished ability to use glycolysis decreases neutrophil survival. In contrast to the response to *P. aeruginosa*, most *Irg1* expression in the setting of *S. aureus* pneumonia is due to neutrophils, whereas both monocyte and neutrophil populations increase *Irg1* expression in *P. aeruginosa* infection. Thus effects of itaconate on neutrophil function can interfere with efficient *S. aureus* clearance from the respiratory tract.

The actual killing of staphylococci is dependent upon the neutrophil oxidative burst, the product of NADPH complex activity [72]. Although the host replenishes neutrophil populations that are expended over the course of *S. aureus* infection, itaconate appears to hinder the efficiency of neutrophil killing [71]. Itaconate significantly decreases the oxygen consumption rate in *S aureus*-infected neutrophils and generation of the oxidative burst, likely through posttranslational modification of the NADPH complex by itaconate [71]. This observation is consistent with impaired staphylococcal killing by WT as compared to $Irg1-/-$ neutrophils. These specific effects of itaconate on neutrophil function are in addition to the global antiinflammatory consequences of the immunometabolite on the inflammasome and its association with Nrf2-dependent antioxidant pathways, as discussed above.

Itaconate and Staphylococcus aureus *biofilm production*

Whereas effects of itaconate on host immune function are expected, itaconate also has direct effects on *S. aureus* metabolism. Unlike *P. aeruginosa*, *S. aureus* does not metabolize itaconate but nonetheless appears to take up the immunometabolite. A major effect of itaconate is the posttranslational modification of both host and bacterial targets, by targeting accessible cysteine residues. As was first described for eukaryotic cells, itaconate inhibits *S. aureus* aldolase activity, a key enzyme in glycolysis, limiting ATP generation by *S. aureus* through this preferred metabolic pathway [73]. The metabolic stress caused by itaconate suppresses the expression of several proteins expected to be involved in pathogenesis, such as the a-hemolysin [73]. In addition, there is substantial metabolic rewiring to enable the bacteria to cope with the increased local oxidant stress. A major component of this stress response is the generation of extracellular polysaccharides which make up biofilm. While glycolysis is inhibited by itaconate, gluconeogenesis is increased, and products are shunted into uridine diphosphate (UTP) and *N*-acetyl glucosamine which are building blocks of biofilm. These metabolic changes can be observed in clinical isolates of *S. aureus* from chronic infections that display increased biofilm formation in the presence of itaconate. To survive in this environment, *S. aureus* use the pentose phosphate shunt to generate biofilm, which itself has antioxidant properties, as well as helping the organisms to avoid phagocytic clearance.

The net effect of itaconate on *S. aureus* in the airway is twofold, interfering with neutrophil function that is essential for efficient clearance, and then imposing substantial metabolic stress driving bacterial metabolic adaptation [71]. Neutrophil production of itaconate in this setting contributes to *S. aureus* persistence by limiting glycolysis and the generation of ROS to kill the pathogens [71]. Moreover, the recruitment of neutrophils to the site of *S. aureus* proliferation contributes to ongoing airway damage and repair mechanisms, including proline biosynthesis which fuels *S. aureus* infection (Fig. 2.3).

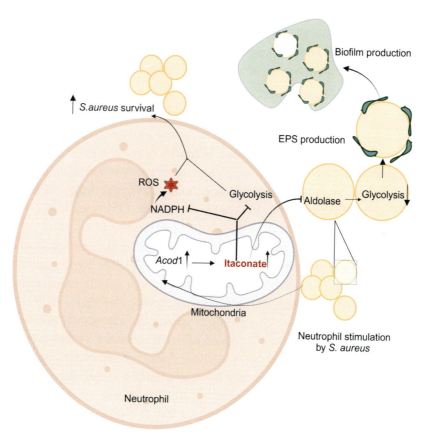

Figure 2.3
Itaconate modifies both neutrophil and *Staphylococcus aureus* metabolism.

The behaviors of *S. aureus* and *P. aeruginosa* have been extensively examined due to their importance in CF and the availability of longitudinal collections of well-characterized clinical isolates to follow the course of infection. For both of these species, itaconate in particular drives biofilm formation and functions to limit the intensity of the immune response that contributes to bacterial killing but also causes host damage. Other airway pathogens must similarly adapt to the immunometabolites in the airway, but each species has its own patterns of gene expression and responses.

Klebsiella pneumoniae *pathotypes direct the immunometabolic response in the lung*

K. pneumoniae is a common Gram-negative pathogen and, globally, an increasingly important cause of a variety of health care associated infections, including pneumonia. It is now included as an organism of concern by the World Health Organization (WHO), not only for its potential virulence but for its alarming resistance to many if not all available classes of antimicrobial agents [74]. *K. pneumoniae* are nonmotile and lack many of the well-characterized virulence factors expressed by other pathogens. It is notable for a copious capsular polysaccharide giving it mucoid appearance in vitro.

In contrast to *S. aureus*, which is often characterized by antimicrobial susceptibility, as MRSA or MSSA, *K. pneumoniae* fall into two distinct pathotypes that differ in several ways, including the immunometabolic response that they activate. The traditional classification of *Kp*, classical or hypervirulent, primarily hinges on the clinical presentation of associated illnesses and by variations in the accessory genome and distinct epidemiological characteristics of associated infections. The hypervirulent *Kp* strains cause fulminant and rapidly lethal infections in healthy individuals [75] whereas the classical strains typically cause subacute and prolonged infections in immunocompromised patients [76]. Nonetheless, even the more indolent infections frequently become fatal, as is commonly the case with ventilator-associated pneumonia [76]. The hypervirulent strains have been characteristically vulnerable to antibiotics although antimicrobial resistance is increasing [77]. These strains express several virulence-associated genes such as *ent*, *iuc*, *iro*, and *ybt* that encode siderophores, including enterobactin, aerobactin, salmochelin, and yersiniabactin, which are often plasmid encoded [75]. The classical strains are notable for their genetic ability to acquire resistance to multiple classes of antibiotics and spread rapidly worldwide. Since their emergence in the United States in the early 2000s, classical *Kp* strains have been recognized as a global public health concern by both the CDC and WHO [78]. However, the strict categorization of *Kp* into two distinct pathotypes is becoming outmoded given the emergence of convergent strains that are both multidrug-resistant (MDR) and have hypervirulent features [77,79].

The mechanisms through which *K. pneumoniae* manipulates host signaling pathways to avoid immune clearance have been an area of active investigation [80]. It is increasingly appreciated that these pathogens have a profound impact on host metabolism. While some *K. pneumoniae* stains activate the metabolic pathways linked to proinflammatory reactions, other *K. pneumoniae* strains stimulate and exhibit antiinflammatory and immunosuppressive immune responses that help to account for the chronicity and eventual lethality of some *K. pneumoniae* infections [81].

Production of host antiinflammatory metabolites is stimulated by Klebsiella pneumoniae

As a Gram-negative rod, much of the immune response to *Kp* is dependent upon production of LPS, the activation of succinate release from immune cells, and proinflammatory cytokine production. However, some of the more common *Kp* serotypes, such as the MDR (multiply drug-resistant) epidemic ST258 strains, induce an airway immune response that disables bacterial clearance [82]. This response is marked by the early accumulation of immunosuppressive myeloid cells (M2-like macrophages and myeloid-derived suppressor cells (MDSCs) and the production of the antiinflammatory metabolite itaconate by the host [82–84] (Fig. 2.4)). MDSCs are perhaps best characterized in the setting of tumors, in which their production of itaconate and arginase limits proinflammatory immune clearance mechanisms [85]. Itaconate is important in modulating inflammation activated by *Kp*. In mouse model systems, pulmonary infection of Irg1-/- mice resulted in heightened inflammation and a significantly greater *K. pneumoniae* burden [82].

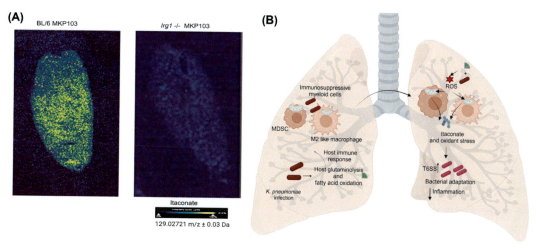

Figure 2.4
Immunometabolic responses to *Klebsiella pneumoniae* during infection.

In addition to stimulating itaconate production, the *Kp* strains associated with persistent infection induce an airway metabolic profile that is clearly distinct from purified LPS or heat-killed bacteria or from hypervirulent strains that cause acute infection [82]. These antibiotic-resistant strains activate glutaminolysis and fatty acid oxidation (FAO), which fuel mitochondrial oxidative phosphorylation (OXPHOS) and the generation of reactive oxygen species (ROS). Glutaminolysis refers to the degradation of the amino acid glutamine into glutamate and α-ketoglutarate, whereas FAO involves the breakdown of fatty acids into acetyl-CoA. Importantly, mitochondrial OXPHOS is closely linked to the activation of antiinflammatory signaling. In animal models, inhibiting host glutaminolysis and FAO is associated with acute infection and a significantly increased bacterial load, inflammation, and immunopathology. These in vivo experiments underscore the pivotal role of these metabolic pathways and itaconate synthesis in fostering the clearance of infection to safeguard the airway integrity and promote host survival.

Airway metabolomic studies illustrate differences in the responses of mice that either survived or succumbed to *Kp* infection [86]. Surviving mice displayed distinct metabolomic profiles featuring D-glucose, glutamine, L-serine, myo-inositol, ethanedioic acid, and lactic acid, in contrast to the mice that succumbed to infection [86]. Pathway enrichment analysis underscores the significance of valine, leucine, and isoleucine biosynthesis in influencing infection outcomes. Subsequent experiments confirmed that administering exogenous L-serine, L-valine, and L-leucine reduced *Kp* burden in the lungs and enhanced survival rates in infected mice. These metabolites enhanced macrophage phagocytosis, highlighting the importance of the metabolic components of a successful host immune response.

Surveys of clinical strains of *K. pneumoniae* confirm the importance of their metabolic adaptation to the host, as has been observed with other ESKAPE pathogens. A recent study demonstrated that 89% of the clinical isolates studied exhibited a marked increase in the uptake and utilization of environmental L-valine in contrast to its limited utilization in laboratory strains [87], although exactly how this alters pathogenicity has yet to be fully defined. Studies utilizing integrated bacterial transcriptional analyses and metabolic simulations underscore the pivotal role of bacterial metabolism itself and its effects on host metabolism in shaping infection dynamics.

Klebsiella pneumoniae *responds to immunometabolic pressure through the type 6 secretion system*

Both host and pathogen metabolic activities are stimulated over the course of pulmonary infection. Just as the host activates immunometabolic defenses, the bacteria also respond to metabolites, especially to reactive oxygen and nitrogen species generated in host defense and by the pathogens themselves. Mice lacking Irg1 were especially susceptible to *Kp* pulmonary infection [82], and itaconate seemed to play a greater role in host defense than against S. *aureus* or *P. aeruginosa*. Under oxidative stress, both in vitro and in vivo *K. pneumoniae* significantly increases the expression of genes involved in maintaining redox balance and the type 6 secretion system (T6SS) [82]. While traditionally known for eliminating bacterial competitors, the T6SS plays an important role in the airways by enhancing antioxidant defenses [88]. The T6SS, resembling a phage-like structure, delivers effector proteins directly into target cells, either bacterial or eukaryotic, using a spike that pierces membranes. In response to environmental stresses, including oxidants [89] T6SS effectors, including catalases and zincophores, are released into the extracellular environment [90–92]. In vivo, the expression of an intact T6SS was required for *K. pneumoniae* survival in the lung under heightened oxidative stress [82]. One of the *K. pneumoniae* T6SS effectors, VgrG4, targets mitochondria, suggesting a potential mechanism for direct manipulation of host metabolism by the T6SS [93]. In the absence of *Irg1*, increased generation of oxidants by the host helps to limit *Kp* infection. Thus in this setting, as was observed with *S. aureus*, the antioxidant effects of itaconate may help to promote infection by these opportunists. As the T6SS is highly conserved throughout Gram-negative species, participation of this secretion system in sensing environmental triggers is likely shared by many pathogens.

Conclusions

Successful opportunistic pathogens that are associated with pulmonary infection have a variety of mechanisms to cope with and exploit environmental conditions that include the accumulation of immunologically active metabolites. As we have illustrated with *P. aeruginosa, S. aureus,* and *K. pneumoniae,* two of the most abundant immunometabolites in the airway, succinate and itaconate, in general, promote infection. These carboxylates can provide a carbon source to fuel proliferation and drive metabolic adaptation in the form of biofilm production which promotes infection recalcitrant to eradication. Airway metabolites have diverse roles in pathogenesis depending upon the stage of infection. While the release of succinate from macrophages activated by LPS and associated proinflammatory signaling is an important part of the acute response to clear infection, the host must also temper these responses with antiinflammatory signaling, such as the release of itaconate to help prevent oxidant damage. This regulation of the immune response and especially the neutrophil oxidant burst serves to enhance bacterial survival, but through suppression of host responses. While immunomodulatory metabolites, such as itaconate, are seemingly important in influencing infection, their overall effect on bacterial clearance is more to prolong infection by driving biofilm formation than to increase susceptibility to acute lethality.

Acknowledgments

The authors are supported by NIH R35GM146776 (SR), K99/R00 HL157550(TW) and RO1HL170129, R35HL135800 (AP).

Disclosures

None

References

[1] Venkateswaran P, Vasudevan S, David H, Shaktivel A, Shanmugam K, Neelakantan P, et al. Revisiting ESKAPE pathogens: virulence, resistance, and combating strategies focusing on quorum sensing. Front Cell Infect Microbiol 2023;13:1159798.

[2] Gelarden I, Nguyen J, Gao J, Chen Q, Morales-Nebreda L, Wunderink R, et al. Comprehensive evaluation of bronchoalveolar lavage from patients with severe COVID-19 and correlation with clinical outcomes. Hum Pathol 2021;113:92–103.

[3] O'Connor JB, Mottlowitz M, Wagner BD, Harris JK, Laguna TA. Metabolomics analysis of bronchoalveolar lavage fluid predicts unique features of the lower airway in pediatric cystic fibrosis. J Cyst Fibros 2024;.

[4] Baker EH, Baines DL. Airway glucose homeostasis: A new target in the prevention and treatment of pulmonary infection. Chest 2018;153(2):507–14.

[5] Riquelme SA, Hopkins BD, Wolfe AL, DiMango E, Kitur K, Parsons R, et al. Cystic fibrosis transmembrane conductance regulator attaches tumor suppressor PTEN to the membrane and promotes anti *Pseudomonas aeruginosa* immunity. Immunity 2017;47(6):1169–81 e7.

[6] Riquelme SA, Liimatta K, Wong Fok Lung T, Fields B, Ahn D, Chen D, et al. *Pseudomonas aeruginosa* utilizes host-derived itaconate to redirect its metabolism to promote biofilm formation. Cell Metab 2020;31(6):1091–106 e6.

[7] Mills E, O'Neill LA. Succinate: a metabolic signal in inflammation. Trends Cell Biol 2014;24(5):313–20.

[8] Madeira VMC. Overview of mitochondrial bioenergetics. Methods Mol Biol 2018;1782:1–6.

[9] Ryan DG, O'Neill LAJ. Krebs cycle reborn in macrophage immunometabolism. Annu Rev Immunol 2020;38:289–313.

[10] Fuhrmann DC, Brune B. Mitochondrial composition and function under the control of hypoxia. Redox Biol 2017;12:208–15.

[11] Montgomery ST, Mall MA, Kicic A, Stick SM, Arest CF. Hypoxia and sterile inflammation in cystic fibrosis airways: mechanisms and potential therapies. Eur Respir J 2017;49(1).

[12] Solaini G, Baracca A, Lenaz G, Sgarbi G. Hypoxia and mitochondrial oxidative metabolism. Biochim Biophys Acta 2010;1797(6-7):1171–7.

[13] Taylor CT, Scholz CC. The effect of HIF on metabolism and immunity. Nat Rev Nephrol 2022;18(9):573–87.

[14] Suresh MV, Aktay S, Yalamanchili G, Solanki S, Sathyarajan DT, Arnipalli MS, et al. Role of succinate in airway epithelial cell regulation following traumatic lung injury. JCI Insight 2023;8(18).

[15] Eckle T, Brodsky K, Bonney M, Packard T, Han J, Borchers CH, et al. HIF1A reduces acute lung injury by optimizing carbohydrate metabolism in the alveolar epithelium. PLoS Biol 2013;11(9):e1001665.

[16] Vohwinkel CU, Burns N, Coit E, Yuan X, Vladar EK, Sul C, et al. HIF1A-dependent induction of alveolar epithelial PFKFB3 dampens acute lung injury. JCI Insight 2022;7(24).

[17] He Y, Han Y, Zou L, Yao T, Zhang Y, Lv X, et al. Succinate promotes pulmonary fibrosis through GPR91 and predicts death in idiopathic pulmonary fibrosis. Sci Rep 2024;14(1):14376.

[18] Wang Z, Chen L, Huang Y, Luo M, Wang H, Jiang Z, et al. Pharmaceutical targeting of succinate dehydrogenase in fibroblasts controls bleomycin-induced lung fibrosis. Redox Biol 2021;46:102082.
[19] Rajesh R, Atallah R, Barnthaler T. Dysregulation of metabolic pathways in pulmonary fibrosis. Pharmacol Ther 2023;246:108436.
[20] Valentini M, Lapouge K. Catabolite repression in *Pseudomonas aeruginosa* PAO1 regulates the uptake of C4-dicarboxylates depending on succinate concentration. Env Microbiol 2013;15(6):1707–16.
[21] Rojo F. Carbon catabolite repression in *Pseudomonas*: optimizing metabolic versatility and interactions with the environment. FEMS Microbiol Rev 2010;34(5):658–84.
[22] Riquelme SA, Lozano C, Moustafa AM, Liimatta K, Tomlinson KL, Britto C, et al. CFTR-PTEN-dependent mitochondrial metabolic dysfunction promotes *Pseudomonas aeruginosa* airway infection. Sci Transl Med 2019;11(499).
[23] Ogger PP, Byrne AJ. Macrophage metabolic reprogramming during chronic lung disease. Mucosal Immunol 2021;14(2):282–95.
[24] Tannahill GM, Curtis AM, Adamik J, Palsson-McDermott EM, McGettrick AF, Goel G, et al. Succinate is an inflammatory signal that induces IL-1beta through HIF-1alpha. Nature 2013;496 (7444):238–42.
[25] Trauelsen M, Hiron TK, Lin D, Petersen JE, Breton B, Husted AS, et al. Extracellular succinate hyperpolarizes M2 macrophages through SUCNR1/GPR91-mediated Gq signaling. Cell Rep 2021;35 (11):109246.
[26] Peruzzotti-Jametti L, Bernstock JD, Vicario N, Costa ASH, Kwok CK, Leonardi T, et al. Macrophage-derived extracellular succinate licenses neural stem cells to suppress chronic neuroinflammation. Cell Stem Cell 2018;22(3):355–68 e13.
[27] Lo Sciuto A, Martorana AM, Fernandez-Pinar R, Mancone C, Polissi A, Imperi F. *Pseudomonas aeruginosa* LptE is crucial for LptD assembly, cell envelope integrity, antibiotic resistance and virulence. Virulence 2018;9(1):1718–33.
[28] Chimalakonda G, Ruiz N, Chng SS, Garner RA, Kahne D, Silhavy TJ. Lipoprotein LptE is required for the assembly of LptD by the beta-barrel assembly machine in the outer membrane of Escherichia coli. Proc Natl Acad Sci U S A 2011;108(6):2492–7.
[29] Tomlinson KL, Chen YT, Junker A, Urso A, Wong Fok Lung T, Ahn D, et al. Ketogenesis promotes tolerance to *Pseudomonas aeruginosa* pulmonary infection. Cell Metab 2023;35(10):1767–81 e6.
[30] Palsson-McDermott EM, O'Neill LA. Signal transduction by the lipopolysaccharide receptor, Toll-like receptor-4. Immunology 2004;113(2):153–62.
[31] McElvaney OJ, Zaslona Z, Becker-Flegler K, Palsson-McDermott EM, Boland F, Gunaratnam C, et al. Specific Inhibition of the NLRP3 Inflammasome as an Antiinflammatory Strategy in Cystic Fibrosis. Am J Respir Crit Care Med 2019;200(11):1381–91.
[32] Elborn JS. Cystic fibrosis. Lancet 2016;388(10059):2519–31.
[33] Ong T, Ramsey BW. Cystic fibrosis: a review. JAMA 2023;329(21):1859–71.
[34] Peace CG, O'Neill LA. The role of itaconate in host defense and inflammation. J Clin Invest 2022;132(2).
[35] Schupp JC, Khanal S, Gomez JL, Sauler M, Adams TS, Chupp GL, et al. Single-cell transcriptional archetypes of airway inflammation in cystic fibrosis. Am J Respir Crit Care Med 2020;202(10):1419–29.
[36] Lampropoulou V, Sergushichev A, Bambouskova M, Nair S, Vincent EE, Loginicheva E, et al. Itaconate links inhibition of succinate dehydrogenase with macrophage metabolic remodeling and regulation of inflammation. Cell Metab 2016;24(1):158–66.
[37] Cordes T, Wallace M, Michelucci A, Divakaruni AS, Sapcariu SC, Sousa C, et al. Immunoresponsive gene 1 and itaconate inhibit succinate dehydrogenase to modulate intracellular succinate levels. J Biol Chem 2016;291(27):14274–84.
[38] He R, Liu B, Xiong R, Geng B, Meng H, Lin W, et al. Itaconate inhibits ferroptosis of macrophage via Nrf2 pathways against sepsis-induced acute lung injury. Cell Death Discov 2022;8(1):43.
[39] Crossley JL, Ostashevskaya-Gohstand S, Comazzetto S, Hook JS, Guo L, Vishlaghi N, et al. Itaconate-producing neutrophils regulate local and systemic inflammation following trauma. JCI Insight 2023;8(20).

[40] Ryan TAJ, Hooftman A, Rehill AM, Johansen MD, Brien ECO, Toller-Kawahisa JE, et al. Dimethyl fumarate and 4-octyl itaconate are anticoagulants that suppress Tissue Factor in macrophages via inhibition of Type I Interferon. Nat Commun 2023;14(1):3513.

[41] Hooftman A, Angiari S, Hester S, Corcoran SE, Runtsch MC, Ling C, et al. The Immunomodulatory metabolite itaconate modifies NLRP3 and inhibits inflammasome activation. Cell Metab 2020;32(3):468–78 e7.

[42] Mills EL, Ryan DG, Prag HA, Dikovskaya D, Menon D, Zaslona Z, et al. Itaconate is an anti-inflammatory metabolite that activates Nrf2 via alkylation of KEAP1. Nature 2018;556(7699):113–17.

[43] Bourner LA, Chung LA, Long H, McGettrick AF, Xiao J, Roth K, et al. Endogenously produced itaconate negatively regulates innate-driven cytokine production and drives global ubiquitination in human macrophages. Cell Rep 2024;43(8):114570.

[44] Luan HH, Medzhitov R. Food fight: Role of itaconate and other metabolites in antimicrobial defense. Cell Metab 2016;24(3):379–87.

[45] Zhu X, Guo Y, Liu Z, Yang J, Tang H, Wang Y. Itaconic acid exerts anti-inflammatory and antibacterial effects via promoting pentose phosphate pathway to produce ROS. Sci Rep 2021;11(1):18173.

[46] Zhang Z, Chen C, Yang F, Zeng YX, Sun P, Liu P, et al. Itaconate is a lysosomal inducer that promotes antibacterial innate immunity. Mol Cell 2022;82(15):2844–57 e10.

[47] Chen M, Sun H, Boot M, Shao L, Chang SJ, Wang W, et al. Itaconate is an effector of a Rab GTPase cell-autonomous host defense pathway against Salmonella. Science 2020;369(6502):450–5.

[48] Hentzer M, Teitzel GM, Balzer GJ, Heydorn A, Molin S, Givskov M, et al. Alginate overproduction affects *Pseudomonas aeruginosa* biofilm structure and function. J Bacteriol 2001;183(18):5395–401.

[49] Kolpen M, Kragh KN, Enciso JB, Faurholt-Jepsen D, Lindegaard B, Egelund GB, et al. Bacterial biofilms predominate in both acute and chronic human lung infections. Thorax 2022;77(10):1015–22.

[50] May TB, Shinabarger D, Maharaj R, Kato J, Chu L, DeVault JD, et al. Alginate synthesis by *Pseudomonas aeruginosa*: a key pathogenic factor in chronic pulmonary infections of cystic fibrosis patients. Clin Microbiol Rev 1991;4(2):191–206.

[51] Pedersen SS, Hoiby N, Espersen F, Koch C. Role of alginate in infection with mucoid *Pseudomonas aeruginosa* in cystic fibrosis. Thorax 1992;47(1):6–13.

[52] Franklin MJ, Nivens DE, Weadge JT, Howell PL. Biosynthesis of the *Pseudomonas aeruginosa* extracellular polysaccharides, alginate, Pel, and Psl. Front Microbiol 2011;2:167.

[53] Sasikaran J, Ziemski M, Zadora PK, Fleig A, Berg IA. Bacterial itaconate degradation promotes pathogenicity. Nat Chem Biol 2014;10(5):371–7.

[54] D'Arpa P, Karna SLR, Chen T, Leung KP. *Pseudomonas aeruginosa* transcriptome adaptations from colonization to biofilm infection of skin wounds. Sci Rep 2021;11(1):20632.

[55] Huang Q, Duan C, Ma H, Nong C, Zheng Q, Zhou J, et al. Structural and functional characterization of itaconyl-CoA hydratase and citramalyl-CoA lyase involved in itaconate metabolism of *Pseudomonas aeruginosa*. Structure 2024;32(7):941–52 e3.

[56] Lundgren BR, Villegas-Penaranda LR, Harris JR, Mottern AM, Dunn DM, Boddy CN, et al. Genetic analysis of the assimilation of C5-dicarboxylic acids in *Pseudomonas aeruginosa* PAO1. J Bacteriol 2014;196(14):2543–51.

[57] Potvin E, Sanschagrin F, Levesque RC. Sigma factors in *Pseudomonas aeruginosa*. FEMS Microbiol Rev 2008;32(1):38–55.

[58] Chevalier S, Bouffartigues E, Bazire A, Tahrioui A, Duchesne R, Tortuel D, et al. Extracytoplasmic function sigma factors in *Pseudomonas aeruginosa*. Biochim Biophys Acta Gene Regul Mech 2019;1862(7):706–21.

[59] Valentini M, Storelli N, Lapouge K. Identification of C(4)-dicarboxylate transport systems in *Pseudomonas aeruginosa* PAO1. J Bacteriol 2011;193(17):4307–16.

[60] Rossi E, La Rosa R, Bartell JA, Marvig RL, Haagensen JAJ, Sommer LM, et al. *Pseudomonas aeruginosa* adaptation and evolution in patients with cystic fibrosis. Nat Rev Microbiol 2021;19(5):331–42.

[61] Rossi E, Falcone M, Molin S, Johansen HK. High-resolution in situ transcriptomics of *Pseudomonas aeruginosa* unveils genotype independent patho-phenotypes in cystic fibrosis lungs. Nat Commun 2018;9(1):3459.

[62] Shao X, Zhang X, Zhang Y, Zhu M, Yang P, Yuan J, et al. RpoN-Dependent Direct Regulation of Quorum Sensing and the Type VI Secretion System in *Pseudomonas aeruginosa* PAO1. J Bacteriol 2018;200(16).

[63] Gabryszewski SJ, Wong Fok Lung T, Annavajhala MK, Tomlinson KL, Riquelme SA, Khan IN, et al. Metabolic Adaptation in Methicillin-Resistant *Staphylococcus aureus* Pneumonia. Am J Respir Cell Mol Biol 2019;61(2):185–97.

[64] Urso AMI, Cheng Y-T, et al. *Staphylococcus aureus* adapts to exploit collagen derived proline during chronic infection. Nat Microbiology 2024;. Available from: https://doi.org/10.1038/s41564-024-01769-9i.

[65] Cheung GYC, Bae JS, Otto M. Pathogenicity and virulence of *Staphylococcus aureus*. Virulence 2021;12(1):547–69.

[66] Sadiku P, Willson JA, Ryan EM, Sammut D, Coelho P, Watts ER, et al. Neutrophils fuel effective immune responses through gluconeogenesis and glycogenesis. Cell Metab 2021;33(5):1062–4.

[67] Lehman MK, Sturd NA, Razvi F, Wellems DL, Carson SD, Fey PD. Proline transporters ProT and PutP are required for *Staphylococcus aureus* infection. PLoS Pathog 2023;19(1):e1011098.

[68] Halsey CR, Lei S, Wax JK, Lehman MK, Nuxoll AS, Steinke L, et al. Amino acid catabolism in *Staphylococcus aureus* and the function of carbon catabolite repression. mBio 2017;8(1).

[69] Wong Fok Lung T, Monk IR, Acker KP, Mu A, Wang N, Riquelme SA, et al. *Staphylococcus aureus* small colony variants impair host immunity by activating host cell glycolysis and inducing necroptosis. Nat Microbiol 2020;5(1):141–53.

[70] Gaupp R, Schlag S, Liebeke M, Lalk M, Gotz F. Advantage of upregulation of succinate dehydrogenase in *Staphylococcus aureus* biofilms. J Bacteriol 2010;192(9):2385–94.

[71] Tomlinson KL, Riquelme SA, Baskota SU, Drikic M, Monk IR, Stinear TP, et al. *Staphylococcus aureus* stimulates neutrophil itaconate production that suppresses the oxidative burst. Cell Rep 2023;42(2):112064.

[72] El-Benna J, Hurtado-Nedelec M, Marzaioli V, Marie JC, Gougerot-Pocidalo MA, Dang PM. Priming of the neutrophil respiratory burst: role in host defense and inflammation. Immunol Rev 2016;273(1):180–93.

[73] Tomlinson KL, Lung TWF, Dach F, Annavajhala MK, Gabryszewski SJ, Groves RA, et al. *Staphylococcus aureus* induces an itaconate-dominated immunometabolic response that drives biofilm formation. Nat Commun 2021;12(1):1399.

[74] Gauba A, Rahman KM. Evaluation of Antibiotic Resistance Mechanisms in Gram-Negative Bacteria. Antibiotics (Basel) 2023;12(11).

[75] Russo TA, Marr CM. Hypervirulent *Klebsiella pneumoniae*. Clin Microbiol Rev 2019;32(3).

[76] Hauck C, Cober E, Richter SS, Perez F, Salata RA, Kalayjian RC, et al. Spectrum of excess mortality due to carbapenem-resistant *Klebsiella pneumoniae* infections. Clin Microbiol Infect 2016;22(6):513–19.

[77] Russo TA, Alvarado CL, Davies CJ, Drayer ZJ, Carlino-MacDonald U, Hutson A, et al. Differentiation of hypervirulent and classical *Klebsiella pneumoniae* with acquired drug resistance. mBio 2024;15(2):e0286723.

[78] European Centre for Disease Prevention and Control Surveillance of antimicrobial resistance in Europe 2018. Antimicrobial resistance surveillance in Europe. 2019.

[79] Kochan TJ, Nozick SH, Valdes A, Mitra SD, Cheung BH, Lebrun-Corbin M, et al. *Klebsiella pneumoniae* clinical isolates with features of both multidrug-resistance and hypervirulence have unexpectedly low virulence. Nat Commun 2023;14(1):7962.

[80] Bengoechea JA, Sa Pessoa J. *Klebsiella pneumoniae* infection biology: living to counteract host defences. FEMS Microbiol Rev 2019;43(2):123–44.

[81] O'Neill LA, Kishton RJ, Rathmell J. A guide to immunometabolism for immunologists. Nat Rev Immunol 2016;16(9):553–65.

[82] Wong Fok Lung T, Charytonowicz D, Beaumont KG, Shah SS, Sridhar SH, Gorrie CL, et al. *Klebsiella pneumoniae* induces host metabolic stress that promotes tolerance to pulmonary infection. Cell Metab 2022;34(5):761–74 e9.

[83] Ahn D, Penaloza H, Wang Z, Wickersham M, Parker D, Patel P, et al. Acquired resistance to innate immune clearance promotes *Klebsiella pneumoniae* ST258 pulmonary infection. JCI Insight 2016;1(17):e89704.

[84] Poe SL, Arora M, Oriss TB, Yarlagadda M, Isse K, Khare A, et al. STAT1-regulated lung MDSC-like cells produce IL-10 and efferocytose apoptotic neutrophils with relevance in resolution of bacterial pneumonia. Mucosal Immunol 2013;6(1):189–99.

[85] Hegde S, Leader AM, Merad M. MDSC: Markers, development, states, and unaddressed complexity. Immunity 2021;54(5):875–84.

[86] Liu S, Zhang P, Liu Y, Gao X, Hua J, Li W. Metabolic regulation protects mice against *Klebsiella pneumoniae* lung infection. Exp Lung Res 2018;44(6):302–11.

[87] Jenior ML, Dickenson ME, Papin JA. Genome-scale metabolic modeling reveals increased reliance on valine catabolism in clinical isolates of *Klebsiella pneumoniae*. NPJ Syst Biol Appl 2022;8(1):41.

[88] Storey D, McNally A, Astrand M, Sa-Pessoa Graca Santos J, Rodriguez-Escudero I, Elmore B, et al. *Klebsiella pneumoniae* type VI secretion system-mediated microbial competition is PhoPQ controlled and reactive oxygen species dependent. PLoS Pathog 2020;16(3):e1007969.

[89] Yu KW, Xue P, Fu Y, Yang L. T6SS mediated stress responses for bacterial environmental survival and host adaptation. Int J Mol Sci 2021;22(2).

[90] Si M, Zhao C, Burkinshaw B, Zhang B, Wei D, Wang Y, et al. Manganese scavenging and oxidative stress response mediated by type VI secretion system in *Burkholderia thailandensis*. Proc Natl Acad Sci U S A 2017;114(11):E2233–42.

[91] Wan B, Zhang Q, Ni J, Li S, Wen D, Li J, et al. Type VI secretion system contributes to Enterohemorrhagic Escherichia coli virulence by secreting catalase against host reactive oxygen species (ROS). PLoS Pathog 2017;13(3):e1006246.

[92] Wang T, Si M, Song Y, Zhu W, Gao F, Wang Y, et al. Type VI secretion system transports Zn2 + to combat multiple stresses and host immunity. PLoS Pathog 2015;11(7):e1005020.

[93] Sa-Pessoa J, Lopez-Montesino S, Przybyszewska K, Rodriguez-Escudero I, Marshall H, Ova A, et al. A trans-kingdom T6SS effector induces the fragmentation of the mitochondrial network and activates innate immune receptor NLRX1 to promote infection. Nat Commun 2023;14(1):871.

CHAPTER 3

Crosstalk between metabolites and myeloid cell biology

Brian P. Goldspiel[1,2,*], Mikel D. Haggadone[3,*], Sunny Shin[3] and Will Bailis[2,4]

[1]Medical Scientist Training Program, Perelman School of Medicine, University of Pennsylvania, Philadelphia, PA, United States, [2]Department of Pathology and Laboratory Medicine, Children's Hospital of Philadelphia, Philadelphia, PA, United States, [3]Department of Microbiology, Perelman School of Medicine, University of Pennsylvania, Philadelphia, PA, United States, [4]Department of Pathology and Laboratory Medicine, Perelman School of Medicine, University of Pennsylvania, Philadelphia, PA, United States

Chapter introduction—metabolites: friend or foe?

Two key functions of the immune system are to survey the environment for disruptions in homeostasis and then adopt the appropriate programming to convey this information to other cells [1–3]. Accordingly, a major focus of research on innate immunity has been to elucidate the key signals that innate cells are sensing and how these specific signals initiate selective programs. A major focus of these efforts has been the identification and study of pattern recognition receptors (PRRs) like the Toll-like receptors (TLRs), which sense conserved pathogen- or damage-associated patterns (PAMPS/DAMPS) and induce inflammatory responses correspondingly [4–7].

Upon engaging their ligands, these PRRs trigger a multitude of signaling pathways, which ultimately converge on two major anabolic biological processes—transcription and translation [1–3,8,9]. Transcription and translation rely on the availability of nucleic acids and amino acids, respectively, not to mention stores of energy in the form of ATP [10–12]. Therefore, in addition to identifying PAMPs or DAMPs in their environment, innate immune cells must also integrate information about the availability of these anabolic metabolites prior to undergoing the functional rewiring dictated by PRRs [2,13–15]. Metabolically sensitive signaling proteins like mammalian target of rapamycin (mTOR) and AMP-activated protein kinase (AMPK) have been shown to serve such a purpose [16–18]. While these metabolic sensors have been extensively studied in other cell types, much less

---

* These authors contributed equally.

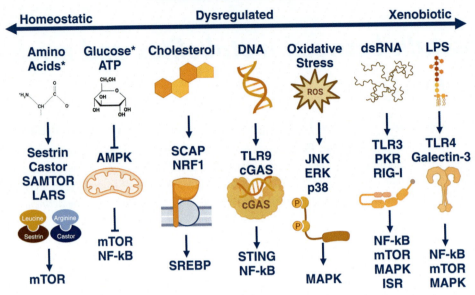

Figure 3.1: Metabolic and innate sensing pathways overlap in the components they sense. Frequently, metabolic and innate immune sensors are considered individual signaling pathways that are sensing either central metabolites or pathogen-associated patterns. However, the molecules that activate these pathways have remarkable overlap. Many such signals may be produced by either host or pathogen, and therefore the sensors required for identifying them have the capacity to communicate to multiple networks simultaneously. Thus, rather than being purely metabolic or inflammatory, we note here that these pathways are capable of sensing molecules on a spectrum, with the capacity to regulate both homeostatic and inflammatory processes simultaneously. Created with BioRender.

is known about how they regulate myeloid cell biology and how metabolic and inflammatory cues are incorporated into a coherent immune response [2,16,19–21].

To unravel the complexity behind this question, let us consider the remarkable overlap that both PRRs and metabolic sensors share in their downstream effectors (Fig. 3.1). For example, TLR4 activation leads to the induction of the mitogen-activated protein kinase (MAPK) pathway, including the kinase extracellular signal-regulated kinase (ERK), which both activates mTOR and coregulates downstream effectors [9]. In this chapter, we will uncover many more ways that these different signaling networks interact. Furthermore, these signaling nodes are often spatially colocalized—a subset of PRRs and mTOR signaling both frequently originate from endolysosomes [22,23]. These features suggest not just crosstalk between inflammatory and metabolic signaling pathways but also a substantial overlap in function. Is this coincidental? Or does this reflect that metabolic and innate immune signaling are part of a single network for coordinating innate immunity?

If we push this concept further, we can begin to see that even the types of molecules that activate PRRs and metabolic networks are ultimately metabolites (Fig. 3.1). When we consider the sources of these activating signals, some may be either host-derived or homeostatic in nature, while others are clearly only made by pathogens and are xenobiotic (Fig. 3.1). Many others still lie somewhere in the middle. Consider, for instance, that cytosolic DNA can activate cyclic GMP-AMP synthase and stimulator of interferon genes (cGAS-STING), whether it be derived from host mitochondrial DNA or a pathogen [24]. Ergo, DNA is neither homeostatic nor xenobiotic, but rather a reflection of an abnormal environment, which we will classify as dysbiotic (Fig. 3.1). It is worth noting that even metabolites we are considering as homeostatic signals, like the amino acids, may reflect dysbiotic states (perhaps related to variations in their concentration—we will discuss this in the next section) [25–28]. Moreover, it is possible that similar biochemical products, like nonproteinogenic amino acids, may be uniquely immunostimulatory [29–31]. Thus, the scale we propose here is flexible and context dependent, but the point still stands—metabolic and immune sensing pathways can be activated by overlapping molecules.

The importance for myeloid cells to differentiate these homeostatic and xenobiotic signals is further underscored by the diversity of metabolic environments that myeloid cells live and work in. Indeed, tissue-resident myeloid cells can reside in metabolically varied tissues like the liver or lung [23,32–34]. Moreover, trafficking myeloid cells experience extreme variations in metabolic availability [32–34]. These cells can leave the metabolically rich blood to enter tissues with broad metabolic perturbations due to various pathologies, like cancers or infections [35–38]. This means that the life of a myeloid cell is inherently one of varied metabolic environments, one in which the cell may encounter a lack or even excess of specific resources in any given inflammatory scenario [38–41]. This presents two critical points. First, myeloid cells are sensitive to dynamic changes in metabolic environments inherent to their lifestyles [28,40]. Second, these cells must adapt to cellular stress [42–44]. Thus, innate signaling, metabolite availability, and cellular stress must be central to regulating the function of myeloid cells.

In this chapter, we will expand on these ideas by considering a few specific myeloid signaling pathways that are central to metabolic and inflammatory regulation. Although there are several signaling molecules we could discuss, for brevity we will focus on three of the most well described in the myeloid cell literature—mTORC1, MAPK, and the sterol regulatory element-binding proteins (SREBPs). First, we will discuss these key nodes in innate and metabolic sensing and the molecules that activate them. Next, we will consider the overlap of metabolic and innate signaling with cellular stress pathways. Lastly, we will explore more recent work aimed at understanding how tissue-specific metabolic environments regulate myeloid cell behaviors. In conclusion, we will reflect on the current state of immunometabolism in innate immunity with a forward-facing lens to our understanding of the signaling pathways that modulate the key functional programs of myeloid cells.

Metabolic and innate immune signaling

Understanding the singular contributions of specific metabolic sensing pathways is made remarkably complex by their overlap [45]. In part, this is due to growth factor and anabolic metabolism signaling converging on cellular biosynthesis and protein production. For the pathways we will discuss in this chapter, this is executed through convergence on functional outputs as well as through substantial crosstalk between signaling nodes (Fig. 3.2). While we will refer to some of the inherent connections between these signaling cascades, we will attempt to simplify this complexity by considering the individual contributions of each specific signaling network. Thus, the goal is to reflect on our current understanding of these sensing pathways by contextualizing their significance for innate immune responses. To do so, we will introduce some of the major cellular sensors and the signals that activate them, while referring to their crosstalk with immune signaling. Lastly, we will reflect on their regulation of specific inflammatory functions.

mTORC1

mTOR is perhaps the best described metabolic sensing network in mammalian cells [46,47]. First identified as the target of the drug rapamycin, the mTOR protein is now known to be part of two major complexes—mTOR complex 1 (mTORC1) and mTOR complex 2 (mTORC2), each with its own roles in regulating cell function and metabolism [48–52]. While mTORC2 certainly has its own importance in myeloid cells, it is primarily understood to be a growth-factor-sensitive complex, whereas mTORC1 plays a direct role in detecting changes in intracellular metabolite levels [47,52]. Indeed, mTORC1's activation induces broad anabolic and functional changes within the cell through both transcriptional and translational mechanisms [21,53–56]. To execute this, mTORC1 regulates the activity of several transcription factors (e.g., transcription factor EB [TFEB] and SREBP, which we will return to), as well as phosphorylation of initiation and elongation factors like S6 kinase (S6K) and eukaryotic translation initiation factor 4 binding protein (4EBP1) to promote translation [57–60]. Simultaneously, mTORC1 activation downregulates catabolic programs, like autophagy, to prevent futile cycling of nutrients [21,46,54,61,62]. In sum, mTORC1 activation licenses cell growth and polypeptide production.

Broadly speaking, mTORC1 can be understood as a rheostat for anabolic permissibility, taking inputs from sensors of a variety of metabolites, growth factors, and activating

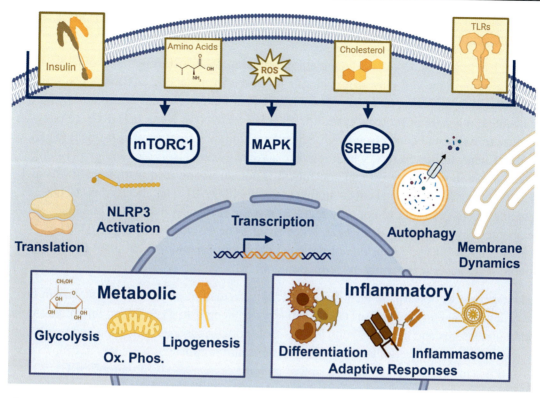

Figure 3.2: Integrators of metabolic and inflammatory signals converge on functional programs in myeloid cells.
Broadly, metabolic and inflammatory signals converge on multiple pathways, including mTORC1, MAPK, and SREBP. These pathways, in turn, regulate central cellular processes, including transcription, translation, inflammation, autophagy, and membrane movement. The sum of these activities is both broad changes in metabolism, including alterations to glycolysis and oxidative phosphorylation, as well as important changes to myeloid cell biology, including their differentiation and immunoregulatory function. These broad connections and shared functional outputs demonstrate the universal aspects of both metabolic and inflammatory signaling. Created with BioRender.

stimuli, including PRR agonism [18,21,63–68]. Among metabolites, mTORC1 is most sensitive to the presence of specific amino acids and lipids, of which leucine is the most extensively studied [18,46,53,69]. Indeed, several specific sensors for leucine have been identified that signal through mTORC1, including SESTRIN2, secretion-associated Ras-related GTPase 1B (SAR1B), leucyl-tRNA synthetase (LARS), and solute carrier family 7 member 5 (SLC7a5) [70–73]. Additionally, leucine catabolism activates mTORC1 via its downstream metabolites [74,75]. Besides leucine, other mTORC1-activating metabolites also have specific sensors (e.g., arginine and S-adenosylmethionine [SAM]), while some others are likely sensed indirectly (e.g., glutamine) or are part of a two-step activation process of mTORC1 [76–80]. This broad sensitivity to amino acids poises mTORC1 as a major integrator of metabolic cues in orchestrating cellular metabolism.

mTORC1 is largely understood to integrate information about cytosolic metabolite contents, but its location in the cell may reflect its role as a broader metabolic environmental sensor. One of the main signaling locations for mTORC1 is around lysosomal membranes, where it is anchored to a suite of proteins called the Ragulator [81–84]. Here, mTORC1 activates in response to lysosomal contents and subsequently inhibits the transcription factor E (TFE) family of transcription factors, which regulate autophagy and lysosome biology [81–86]. Given its role in sensing lysosomal contents, it is not surprising then that phagocytosis and macropinocytosis activate mTORC1 in myeloid cells [87–90]. This means that mTORC1 signaling has the capacity to not only regulate specific responses depending on what metabolites are present but also *where*, whether intra- or extracellular [47,85,91]. This positions mTORC1 at perhaps one of the most important immunological interfaces for professional phagocytes—at the lysosomal membrane.

It should come as no surprise then that mTORC1's regulation plays substantial roles in the life of a myeloid cell. Indeed, mTORC1 activation is central to TLR-driven inflammation in both macrophages and dendritic cells [65,92–94]. Furthermore, its activation and regulation are pivotal to myeloid cell differentiation decisions and, ultimately, their specific functions [94–100]. This plays out in altered adaptive immune responses given that mTORC1 activity is required for antigen presentation [101–103]. These responses are after PRR engagement, but mTORC1 is also likely central to steady-state myeloid cell biology. For instance, rapamycin's activity as an mTORC1 inhibitor has made the drug an active area of aging research. Recent work has suggested that part of rapamycin's geroprotective role is via cytokine signaling, given the key role that sterile inflammation plays in aging [47,104,105]. It then follows that a potential mechanistic explanation for rapamycin's geroprotective effect is via its suppression of myeloid cell-driven inflammation [106]. Indeed, we do see in other forms of sterile inflammation—like atherosclerosis—that rapamycin's inhibition of myeloid cell mTORC1 is protective against pathology [69]. This is all to say, ultimately, that mTORC1 activity is central to innate inflammatory function. How then can myeloid cells use the information conveyed by mTORC1 to orchestrate the immune response?

Studies in the context of bacterial infection may help guide our answer to this question [107]. Let us consider the intracellular pathogen, *Legionella pneumophila*, which can rewire myeloid cells to develop an endoplasmic reticulum (ER)-derived replicative niche called the *Legionella*-containing vacuole (LCV) [108]. Recent work has suggested that one of the central mechanisms allowing it to develop the LCV is by employing bacterial effector proteins that regulate mTORC1 signaling [109–112]. This may be at least in part due to the biosynthetic demand of *Legionella* replication inside the LCV, requiring both host-derived amino acids and lipids [113]. Supporting this, mTORC1 suppression upon *Legionella* infection is protective against the pathogen by destabilizing the LCV, and reversing mTORC1 inhibition is necessary for *Legionella* survival in the LCV [112]. This raises the distinct possibility that *Legionella* consumption of host metabolites is a fundamental cue for enabling a proper immune response to the pathogen [107].

One additional intriguing possibility is that mTORC1 in myeloid cells might be *directly* sensing metabolic variability. There is strong evidence that products of catabolism—like branched-chain amino acid (BCAA)-derived metabolites—have the capacity to activate mTORC1 [74]. Meanwhile, nonessential amino acids, like those that can be synthesized through anabolic metabolism, activate mTORC1 independently of the Ragulator [80]. We also know that macrophages upregulate different metabolic pathways in accordance with their function [29]. It follows then that mTORC1's sensitivity to specific metabolites, particularly those of amino acid catabolism and synthesis whose availability can rapidly change, would be critical to those cells. This suggests that mTORC1 is more than a homeostatic integrator but *also* has the capacity to identify the unique metabolic byproducts of inflammatory or antiinflammatory myeloid cells. More research is needed to explore this critical role for mTORC1 in varied metabolic environments.

In sum, mTORC1 has become of great interest in innate immunity and for good reason—this signaling node is central to many fundamental myeloid cell functions. Much work is needed to better understand how we might integrate the multifaceted roles of mTORC1 in innate immune responses. mTORC1's sensitivity to a multitude of dynamic ranges of metabolites likely contributes to selectivity in immune reactions. Understanding these nuances will allow us to target this specificity in treatments for inflammatory disease. This puts mTORC1 as a distinct node of homeostatic and pathologic myeloid cell signaling.

MAPK

The MAPK family of signaling molecules encompasses a complex signaling network that includes multiple kinases—namely, ERK, p38, and c-jun-N-terminal kinase (JNK) subfamilies [114–116]. Just like mTORC1, these proteins regulate cellular processes of anabolic growth and are responsible for metabolic reprogramming in myeloid cells [114–118]. Illustrating their functional overlap, they can be activated by some of the same metabolic sensors (e.g., LAMTOR) and regulate cellular biology through shared targets (e.g., S6 and eukaryotic translation initiation factor 4b [eIF4b]) [119–121]. However, MAPK signaling also orchestrates these metabolic shifts through unique downstream effectors, as dictated by the activation of specific subfamilies [114–116]. Additionally, MAPK signaling plays a central role in cellular stress responses and cell death decisions [45,116,122–124]. While MAPK signaling is necessary for anabolic growth, it also contributes substantially to cell survival [45,114–116]. These specific functions make the MAP kinases indispensable regulators of myeloid cell activity.

The MAP kinases are exquisitely sensitive to both extracellular and intracellular signals downstream of a broad array of sensors [45,114,116,125]. These sensors include PRRs like the TLRs, cytokine receptors, hypoxia, and hormone receptors like those for insulin [114,126]. In addition, the MAP kinases are activated upon exposure to reactive oxygen species (ROS) [127–129]. For myeloid cells, ROS are both a natural product of myeloid cell metabolism and, for nitric oxide in particular, important mediators of pathogen clearance [29,130]. Moreover, ROS themselves play substantial roles in regulating both the physiological and inflammatory metabolism of myeloid cells [131–133]. The importance of ROS in myeloid metabolism implies that the MAP kinases are poised not just as mediators of inflammatory signaling but metabolic signaling as well. We will return to this idea shortly.

Much of our understanding of these kinases' roles in myeloid cells stems from their activation downstream of TLR signaling. Indeed, MAPK activation is necessary for the transcription and translation of inflammatory cytokines in both macrophages and dendritic cells [65,100,114]. This is tunable depending on which of the MAP kinases are activated, but broadly, MAPK signaling skews cells towards inflammatory phenotypes and induces the production of pro-inflammatory cytokines [134–136]. As a result, MAPK activity plays multiple roles in regulating innate immune responses, including its roles in both adaptive immunity and tumorigenesis [94,137–141]. Moreover, the influence of ROS on myeloid cell biology underscores the important functional roles of the MAPK signaling pathway. For one, ROS-mediated activation of the MAP kinases is essential for macrophage differentiation [142,143]. Additionally, ROS are central to both dendritic cell function and antigen presentation to adaptive immune cells [144]. Ergo, MAP kinase sensing of metabolism through ROS is critical to its role in myeloid cells.

Notably, ROS are not the only forms of metabolic stress that activate the MAPK pathway. Another strong trigger of MAPK signaling is ribotoxic stress, which is sensed through the sterile alpha motif and leucine zipper-containing kinase (ZAKα) [145]. Broadly, ribotoxic stress is triggered by ribosomal dysfunction downstream of a variety of insults, including amino acid deprivation and UV light [145,146]. Therefore, this sensor stands at the crossroads of metabolic and stress signaling, which is in turn elaborated by the MAP kinases. Importantly, activation of this pathway also orchestrates key functional programs in myeloid cells—UV-triggered ZAKα activation promotes assembly of the NOD-like receptor protein 1 (NLRP1) inflammasome in human monocytes [146]. It remains unknown if ribotoxic stress downstream of metabolic cues also tunes inflammasome function in myeloid cells, but these connections illustrate the intimate nature of MAPK sensing of environmental metabolites and its resulting regulation of innate immunity.

One of the main mechanisms through which these signaling pathways regulate myeloid cell function is through their activation of glycolysis [147–149]. Indeed, the glycolytic burst downstream of MAPK signaling is required in both macrophages and dendritic cells for early immune responses [147–149]. Notably, glucose is used as a key determinant of myeloid cell programming and function [29,150]. The MAP kinases accomplish this through both the upregulation of glycolytic enzymes and glucose transporters [148]. It is intriguing then that among the diversity of cell types that inhabit tumor microenvironments (TMEs), myeloid cells display the greatest capacity for taking up exogenous glucose [151]. Notably, the TME is known as a stressful environment, where hypoxia and high levels of ROS could potentiate MAPK activity [152–155]. These connections suggest that metabolic sensitivity to ROS via the MAP kinases could be responsible for a myeloid cell's dependence on glucose in the TME, but this remains unproven. Nevertheless, the implications of these findings are that MAP kinase sensitivity to ROS is crucial to innate immune cells in the TME, in part due to its influence on glucose metabolism.

One potential application for this relationship would be to target myeloid-derived suppressor cells (MDSCs) found within TMEs, which support tumor growth and metastasis through the production of antiinflammatory signals [156,157]. Reversal of MDSCs into a pro-inflammatory phenotype has been shown to aid in tumor clearance, making these cells a particular area of interest in cancer therapeutics [156–158]. To this end, MAPK inhibitors are a potential approach to reverse MDSC phenotypes [140,159]. More exploration is needed to understand the specific contribution of the MAPK pathway to MDSC function, but the results are promising and support the idea that metabolic cues through the MAP kinases are essential for regulating innate cell-driven inflammation.

To summarize, the MAP kinases are broadly sensitive to specific metabolic signals, including ROS and ribotoxic stress, downstream of metabolic dysfunction. In turn, the MAP kinases play central roles in altering both the inflammatory function and metabolism of myeloid cells. This means that MAPK activity is not only a central regulator of immune and metabolic function but is also deeply connected to the metabolic environment. This presents us with a bit of a chicken or egg conundrum. Is MAPK activity required for metabolism rewiring in myeloid cells or does metabolism rewiring regulate MAPK functions? The answer to both is likely yes, but more pertinently, it means that the MAP kinases are key cellular regulators in inflammatory cells, including their metabolic needs. We are just beginning to understand the complexity of these networks and the mechanisms through which they enact the specificity of their programs, but one thing is clear—the MAP kinases are neither simply immune nor metabolic, but rather broader pathways for regulating myeloid cell biology.

SREBP

Phagocytosis and membrane trafficking are fundamental to a myeloid cell's capacity for sensing their environment and clearing environmental hazards like pathogens or apoptotic debris [160–164]. These processes necessitate an ample pool of lipids and related membrane components like cholesterol [165]. A key mechanism that cells use to regulate lipid biogenesis and homeostasis is through the SREBP family of transcription factors [166,167]. Broadly, these proteins regulate lipid biogenesis and cellular metabolism through the upregulation of lipid and cholesterol biosynthetic pathways [166,167]. The SREBP proteins remain inactive on the ER until signals lead to their cleavage and transport to the nucleus where they activate a transcriptional program to drive cellular processes like lipogenesis and autophagy [168,169].

SREBPs are triggered through the activity of the signaling cascades we have already discussed, including MAPK and mTORC1 [170]. In addition to these, the SREBPs are induced more directly downstream of lipid bioavailability [171,172]. Briefly, SREBPs become activated when the chaperone protein SREBP cleavage-activating protein (SCAP) brings SREBP from the ER to the Golgi, where it is cleaved and released [173]. In the presence of cholesterols, however, this process is inhibited by the insulin-induced gene (INSIG) proteins, which bind SCAP and prevent SREBP from leaving the ER [174,175]. Intriguingly, INSIG can signal to multiple pathways in the cell, including the antiviral protein STING [176]. This functional overlap in cholesterol sensing, lipid metabolism, and antiviral immunity illustrates the inherent connection of lipid biology and innate immunity.

Their capacity for regulating unique and specific responses can be seen in their time-dependent effects on myeloid cell function. Early after TLR4 activation, SREBP is necessary in macrophages for TLR4 signaling by increasing phagocytosis and driving inflammasome-triggered interleukin (IL)-1β production [177]. Later, however, SREBP activity suppresses inflammation by driving the production of antiinflammatory cytokines like IL-10 [178]. The difference in requirements for SREBP in inflammation and its resolution suggests that the cell could be utilizing different lipid signals from its environment. SREBP may accomplish this through sensing specific lipid species. Indeed, SREBP is known to be uniquely sensitive to specific species of oxylipins, components of the cell membrane and lipid metabolism generated as part of inflammation [179,180]. Intriguingly, the composition of these oxylipins differs depending on the initiating inflammatory context, with roles in regulating both the microbiome and pathogenic immune responses [181]. We do not know the extent to which certain oxylipins regulate specific immune responses, and deeper investigation is warranted.

Many bacterial and viral pathogens trigger rapid changes in membrane dynamics, highlighting the importance of lipid species in innate immune responses [163,182–184]. For myeloid cells, changes in membrane lipid composition are sensed by SREBP, and this information is used to ultimately regulate myeloid cell function [185]. To this end, mice given high-fat diets have increased myeloid cell inflammation even after returning to regular chow, in part due to inflammasome-mediated trained immunity [186]. Intriguingly,

SREBP and SCAP activation downstream of cholesterol biosynthesis signaling has been shown to promote NOD-, LRR-, and pyrin domain-containing protein 3 (NLRP3) translocation to the Golgi, and in turn, inflammasome activation [187]. These studies would suggest that the lipid-sensing activities of the SREBP pathway are paramount to its ability to regulate myeloid cell inflammation and likely exist at the nexus of metabolism and immunity.

Given the central roles that lipid and cholesterol metabolism play in a myeloid cell's lifestyle, it remains an intriguing possibility that select lipid species are sensed through SREBP and confer specificity in tuning the immune response. We know that lipid species made by macrophages vary greatly depending on which TLR ligand is being sensed [188,189]. Moreover, lipid sensing through SREBP is known to be central to interferon responses and even resistance against bacterial toxins [173,190]. Therefore it is possible that specific lipidomes shaped by individual TLR ligands are integrated at the level of SREBP.

In sum, SREBP signaling is central to myeloid cell biology. This transcription factor and cholesterol rheostat ultimately regulates several fundamental aspects of innate immunity, including NLRP3 localization and interferon production. We are beginning to understand how specificity may be conferred through SREBP's activation downstream of distinct lipid species, but it places this signaling pathway at the center of lipid signaling and inflammation. Through the sum of its activities, SREBP is a necessary and central part of both myeloid cell function and metabolism.

With these various sensors in place, myeloid cells can respond to a variety of environmental challenges. However, with the challenges inherent to a myeloid cell's life comes stress on the cell—metabolic starvation, ROS, and unfolded proteins. The pathways we have already discussed (particularly MAPK) are part of the response to cellular stress, but still there are unique cellular stressors that MAPK cannot sense, which require specific sensors. Thus, it is not so simple to just sense their environment, but these cells must also be ready to handle the dangers of their complex lifestyles.

Stress responses in myeloid cells

Cellular stress is unavoidable for myeloid cells. For one, these cells rely on ROS as part of their role in clearing pathogens. Additionally, they experience rapid variations in protein synthesis, leading to protein and ribosomal stress. Lastly, they are dynamic cells that can enter metabolically depleted environments. Some of the pathways we have already discussed—like the MAP kinases—sense and respond to these stressors [191–193]. However, among these stress-adaptive pathways, the integrated stress response (ISR) appears to be particularly relevant for straddling immune and metabolic signaling.

The ISR consists of four kinases—general control nonderepressible 2 (GCN2), protein kinase R-like ER kinase (PERK), protein kinase R-activated (PKR), and heme-regulated inhibitor (HRI) [194]. These four kinases are sensitive to different intracellular stressors: uncharged tRNAs, ER stress, double-stranded (ds)RNAs, and heme, respectively [194]. Upon activation, these kinases phosphorylate eukaryotic translation initiation factor 2 A (eIF2A), which inhibits cap-dependent translation and licenses a transcriptional adaptation program through the selective translation of transcription factors such as activating transcription factor 4 (ATF4) [194–196]. Although this is not currently well understood, it does appear that despite the overlapping signaling pathways shared by these four kinases, there may be unique contributions and sensitivities that provide specificity depending on the kinase triggered [197–199].

We know that ISR kinases span a broad range of molecules that they are sensitive to, but this illustrates the same theme as the signaling pathways discussed previously—the ISR typifies the idea that immune and metabolic sensors share overlapping functions. First, let's consider the kinase PKR, which is known as a central sensor for dsRNAs [200–202]. dsRNAs can be products of viral infections, reflecting the kinase's capacity as a PRR, but dsRNAs are also generated during metabolic stress in cells under sterile conditions [203–205]. There is some, albeit limited, data suggesting that host-derived dsRNAs under metabolic stress have the capacity to activate PKR, although the extent to which this occurs in myeloid cells is not known [206]. However, what this suggests is that viral sensing by the ISR may also be equally attuned to metabolic stress.

PKR, however, is not the only possible metabolic sensor in the ISR. GCN2 is a sensor for uncharged tRNAs and therefore responds to metabolic stress via the absence of amino acids [194]. In addition to PKR, GCN2 is well appreciated as a regulator of myeloid cell inflammation. For example, GCN2 activation promotes antigen presentation by dendritic cells and the subsequent adaptive immune response post-vaccination [207]. Further, GCN2 activation is necessary for immunosuppression in the context of both inflammatory bowel disease and cancer through its inhibition of inflammasome activity [208–210]. Mechanistically, this may be at least in part due to sequestration of the pro-inflammatory cytokine produced by the inflammasome, IL-1β, into stress granules [208,211]. Curiously, and in contrast to GCN2, PKR appears to be an activator of the inflammasome [202]. This once again suggests some specificity depending on the ISR kinase that is activated, but in either case, both are indications of metabolic dysregulation.

While the ISR clearly responds to stressful environmental cues, this pathway stands at the interface of both pathogenic and metabolic signals. The activity of these kinases illustrates the overlapping functions that this pathway shares with those already discussed. More specifically, it integrates these various cues and ultimately converges on myeloid cell biology to modify cellular functions, likely in an ISR kinase-dependent manner. The summative impact of this stress-responsive pathway is to survey environmental cues and tune myeloid cell function accordingly.

Broadly, stress responses are fundamental aspects of myeloid biology, in part due to these cells' lifestyles. Part of that lifestyle is living in remarkably different metabolic environments. Indeed, tissue-resident macrophages (TRMs) must adapt to their local environments and ideally carry out their functions even with the distinct stressors and signals these cells will receive. Now that we have covered some of the overlapping features of metabolic, inflammatory, and stress sensing, we will next explore the unique attributes of tissue environments that converge on these pathways to modify myeloid cell biology.

Crosstalk between tissue microenvironment and tissue-resident macrophage metabolism

Given their prominent role as environmental sensors, macrophages reside in virtually every organ of the body where they perform tissue-specific functions that are programmed according to the demands imposed by their niche [212]. Therefore, in addition to serving as sentinel cells that guard against infection, TRMs carry out diverse tasks to maintain homeostasis in physiologically and metabolically unique environments [28]. Although different adult TRM populations derive from ontogenically distinct precursor cells (reviewed extensively [213,214]), their functional specialization appears to be, in part, imprinted by signals present in their niche [215]. This is evident in the observation that TRM depletion yields their replenishment by circulating monocytes that can ultimately adopt the original population's phenotypic and functional program [216–218]. Although these microenvironmental signals include secreted cytokines and growth factors that define a unique transcription factor signature [219–222], an emerging body of evidence suggests that tissue-specific metabolism also fundamentally tunes the distinct biology of different TRMs [223]. Therefore, steady-state nutrient sensing and handling shape how macrophages functionally fulfill the homeostatic requirements of their environment. Further, sterile and/or infectious perturbations that alter a tissue's metabolite composition can profoundly alter TRM metabolism to drive immunopathology.

Metabolic and functional specialization of macrophages during homeostasis

This paradigm is evident in one of the body's most metabolically unique microenvironments containing TRMs with an extreme bioenergetic phenotype: alveolar macrophages (AMs) in the distal lung. As the site of gas exchange between inspired air and the blood, the alveolar space is rich in pulmonary surfactant, a lipid–protein complex mainly comprising phospholipids and cholesterol that is homeostatically recycled by AMs

[219]. Furthermore, AMs in the steady-state lung are exposed to low glucose levels due to glucose transporter activity in the surrounding epithelium [224–226]. Given these metabolic constraints, it is therefore unsurprising that AMs display a unique metabolism that is poised for lipid catabolism and handling [223] but restrained in glycolytic capacity [227,228].

A defining feature of AMs is their developmental requirement for peroxisome proliferator-activated receptor gamma (PPARγ), a master regulator of lipid catabolism whose expression in AMs is orchestrated by the essential growth factors granulocyte-macrophage colony-stimulating factor (GM-CSF) and transforming growth factor beta (TGF-β) [222,229]. Accordingly, loss of PPARγ expression not only elevates intracellular lipid levels in, and compromises cholesterol efflux from, AMs, but it also dramatically disrupts their gene expression signature and abundance in vivo [222,229,230]. This underscores that AM development and maintenance is fundamentally shaped by residence in a surfactant-rich milieu, as AM bioenergetics are uniquely driven by these cells' need to handle, traffic, and catabolize large amounts of lipid. Among all the distinct TRM populations, AMs display the most extreme dependency on mitochondrial oxidative phosphorylation (OXPHOS) for their homeostatic maintenance [223]. In line with this, disrupting mitochondrial metabolism dramatically reduces AM numbers in the lung, but not because of ATP depletion. Rather, impeding the ability of AMs to process lipids and cholesterol via mitochondrial oxidative processes yields toxic buildup of these surfactant-derived metabolites, thus triggering stress responses that suppress AM proliferation and promote apoptosis [223]. As further evidence that pulmonary TRM metabolism is fundamentally shaped by these cells' nutrient environment, mTORC1 signaling is tissue-specifically purposed to support SREBP-dependent lipid metabolism in AMs and other myeloid cells in the lung [231]. The same is true for oxygen sensing metabolism, which is required for imprinting AM lipid handling during these cells' development in an oxygen-rich niche [232]. These findings highlight the profound influence of tissue nutrient environment on TRM identity, with AM development and metabolism biased toward a lipid-recycling program that is appropriately suited for residence in the surfactant-producing alveolar space.

Parallel to the unique capacity for AMs to handle and metabolize lipids, these cells concomitantly display suppressed capacity for glycolytic metabolism, a phenotype suited for their glucose-deprived niche in the healthy distal lung [233,234]. Such glycolytic suppression is not an intrinsic quality of AMs themselves but rather a metabolic phenotype imprinted by these cells' environment. Accordingly, ex vivo culture of AMs outside of their niche enhances glucose metabolism, whereas instillation of nonpulmonary macrophages into the lung inhibits their glycolytic rate [227]. The net result of a metabolic phenotype rich in fatty acid oxidation (FAO) and void of glucose utilization is a functional program that supports inflammatory quiescence in the distal airways. OXPHOS-dominant metabolism in AMs makes them more permissive to pathogen replication relative to neighboring macrophages that reside in the pulmonary interstitium, which exhibit higher steady-state rates of glycolysis [235]. Viral exposure can release this brake on AM glucose utilization, a metabolic "training" event that consequently augments these cells' antibacterial and antitumor inflammatory activity [236,237]. AMs with enhanced glycolytic activity also lose their hyporesponsiveness to type 2 cytokines [227] and are unable to secrete suppression of cytokine signaling proteins [238] that homeostatically restrain inflammatory signaling in the surrounding alveolar epithelium [239]. Further, a glycolytic signature in AMs is observed during both sterile (e.g., lung fibrosis [240]) and infectious [241] inflammatory insults. Therefore the extant body of evidence suggests that glucose restriction in the alveolar niche and the corresponding suppression of glycolysis in AMs endow these cells with their functional quiescence. On the contrary, environmental perturbations that increase glucose availability in the distal lung [242,243] appear to support a metabolic shift favoring glucose metabolism and the consequent polarization of AMs toward a more inflammatory phenotype. These findings underscore the dynamically synchronized interplay between tissue and cellular metabolism.

However, although much is known about the influence of lipid and glucose availability on AM metabolism, less is known about the availability and biological impact of other major nutrient classes in the alveolar space. Metabolic profiling of bronchial wash versus bronchoalveolar lavage fluid samples collected from human donors has suggested that, on average, amino acids are more abundantly represented in the upper versus lower airways [244]. If and how limited amino acid availability tunes the biology of AMs remains unknown, though as discussed in this chapter, it likely imprints a unique nutrient sensing program with tissue-specific functional outputs. Given their residence at a major mucosal barrier site, AMs are also exposed to myriad microbiota-derived metabolites. The airways and alveoli are colonized primarily by proteobacteria, bacteroidetes, and firmicutes [245,246], all of which produce large amounts of short-chain fatty acids with known immunomodulatory properties [247]. Further, commensal bacteria are known to serve—with remarkable selectivity—as both sources and sinks of amino acids to the host [248]. Therefore the tissue-specific microbiota integrates with and shapes the metabolic environment of barrier sites such as the lung; however, its influence on the collection of metabolic signals available to, and functional regulation of, TRMs during homeostasis and pathology remains poorly understood.

Although AMs comprise arguably the most metabolically extreme population of TRMs, macrophages that reside in other body sites similarly assume distinctive phenotypic programs driven by the need to handle specific nutrients in their environment. For example, TRMs present in the spleen and liver are not only poised to guard against bloodborne pathogens but must also fulfill the key physiologic function of storing, recycling, and metabolizing large amounts of circulating iron [249,250]. In the spleen, this task is carried out by its most abundant TRM population, red pulp macrophages (RPMs), which homeostatically clear erythrocytes and platelets by phagocytosis [251]. In the liver, this is performed by the largest TRM population in the body, Kupffer cells (KCs) [252]. Given these functions, RPMs and KCs share many phenotypic characteristics that molecularly endow these cells with their iron-handling capabilities, including expression of heme oxygenase 1 (HO-1), ferroportin, and ferritin [253,254]. This metabolic program, defined by the expression of nuclear factor erythroid 2-related factor (NRF2) and Spi-C transcription factors [254,255], thematically parallels the environmental imprinting described above for AMs, as RPM turnover and niche replenishment by circulating monocytes are driven by heme sensing and the consequent induction of Spi-C expression [256]. Correspondingly, the loss of Spi-C expression hinders RPM development and phagocytic clearing of erythrocytes [255]. Further, HO-1 deficiency severely compromises macrophage numbers in the spleen and liver [257]. In parallel, and like AMs, both spleen and liver macrophages exhibit a transcriptional signature indicative of lipid metabolism, including expression of PPARγ [32,220]. Although the functional significance of lipid handling in RPMs and KCs remains incompletely understood, evidence suggests a role for these TRMs in mediating systemic lipid homeostasis [258]. Such findings further underscore how a TRM's phenotypic and functional program is profoundly shaped by the nutrient-handling pressures of its niche. Here, TRMs that homeostatically interface with the blood are uniquely poised to handle and process metabolites enriched in the circulation.

Tissue fuels as drivers of inflammation

It is therefore evident that microenvironmental nutrient composition metabolically and functionally imprints macrophages to ensure homeostasis in diverse body sites with different physiologic needs. However, akin to the interplay between glucose availability and AM inflammatory function described above, there is also substantial evidence suggesting that tissue-specific changes in nutrient availability drive inflammatory processes during pathologic insults. This is perhaps most evident during nutritional challenges imposed on adipose tissue macrophages (ATMs) during metabolic dysregulation. Homeostatic white adipose tissue (WAT) contains distinct TRMs, primarily of embryonic origin but with some contribution by bone marrow-derived macrophages, that are distinguished by different phenotypic and functional features [259]. At steady state, these bonafide TRMs exhibit a quiescent metabolism with low OXPHOS and glycolysis activity [260] and are unaffected by disruptions to their mitochondrial metabolism [223]. However, upon overnutrition, bone marrow-derived macrophages are recruited into the niche where they proliferate around dying adipocytes to form crown-like structures [261]. Given the abundance of extracellular lipids released from dying adipocytes, these newly recruited macrophages act as lipid reservoirs [262] and become bioenergetically activated in a manner that supports their pro-inflammatory function [260,263]. Further, the microenvironmental pressure to handle excess lipids forces these macrophages to rely on OXPHOS metabolism for supporting fatty acid catabolism. Accordingly, unlike homeostatic ATMs, which do not require intact mitochondrial function for their maintenance, pro-inflammatory ATMs are extremely vulnerable to mitochondrial perturbations that disrupt lipid processing [223]. Such observations highlight the tissue-specific functional consequences of nutrient utilization: whereas lipid handling in AMs promotes homeostasis via surfactant recycling in the lung, it conversely drives metabolic dysfunction by supporting the pro-inflammatory actions of macrophages during obesity (Fig. 3.3).

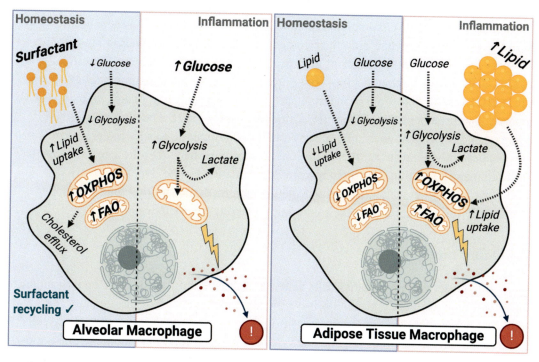

Figure 3.3: Microenvironmental nutrient sensing imprints TRM metabolism and function. TRMs dynamically respond to their metabolic niche during homeostasis and inflammation. Given their residence in the surfactant-rich, glucose-restricted alveolar space, steady-state AMs are metabolically poised to process and handle large amounts of lipid and cholesterol. This function is supported by high OXPHOS metabolism, which homeostatically promotes surfactant recycling in the healthy lung. Conversely, environmental insults that elevate alveolar glucose levels appear to drive glycolytic metabolism in AMs, thus promoting their inflammatory function. In contrast, whereas lipid handling supports inflammatory quiescence in TRMs resident to the lung, elevated lipid uptake and OXPHOS metabolism instead promote the inflammatory phenotype of ATMs during adipose tissue hypertrophy. Therefore TRM functions are uniquely and, in some cases, divergently tuned by their distinct metabolic environments. Created with BioRender. *AM*, Alveolar macrophages; *TRM*, tissue-resident macrophage.

Hypercholesterolemia represents another pathology where specific nutrient pressures drive the pro-inflammatory functions of macrophages resident within the atherosclerotic plaque. Through various means of uptake, macrophages in atherosclerotic lesions acquire environmental lipids and fatty acids (e.g., oxidized phospholipids and low-density lipoprotein [LDL]) that profoundly alter these cells' bioenergetic state. One such component of the LDL aggregate that promotes atherosclerosis is an oxidized phospholipid, 1-palmitoyl-2-arachidonoyl-*sn*-glycero-3-phosphorylcholine (oxPAPC) [264]. oxPAPC sensing by macrophages drives glucose and glutamine metabolism [265] to promote a unique "hyperactivated" phenotype whereby IL-1β is durably and robustly released without cell death [266]. Owing to the pathophysiologic importance of this lipid-sensing pathway, inhibition of these oxPAPC-stimulated metabolic changes hinders IL-1β-mediated atherosclerosis [265]. Beyond pro-atherogenic lipids, the sensing of specific amino acids represents another metabolic driver of atherosclerotic plaque development. Specifically, elevated levels of circulating leucine—but not other dietarily tunable amino acids—dictate an mTORC1 sensing threshold in macrophages [69] to suppress mitophagy, trigger apoptosis, and promote necrotic core formation in plaques [267]. The above-described findings demonstrate that aberrantly elevated metabolites can be locally integrated by macrophages with exquisite sensitivity to fundamentally reshape their homeostatic versus pro-inflammatory function. Further, they provide evidence for the dynamic interplay between microenvironmental and cellular metabolism by demonstrating that macrophages are internally tuned according to their external metabolic microenvironment.

Concluding thoughts

Although the discovery of myeloid cells as tissue sentinels far preceded our understanding of their profound metabolic plasticity, it is now abundantly clear that the capacity for integrating homeostatic and inflammatory information is inextricably linked to these cells' nutrient environment and bioenergetic state. As discussed herein, this phenomenon is most fundamentally evident in the molecular convergence of innate immune and metabolic intracellular signaling pathways. It is further underscored by the observation that changes in metabolism and nutrient consumption are not only coincident with but also indispensable for shaping myeloid cell function. Beyond these cell-intrinsic phenomena, a burgeoning body of work has further demonstrated the exquisitely synchronized interplay between a myeloid cell and its metabolic environment, whereby tissue-specific nutrients impose functional demands that shape cellular identity. Despite these exciting advances, we are, nevertheless, only beginning our exploration into the complexity of this interplay between metabolism and innate immunity. For example, among the myriad nutrients present in a myeloid cell's environment at any given time, what determines primacy for the specific metabolic cues that are sensed and/or integrated to consequently shape cellular function? How is this primacy programmed in different tissues and in response to different microenvironmental signals? How does the resulting convergence of distinct metabolic signaling events then yield functional outputs that dictate these cells' homeostatic and inflammatory biology? Future experiments unraveling this complexity will help us better understand the basic biochemical regulators of myeloid cell function. In turn, understanding this biochemistry holds immense potential for therapeutically targeting immunometabolism to treat inflammatory and infectious diseases.

References

[1] Saini A, Ghoneim HE, Lio CWJ, Collins PL, Oltz EM. Gene regulatory circuits in innate and adaptive immune cells. Annu Rev Immunology 2022;40:387—411. Available from: https://doi.org/10.1146/annurev-immunol-101320-025949, http://www.annualreviews.org/journal/immunol.

[2] Tsalikis J, Croitoru DO, Philpott DJ, Girardin SE. Nutrient sensing and metabolic stress pathways in innate immunity. Cell Microbiol 2013;15(10):1632—41. Available from: https://doi.org/10.1111/cmi.12165.

[3] Zhong B, Tien P, Shu HB. Innate immune responses: crosstalk of signaling and regulation of gene transcription. Virology 2006;352(1):14—21. Available from: https://doi.org/10.1016/j.virol.2006.04.029.

[4] Arancibia SA, Beltrán CJ, Aguirre IM, Silva P, Peralta AL, Malinarich F, et al. Toll-like receptors are key participants in innate immune responses. Biol Res 2007;40(2):97—112. Available from: https://doi.org/10.4067/S0716-97602007000200001, http://biolres.biomedcentral.com/.

[5] Gong T, Liu L, Jiang W, Zhou R. DAMP-sensing receptors in sterile inflammation and inflammatory diseases. Nat Rev Immunol 2020;20(2):95—112. Available from: https://doi.org/10.1038/s41577-019-0215-7, http://www.nature.com/nri/index.html.

[6] Kawai T, Akira S. The role of pattern-recognition receptors in innate immunity: update on Toll-like receptors. Nat Immunol 2010;11(5):373—84. Available from: https://doi.org/10.1038/ni.1863.

[7] Kawai T, Akira S. TLR signaling. SemImmunology 2007;19(1):24—32. Available from: https://doi.org/10.1016/j.smim.2006.12.004.

[8] Carpenter S, Ricci EP, Mercier BC, Moore MJ, Fitzgerald KA. Post-transcriptional regulation of gene expression in innate immunity. Nat Rev Immunol 2014;14(6):361—76. Available from: https://doi.org/10.1038/nri3682.

[9] López-Pelaéz M, Fumagalli S, Sanz C, Herrero C, Guerra S, Fernandez M, et al. Cot/tpl2-MKK1/2-Erk1/2 controls mTORC1-mediated mRNA translation in Toll-like receptor—activated macrophages. Mol Biol Cell 2012;23(15):2982—92. Available from: https://doi.org/10.1091/mbc.e12-02-0135.

[10] Hu XP, Yang Y, Ma BG. Amino acid flux from metabolic network benefits protein translation: the role of resource availability. Sci Rep 2015;5. Available from: https://doi.org/10.1038/srep11113, www.nature.com/srep/index.html.

[11] Lane AN, Fan TWM. Regulation of mammalian nucleotide metabolism and biosynthesis. Nucleic Acids Res 2015;43(4):2466—85. Available from: https://doi.org/10.1093/nar/gkv047, http://nar.oxfordjournals.org/.

[12] Lee CD, Tu BP. Metabolic influences on RNA biology and translation. Crit Rev Biochem Mol Biol 2017;52(2):176—84. Available from: https://doi.org/10.1080/10409238.2017.1283294.

[13] Halaby MJ, McGaha TL. Amino acid transport and metabolism in myeloid function. Front Immunology 2021;12. Available from: https://doi.org/10.3389/fimmu.2021.695238, https://www.frontiersin.org/journals/immunology#.

[14] O'Neill LAJ, Pearce EJ. Immunometabolism governs dendritic cell and macrophage function. J Exp Med 2016;213(1):15—23. Available from: https://doi.org/10.1084/jem.20151570, http://jem.rupress.org/content/213/1/15.full.pdf.

[15] Wang M, Flaswinkel H, Joshi A, Napoli M, Masgrau-Alsina S, Kamper JM, et al. Phosphorylation of PFKL regulates metabolic reprogramming in macrophages following pattern recognition receptor activation. Nat Commun 2024;15(1). Available from: https://doi.org/10.1038/s41467-024-50104-7.

[16] Kemp BE, Mitchelhill KI, Stapleton D, Michell BJ, Chen ZP, Witters LA. Dealing with energy demand: the AMP-activated protein kinase. Trends Biochem Sci 1999;24(1):22–5. Available from: https://doi.org/10.1016/S0968-0004(98)01340-1.

[17] Yan L, Mieulet V, Lamb RF. Nutrient regulation of mTORC1 and cell growth. Cell Cycle 2010;9(13):2473–4. Available from: https://doi.org/10.4161/cc.9.13.12124, http://www.landesbioscience.com/journals/cc/article/YanCC9-13.pdf.

[18] Yue S, Li G, He S, Li T. The central role of mTORC1 in amino acid sensing. Cancer Res 2022;82(17):2964–74. Available from: https://doi.org/10.1158/0008-5472.can-21-4403.

[19] Byles V, Covarrubias AJ, Ben-Sahra I, Lamming DW, Sabatini DM, Manning BD, et al. The TSC-mTOR pathway regulates macrophage polarization. Nat Commun 2013;4. Available from: https://doi.org/10.1038/ncomms3834, http://www.nature.com/ncomms/index.html.

[20] Collins SL, Oh MH, Sun IH, Chan-Li Y, Zhao L, Powell JD, et al. MTORC1 signaling regulates proinflammatory macrophage function and metabolism. J Immunology 2021;207(3):913–22. Available from: https://doi.org/10.4049/jimmunol.2100230, https://www.jimmunol.org/content/207/3/913.

[21] Goul C, Peruzzo R, Zoncu R. The molecular basis of nutrient sensing and signalling by mTORC1 in metabolism regulation and disease. Nat Rev Mol Cell Biol 2023;24(12):857–75. Available from: https://doi.org/10.1038/s41580-023-00641-8.

[22] Inpanathan S, Botelho RJ. The lysosome signaling platform: adapting with the Times. Front Cell Developmental Biol 2019;7. Available from: https://doi.org/10.3389/fcell.2019.00113, https://www.frontiersin.org/journals/cell-and-developmental-biology#.

[23] Jones RG, Pearce EJ. MenTORing immunity: mTOR signaling in the development and function of tissue-resident immune cells. Immunity 2017;46(5):730–42. Available from: https://doi.org/10.1016/j.immuni.2017.04.028, www.immunity.com.

[24] Hopfner KP, Hornung V. Molecular mechanisms and cellular functions of cGAS–STING signalling. Nat Rev Mol Cell Biol 2020;21(9):501–21. Available from: https://doi.org/10.1038/s41580-020-0244-x, http://www.nature.com/molcellbio.

[25] Tome D. Amino acid metabolism and signalling pathways: potential targets in the control of infection and immunity. Nutr Diabetes 2021;11(1).

[26] Olive AJ, Sassetti CM. Metabolic crosstalk between host and pathogen: Sensing, adapting and competing. Nat Rev Microbiology 2016;14(4):221–34. Available from: https://doi.org/10.1038/nrmicro.2016.12, http://www.nature.com/nrmicro/index.html.

[27] Ren W, Rajendran R, Zhao Y, Tan B, Wu G, Bazer FW, et al. Amino acids as mediators of metabolic cross talk between host and pathogen. Front Immunology 2018;9. Available from: https://doi.org/10.3389/fimmu.2018.00319, https://www.frontiersin.org/articles/10.3389/fimmu.2018.00319/full.

[28] Wculek SK, Dunphy G, Heras-Murillo I, Mastrangelo A, Sancho D. Metabolism of tissue macrophages in homeostasis and pathology. Cell Mol Immunology 2022;19(3):384–408. Available from: https://doi.org/10.1038/s41423-021-00791-9, https://www.nature.com/cmi/.

[29] Jha AK, Huang SCC, Sergushichev A, Lampropoulou V, Ivanova Y, Loginicheva E, et al. Network integration of parallel metabolic and transcriptional data reveals metabolic modules that regulate macrophage polarization. Immunity 2015;42(3):419–30. Available from: https://doi.org/10.1016/j.immuni.2015.02.005, www.immunity.com.

[30] Puleston DJ, Buck MD, Klein Geltink RI, Kyle RL, Caputa G, O'Sullivan D, et al. Polyamines and eIF5A hypusination modulate mitochondrial respiration and macrophage activation. Cell Metab 2019;30(2):352. Available from: https://doi.org/10.1016/j.cmet.2019.05.003, http://www.cellmetabolism.org/.

[31] Rapovy SM, Zhao J, Bricker RL, Schmidt SM, Setchell KDR, Qualls JE. Differential requirements for L-citrulline and L-arginine during antimycobacterial macrophage activity. J Immunol 2015;195(7):3293–300. Available from: https://doi.org/10.4049/jimmunol.1500800, http://www.jimmunol.org/content/195/7/3293.full.pdf + html.

[32] Gautier EL, Shay T, Miller J, Greter M, Jakubzick C, Ivanov S, et al. Gwendalyn J Randolph, Gene-expression profiles and transcriptional regulatory pathways that underlie the identity and diversity of

mouse tissue macrophages. Nat Immunol 2012;13(11):1118−28. Available from: https://doi.org/10.1038/ni.2419.
[33] Ivanisevic J, Elias D, Deguchi H, Averell PM, Kurczy M, Johnson CH, et al. Blood metabolomics: a readout of intra-tissue metabostasis. Sci Rep 2015;5.
[34] Saoi M, Britz-McKibbin P. New Advances in Tissue Metabolomics: A Review. Metabolites 2021;11 (10):672. Available from: https://doi.org/10.3390/metabo11100672.
[35] Elia I, Haigis MC. Metabolites and the tumour microenvironment: from cellular mechanisms to systemic metabolism. Nat Metab 2021;3(1):21−32. Available from: https://doi.org/10.1038/s42255-020-00317-z, https://www.nature.com/natmetab/.
[36] Manchester M, Anand A. Metabolomics: strategies to define the role of metabolism in virus infection and pathogenesis. Adv Virus Res 2017;98:57−81. Available from: https://doi.org/10.1016/bs.aivir.2017.02.001, http://www.elsevier.com/wps/find/bookdescription.cws_home/704107/description#description.
[37] Mayers JR, Varon J, Zhou RR, Daniel-Ivad M, Beaulieu C, Bhosle A, et al. A metabolomics pipeline highlights microbial metabolism in bloodstream infections. Cell 2024;187(15):4095. Available from: https://doi.org/10.1016/j.cell.2024.05.035, https://www.sciencedirect.com/science/journal/00928674.
[38] Yang H, Kim C, Zou W. Metabolism and macrophages in the tumor microenvironment. Curr OpImmunology 2024;91:102491. Available from: https://doi.org/10.1016/j.coi.2024.102491.
[39] Diray-Arce J, Conti MG, Petrova B, Kanarek N, Angelidou A, Levy O. Integrative metabolomics to identify molecular signatures of responses to vaccines and infections. Metabolites 2020;10(12):1−18. Available from: https://doi.org/10.3390/metabo10120492, https://www.mdpi.com/2218-1989/10/12/492/pdf.
[40] Guo C, Chi H. Immunometabolism of dendritic cells in health and disease. Elsevier BV; 2023. p. 83−116. Available from: https://doi.org/10.1016/bs.ai.2023.10.002.
[41] Rattigan KM, Pountain AW, Regnault C, Achcar F, Vincent IM, Goodyear CS, et al. Metabolomic profiling of macrophages determines the discrete metabolomic signature and metabolomic interactome triggered by polarising immune stimuli. PLoS ONE 2018;13(3). Available from: https://doi.org/10.1371/journal.pone.0194126, http://journals.plos.org/plosone/article/file?id = 10.1371/journal.pone.0194126&type = printable.
[42] Møller SH, Wang L, Ho PC. Metabolic programming in dendritic cells tailors immune responses and homeostasis. Cell Mol Immunology 2022;19(3):370−83. Available from: https://doi.org/10.1038/s41423-021-00753-1, https://www.nature.com/cmi/.
[43] Shan B, Wang X, Wu Y, Xu C, Xia Z, Dai J, et al. The metabolic ER stress sensor IRE1α suppresses alternative activation of macrophages and impairs energy expenditure in obesity. Nat Immunology 2017;18(5):519−29. Available from: https://doi.org/10.1038/ni.3709.
[44] Viola A, Munari F, Sánchez-Rodríguez R, Scolaro T, Castegna A. The metabolic signature of macrophage responses. Front Immunology 2019;10(JULY). Available from: https://doi.org/10.3389/fimmu.2019.01462.
[45] Hotamisligil GS, Davis RJ. Cell signaling and stress responses. Cold Spring Harb Perspect Biol 2016;8 (10). Available from: https://doi.org/10.1101/cshperspect.a006072, http://cshperspectives.cshlp.org/content/8/10/a006072.full.pdf.
[46] Condon KJ, Sabatini DM. Nutrient regulation of mTORC1 at a glance. J Cell Sci 2019;132(21). Available from: https://doi.org/10.1242/JCS.222570, https://jcs.biologists.org/content/joces/132/21/jcs222570.full.pdf.
[47] Saxton RA, Sabatini DM. mTOR signaling in growth, metabolism, and disease. Cell 2017;169 (2):361−71. Available from: https://doi.org/10.1016/j.cell.2017.03.035.
[48] Heitman J, Movva NR, Hall MN. Targets for cell cycle arrest by the immunosuppressant rapamycin in yeast. Science 1991;253(5022):905−9. Available from: https://doi.org/10.1126/science.1715094.
[49] Jhanwar-Uniyal M, Wainwright JV, Mohan AL, Tobias ME, Murali R, Gandhi CD, et al. Diverse signaling mechanisms of mTOR complexes: mTORC1 and mTORC2 in forming a formidable relationship. Adv Biol Regul 2019;72:51−62. Available from: https://doi.org/10.1016/j.jbior.2019.03.003, http://www.sciencedirect.com/science/journal/22124926.
[50] Li J, Kim SG, Blenis J. Rapamycin: one drug, many effects. Cell Metab 2014;19(3):373−9. Available from: https://doi.org/10.1016/j.cmet.2014.01.001.

[51] Ragupathi A, Kim C, Jacinto E. The mTORC2 signaling network: targets and cross-talks. Biochem J 2024;481(2):45–91. Available from: https://doi.org/10.1042/bcj20220325.

[52] Szwed A, Kim E, Jacinto E. Regulation and metabolic functions of mTORC1 and mTORC2. Physiological Rev 2021;101(3):1371–426. Available from: https://doi.org/10.1152/physrev.00026.2020.

[53] Ben-Sahra I, Manning BD. mTORC1 signaling and the metabolic control of cell growth. Curr OpCell Biol 2017;45:72–82. Available from: https://doi.org/10.1016/j.ceb.2017.02.012, http://www.elsevier.com/locate/ceb.

[54] Laplante M, Sabatini DM. Regulation of mTORC1 and its impact on gene expression at a glance. J Cell Sci 2013;126(8):1713–19. Available from: https://doi.org/10.1242/jcs.125773, http://jcs.biologists.org/content/126/8/1713.full.pdf. Canada.

[55] Laribee RN. Transcriptional and epigenetic regulation by the mechanistic target of rapamycin complex 1 pathway. J Mol Biol 2018;430(24):4874–90. Available from: https://doi.org/10.1016/j.jmb.2018.10.008, https://www.journals.elsevier.com/journal-of-molecular-biology.

[56] Thoreen CC. The molecular basis of mTORC1-regulated translation. Biochemical Soc Trans 2017;45(1):213–21. Available from: https://doi.org/10.1042/BST20160072, http://www.biochemsoctrans.org/content/45/1/213.full-text.pdf.

[57] Lewis CA, Griffiths B, Santos CR, Pende M, Schulze A. Regulation of the SREBP transcription factors by mTORC1. Biochemical Soc Trans 2011;39(2):495–9. Available from: https://doi.org/10.1042/BST0390495, http://www.biochemsoctrans.org/bst/039/0495/0390495.pdf. United Kingdom.

[58] Magnuson B, Ekim B, Fingar DC. Regulation and function of ribosomal protein S6 kinase (S6K) within mTOR signalling networks. Biochemical J 2012;441(1):1–21. Available from: https://doi.org/10.1042/BJ20110892, http://www.biochemj.org/bj/441/0001/4410001.pdf. United States.

[59] Proud CG. mTORC1 signalling and mRNA translation. Biochem Soc Trans 2009;37:227–31.

[60] Tan A, Prasad R, Lee C, Jho Eh. Past, present, and future perspectives of transcription factor EB (TFEB): mechanisms of regulation and association with disease. Cell Death Differ 2022;29(8):1433–49. Available from: https://doi.org/10.1038/s41418-022-01028-6, http://www.nature.com/cdd/index.html.

[61] Deleyto-Seldas N, Efeyan A. The mTOR-Autophagy Axis and the Control of Metabolism. Front Cell Dev Biol 2021;9.

[62] Rabanal-Ruiz Y, Otten EG, Korolchuk VI. MTORC1 as the main gateway to autophagy. Essays Biochem 2017;61(6):565–84. Available from: https://doi.org/10.1042/EBC20170027, http://essays.biochemistry.org/content/61/6/565.full-text.pdf.

[63] Coillard A, Guyonnet L, De Juan A, Cros A, Segura E. TLR or NOD receptor signaling skews monocyte fate decision via distinct mechanisms driven by mTOR and miR-155. Proc Natl Acad Sci 2021;118(43). Available from: https://doi.org/10.1073/pnas.2109225118.

[64] Dibble CC, Cantley LC. Regulation of mTORC1 by PI3K signaling. Cell Biol 2015;25(9):545–55. Available from: https://doi.org/10.1016/j.tcb.2015.06.002, www.elsevier.com/locate/tcb.

[65] Gajanayaka N, Dong SXM, Ali H, Iqbal S, Mookerjee A, Lawton DA, et al. TLR-4 agonist induces IFN-γ production selectively in proinflammatory human M1 macrophages through the PI3K-mTOR– and JNK-MAPK–activated p70S6K pathway. J Immunol 2021;207(9):2310–24. Available from: https://doi.org/10.4049/jimmunol.2001191.

[66] Kobayashi T, Nguyen-Tien D, Sorimachi Y, Sugiura Y, Suzuki T, Karyu H, et al. SLC15A4 mediates M1-prone metabolic shifts in macrophages and guards immune cells from metabolic stress. Proc Natl Acad Sci USA 2021;118(33). Available from: https://doi.org/10.1073/pnas.2100295118.

[67] Sanchez-Garrido J, Shenoy AR. Regulation and repurposing of nutrient sensing and autophagy in innate immunity. Autophagy 2021;17(7):1571–91. Available from: https://doi.org/10.1080/15548627.2020.1783119.

[68] Valvezan AJ, Manning BD. Molecular logic of mTORC1 signalling as a metabolic rheostat. Nat Metab 2019;1(3):321–33. Available from: https://doi.org/10.1038/s42255-019-0038-7, https://www.nature.com/natmetab/.

[69] Zhang X, Kapoor D, Jeong SJ, Fappi A, Stitham J, Shabrish V, et al. Identification of a leucine-mediated threshold effect governing macrophage mTOR signalling and cardiovascular risk. Nat Metab 2024;6

[70] Chen J, Ou Y, Luo R, Wang J, Wang D, Guan J, et al. SAR1B senses leucine levels to regulate mTORC1 signalling. Nature 2021;596(7871):281–4. Available from: https://doi.org/10.1038/s41586-021-03768-w.

[71] Kim S, Yoon I, Son J, Park J, Kim K, Lee J-H, et al. Leucine-sensing mechanism of leucyl-tRNA synthetase 1 for mTORC1 activation. Cell Rep 2021;35(4):109031. Available from: https://doi.org/10.1016/j.celrep.2021.109031.

[72] Nicklin P, Bergman P, Zhang B, Triantafellow E, Wang H, Nyfeler B, et al. Bidirectional transport of amino acids regulates mTOR and autophagy. Cell 2009;136(3):521–34. Available from: https://doi.org/10.1016/j.cell.2008.11.044.

[73] Wolfson RL, Chantranupong L, Saxton RA, Shen K, Scaria SM, Cantor JR, et al. Sestrin2 is a leucine sensor for the mTORC1 pathway. Science 2016;351(6268):43–8. Available from: https://doi.org/10.1126/science.aab2674, http://www.sciencemag.org/content/351/6268/43.full.pdf.

[74] Son SM, Park SJ, Lee H, Siddiqi F, Lee JE, Menzies FM, et al. Leucine signals to mTORC1 via its metabolite acetyl-coenzyme A. Cell Metab 2019;29(1):192. Available from: https://doi.org/10.1016/j.cmet.2018.08.013, http://www.cellmetabolism.org/.

[75] Son SM, Park SJ, Stamatakou E, Vicinanza M, Menzies FM, Rubinsztein DC. Leucine regulates autophagy via acetylation of the mTORC1 component raptor. Nat Commun 2020;11(1). Available from: https://doi.org/10.1038/s41467-020-16886-2, http://www.nature.com/ncomms/index.html.

[76] Chantranupong L, Scaria SM, Saxton RA, Gygi MP, Shen K, Wyant GA, et al. The CASTOR proteins are arginine sensors for the mTORC1 pathway. Cell 2016;165(1):153–64. Available from: https://doi.org/10.1016/j.cell.2016.02.035, https://www.sciencedirect.com/journal/cell.

[77] Durán RV, Oppliger W, Robitaille AM, Heiserich L, Skendaj R, Gottlieb E, et al. Glutaminolysis activates Rag-mTORC1 signaling. Mol Cell 2012;47(3):349–58. Available from: https://doi.org/10.1016/j.molcel.2012.05.043.

[78] Gu X, Orozco JM, Saxton RA, Condon KJ, Liu GY, Krawczyk PA, et al. SAMTOR is an S-adenosylmethionine sensor for the mTORC1 pathway. Science 2017;358(6364):813–18. Available from: https://doi.org/10.1126/science.aao3265, http://science.sciencemag.org/content/sci/358/6364/813.full.pdf.

[79] Jewell JL, Kim YC, Russell RC, Yu FX, Park HW, Plouffe SW, et al. Differential regulation of mTORC1 by leucine and glutamine. Science 2015;347(6218):194–8. Available from: https://doi.org/10.1126/science.1259472, http://www.sciencemag.org/content/347/6218/194.full.pdf.

[80] Meng D, Yang Q, Wang H, Melick CH, Navlani R, Frank AR, et al. Glutamine and asparagine activate mTORC1 independently of Rag GTPases. J Biol Chem 2020;295(10):2890–9. Available from: https://doi.org/10.1074/jbc.AC119.011578, https://www.jbc.org/content/295/10/2890.full.pdf.

[81] Cui Z, Napolitano G, de Araujo MEG, Esposito A, Monfregola J, Huber LA, et al. Structure of the lysosomal mTORC1–TFEB–Rag–Ragulator megacomplex. Nature 2023;614(7948):572–9. Available from: https://doi.org/10.1038/s41586-022-05652-7, https://www.nature.com/nature/.

[82] Dyachok J, Earnest S, Iturraran EN, Cobb MH, Ross EM. Amino acids regulate mTORC1 by an obligate two-step mechanism. J Biol Chem 2016;291(43):22414–26. Available from: https://doi.org/10.1074/jbc.M116.732511, http://www.jbc.org/content/291/43/22414.full.pdf.

[83] Hesketh GG, Papazotos F, Pawling J, Rajendran D, Knight JDR, Martinez S, et al. The GATOR-Rag GTPase pathway inhibits mTORC1 activation by lysosome-derived amino acids. Science 2020;370(6514):351–6. Available from: https://doi.org/10.1126/science.aaz0863, https://science.sciencemag.org/content/370/6514/351.

[84] Sancak Y, Bar-Peled L, Zoncu R, Markhard AL, Nada S, Sabatini DM. Ragulator-rag complex targets mTORC1 to the lysosomal surface and is necessary for its activation by amino acids. Cell 2010;141(2):290–303. Available from: https://doi.org/10.1016/j.cell.2010.02.024, https://www.sciencedirect.com/journal/cell.

[85] Napolitano G, Di Malta C, Ballabio A. Non-canonical mTORC1 signaling at the lysosome. Trends Cell Biol 2022;32(11):920–31. Available from: https://doi.org/10.1016/j.tcb.2022.04.012.

[86] Settembre C, Zoncu R, Medina DL, Vetrini F, Erdin S, Erdin S, et al. A lysosome-to-nucleus signalling mechanism senses and regulates the lysosome via mTOR and TFEB. EMBO J 2012;31(5):1095–108. Available from: https://doi.org/10.1038/emboj.2012.32.

[87] Li Q, Cheng H, Liu Y, Wang X, He F, Tang L. Activation of mTORC1 by LSECtin in macrophages directs intestinal repair in inflammatory bowel disease. Cell Death Dis 2020;11(10). Available from: https://doi.org/10.1038/s41419-020-03114-4, https://www.nature.com/cddis/.

[88] Mendel ZI, Reynolds MB, Abuaita BH, O'Riordan MX, Swanson JA. Amino acids suppress macropinocytosis and promote release of CSF1 receptor in macrophages. J Cell Sci 2022;135(4). Available from: https://doi.org/10.1242/jcs.259284, https://journals.biologists.com/jcs/article/135/4/jcs259284/274458/Amino-acids-suppress-macropinocytosis-and-promote.

[89] Pacitto R, Gaeta I, Swanson JA, Yoshida S. CXCL12-induced macropinocytosis modulates two distinct pathways to activate mTORC1 in macrophages. J Leukoc Biol 2017;101(3):683–92. Available from: https://doi.org/10.1189/jlb.2A0316-141RR, http://www.jleukbio.org/content/101/3/683.full.pdf.

[90] Yoshida S, Pacitto R, Inoki K, Swanson J. Macropinocytosis, mTORC1 and cellular growth control. Cell Mol Life Sci 2018;75(7):1227–39. Available from: https://doi.org/10.1007/s00018-017-2710-y.

[91] Fernandes SA, Angelidaki DD, Nüchel J, Pan J, Gollwitzer P, Elkis Y, et al. Spatial and functional separation of mTORC1 signalling in response to different amino acid sources. Nat Cell Biol 2024. Available from: https://doi.org/10.1038/s41556-024-01523-7, https://www.nature.com/ncb/.

[92] Amiel E, Everts B, Freitas TC, King IL, Curtis JD, Pearce EL, et al. Inhibition of mechanistic target of rapamycin promotes dendritic cell activation and enhances therapeutic autologous vaccination in mice. J Immunol 2012;189(5):2151–8. Available from: https://doi.org/10.4049/jimmunol.1103741, http://www.jimmunol.org/content/189/5/2151.full.pdf+html. United States.

[93] Krawczyk CM, Holowka T, Sun J, Blagih J, Amiel E, DeBerardinis RJ, et al. Toll-like receptor-induced changes in glycolytic metabolism regulate dendritic cell activation. Blood 2010;115(23):4742–9. Available from: https://doi.org/10.1182/blood-2009-10-249540, http://bloodjournal.hematologylibrary.org/cgi/reprint/115/23/4742.

[94] Zhang M, Liu F, Zhou P, Wang Q, Xu C, Li Y, et al. The MTOR signaling pathway regulates macrophage differentiation from mouse myeloid progenitors by inhibiting autophagy. Autophagy 2019;15(7):1150–62. Available from: https://doi.org/10.1080/15548627.2019.1578040.

[95] Adamik J, Munson PV, Hartmann FJ, Combes AJ, Pierre P, Krummel MF, et al. Distinct metabolic states guide maturation of inflammatory and tolerogenic dendritic cells. Nat Commun 2022;13(1). Available from: https://doi.org/10.1038/s41467-022-32849-1, https://www.nature.com/ncomms/.

[96] Covarrubias AJ, Aksoylar HI, Horng T. Control of macrophage metabolism and activation by mTOR and Akt signaling. SemImmunology 2015;27(4):286–96. Available from: https://doi.org/10.1016/j.smim.2015.08.001, http://www.elsevier.com/inca/publications/store/6/2/2/9/4/5/index.htt.

[97] Covarrubias AJ, Aksoylar HI, Yu J, Snyder NW, Worth AJ, Iyer SS, et al. Akt-mTORC1 signaling regulates Acly to integrate metabolic input to control of macrophage activation. eLife 2016;5:2016. Available from: https://doi.org/10.7554/eLife.11612, http://elifesciences.org/content/5/e11612.full.pdf.

[98] Erra Díaz F, Ochoa V, Merlotti A, Dantas E, Mazzitelli I, Gonzalez Polo V, et al. Extracellular acidosis and mTOR inhibition drive the differentiation of human monocyte-derived dendritic cells. Cell Rep 2020;31(5):107613. Available from: https://doi.org/10.1016/j.celrep.2020.107613.

[99] Haidinger M, Poglitsch M, Geyeregger R, Kasturi S, Zeyda M, Zlabinger GJ, et al. A versatile role of mammalian target of rapamycin in human dendritic cell function and differentiation. J Immunol 2010;185(7):3919–31. Available from: https://doi.org/10.4049/jimmunol.1000296, http://www.jimmunol.org/content/185/7/3919.full.pdf+html. Austria.

[100] Labonte AC, Tosello-Trampont AC, Hahn YS. The role of macrophage polarization in infectious and inflammatory diseases. Mol Cell 2014;37(4):275–85. Available from: https://doi.org/10.14348/molcells.2014.2374, http://pdf.medrang.co.kr/KSMCB/2014/037/molcell-37-4-275-1.pdf.

[101] Bader JE, Wolf MM, Lupica-Tondo GL, Madden MZ, Reinfeld BI, Arner EN, et al. Obesity induces PD-1 on macrophages to suppress anti-tumour immunity. Nature 2024;630(8018):968–75. Available from: https://doi.org/10.1038/s41586-024-07529-3, https://www.nature.com/nature/.

[102] Luo Y, Li W, Yu G, Yu J, Han L, Xue T, et al. Tsc1 expression by dendritic cells is required to preserve T-cell homeostasis and response. Cell Death Dis 2017;8(1). Available from: https://doi.org/10.1038/cddis.2016.487, http://www.nature.com/cddis/marketing/index.html.

[103] Rosborough BR, Raïch-Regué D, Matta BM, Lee K, Gan B, DePinho RA, et al. Murine dendritic cell rapamycin-resistant and rictor-independent mTOR controls IL-10, B7-H1, and regulatory T-cell induction. Blood 2013;121(18):3619−30. Available from: https://doi.org/10.1182/blood-2012-08-448290, http://bloodjournal.org/content/121/18/3619.full-text.pdf + html.

[104] Shaw AC, Goldstein DR, Montgomery RR. Age-dependent dysregulation of innate immunity. Nat Rev Immunol 2013;13(12):875−87. Available from: https://doi.org/10.1038/nri3547.

[105] Widjaja AA, Lim WW, Viswanathan S, Chothani S, Corden B, Dasan CM, et al. Inhibition of IL-11 signalling extends mammalian healthspan and lifespan. Nature 2024;632(8023):157−65. Available from: https://doi.org/10.1038/s41586-024-07701-9, https://www.nature.com/nature/.

[106] Lee DJW, Hodzic Kuerec A, Maier AB. Targeting ageing with rapamycin and its derivatives in humans: a systematic review. Lancet Healthy Longev 2024;5(2):e152. Available from: https://doi.org/10.1016/S2666-7568(23)00258-1, https://www.sciencedirect.com/science/journal/26667568.

[107] Nouwen LV, Everts B. Pathogens menTORing macrophages and dendritic cells: manipulation of mTOR and cellular metabolism to promote immune escape. Cells 2020;9(1). Available from: https://doi.org/10.3390/cells9010161, https://www.mdpi.com/2073-4409/9/1/161/pdf.

[108] Mondino S, Schmidt S, Rolando M, Escoll P, Gomez-Valero L, Buchrieser C. Legionnaires' disease: state of the art knowledge of pathogenesis mechanisms of legionella. Annu Rev Pathology: Mechanisms Dis 2020;15(1):439−66. Available from: https://doi.org/10.1146/annurev-pathmechdis-012419-032742.

[109] Abshire CF, Dragoi A-M, Roy CR, Ivanov SS, Coers J. MTOR-Driven Metabolic Reprogramming Regulates Legionella pneumophila Intracellular Niche Homeostasis. PLOS Pathog 2016;12(12): e1006088. Available from: https://doi.org/10.1371/journal.ppat.1006088.

[110] De Leon JA, Qiu J, Nicolai CJ, Counihan JL, Barry KC, Xu L, et al. Positive and negative regulation of the master metabolic regulator mTORC1 by two families of *Legionella pneumophila* effectors. Cell Rep 2017;21(8):2031−8. Available from: https://doi.org/10.1016/j.celrep.2017.10.088, http://www.sciencedirect.com/science/journal/22111247.

[111] Ivanov SS. The tug-of-war over MTOR in Legionella infections. Microb Cell 2017;4(2):67−8. Available from: https://doi.org/10.15698/mic2017.02.559, http://microbialcell.com/wordpress/wp-content/uploads/2017/01/2017A-Ivanov-Microbial-Cell.pdf.

[112] Ondari E, Wilkins A, Latimer B, Dragoi AM, Ivanov SS. Cellular cholesterol licenses Legionella pneumophila intracellular replication in macrophages. Microb Cell 2023;10(1):1−17. Available from: https://doi.org/10.15698/mic2023.01.789, http://microbialcell.com/wordpress/wp-content/uploads/2022A-Ondari-Microbial-Cell.pdf.

[113] Price CTD, Al-Quadan T, Santic M, Rosenshine I, Abu Kwaik Y. Host proteasomal degradation generates amino acids essential for intracellular bacterial growth. Science 2011;334(6062):1553−7. Available from: https://doi.org/10.1126/science.1212868.

[114] Arthur JSC, Ley SC. Mitogen-activated protein kinases in innate immunity. Nat Rev Immunology 2013;13(9):679−92. Available from: https://doi.org/10.1038/nri3495.

[115] Cargnello M, Roux PP. Activation and function of the MAPKs and their substrates, the MAPK-activated protein kinases. Microbiology Mol Biol Rev 2011;75(1):50−83. Available from: https://doi.org/10.1128/MMBR.00031-10Canada, http://mmbr.asm.org/cgi/reprint/75/1/50.

[116] Kim EK, Choi EJ. Pathological roles of MAPK signaling pathways in human diseases. Biochim Biophys Acta - Mol Basis Dis 2010;1802(4):396−405. Available from: https://doi.org/10.1016/j.bbadis.2009.12.009.

[117] Liu Y, Shepherd EG, Nelin LD. MAPK phosphatases - regulating the immune response. Nat Rev Immunol 2007;7(3):202−12. Available from: https://doi.org/10.1038/nri2035.

[118] Schultze SI, Hemmings DA, Niessen M, Tschopp O. PI3K/AKT, signalling. Expert Rev Mol Med 2012;14.

[119] Lamberti G, De Smet CH, Angelova M, Kremser L, Taub N, Herrmann C, et al. LAMTOR/Ragulator regulates lipid metabolism in macrophages and foam cell differentiation. FEBS Lett 2020;594(1):31−42. Available from: https://doi.org/10.1002/1873-3468.13579, http://onlinelibrary.wiley.com/journal/10.1002/(ISSN)1873-3468.

[120] Liebscher G, Vujic N, Schreiber R, Heine M, Krebiehl C, Duta-Mare M, et al. The lysosomal LAMTOR / Ragulator complex is essential for nutrient homeostasis in brown adipose tissue. Mol Metab 2023;71:101705. Available from: https://doi.org/10.1016/j.molmet.2023.101705.

[121] Shahbazian D, Roux PP, Mieulet V, Cohen MS, Raught B, Taunton J, et al. The mTOR/PI3K and MAPK pathways converge on eIF4B to control its phosphorylation and activity. EMBO J 2006;25(12):2781−91. Available from: https://doi.org/10.1038/sj.emboj.7601166.

[122] Boccuni L, Podgorschek E, Schmiedeberg M, Platanitis E, Traxler P, Fischer P, et al. Stress signaling boosts interferon-induced gene transcription in macrophages. Sci Signal 2022;15(764). Available from: https://doi.org/10.1126/scisignal.abq5389.

[123] Rezatabar S, Karimian A, Rameshknia V, Parsian H, Majidinia M, Kopi TA, et al. RAS/MAPK signaling functions in oxidative stress, DNA damage response and cancer progression. J Cell Physiol 2019;234(9):14951−65. Available from: https://doi.org/10.1002/jcp.28334, http://onlinelibrary.wiley.com/journal/10.1002/(ISSN)1097-4652.

[124] Rincón M, Davis RJ. Regulation of the immune response by stress-activated protein kinases. Immunol Rev 2009;228(1):212−24. Available from: https://doi.org/10.1111/j.1600-065X.2008.00744.x.

[125] Ashwell JD. The many paths to p38 mitogen-activated protein kinase activation in the immune system. Nat Rev Immunol 2006;6(7):532−40. Available from: https://doi.org/10.1038/nri1865.

[126] Fitzgerald KA, Kagan JC. Toll-like receptors and the control of immunity. Cell 2020;180(6):1044−66. Available from: https://doi.org/10.1016/j.cell.2020.02.041, https://www.sciencedirect.com/journal/cell.

[127] Canovas B, Nebreda AR. Diversity and versatility of p38 kinase signalling in health and disease. Nat Rev Mol Cell Biol 2021;22(5):346−66. Available from: https://doi.org/10.1038/s41580-020-00322-w, http://www.nature.com/molcellbio.

[128] Son Y, Cheong Y-K, Kim N-H, Chung H-T, Kang DG, Pae H-O. Mitogen-activated protein kinases and reactive oxygen species: how can ROS activate MAPK pathways? J Signal Transduct 2011;2011:1−6. Available from: https://doi.org/10.1155/2011/792639.

[129] Zhang J, Wang X, Vikash V, Ye Q, Wu D, Liu Y, et al. ROS and ROS-mediated cellular signaling. Oxid Med Cell Longev 2016;2016. Available from: https://doi.org/10.1155/2016/4350965, http://www.hindawi.com/journals/oximed/.

[130] Palmieri EM, McGinity C, Wink DA, McVicar DW. Nitric oxide in macrophage immunometabolism: hiding in plain sight. Metabolites 2020;10(11):1−34. Available from: https://doi.org/10.3390/metabo10110429, https://www.mdpi.com/2218-1989/10/11/429/pdf.

[131] Forrester SJ, Kikuchi DS, Hernandes MS, Xu Q, Griendling KK. Reactive oxygen species in metabolic and inflammatory signaling. Circulation Res 2018;122(6):877−902. Available from: https://doi.org/10.1161/CIRCRESAHA.117.311401, http://circres.ahajournals.org.

[132] Muri J, Kopf M. Redox regulation of immunometabolism. Nat Rev Immunology 2021;21(6):363−81. Available from: https://doi.org/10.1038/s41577-020-00478-8.

[133] Rendra E, Riabov V, Mossel DM, Sevastyanova T, Harmsen MC, Kzhyshkowska J. Reactive oxygen species (ROS) in macrophage activation and function in diabetes. Immunobiology 2019;224(2):242−53. Available from: https://doi.org/10.1016/j.imbio.2018.11.010, www.urbanfischer.de/journals/immunobiol/i_biol.htm.

[134] Lumeng CN, Bodzin JL, Saltiel AR. Obesity induces a phenotypic switch in adipose tissue macrophage polarization. J Clin Investigation 2007;117(1):175−84. Available from: https://doi.org/10.1172/JCI29881, http://www.jci.org/cgi/reprint/117/1/175. United States.

[135] Youssif C, Cubillos-Rojas M, Comalada M, Llonch E, Perna C, Djouder N, et al. Myeloid p38alpha signaling promotes intestinal IGF-1 production and inflammation-associated tumorigenesis. EMBO Mol Med 2018;10(7).

[136] Zhou D, Huang C, Lin Z, Zhan S, Kong L, Fang C, et al. Macrophage polarization and function with emphasis on the evolving roles of coordinated regulation of cellular signaling pathways. Cell Signal 2014;26(2):192–7. Available from: https://doi.org/10.1016/j.cellsig.2013.11.004.

[137] Chen HH, Yu YR, Hsiao YL, Chen SH, Lee CK. Plasmacytoid Dendritic Cells Enhance T-Independent B Cell Response through a p38 MAPK-STAT1 Axis. J Immunology 2023;211(4):576–90. Available from: https://doi.org/10.4049/jimmunol.2200210, https://journals.aai.org/jimmunol/article/211/4/576/265772/Plasmacytoid-Dendritic-Cells-Enhance-T-Independent.

[138] Hato L, Vizcay A, Eguren I, Pérez-Gracia JL, Rodríguez J, Gállego Pérez-Larraya J, et al. Dendritic cells in cancer immunology and immunotherapy. Cancers 2024;16(5):981. Available from: https://doi.org/10.3390/cancers16050981.

[139] Neophytou CM, Pierides C, Christodoulou MI, Costeas P, Kyriakou TC, Papageorgis P. The role of tumor-associated myeloid cells in modulating cancer therapy. Front Oncol 2020;10. Available from: https://doi.org/10.3389/fonc.2020.00899, http://www.frontiersin.org/Oncology/about.

[140] Yu J, Li H, Zhang Z, Lin W, Wei X, Shao B. Targeting the MDSCs of tumors in situ with inhibitors of the MAPK signaling pathway to promote tumor regression. Front Oncol 2021;11. Available from: https://doi.org/10.3389/fonc.2021.647312.

[141] Zheng T, Zhang B, Chen C, Ma J, Meng D, Huang J, et al. Protein kinase p38alpha signaling in dendritic cells regulates colon inflammation and tumorigenesis. Proc Natl Acad Sci USA 2018;115(52).

[142] Tan H-Y, Wang N, Li S, Hong M, Wang X, Feng Y, et al. The reactive oxygen species in macrophage polarization: reflecting its dual role in progression and treatment of human diseases. Oxid Med Cell Longev 2016;2016(1). Available from: https://doi.org/10.1155/2016/2795090.

[143] Zhang Y, Choksi S, Chen K, Pobezinskaya Y, Linnoila I, Liu ZG. ROS play a critical role in the differentiation of alternatively activated macrophages and the occurrence of tumor-associated macrophages. Cell Res 2013;23(7):898–914. Available from: https://doi.org/10.1038/cr.2013.75.

[144] Al-Huseini LMA, Aw Yeang HX, Hamdam JM, Sethu S, Alhumeed N, Wong W, et al. Heme oxygenase-1 regulates dendritic cell function through modulation of p38 MAPK-CREB/ATF1 signaling. J Biol Chem 2014;289(23):16442–51. Available from: https://doi.org/10.1074/jbc.m113.532069.

[145] Snieckute G, Genzor AV, Vind AC, Ryder L, Stoneley M, Chamois S, et al. Ribosome stalling is a signal for metabolic regulation by the ribotoxic stress response. Cell Metab 2022;34(12):2036. Available from: https://doi.org/10.1016/j.cmet.2022.10.011, http://www.cellmetabolism.org/.

[146] Robinson KS, Toh GA, Rozario P, Chua R, Bauernfried S, Sun Z, et al. ZAKα-driven ribotoxic stress response activates the human NLRP1 inflammasome. Science 2022;377(6603):328–35. Available from: https://doi.org/10.1126/science.abl6324, https://www.science.org/doi/10.1126/science.abl6324.

[147] Mager CE, Mormol JM, Shelton ED, Murphy PR, Bowman BA, Barley TJ, et al. p38 MAPK and MKP-1 control the glycolytic program via the bifunctional glycolysis regulator PFKFB3 during sepsis. J Biol Chem 2023;299(4). Available from: https://doi.org/10.1016/j.jbc.2023.103043, https://www.sciencedirect.com/journal/journal-of-biological-chemistry.

[148] Papa S, Choy PM, Bubici C. The ERK and JNK pathways in the regulation of metabolic reprogramming. Oncogene 2019;38(13):2223–40. Available from: https://doi.org/10.1038/s41388-018-0582-8, http://www.nature.com/onc/index.html.

[149] Perrin-Cocon L, Aublin-Gex A, Diaz O, Ramière C, Peri F, André P, et al. Toll-like receptor 4-induced glycolytic burst in human monocyte-derived dendritic cells results from p38-dependent stabilization of HIF-1α and increased hexokinase II Expression. J Immunology 2018;201(5):1510–21. Available from: https://doi.org/10.4049/jimmunol.1701522, http://www.jimmunol.org/content/jimmunol/201/5/1510.full.pdf.

[150] Du X, Chapman NM, Chi H. Emerging roles of cellular metabolism in regulating dendritic cell subsets and function. Front Cell Developmental Biol 2018;6. Available from: https://doi.org/10.3389/fcell.2018.00152, https://www.frontiersin.org/articles/10.3389/fcell.2018.00152/full.

[151] Reinfeld BI, Madden MZ, Wolf MM, Chytil A, Bader JE, Patterson AR, et al. Cell-programmed nutrient partitioning in the tumour microenvironment. Nature 2021;593(7858):282–8. Available from: https://doi.org/10.1038/s41586-021-03442-1, http://www.nature.com/nature/index.html.

[152] Huang J, Zhao Y, Zhao K, Yin K, Wang S. Function of reactive oxygen species in myeloid-derived suppressor cells. Front Immunology 2023;14. Available from: https://doi.org/10.3389/fimmu.2023.1226443.

[153] Tafani M, Sansone L, Limana F, Arcangeli T, De Santis E, Polese M, et al. The Interplay of reactive oxygen species, hypoxia, inflammation, and sirtuins in cancer initiation and progression. Oxid Med Cell Longev 2016;2016(1). Available from: https://doi.org/10.1155/2016/3907147.

[154] Wang B, Zhao Q, Zhang Y, Liu Z, Zheng Z, Liu S, et al. Targeting hypoxia in the tumor microenvironment: a potential strategy to improve cancer immunotherapy. J Exp & Clin Cancer Res 2021;40(1). Available from: https://doi.org/10.1186/s13046-020-01820-7.

[155] Weinberg F, Ramnath N, Nagrath D. Reactive oxygen species in the tumor microenvironment: an overview. Cancers 2019;11(8):1191. Available from: https://doi.org/10.3390/cancers11081191.

[156] Hegde S, Leader AM, Merad M. MDSC: markers, development, states, and unaddressed complexity. Immunity 2021;54(5):875−84. Available from: https://doi.org/10.1016/j.immuni.2021.04.004, www.immunity.com.

[157] Veglia F, Perego M, Gabrilovich D. Myeloid-derived suppressor cells coming of age. Nat Immunol 2018;19(2):108−19. Available from: https://doi.org/10.1038/s41590-017-0022-x.

[158] Lasser SA, Ozbay Kurt FG, Arkhypov I, Utikal J, Umansky V. Myeloid-derived suppressor cells in cancer and cancer therapy. Nat Rev Clin Oncol 2024;21(2):147−64. Available from: https://doi.org/10.1038/s41571-023-00846-y, https://www.nature.com/nrclinonc/archive/.

[159] Zhang P, Guan H, Yuan S, Cheng H, Zheng J, Zhang Z, et al. Targeting myeloid derived suppressor cells reverts immune suppression and sensitizes BRAF-mutant papillary thyroid cancer to MAPK inhibitors. Nat Commun 2022;13(1). Available from: https://doi.org/10.1038/s41467-022-29000-5.

[160] Maschalidi S, Mehrotra P, Keçeli BN, De Cleene HKL, Lecomte K, Van der Cruyssen R, et al. Targeting SLC7A11 improves efferocytosis by dendritic cells and wound healing in diabetes. Nature 2022;606(7915):776−84. Available from: https://doi.org/10.1038/s41586-022-04754-6, http://www.nature.com/nature/index.html.

[161] Razi S, Yaghmoorian Khojini J, Kargarijam F, Panahi S, Tahershamsi Z, Tajbakhsh A, et al. Macrophage efferocytosis in health and disease. Cell Biochem Funct 2023;41(2):152−65. Available from: https://doi.org/10.1002/cbf.3780.

[162] Savina A, Amigorena S. Phagocytosis and antigen presentation in dendritic cells. Immunological Rev 2007;219(1):143−56. Available from: https://doi.org/10.1111/j.1600-065x.2007.00552.x.

[163] Winer BY, Settle AH, Yakimov AM, Jeronimo C, Lazarov T, Tipping M, et al. Plasma membrane abundance dictates phagocytic capacity and functional cross-talk in myeloid cells. Sci Immunology 2024;9(96). Available from: https://doi.org/10.1126/sciimmunol.adl2388, https://www.science.org/doi/10.1126/sciimmunol.adl2388.

[164] You Z, Chi H. Lipid metabolism in dendritic cell biology. Immunological Rev 2023;317(1):137−51. Available from: https://doi.org/10.1111/imr.13215.

[165] Schumann J. It is all about fluidity: fatty acids and macrophage phagocytosis. Eur J Pharmacology 2016;785:18−23. Available from: https://doi.org/10.1016/j.ejphar.2015.04.057.

[166] Shao W, Espenshade PJ. Expanding roles for SREBP in metabolism. Cell Metab 2012;16(4):414−19. Available from: https://doi.org/10.1016/j.cmet.2012.09.002.

[167] Shimano H, Sato R. SREBP-regulated lipid metabolism: convergent physiology—divergent pathophysiology. Nat Rev Endocrinol 2017;13(12):710−30. Available from: https://doi.org/10.1038/nrendo.2017.91.

[168] Geng F, Zhong Y, Su H, Lefai E, Magaki S, Cloughesy TF, et al. SREBP-1 upregulates lipophagy to maintain cholesterol homeostasis in brain tumor cells. Cell Rep 2023;42(7):112790. Available from: https://doi.org/10.1016/j.celrep.2023.112790.

[169] Horton JD, Goldstein JL, Brown MS. SREBPs: Activators of the complete program of cholesterol and fatty acid synthesis in the liver. J Clin Investigation 2002;109(9):1125−31. Available from: https://doi.org/10.1172/JCI0215593, http://www.jci.org.

[170] Peterson TR, Sengupta SS, Harris TE, Carmack AE, Kang SA, Balderas E, et al. MTOR complex 1 regulates lipin 1 localization to control the srebp pathway. Cell 2011;146(3):408−20. Available from: https://doi.org/10.1016/j.cell.2011.06.034, https://www.sciencedirect.com/journal/cell.

[171] Dobrosotskaya IY, Seegmiller AC, Brown MS, Goldstein JL, Rawson RB. Regulation of SREBP processing and membrane lipid production by phospholipids in Drosophila. Science 2002;296 (5569):879−83. Available from: https://doi.org/10.1126/science.1071124.

[172] Sakai J, Duncan EA, Rawson RB, Hua X, Brown MS, Goldstein JL. Sterol-regulated release of SREBP-2 from cell membranes requires two sequential cleavages, one within a transmembrane segment. Cell 1996;85(7):1037−46. Available from: https://doi.org/10.1016/S0092-8674(00)81304-5, https://www.sciencedirect.com/journal/cell.

[173] York AG, Williams KJ, Argus JP, Zhou QD, Brar G, Vergnes L, et al. Limiting cholesterol biosynthetic flux spontaneously engages type i IFN signaling. Cell 2015;163(7):1716−29. Available from: https://doi.org/10.1016/j.cell.2015.11.045, https://www.sciencedirect.com/journal/cell.

[174] Engelking LJ, Kuriyama H, Hammer RE, Horton JD, Brown MS, Goldstein JL, et al. Overexpression of Insig-1 in the livers of transgenic mice inhibits SREBP processing and reduces insulin-stimulated lipogenesis. J Clin Invest 2004;113(8):1168−75. Available from: https://doi.org/10.1172/JCI20978, http://www.jci.org.

[175] Yabe D, Brown MS, Goldstein JL. Insig-2, a second endoplasmic reticulum protein that binds SCAP and blocks export of sterol regulatory element-binding proteins. Proc Natl Acad Sci U S Am 2002;99 (20):12753−8. Available from: https://doi.org/10.1073/pnas.162488899.

[176] Wang Q, Liu X, Cui Y, Tang Y, Chen W, Li S, et al. The E3 ubiquitin ligase AMFR and INSIG1 bridge the activation of TBK1 kinase by modifying the adaptor STING. Immunity 2014;41(6):919−33. Available from: https://doi.org/10.1016/j.immuni.2014.11.011.

[177] Im SS, Yousef L, Blaschitz C, Liu JZ, Edwards RA, Young SG, et al. Linking lipid metabolism to the innate immune response in macrophages through sterol regulatory element binding protein-1a. Cell Metab 2011;13(5):540−9. Available from: https://doi.org/10.1016/j.cmet.2011.04.001.

[178] Bidault G, Virtue S, Petkevicius K, Jolin HE, Dugourd A, Guénantin AC, et al. SREBP1-induced fatty acid synthesis depletes macrophages antioxidant defences to promote their alternative activation. Nat Metab 2021;3(9):1150−62. Available from: https://doi.org/10.1038/s42255-021-00440-5, https://www.nature.com/natmetab/.

[179] Roh K, Noh J, Kim Y, Jang Y, Kim J, Choi H, et al. Lysosomal control of senescence and inflammation through cholesterol partitioning. Nat Metab 2023;5(3):398−413. Available from: https://doi.org/10.1038/s42255-023-00747-5.

[180] Serhan CN, Chiang N, Van Dyke TE. Resolving inflammation: dual anti-inflammatory and pro-resolution lipid mediators. Nat Rev Immunology 2008;8(5):349−61. Available from: https://doi.org/10.1038/nri2294.

[181] Brown EM, Clardy J, Xavier RJ. Gut microbiome lipid metabolism and its impact on host physiology. Cell Host Microbe 2023;31(2):173−86. Available from: https://doi.org/10.1016/j.chom.2023.01.009.

[182] Gruenberg J. Viruses and endosome membrane dynamics. Curr Opin Cell Biol 2009;21(4):582−8. Available from: https://doi.org/10.1016/j.ceb.2009.03.008.

[183] Hilbi H, Nagai H, Kubori T, Roy CR. Subversion of host membrane dynamics by the legionella Dot/Icm Type IV secretion system. Current Topics in Microbiology and Immunology 2017;413:221−42. Available from: https://doi.org/10.1007/978-3-319-75241-9_9, http://www.springer.com/series/82.

[184] Stavru F, Bouillaud F, Sartori A, Ricquier D, Cossart P. Listeria monocytogenes transiently alters mitochondrial dynamics during infection. Proc Natl Acad Sci USA 2011;108(9):3612−17. Available from: https://doi.org/10.1073/pnas.1100126108.

[185] Heisler DB, Johnson KA, Ma D, Ohlson MB, Zhang L, Tran M, et al. A concerted mechanism involving ACAT and SREBPs by which oxysterols deplete accessible cholesterol to restrict microbial infection. eLife 2023;12. Available from: https://doi.org/10.7554/eLife.83534, https://elifesciences.org/articles/83534.

[186] Christ A, Günther P, Lauterbach MAR, Duewell P, Biswas D, Pelka K, et al. Western Diet Triggers NLRP3-Dependent Innate Immune Reprogramming. Cell Press, Ger Cell 2018;172(1-2):162. Available from: https://doi.org/10.1016/j.cell.2017.12.013, https://www.sciencedirect.com/journal/cell.

[187] Guo C, Chi Z, Jiang D, Xu T, Yu W, Wang Z, et al. Cholesterol Homeostatic Regulator SCAP-SREBP2 Integrates NLRP3 Inflammasome Activation and Cholesterol Biosynthetic Signaling in Macrophages. Immunity 2018;49(5):842. Available from: https://doi.org/10.1016/j.immuni.2018.08.021.

[188] Hsieh WY, Zhou QD, York AG, Williams KJ, Scumpia PO, Kronenberger EB, et al. Toll-like receptors induce signal-specific reprogramming of the macrophage lipidome. Cell Metab 2020;32(1):128. Available from: https://doi.org/10.1016/j.cmet.2020.05.003, http://www.cellmetabolism.org/.

[189] Leslie DS, Dascher CC, Cembrola K, Townes MA, Hava DL, Hugendubler LC, et al. Serum lipids regulate dendritic cell CD1 expression and function. Immunology 2008;125(3):289–301. Available from: https://doi.org/10.1111/j.1365-2567.2008.02842.x.

[190] Zhou QD, Chi X, Lee MS, Hsieh WY, Mkrtchyan JJ, Feng AC, et al. Interferon-mediated reprogramming of membrane cholesterol to evade bacterial toxins. Nat Immunology 2020;21(7):746–55. Available from: https://doi.org/10.1038/s41590-020-0695-4, http://www.nature.com/ni.

[191] Cubillos-Ruiz JR, Silberman PC, Rutkowski MR, Chopra S, Perales-Puchalt A, Song M, et al. ER stress sensor XBP1 controls anti-tumor immunity by disrupting dendritic cell homeostasis. Cell 2015;161(7):1527–38. Available from: https://doi.org/10.1016/j.cell.2015.05.025, https://www.sciencedirect.com/journal/cell.

[192] Di Conza G, Ho P-C. ER stress responses: an emerging modulator for innate immunity. Cells 2020;9(3):695. Available from: https://doi.org/10.3390/cells9030695.

[193] Koelwyn GJ, Corr EM, Erbay E, Moore KJ. Regulation of macrophage immunometabolism in atherosclerosis. Nat Immunol 2018;19(6):526–37. Available from: https://doi.org/10.1038/s41590-018-0113-3, http://www.nature.com/ni.

[194] Pakos-Zebrucka K, Koryga I, Mnich K, Ljujic M, Samali A, Gorman AM. The integrated stress response. EMBO Rep 2016;17(10):1374–95. Available from: https://doi.org/10.15252/embr.201642195, http://embor.embopress.org/.

[195] Klann K, Tascher G, Münch C. Functional translatome proteomics reveal converging and dose-dependent regulation by mTORC1 and eIF2α. Mol Cell 2020;77(4):913. Available from: https://doi.org/10.1016/j.molcel.2019.11.010.

[196] Mukhopadhyay S, Amodeo ME, Lee ASY. eIF3d controls the persistent integrated stress response. Mol Cell 2023;83(18):3303. Available from: https://doi.org/10.1016/j.molcel.2023.08.008, www.molecule.org.

[197] Dang Do AN, Kimball SR, Cavener DR, Jefferson LS. eIF2α kinases GCN2 and PERK modulate transcription and translation of distinct sets of mRNAs in mouse liver. Physiol Genom 2009;38(3):328–41. Available from: https://doi.org/10.1152/physiolgenomics.90396.2008, http://physiolgenomics.physiology.org/cgi/reprint/38/3/328. United States.

[198] Szaruga M, Janssen DA, de Miguel C, Hodgson G, Fatalska A, Pitera AP, et al. Activation of the integrated stress response by inhibitors of its kinases. Nat Commun 2023;14(1). Available from: https://doi.org/10.1038/s41467-023-40823-8, https://www.nature.com/ncomms/.

[199] Wanders D, Stone KP, Forney LA, Cortez CC, Dille KN, Simon J, et al. Role of GCN2-independent signaling through a noncanonical PERK/NRF2 pathway in the physiological responses to dietary methionine restriction. Diabetes. 2016;65(6):1499–510. Available from: https://doi.org/10.2337/db15-1324, http://diabetes.diabetesjournals.org/content/diabetes/65/6/1499.full.pdf.

[200] Guo Y-L, Gurung C, Fendereski M, Huang F. Dicer and PKR as novel regulators of embryonic stem cell fate and antiviral innate immunity. J Immunology 2022;208(10):2259–66. Available from: https://doi.org/10.4049/jimmunol.2200042.

[201] Kang R, Tang D. PKR-dependent inflammatory signals. Sci Signal 2012;5(247). Available from: https://doi.org/10.1126/scisignal.2003511.

[202] Lu B, Nakamura T, Inouye K, Li J, Tang Y, Lundbäck P, et al. Novel role of PKR in inflammasome activation and HMGB1 release. Nature 2012;488(7413):670–4. Available from: https://doi.org/10.1038/nature11290.

[203] Chen YG, Hur S. Cellular origins of dsRNA, their recognition and consequences. Nat Rev Mol Cell Biol 2022;23(4):286–301. Available from: https://doi.org/10.1038/s41580-021-00430-1, https://www.nature.com/molcellbio.

[204] Goh KC, DeVeer MJ, Williams BRG. The protein kinase PKR is required for p38 MAPK activation and the innate immune response to bacterial endotoxin. EMBO J 2000;19(16):4292–7. Available from: https://doi.org/10.1093/emboj/19.16.4292, http://emboj.embopress.org/.

[205] Nakamura T, Furuhashi M, Li P, Cao H, Tuncman G, Sonenberg N, et al. Double-stranded RNA-dependent protein kinase links pathogen sensing with stress and metabolic homeostasis. Cell 2010;140(3):338–48. Available from: https://doi.org/10.1016/j.cell.2010.01.001.

[206] Youssef OA, Safran SA, Nakamura T, Nix DA, Hotamisligil GS, Bass BL. Potential role for snoRNAs in PKR activation during metabolic stress. Proc Natl Acad Sci USA 2015;112(16):5023–8. Available from: https://doi.org/10.1073/pnas.1424044112.

[207] Ravindran R, Khan N, Nakaya HI, Li S, Loebbermann J, Maddur MS, et al. Vaccine activation of the nutrient sensor GCN2 in dendritic cells enhances antigen presentation. Science 2014;343(6168):313–17. Available from: https://doi.org/10.1126/science.1246829, http://www.sciencemag.org/content/343/6168/313.full.pdf.

[208] Battu S, Afroz S, Giddaluru J, Naz S, Huang W, Khumukcham SS, et al. Amino acid starvation sensing dampens IL-1β production by activating riboclustering and autophagy. PLOS Biol 2018;16(4):e2005317. Available from: https://doi.org/10.1371/journal.pbio.2005317.

[209] Halaby MJ, Hezaveh K, Lamorte S, Ciudad MT, Kloetgen A, MacLeod BL, et al. GCN2 drives macrophage and MDSC function and immunosuppression in the tumor microenvironment. Sci Immunol 2019;4(42). Available from: https://doi.org/10.1126/sciimmunol.aax8189, https://www.science.org/doi/epdf/10.1126/sciimmunol.aax8189.

[210] Ravindran R, Loebbermann J, Nakaya HI, Khan N, Ma H, Gama L, et al. The amino acid sensor GCN2 controls gut inflammation by inhibiting inflammasome activation. Nature 2016;531(7595):523–7. Available from: https://doi.org/10.1038/nature17186, http://www.nature.com/nature/index.html.

[211] Naz S, Battu S, Khan RA, Afroz S, Giddaluru J, Vishwakarma SK, et al. Activation of integrated stress response pathway regulates IL-1β production through posttranscriptional and translational reprogramming in macrophages. Eur J Immunol 2019;49(2):277–89. Available from: https://doi.org/10.1002/eji.201847513, http://onlinelibrary.wiley.com/journal/10.1002/(ISSN)1521-4141.

[212] Park MD, Silvin A, Ginhoux F, Merad M. Macrophages in health and disease. Cell 2022;185(23):4259–79. Available from: https://doi.org/10.1016/j.cell.2022.10.007.

[213] Ginhoux F, Guilliams M. Tissue-resident macrophage ontogeny and homeostasis. Immunity 2016;44(3):439–49. Available from: https://doi.org/10.1016/j.immuni.2016.02.024.

[214] Mass E, Nimmerjahn F, Kierdorf K, Schlitzer A. Tissue-specific macrophages: how they develop and choreograph tissue biology. Nat Rev Immunology 2023;23(9):563–79. Available from: https://doi.org/10.1038/s41577-023-00848-y.

[215] Blériot C, Chakarov S, Ginhoux F. Determinants of resident tissue macrophage identity and function. Immunity 2020;52(6):957–70. Available from: https://doi.org/10.1016/j.immuni.2020.05.014.

[216] Bellomo A, Mondor I, Spinelli L, Lagueyrie M, Stewart BJ, Brouilly N, et al. Reticular fibroblasts expressing the transcription factor WT1 define a stromal niche that maintains and replenishes splenic red pulp macrophages. Immunity 2020;53(1):127. Available from: https://doi.org/10.1016/j.immuni.2020.06.008, www.immunity.com.

[217] Bonnardel J, T'Jonck W, Gaublomme D, Browaeys R, Scott CL, Martens L, et al. Stellate cells, hepatocytes, and endothelial cells imprint the kupffer cell identity on monocytes colonizing the liver macrophage niche. Immunity 2019;51(4):638. Available from: https://doi.org/10.1016/j.immuni.2019.08.017, www.immunity.com.

[218] Sakai M, Troutman TD, Seidman JS, Ouyang Z, Spann NJ, Abe Y, et al. Liver-derived signals sequentially reprogram myeloid enhancers to initiate and maintain kupffer cell identity. Immunity 2019;51(4):655. Available from: https://doi.org/10.1016/j.immuni.2019.09.002, www.immunity.com.

[219] Dranoff G, Crawford AD, Sadelain M, Ream B, Rashid A, Bronson RT, et al. Involvement of granulocyte-macrophage colony-stimulating factor in pulmonary homeostasis. Science 1994;264 (5159):713−16. Available from: https://doi.org/10.1126/science.8171324, www.sciencemag.org.

[220] Lavin Y, Winter D, Blecher-Gonen R, David E, Keren-Shaul H, Merad M, et al. Tissue-resident macrophage enhancer landscapes are shaped by the local microenvironment. Cell 2014;159(6):1312−26. Available from: https://doi.org/10.1016/j.cell.2014.11.018.

[221] van de Laar L, Saelens W, De Prijck S, Martens L, Scott CL, Van Isterdael G, et al. Fetal liver, and adult monocytes can colonize an empty niche and develop into functional tissue-resident macrophages. Immunity 2016;44(4):755−68. Available from: https://doi.org/10.1016/j.immuni.2016.02.017, www.immunity.com.

[222] Yu X, Buttgereit A, Lelios I, Utz SG, Cansever D, Becher B, et al. The Cytokine TGF-beta promotes the development and homeostasis of alveolar macrophages. Immunity 2017;47(5):903−12.

[223] Wculek SK, Heras-Murillo I, Mastrangelo A, Mañanes D, Galán M, Miguel V, et al. Oxidative phosphorylation selectively orchestrates tissue macrophage homeostasis. Immunity 2023;56(3):516. Available from: https://doi.org/10.1016/j.immuni.2023.01.011, www.immunity.com.

[224] Barker PM, Boyd CA, Ramsden CA, Strang LB, Walters DV. Pulmonary glucose transport in the fetal sheep. J Physiol 1989;409(1):15−27. Available from: https://doi.org/10.1113/jphysiol.1989.sp017482.

[225] Garnett JP, Baker EH, Baines DL. Sweet talk: insights into the nature and importance of glucose transport in lung epithelium. Eur Respiratory J 2012;40(5):1269−76. Available from: https://doi.org/10.1183/09031936.00052612.

[226] Saumon G, Martet G, Loiseau P. Glucose transport and equilibrium across alveolar-airway barrier of rat. Am J Physiol-Lung Cell Mol Physiology 1996;270(2):L183. Available from: https://doi.org/10.1152/ajplung.1996.270.2.l183.

[227] Svedberg FR, Brown SL, Krauss MZ, Campbell L, Sharpe C, Clausen M, et al. The lung environment controls alveolar macrophage metabolism and responsiveness in type 2 inflammation. Nat Immunology 2019;20(5):571−80. Available from: https://doi.org/10.1038/s41590-019-0352-y, http://www.nature.com/ni.

[228] Woods PS, Kimmig LM, Meliton AY, Sun KA, Tian Y, O'Leary EM, et al. Tissue-resident alveolar macrophages do not rely on glycolysis for LPS-induced inflammation. Am J Respiratory Cell Mol Biol 2020;62(2):243−55. Available from: https://doi.org/10.1165/rcmb.2019-0244OC, https://www.atsjournals.org/doi/pdf/10.1165/rcmb.2019-0244OC.

[229] Schneider C, Nobs SP, Kurrer M, Rehrauer H, Thiele C, Kopf M. Induction of the nuclear receptor PPAR-γ 3 by the cytokine GM-CSF is critical for the differentiation of fetal monocytes into alveolar macrophages. Nat Immunol 2014;15(11):1026−37. Available from: https://doi.org/10.1038/ni.3005, http://www.nature.com/ni.

[230] Baker AD, Malur A, Barna BP, Ghosh S, Kavuru MS, Malur AG, et al. Targeted PPARγ deficiency in alveolar macrophages disrupts surfactant catabolism. J Lipid Res 2010;51(6):1325−31. Available from: https://doi.org/10.1194/jlr.M001651, http://www.jlr.org/cgi/reprint/51/6/1325. United States.

[231] Sinclair C, Bommakanti G, Gardinassi L, Loebbermann J, Johnson MJ, Hakimpour P, et al. MTOR regulates metabolic adaptation of APCs in the lung and controls the outcome of allergic inflammation. Science 2017;357(6355):1014−21. Available from: https://doi.org/10.1126/science.aaj2155, http://science.sciencemag.org/content/sci/357/6355/1014.full.pdf.

[232] Izquierdo HM, Brandi P, Gómez MJ, Conde-Garrosa R, Priego E, Enamorado M, et al. Von Hippel-Lindau protein is required for optimal alveolar macrophage terminal differentiation, self-renewal, and function. Cell Rep 2018;24(7):1738−46. Available from: https://doi.org/10.1016/j.celrep.2018.07.034, http://www.sciencedirect.com/science/journal/22111247.

[233] Lavrich KS, Speen AM, Ghio AJ, Bromberg PA, Samet JM, Alexis NE. Macrophages from the upper and lower human respiratory tract are metabolically distinct. Am J Physiol - Lung Cell Mol Physiol 2018;315(5):L752. Available from: https://doi.org/10.1152/ajplung.00208.2018, https://www.physiology.org/doi/pdf/10.1152/ajplung.00208.2018.

[234] Mould KJ, Barthel L, Mohning MP, Thomas SM, McCubbrey AL, Danhorn T, et al. Cell origin dictates programming of resident versus recruited macrophages during acute lung injury. Am J Respiratory Cell Mol Biol 2017;57(3):294–306. Available from: https://doi.org/10.1165/rcmb.2017-0061OC, http://www.atsjournals.org/doi/pdf/10.1165/rcmb.2017-0061OC.

[235] Huang L, Nazarova EV, Tan S, Liu Y, Russell DG. Growth of Mycobacterium tuberculosis in vivo segregates with host macrophage metabolism and ontogeny. J Exp Med 2018;215(4):1135–52. Available from: https://doi.org/10.1084/jem.20172020, http://jem.rupress.org/content/jem/215/4/1135.full.pdf.

[236] Wang T, Zhang J, Wang Y, Li Y, Wang L, Yu Y, et al. Influenza-trained mucosal-resident alveolar macrophages confer long-term antitumor immunity in the lungs. Nat Immunology 2023;24(3):423–38. Available from: https://doi.org/10.1038/s41590-023-01428-x.

[237] Yao Y, Jeyanathan M, Haddadi S, Barra NG, Vaseghi-Shanjani M, Damjanovic D, et al. Induction of autonomous memory alveolar macrophages requires T cell help and is critical to trained immunity. Cell 2018;175(6):1634. Available from: https://doi.org/10.1016/j.cell.2018.09.042, https://www.sciencedirect.com/journal/cell.

[238] Haggadone MD, Speth J, Hong HS, Penke LR, Zhang E, Lyssiotis CA, et al. ATP citrate lyase links increases in glycolysis to diminished release of vesicular suppressor of cytokine signaling 3 by alveolar macrophages. Biochim Biophysica Acta (BBA) - Mol Basis Dis 2022;1868(10):166458. Available from: https://doi.org/10.1016/j.bbadis.2022.166458.

[239] Bourdonnay E, Zasłona Z, Penke LRK, Speth JM, Schneider DJ, Przybranowski S, et al. Transcellular delivery of vesicular SOCS proteins from macrophages to epithelial cells blunts inflammatory signaling. J Exp Med 2015;212(5):729–42. Available from: https://doi.org/10.1084/jem.20141675.

[240] Xie N, Cui H, Ge J, Banerjee S, Guo S, Dubey S, et al. Metabolic characterization and RNA profiling reveal glycolytic dependence of profibrotic phenotype of alveolar macrophages in lung fibrosis. Am J Physiol-Lung Cell Mol Physiology 2017;313(5):L834. Available from: https://doi.org/10.1152/ajplung.00235.2017.

[241] Gleeson LE, Sheedy FJ, Palsson-McDermott EM, Triglia D, O'Leary SM, O'Sullivan MP, et al. Cutting edge: Mycobacterium tuberculosis induces aerobic glycolysis in human alveolar macrophages that is required for control of intracellular bacillary replication. J Immunology 2016;196(6):2444–9. Available from: https://doi.org/10.4049/jimmunol.1501612, http://www.jimmunol.org/content/196/6/2444.full.pdf+html.

[242] Baker EH, Baines DL. Airway glucose homeostasis: a new target in the prevention and treatment of pulmonary infection. Chest 2018;153(2):507–14. Available from: https://doi.org/10.1016/j.chest.2017.05.031, http://www.chestjournal.org/.

[243] Baker EH, Clark N, Brennan AL, Fisher DA, Gyi KM, Hodson ME, et al. Hyperglycemia and cystic fibrosis alter respiratory fluid glucose concentrations estimated by breath condensate analysis. J Appl Physiol 2007;102(5):1969–75. Available from: https://doi.org/10.1152/japplphysiol.01425.2006, http://jap.physiology.org/cgi/reprint/102/5/1969.pdf. United Kingdom.

[244] Surowiec I, Karimpour M, Gouveia-Figueira S, Wu J, Unosson J, Bosson JA, et al. Multi-platform metabolomics assays for human lung lavage fluids in an air pollution exposure study. Anal Bioanal Chem 2016;408(17):4751–64. Available from: https://doi.org/10.1007/s00216-016-9566-0, link.springer.de/link/service/journals/00216/index.htm.

[245] Huffnagle GB, Dickson RP, Lukacs NW. The respiratory tract microbiome and lung inflammation: a two-way street. Mucosal Immunology 2017;10(2):299–306. Available from: https://doi.org/10.1038/mi.2016.108.

[246] Invernizzi R, Lloyd CM, Molyneaux PL. Respiratory microbiome and epithelial interactions shape immunity in the lungs. Immunology 2020;160(2):171–82. Available from: https://doi.org/10.1111/imm.13195, http://onlinelibrary.wiley.com/journal/10.1111/(ISSN)1365-2567.

[247] Postler TS, Ghosh S. Understanding the holobiont: how microbial metabolites affect human health and shape the immune system. Cell Metab 2017;26(1):110–30. Available from: https://doi.org/10.1016/j.cmet.2017.05.008.

[248] Li TT, Chen X, Huo D, Arifuzzaman M, Qiao S, Jin WB, et al. Microbiota metabolism of intestinal amino acids impacts host nutrient homeostasis and physiology. Cell Host Microbe 2024;32(5):661. Available from: https://doi.org/10.1016/j.chom.2024.04.004, https://www.sciencedirect.com/science/journal/19313128.

[249] A-Gonzalez N, Castrillo A. Origin and specialization of splenic macrophages. Cell Immunol 2018;330:151−8. Available from: https://doi.org/10.1016/j.cellimm.2018.05.005.

[250] Scott CL, Guilliams M. The role of Kupffer cells in hepatic iron and lipid metabolism. J Hepatol 2018;69(5):1197−9. Available from: https://doi.org/10.1016/j.jhep.2018.02.013.

[251] Korolnek T, Hamza I. Macrophages and iron trafficking at the birth and death of red cells. Blood 2015;125(19):2893−7. Available from: https://doi.org/10.1182/blood-2014-12-567776.

[252] Kondo H, Saito K, Grasso JP, Aisen P. Iron metabolism in the erythrophagocytosing Kupffer cell. Hepatology 1988;8(1):32−8. Available from: https://doi.org/10.1002/hep.1840080108.

[253] Kim KS, Zhang DL, Kovtunovych G, Ghosh MC, Ollivierre H, Eckhaus MA, et al. Infused wild-type macrophages reside and self-renew in the liver to rescue the hemolysis and anemia of Hmox1-deficient mice. Blood Adv 2018;2(20):2732−43. Available from: https://doi.org/10.1182/bloodadvances.2018019737, http://www.bloodadvances.org/content/bloodoa/2/20/2732.full.pdf.

[254] Theurl I, Hilgendorf I, Nairz M, Tymoszuk P, Haschka D, Asshoff M, et al. On-demand erythrocyte disposal and iron recycling requires transient macrophages in the liver. Nat Med 2016;22(8):945−51. Available from: https://doi.org/10.1038/nm.4146.

[255] Kohyama M, Ise W, Edelson BT, Wilker PR, Hildner K, Mejia C, et al. Role for Spi-C in the development of red pulp macrophages and splenic iron homeostasis. Nature 2009;457(7227):318−21. Available from: https://doi.org/10.1038/nature07472.

[256] Haldar M, Kohyama M, So AY-L, KC W, Wu X, Briseño CG, et al. Heme-Mediated SPI-C induction promotes monocyte differentiation into iron-recycling macrophages. Cell 2014;156(6):1223−34. Available from: https://doi.org/10.1016/j.cell.2014.01.069.

[257] Kovtunovych G, Eckhaus MA, Ghosh MC, Ollivierre-Wilson H, Rouault TA. Dysfunction of the heme recycling system in heme oxygenase 1-deficient mice: Effects on macrophage viability and tissue iron distribution. Blood 2010;116(26):6054−62. Available from: https://doi.org/10.1182/blood-2010-03-272138, http://bloodjournal.hematologylibrary.org/cgi/reprint/116/26/6054.

[258] Di Nunzio G, Hellberg S, Zhang Y, Ahmed O, Wang J, Zhang X, et al. Kupffer cells dictate hepatic responses to the atherogenic dyslipidemic insult. Nat Cardiovascular Res 2024;3(3):356−71. Available from: https://doi.org/10.1038/s44161-024-00448-6.

[259] Jacks RD, Lumeng CN. Macrophage and T cell networks in adipose tissue. Nat Rev Endocrinol 2024;20(1):50−61. Available from: https://doi.org/10.1038/s41574-023-00908-2, https://www.nature.com/nrendo/.

[260] Serbulea V, Upchurch CM, Schappe MS, Voigt P, DeWeese DE, Desai BN, et al. Macrophage phenotype and bioenergetics are controlled by oxidized phospholipids identified in lean and obese adipose tissue. Proc Natl Acad Sci U S Am 2018;115(27):E6254. Available from: https://doi.org/10.1073/pnas.1800544115, http://www.pnas.org/content/pnas/115/27/E6254.full.pdf.

[261] Cinti S, Mitchell G, Barbatelli G, Murano I, Ceresi E, Faloia E, et al. Adipocyte death defines macrophage localization and function in adipose tissue of obese mice and humans. J Lipid Res 2005;46(11):2347−55. Available from: https://doi.org/10.1194/jlr.m500294-jlr200.

[262] Xu X, Grijalva A, Skowronski A, Van Eijk M, Serlie MJ, Ferrante AW. Obesity activates a program of lysosomal-dependent lipid metabolism in adipose tissue macrophages independently of classic activation. Cell Metab 2013;18(6):816−30. Available from: https://doi.org/10.1016/j.cmet.2013.11.001.

[263] Sharma M, Boytard L, Hadi T, Koelwyn G, Simon R, Ouimet M, et al. Enhanced glycolysis and HIF-1alpha activation in adipose tissue macrophages sustains local and systemic interleukin-1beta production in obesity. Sci Rep 2020;10(1).

[264] Que X, Hung MY, Yeang C, Gonen A, Prohaska TA, Sun X, et al. Oxidized phospholipids are proinflammatory and proatherogenic in hypercholesterolaemic mice. Nature 2018;558(7709):301−6. Available from: https://doi.org/10.1038/s41586-018-0198-8, http://www.nature.com/nature/index.html.

[265] Di Gioia M, Spreafico R, Springstead JR, Mendelson MM, Joehanes R, Levy D, et al. Endogenous oxidized phospholipids reprogram cellular metabolism and boost hyperinflammation. Nat Immunology 2020;21(1):42–53. Available from: https://doi.org/10.1038/s41590-019-0539-2, http://www.nature.com/ni.

[266] Zanoni I, Tan Y, Di Gioia M, Springstead JR, Kagan JC. By Capturing Inflammatory Lipids Released from Dying Cells, the Receptor CD14 Induces Inflammasome-Dependent Phagocyte Hyperactivation. Immunity 2017;47(4):697. Available from: https://doi.org/10.1016/j.immuni.2017.09.010, www.immunity.com.

[267] Zhang X, Sergin I, Evans TD, Jeong SJ, Rodriguez-Velez A, Kapoor D, et al. High-protein diets increase cardiovascular risk by activating macrophage mTOR to suppress mitophagy. Nat Metab 2020;2(1):110–25. Available from: https://doi.org/10.1038/s42255-019-0162-4, https://www.nature.com/natmetab/.

CHAPTER 4

Immunometabolism in macrophage cell death

Sara Cahill, Laurel Stine and Fiachra Humphries
Division of Innate Immunity, Department of Medicine, UMass Chan Medical School, Worcester, MA, United States

Introduction

Macrophages are phagocytic cells of the innate immune system that play a crucial role in immune responses and maintaining tissue homeostasis. Macrophages are heterogenous cell types; circulating monocytes in the blood give rise to macrophages, while tissue-resident cells occupy most tissues throughout the body and exhibit different phenotypes depending on their localization and environmental cues [1]. More generally, macrophages are important for detecting and eliminating pathogens, clearing cellular debris, contributing to nutrient metabolism, and modulating the inflammatory response [2–4].

The metabolic state of macrophages plays a significant role in the activation state and phenotype of the cell. Macrophages exhibit a highly plastic metabolic profile that can be adjusted to changing oxygen and nutrient concentrations [5,6]. Metabolic shifts and the accumulation of key metabolites alter gene transcription and the macrophage transcriptional profile. For example, increased dependence on glycolysis is associated with a more inflammatory transcriptional profile, while macrophages exhibiting a preference for oxidative phosphorylation tend to adopt an antiinflammatory, pro-tissue repair phenotype [4]. Furthermore, macrophages' metabolic state can impact the cell's susceptibility to different forms of programmed cell death.

Macrophages can undergo several forms of programmed cell death in response to intrinsic and extrinsic signals. Each form of programmed cell death has specific consequences within a tissue which impacts the duration and severity of the immune response. Indeed, apoptotic cell death is immunogenetically silent, while necroptosis, pyroptosis, and ferroptosis can propagate inflammation. During viral infection, macrophage pyroptosis promotes lung inflammation and significantly contributes to lung pathology and disease severity [7]. Similarly, ferroptosis in the lung is connected to severe COVID-19 disease and inflammatory lung pathology [8]. In addition to impacting viral infection outcomes, pyroptotic macrophages drive antitumor immune responses by releasing inflammatory cytokines in the tumor microenvironment (TME) [9,10]. Likewise, ferroptosis macrophages in the TME differentially kill pro-tumorigenic macrophages and promote an anticancer immune response [11,12].

Recent studies have highlighted the key roles macrophage metabolism plays in regulating programmed cell death. Here we review the recent findings in the field and highlight the key metabolites that impact macrophage programmed cell death.

Macrophage programmed cell death

Apoptosis, necroptosis, and pyroptosis are three forms of programmed cell death that occur in macrophages subjected to immune, pathogenic, or cellular stimuli [13–15] (see Fig. 4.1).

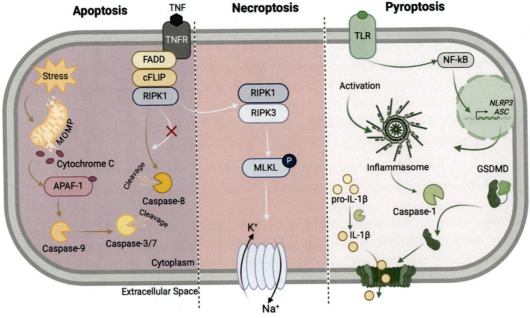

Figure 4.1: Pathways involved in macrophage programmed cell death.
(Left) Apoptosis can be induced by cellular stress via induction of MOMP and release of cytochrome c. Cytoplasmic cytochrome c binds APAF-1 and activates caspase-9. Active caspase-9 cleaves and activates caspases-3 and -7, which cleave a wide variety of substrates and drive apoptosis. Alternatively, activation of the TNFR can activate caspase-8 through the FADD/cFLIP/RIPK1 inducing widespread cleavage events. (Middle) Alternatively, in the absence of caspase-8 activation, RIPK1 can associate with RIPK3 and phosphorylate MLKL to drive necroptosis through pore formation and ion efflux. (Right) Pyroptosis begins with a priming and activation signal. TLR priming signals drive expression of inflammasome components NLRP3 and ASC via NF-κB activation. Then, activation signals induce the formation of the NLRP3 inflammasome and activation of caspase-1. Caspase-1 cleaves GSDMD releasing N-terminal fragments to oligomerize into membrane pores and pro-IL-1β resulting in mature IL-1β excretion through GSDMD membrane pores. Created with BioRender.com.

Pyroptosis and necroptosis are inflammatory forms of lytic cell death, while apoptosis is typically a silent form of cell death to facilitate the noninflammatory elimination of a dying cell. During apoptosis, mitochondrial signaling events initiate mitochondrial outer membrane permeabilization (MOMP). Once MOMP occurs, mitochondria release cytochrome c, which binds to apoptotic peptidase activating factor-1 (APAF-1) [16]. The complex of cytochrome c and APAF-1 then oligomerizes with pro-caspase-9 to form the apoptosome. Apoptosome formation triggers the cleavage and activation of caspase-9 [17–19]. Active caspase-9 cleaves and activates effector caspases, caspase-3 and caspase-7, which have over 1,300 different substrates. Caspase-3 is specifically essential for condensing chromatin, fragmenting DNA, dismantling the nuclear machinery of the cells, and inducing the formation of apoptotic bodies. These apoptotic bodies restrict the release of intracellular content such as damage-associated molecular patterns (DAMPs) and inflammatory cytokines [20,21].

Macrophage apoptosis can also occur in response to tumor necrosis factor (TNF). Following ligation of the TNF receptor (TNFR), TNF-a stimulates the recruitment of complex I containing Fas-associated death domain (FADD), TNFR-associated death domain (TRADD), TNFR-associated factors (TRAFs), cellular inhibitor of apoptosis protein (cIAP), and receptor-interacting protein kinase 1 (RIPK1) [22]. Complex I formation initiates a ubiquitination and phosphorylation cascade that leads to the activation of nuclear factor (NF-kB) and induction of pro-inflammatory cytokines and pro-survival genes [23]. Similarly, when RIPK1 is deubiquitinated, it can form a second complex with FADD, cellular FLICE-like inhibitory protein (cFLIP), and caspase-8, which initiates apoptosis [24,25]. TNF-stimulated macrophages undergo a switch from an inflammatory pro-survival profile to an apoptotic response when complex I is impaired [26]. Additionally, when caspase-8 is blocked or inactivated, macrophages will undergo another form of programmed cell death termed necroptosis [27].

Necroptosis is a caspase-independent lytic form of cell death directed by RIPK3 and its substrate, mixed lineage kinase-like (MLKL). In the absence of caspase-8, TNF-a stimulation promotes the interaction of RIPK1 with RIPK3 via the RIP homotypic interaction motif (RHIM) to form the necrosome. The lack of caspase-8 activity is critical for necroptosis; otherwise, caspase-8 would cleave RIPK1 and RIPK3, and the necrosome would not form [28]. In the necrosome, RIPK3 auto-phosphorylates and recruits MLKL through the interaction of MLKL's kinase-like domain (KLD) and RIPK3's kinase domain. RIPK3 then phosphorylates and activates MLKL [29,30]. Once phosphorylated, MLKL oligomerizes and translocates to the plasma membrane. At the cell membrane, MLKL interacts with surrounding phosphatidylinositol phosphates (PIPs) through the positively charged surface of its four-helical bundle domain (4HBD) to form pores in the plasma membrane [31]. The pores cause a flux of ions, swelling of the cell and, eventually, cell lysis [32–34].

Necroptosis can also be initiated by toll-like receptor (TLR) stimulation in macrophages. Indeed, TLR3 and TLR4 can interact with RIPK1 and RIPK3 and initiate MLKL-executed necroptosis [35]. TLR3 is located on intracellular endosomes, and once stimulated by double-stranded RNA, TLR3 can interact directly with RIPK1 and RIPK3 through Toll/interleukin-1 receptor (TIR) domain-containing adaptor protein inducing interferon-beta (TRIF) [36,37]. In addition, TLR4 translocation to the endosome can cause loss of mitochondrial transmembrane potential (Djm). Djm then drives necroptosis when caspase-8 is inhibited [38]. Interestingly, all TLRs have shown potential to initiate necroptosis [37]. However, certain criteria, such as caspase-8 inhibition, must be fulfilled to drive programmed cell death specifically toward necroptosis and not apoptosis, or a third form of cell death, pyroptosis.

Pyroptosis is distinct from other forms of programmed cell death, such as apoptosis and necrosis, because it is associated with a stronger inflammatory response. Several inflammatory diseases, such as inflammatory bowel disease, cardiovascular disease, multiple sclerosis, Parkinson's disease, Alzheimer's disease, and stroke, have all been linked to aberrant pyroptosis [39,40]. Excessive or dysregulated pyroptosis can also contribute to tissue damage and organ dysfunction [41]. Pyroptosis is triggered downstream of inflammasome activation. Inflammasomes are multimeric signaling complexes, which are activated in response to damage signals and cellular stress [42,43]. During initial assembly, inflammasome complexes facilitate the activation of pro-caspase-1. Active caspase-1 cleaves gasdermin D (GSDMD) to release an active N-terminal fragment that oligomerizes and forms membrane pores [44,45]. Active caspase-1 also triggers the maturation and release of interleukin-1b (IL-1β) and IL-18, pro-inflammatory cytokines, which further amplify the inflammatory response [46]. Alternatively, the noncanonical inflammasome is activated by caspase-4/5/11 following the detection of cytosolic LPS. Specifically, when caspase-11 binds LPS, caspase-11 cleaves itself, activates, and cleaves GSDMD. Once translocated to the plasma membrane, GSDMD forms pores that cause potassium efflux which stimulates nod-like receptor (NLR) family pyrin domain-containing 3 (NLRP3), caspase-1 activity, and the maturation of IL-1β and IL-18 [47].

While the activation of GSDMD and IL-1β release has been extensively studied, recent studies have identified an additional player during pyroptosis. Ninjurin-1 (NINJ1) is a cell adhesion molecule that is expressed in a variety of tissues and cell types, including neurons, immune cells, and cancer cells [48]. As a transmembrane protein, NINJ1 comprises two extracellular domains, a single transmembrane domain, and a short cytoplasmic tail [49]. The N-terminal extracellular domain of NINJ1 contains a conserved alpha-helix that mediates homophilic and heterophilic interactions with other molecules, including integrins and extracellular matrix proteins. In addition to its role in axonal outgrowth and guidance, NINJ1 has also been implicated in immune cell activation and migration, as well as tumor progression and metastasis [48,50]. NINJ1 acts downstream of GSDMD, where it oligomerizes to form higher-order fibril-like structures that break the plasma membrane releasing pro-inflammatory molecules [51]. Thus NINJ1 plays a crucial role in the final steps of pyroptosis to amplify the release of intracellular contents.

Ferroptosis

In addition to these classical forms of programmed cell death, researchers have identified a caspase-independent, iron-dependent form of cell death termed ferroptosis. Ferroptosis is an important regulator of inflammation and tumorigenesis and is mediated by the cellular metabolic machinery (Fig. 4.2). Ferroptosis, initially termed oxytosis, is driven by iron-dependent generation and accumulation of oxidatively damaged phospholipids within the cell [52,53]. Free cytoplasmic iron can drive lipid peroxidation through the Fenton reaction, in which Fe^{2+} reacts

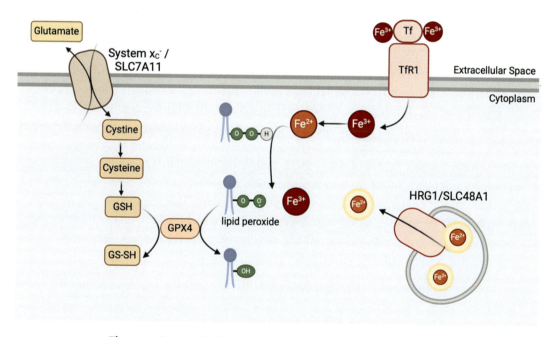

Figure 4.2: Metabolic pathways mediating lipid peroxidation.
The amount of lipid peroxide in the cell depends on the activity of enzyme GPX4, which uses GSH as an electron donor to reduce lipid peroxide groups into alcohol groups. GSH availability is dictated by system xc^-, and its subunit SLC7A11. This transport system exports glutamate from the cytoplasm and imports cystine into the cell, which is readily converted into cysteine and GSH. Intracellular iron gets channeled into macrophages by transferrin receptor TfR1, which imports free Fe^{3+}, and HRG1/SLC48A1, which transports heme molecules from endosomes into the cytoplasm. Intracellular Fe^{2+}, which is rapidly produced from Fe^{3+}, can mediate the production of lipid peroxides by reducing free LOOH groups into reactive free radicals. Created with BioRender.com.

with lipid hydroperoxide (LOOH) to form lipid-associated oxygen free radicals [54,55]. Iron is also a critical component of lipoxygenases (LOX), which contributes to the production of lipid peroxides [56]. The cellular availability and metabolism of iron impact the likelihood of ferroptosis; chelation of cellular iron decreases ferroptosis cell death while iron supplementation increases occurrence [53].

Transferrin receptor 1 (TfR1) is an important receptor for cellular uptake of free iron. TfR1 binds transferrin, a soluble protein that binds and facilitates the uptake of free iron and carries free iron into the cytoplasm via receptor-mediated endocytosis [57]. Increased expression of TfR1 increases susceptibility to ferroptosis [58]. Macrophages can also recycle iron from phagocytosed erythrocytes; heme-responsive gene 1 (HRG1/SLC48A1) transports heme from phagolysosomes into the cytoplasm for cellular recycling [59–61]. *HRG1* expression is controlled by the transcription factor nuclear factor erythroid 2 (NRF2) and is induced by oxidative stress and changes in cellular metabolism [62].

In addition to iron availability, the activity of enzyme glutathione peroxidase 4 (GPX4) regulates ferroptosis. GPX4 converts toxic peroxide groups on phospholipids to innocuous alcohol groups. Thus inactivated GPX4 contributes to the accumulation of lipid peroxides leading to ferroptosis [63–65]. GPX4 reduces lipid peroxides by oxidizing molecules of reduced glutathione (GSH) to generate nontoxic lipids and glutathione disulfide (GS-SG) [64,66]. The production of GSH is limited by the levels of cytoplasmic cysteine, which is in part regulated by amino acid metabolism, a glutamate/cysteine antiporter system x_c^-, and the active protein subunit xCT/SLC7A11 [67]. Inhibition of system x_c^- with the small-molecule erastin depletes intracellular cystine and limits GPX4, driving ferroptosis [53]. Furthermore, cellular energetic stress can regulate ferroptosis. The adenosine monophosphate (AMP) sensor, AMP-activated protein kinase (AMPK), can phosphorylate and inactivate acetyl CoA-carboxylase (ACC), which significantly reduces fatty acid synthesis and limits the availability of lipids for peroxidation [68].

Oncogenic cancer cells exhibit increased susceptibility to ferroptosis compared to nontransformed cells. This sensitivity was first observed in oncogenic cells overexpressing Ras genes; when treated with erastin, cancer cells underwent ferroptosis at a significantly higher rate compared to noncancerous cells [69]. Commonly mutated oncogene p53 also sensitizes cancer cells to ferroptosis. p53 downregulates the x_c^- system component SLC7A11 via transcription factor arachidonate 12-lipoxygenase (ALOX12) reducing cystine transport into the cell [70,71]. Epigenetic regulator mixed lineage leukemia 4 (MLL4) is another frequently mutated oncogene that activates ALOX12 through epigenetic modifications and further contributes to the sensitization of cancer cells to ferroptosis [72,73]. There is growing interest in the field to exploit this vulnerability and to target cancer cells via induction of ferroptosis.

The Warburg effect primes macrophage activation

Immune stimulation of macrophages triggers an essential metabolic shift to facilitate a transcriptional inflammatory response. LPS-treated macrophages reprogram their metabolism to generate adenosine triphosphate (ATP) via the glycolytic machinery. This metabolic switch is known as the Warburg effect. The Warburg effect was first described in tumor cells; it was observed that tumor cells consume significantly more glucose than nontransformed cells and produce lactate at very high rates. Tumor cells favor anaerobic glycolysis for rapid energetic payoff and to reduce dependence on oxygen instead of oxidative phosphorylation. This metabolic switch was termed the Warburg effect [74]. However, this phenomenon is not specific to cancer cells. In macrophages, LPS exposure stimulates the glycolytic response to yield higher levels of ATP, reactive oxygen species (ROS), and increased cytokine production [75–77].

Macrophage metabolic shifts interrupt the tricarboxylic acid (TCA) cycle, and immunomodulatory metabolites, such as succinate, itaconate, and fumarate, accumulate in the cytosol. Accumulation of succinate increases expression of pro-inflammatory genes, including IL-1β [78]. Oxidation of succinate-by-succinate dehydrogenase (SDH) also increases production of mitochondrial reactive oxygen species (mROS), which drives pro-inflammatory gene expression through activation of transcription factor hypoxia-inducible factor-1 (HIF-1α) [75]. In addition, itaconate accumulates to mM levels in activated macrophages. Itaconate is synthesized from *cis*-aconitate shunted from the TCA cycle. The immune-responsive gene 1 (Irg1), also known as aconitate decarboxylase 1 (Acod1), is upregulated in activated macrophages and catalyzes the conversion of aconitate to itaconate [79,80]. Itaconate serves as an antiinflammatory negative feedback loop to resolve inflammatory responses. The electrophilic nature of itaconate can stimulate the stabilization of NRF2 via the inhibition of kelch-like ECH-associated protein-1 (KEAP1). Itaconate also displays potent antibacterial activity and can limit salmonella replication [81,82].

Cytosolic levels of the TCA intermediate fumarate also increase following macrophage stimulation and activation. The TCA-cycle enzyme, fumarate hydratase (FH), controls the intracellular levels of fumarate by catalyzing the hydration of fumarate to malate [83]. Additionally, FH can act as a tumor suppressor; mutations in FH are the underlying cause of hereditary leiomyomatosis and renal cell cancer (HLRCC) [84]. Furthermore, FH regulates inflammatory responses via the arginosuccinate shunt in LPS-activated macrophages [85]. Activated macrophages also exhibit increased expression of arginosuccinate synthase (ASS1), which is responsible for producing arginosuccinate that is readily broken down to produce fumarate [86]. Additionally, increases in cytosolic fumarate impact mitochondrial morphology, membrane potential, and release of mitochondrial RNA and DNA (mtRNA and mtDNA) into the cytoplasm. Once in the cytosol, mtRNA and mtDNA can trigger an inflammatory response through intracellular nucleic acid sensors; mtRNA can trigger TLR7, RIG-I, and MDA5, while mtDNA activates the inflammatory cGAS-STING pathway [86,87]. Thus the fumarate that accumulates in macrophages following stimulation contributes to cell activation and induces an inflammatory response.

In a type I interferon (IFN)-dependent manner, LPS can also drive the synthesis of tissue factor (TF), a crucial component of the coagulation cascade released from macrophages during pyroptosis [88,89]. TF release is inhibited by itaconate and fumarate via suppression of type I IFN and caspase activation [90]. Accumulation of metabolites can also exert their immunomodulatory roles on macrophage transcription by inducing epigenetic changes through histone modifications [91]. Lactic acid, a by-product of anaerobic glycolysis increased by the Warburg effect, modifies the epigenome by lactylation of lysine residues on histones. Lactate modifications on histones can increase transcription of modified chromatin [92].

Metabolic regulation of cell death

A significant number of studies have characterized the key metabolic changes after macrophage activation that drive the pro-inflammatory transcriptional responses. However, it was unclear how immunomodulatory metabolites regulate secondary responses, such as cell death. Recently, several studies have characterized how electrophilic metabolites, such as fumarate and itaconate, can impact cell death events by targeting and inactivating thiol groups on functionally important cysteine residues [93]. Further, studies show that mROS regulates GSDMD biology by stimulating the activity of GSDM family members through enhanced palmitoylation [94–96]. Together, these studies indicate that metabolic signals modulate key effector proteins during pyroptosis when metabolic signals accumulate during the priming events that precede pyroptosis.

Regulation of pyroptosis by fumarate

Following LPS stimulation, macrophages accumulate the TCA intermediate fumarate. Fumarate is an electrophilic metabolite that can modify cysteine residues with a nonenzymatic post-translational modification known as succination [97]. Succination modifications form when fumarate reacts with the thiol group in a cysteine residue to form an S-(2-succino)-cysteine (2SC) adduct [98]. FH, which is essential for controlling cytosolic fumarate levels, is downregulated following LPS stimulation in macrophages [83,85]. Loss-of-function mutations in FH result in the intracellular accumulation of fumarate. Intracellular fumarate accumulation creates excessive succination of target cysteine residues. Fumarate accumulation can also stabilize HIF-1α and activate pro-tumorigenic HIF-dependent pathways. Additionally, fumarate accumulation activates NRF2, elevates mROS levels, and inhibits TCA enzyme aconitase, which limits aconitate availability for conversion into itaconate [99,100]. Succination can also impair inflammatory responses by inactivating the glycolytic enzyme glyceraldehyde 3-phosphate dehydrogenase (GAPDH) [85,101].

The therapeutic analog of fumarate, dimethyl fumarate (DMF, tradename Tecfidera), is a frontline treatment for multiple sclerosis [102]. Following oral administration, DMF is rapidly reduced to its active form monomethyl fumarate (MMF), which can form a +130 Da 2-monomethyl succinyl cysteine adduct [97,98]. In a recent study, fumarate and DMF potently inhibit pyroptosis by succinating GSDMD [93,102]. When fumarate accumulates, it limits GSDMD oligomerization and pore formation by targeting Cys^{191} on GSDMD during inflammasome activation. In macrophages treated with DMF, there was significantly less cell membrane permeabilization than with other metabolites such as succinate and itaconate. Mechanistically fumarate succinated Cys^{191} on GSDMD to form a S-(2-succinyl)-cysteine adduct. Succination of GSDMD impaired GSDMD oligomerization, thus inhibiting pyroptosis [93]. Additional studies have also implicated fumarate in regulating apoptosis-associated speck-like protein (ASC) and NLRP3, thus preventing inflammasome formation via succination of the Cys^{673} residue on NLRP3 [103] (see Fig. 4.3).

Fumarate accumulation can also drive other modes of programmed cell death such as apoptosis and necroptosis. Before apoptosis begins, fumarate blocks thioredoxin-1 (Trx1) [104]. Trx1 is essential for NF-kB binding and facilitates the transcription of antiapoptotic genes [105,106]. Once fumarate blocks Trx1, pro-apoptotic proteins outweigh cell death suppressor proteins shifting the cell toward apoptosis. Specifically, DMF blocks Trx1 by succinating a key regulatory cystine, Cys^{73}, which inhibits Trx1's interaction with NF-kB. This can lead to ripoptosome formation and decreases in antiapoptotic proteins such as cFLIP [104]. Fumarate can also deplete glutathione (GSH), increase cellular ROS, and activate mitogen-activated protein kinases (MAPKs) to promote necroptosis [107].

Itaconation in cell death and tolerance

In addition to fumarate, itaconate can also react with thiol groups in cysteine residues via a modification termed itaconation. Two recent studies identified key roles for itaconate and the itaconate analog, 4-ocytl itaconate (4-OI), as inhibitors of pyroptosis by targeting GSDMD and NLRP3, respectively [86,108] (see Fig. 4.4). In the first step of inflammasome assembly, activated NLRP3 must first complex with NIMA-related kinase 7 (NEK-7) to recruit ASC and pro-caspase-1 [109]. 4-OI inhibits the interaction between NLRP3 and NEK-7 by modifying Cys^{548}, on NLRP3, thus impairing NLRP3 inflammasome assembly, IL-1β and IL-18 maturation, and induction of pyroptosis [86]. Interestingly, peripheral blood mononuclear cells (PBMCs) from cryopyrin-associated periodic syndrome (CAPS)

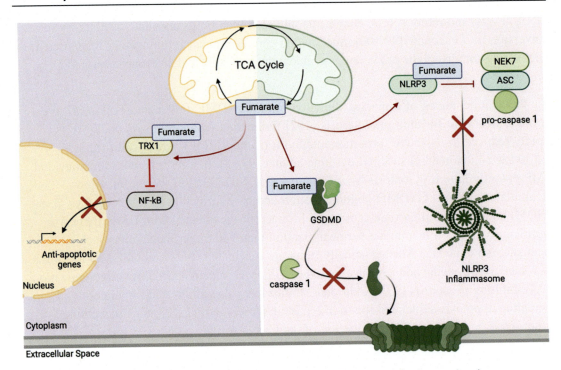

Figure 4.3: Fumarate regulation of apoptosis and pyroptosis via succination.
Fumarate is produced during the TCA cycle and is an intermediate metabolite of the pathway. Shunted fumarate can induce apoptosis by succinating Trx1, a protein that binds NF-κB, to facilitate its activity as a transcription factor. Succination of Trx1 inhibits interaction with NF-κB and disrupts its activity, resulting in reduced transcription of antiapoptotic genes. Conversely, fumarate inhibits pyroptosis via independent succination of NLRP3 and GSDMD. Modification of NLRP3 inhibits inflammasome formation and caspase-1 activation by blocking NLRP3 interactions with the other inflammasome components. Modification of GSDMD inhibits caspase-1-mediated cleavage such that the N-terminal fragment does not oligomerize into pores, inhibiting pyroptosis. Created with BioRender.com.

patients, a disease characterized by mutations in the NLRP3 gene, incubated with 4-OI exhibit constitutive NLRP3 activation and inhibit IL-1β release [86,110,111].

In another study, the accumulation of itaconate acts as a key tolerizing metabolite by targeting GSDMD. Canonical inflammasome activation and assembly occur in a two-step process. First, a transcriptional priming event, usually mediated by a TLR-dependent signal, is followed by a secondary DAMP sensed by NLR receptors, such as NLRP3 [112–115]. Macrophages exposed to prolonged LPS priming failed to undergo pyroptosis following treatment with the NLRP3 activator, nigericin, because of itaconate-mediated tolerance. This tolerizing effect was lost in *Irg1*-deficient macrophages. Further, reconstitution of

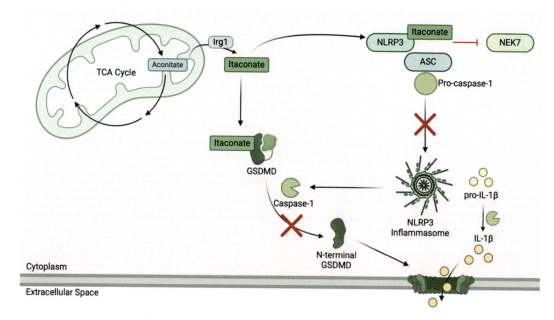

Figure 4.4: Inhibition of pyroptosis via itaconation.
Intermediate TCA metabolite aconitate is converted into itaconate by the enzyme Irg1. Itaconate can modify NLRP3 post-translationally, which inhibits NLRP3 and NEK-7 interaction and subsequently ASC and pro-caspase-1 interaction. Disrupting these interactions inhibits formation of the NLRP3 inflammasome and activation of caspase-1. Independently, GSDMD can be directly modified via itaconation, impairing its cleavage by caspase-1 and oligomerization into plasma membrane pores. Created with BioRender.com.

Irg1-deficient cells with exogenous itaconate rescued the tolerizing effect and suppressed late inflammasome formation. Mechanistically, itaconate accumulation over time causes direct itaconation of GSDMD on Cys^{77}. Although Cys^{77} is indispensable for oligomerization and pore formation, Cys^{77} may facilitate the association of GSDMD and caspase-1 [108]. Further studies evaluating GSDMD-Cys^{77} in GSDMD function will provide additional insights into the late inflammasome [116]. Thus the kinetics of itaconate accumulation is an important consideration when evaluating post-transcriptional responses, such as cell death, in macrophages.

Mitochondrial reactive oxygen species prime pyroptosis

Given the sensitivity of GSDMD to cysteine ligands, additional studies have probed the redox sensitivity of GSDMD activity and its proclivity for modifications on functionally important cysteines. mROS is produced as a by-product of cellular respiration within the mitochondria. mROS is primarily generated in the mitochondrial electron transport chain during ATP production. Specifically, electrons leak from complexes I and III of the electron transport chain (ETC), which can react with molecular oxygen to form superoxide anions. Other mitochondrial enzymes, such as monoamine oxidase and alpha-ketoglutarate dehydrogenase, also contribute to mROS production. mROS formed in mitochondria is quickly converted to hydrogen peroxide (H_2O_2) by the detoxifying enzyme superoxide dismutase (SOD). H_2O_2 diffuses through membranes and reacts with metal ions to form hydroxyl radicals. Hydroxyl radicals are highly reactive and damaging to cellular components. Excessive levels of mROS have been implicated in driving cell death responses, including apoptosis and pyroptosis. To counter these damaging effects, macrophages have antioxidant systems to remove intracellular mROS and reduce oxidative stress. Indeed, mitochondria and peroxisomes have robust antioxidant defenses, including enzymes like SOD, catalase, and glutathione peroxidase. Numerous studies have recently identified key signaling nodes between mROS and the GSDM family that mediate the induction of pyroptosis.

In addition to cell membrane pores, GSDMD also forms pores at the mitochondrial membrane. Following activation of GSDMD, the N-terminal pore-forming fragment relocalizes at the mitochondria. Here, it creates pores on the inner and outer mitochondrial membranes (OMMs), resulting in a loss of membrane potential and an increase in mROS release [117,118]. Importantly, mitochondrial pores are formed before plasma membrane damage and are dependent on binding to cardiolipin. Interestingly, deletion of cardiolipin synthase (Crls1) or scramblase (Plscr3) that transports cardiolipin to the OMM abrogated GSDMD pore formation. Thus GSDMD pores act as a conduit for metabolic DAMP release from the mitochondria. Additional studies have shown direct interactions between GSDMD and mROS. Indeed, mROS accumulation during pyroptosis can oxidize $Cys^{191/192}$ to promote GSDMD oligomerization and pore formation [119].

In line with these findings, a further three studies identify GSDMD-$Cys^{191/192}$ as a target of S-palmitoylation [94–96]. Remarkably, palmitoylation does not affect GSDMD caspase cleavage, and palmitoylation is enhanced by mROS release. Most strikingly, full-length GSDMD subjected to palmitoylation exhibits pore-forming activity. Mechanistically, the palmitoyl transferases ZDHHC5 and ZDHHC9 mediate GSDMD palmitoylation. ZDHHC5 and ZDHHC9 expressions are upregulated when macrophages are exposed to DAMPs and mROS [95] (see Fig. 4.5). Additionally, palmitoylation is not limited to GSDMD; all GSDM family members are sensitive to N-terminal palmitoylation. Thus GSDMD palmitoylation is a vital regulatory mechanism for controlling GSDMD membrane localization and activation, presenting a potential target for modulating cell death for the treatment of inflammatory diseases. Intriguingly, given that fumarate also targets $Cys^{191/192}$ to succinate and inactivate GSDMD, fumarate-mediated inhibition of GSDMD oligomerization may compete with the palmitoylation site to limit GSDMD activity. Further investigation of this interplay will be of great interest to the field.

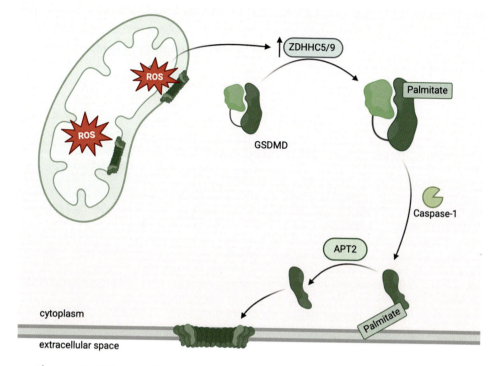

Figure 4.5: Priming of pyroptotic cell death by mROS-induced palmitoylation.
mROS produced in the mitochondria is released into the cytoplasm through GSDMD pores in both inner and outer mitochondrial membranes. mROS induces upregulation of ZDHHC5 and ZDHHC9 expression which mediate palmitoylation of GSDMD. Once palmitoylated, GSDMD can be cleaved by active caspase-1, and the N-terminal fragment can localize to the plasma membrane. APT2 catalyzes the removal of the palmitate from the fragment, and the monomers can oligomerize into membrane pores. Created with BioRender.com.

Summary and future directions

Macrophages have well-documented plasticity and can adjust their metabolic pathways based on their environment and intercellular signals. Their shifts in metabolic pathways were considered a passive process, but it is now established that the metabolic machinery and changes to macrophage metabolism following immune stimulation play a critical role in initiating transcriptional changes and programmed cell death pathways. In this chapter, we have described four different types of programmed cell death in macrophages: apoptosis, necroptosis, pyroptosis, and ferroptosis, and how accumulation of cellular metabolites can affect the trajectory of cell death. An emerging trend suggests that macrophages accumulate metabolites to engage with cell death executioner proteins and regulate their function. Indeed, functionally indispensable cysteine residues are frequently targeted by electrophilic metabolites to both activate and inactivate cell death. Given that specific metabolites target the same cystine residues, it will be of great interest to explore the interplay and pharmacology of how these modifications occur and their competition for occupying cysteine sites. In addition, these studies reveal that metabolic modification of cysteine residues can be leveraged therapeutically.

References

[1] Davies LC, et al. Tissue-resident macrophages. Nat Immunol 2013;14(10):986–95.
[2] Aderem A, Underhill DM. Mechanisms of phagocytosis in macrophages. Annu Rev Immunol 1999;17:593–623.
[3] Biswas SK, Mantovani A. Orchestration of metabolism by macrophages. Cell Metab 2012;15(4):432–7.
[4] Mills CD, et al. M-1/M-2 macrophages and the Th1/Th2 paradigm. J Immunol 2000;164(12):6166–73.
[5] Jha AK, et al. Network integration of parallel metabolic and transcriptional data reveals metabolic modules that regulate macrophage polarization. Immunity 2015;42(3):419–30.
[6] Zhu X, et al. Stimulating pyruvate dehydrogenase complex reduces itaconate levels and enhances TCA cycle anabolic bioenergetics in acutely inflamed monocytes. J Leukoc Biol 2020;107(3):467–84.
[7] Sefik E, et al. Inflammasome activation in infected macrophages drives COVID-19 pathology. Nature 2022;606(7914):585–93.
[8] Qiu B, et al. Fatal COVID-19 pulmonary disease involves ferroptosis. Nat Commun 2024;15(1):3816.
[9] Hage C, et al. Sorafenib induces pyroptosis in macrophages and triggers natural killer cell-mediated cytotoxicity against hepatocellular carcinoma. Hepatology 2019;70(4):1280–97.
[10] Okondo MC, et al. DPP8 and DPP9 inhibition induces pro-caspase-1-dependent monocyte and macrophage pyroptosis. Nat Chem Biol 2017;13(1):46–53.
[11] Gu Z, et al. Ferroptosis-strengthened metabolic and inflammatory regulation of tumor-associated macrophages provokes potent tumoricidal activities. Nano Lett 2021;21(15):6471–9.
[12] Hao X, et al. Inhibition of APOC1 promotes the transformation of M2 into M1 macrophages via the ferroptosis pathway and enhances anti-PD1 immunotherapy in hepatocellular carcinoma based on single-cell RNA sequencing. Redox Biol 2022;56:102463.
[13] Kerr JF, Wyllie AH, Currie AR. Apoptosis: a basic biological phenomenon with wide-ranging implications in tissue kinetics. Br J Cancer 1972;26(4):239–57.
[14] Zychlinsky A, Prevost MC, Sansonetti PJ. Shigella flexneri induces apoptosis in infected macrophages. Nature 1992;358(6382):167–9.
[15] Holler N, et al. Fas triggers an alternative, caspase-8-independent cell death pathway using the kinase RIP as effector molecule. Nat Immunol 2000;1(6):489–95.
[16] Li P, et al. Cytochrome c and dATP-dependent formation of Apaf-1/caspase-9 complex initiates an apoptotic protease cascade. Cell 1997;91(4):479–89.
[17] Hu Y, et al. Role of cytochrome c and dATP/ATP hydrolysis in Apaf-1-mediated caspase-9 activation and apoptosis. EMBO J 1999;18(13):3586–95.
[18] Cain K, et al. Apaf-1 oligomerizes into biologically active approximately 700-kDa and inactive approximately 1.4-MDa apoptosome complexes. J Biol Chem 2000;275(9):6067–70.
[19] Bratton SB, et al. Recruitment, activation and retention of caspases-9 and -3 by Apaf-1 apoptosome and associated XIAP complexes. EMBO J 2001;20(5):998–1009.
[20] Crawford ED, et al. The DegraBase: a database of proteolysis in healthy and apoptotic human cells. Mol Cell Proteomics 2013;12(3):813–24.
[21] Singh R, Letai A, Sarosiek K. Regulation of apoptosis in health and disease: the balancing act of BCL-2 family proteins. Nat Rev Mol Cell Biol 2019;20(3):175–93.
[22] Welz PS, et al. FADD prevents RIP3-mediated epithelial cell necrosis and chronic intestinal inflammation. Nature 2011;477(7364):330–4.

[23] Kearney CJ, et al. Necroptosis suppresses inflammation via termination of TNF- or LPS-induced cytokine and chemokine production. Cell Death Differ 2015;22(8):1313–27.

[24] Wang L, Du F, Wang X. TNF-alpha induces two distinct caspase-8 activation pathways. Cell 2008;133(4):693–703.

[25] Tran TM, et al. TNFalpha-induced macrophage death via caspase-dependent and independent pathways. Apoptosis 2009;14(3):320–32.

[26] Micheau O, Tschopp J. Induction of TNF receptor I-mediated apoptosis via two sequential signaling complexes. Cell 2003;114(2):181–90.

[27] Oberst A, et al. Catalytic activity of the caspase-8-FLIP(L) complex inhibits RIPK3-dependent necrosis. Nature 2011;471(7338):363–7.

[28] Orozco S, et al. RIPK1 both positively and negatively regulates RIPK3 oligomerization and necroptosis. Cell Death Differ 2014;21(10):1511–21.

[29] Wu XN, et al. Distinct roles of RIP1-RIP3 hetero- and RIP3-RIP3 homo-interaction in mediating necroptosis. Cell Death Differ 2014;21(11):1709–20.

[30] Sun L, et al. Mixed lineage kinase domain-like protein mediates necrosis signaling downstream of RIP3 kinase. Cell 2012;148(1-2):213–27.

[31] Dondelinger Y, et al. MLKL compromises plasma membrane integrity by binding to phosphatidylinositol phosphates. Cell Rep 2014;7(4):971–81.

[32] Cai Z, et al. Plasma membrane translocation of trimerized MLKL protein is required for TNF-induced necroptosis. Nat Cell Biol 2014;16(1):55–65.

[33] Wang H, et al. Mixed lineage kinase domain-like protein MLKL causes necrotic membrane disruption upon phosphorylation by RIP3. Mol Cell 2014;54(1):133–46.

[34] Chen X, et al. Translocation of mixed lineage kinase domain-like protein to plasma membrane leads to necrotic cell death. Cell Res 2014;24(1):105–21.

[35] He S, et al. Toll-like receptors activate programmed necrosis in macrophages through a receptor-interacting kinase-3-mediated pathway. Proc Natl Acad Sci U S A 2011;108(50):20054–9.

[36] Buchrieser J, et al. RIPK1 is a critical modulator of both tonic and TLR-responsive inflammatory and cell death pathways in human macrophage differentiation. Cell Death Dis 2018;9(10):973.

[37] Kaiser WJ, et al. Toll-like receptor 3-mediated necrosis via TRIF, RIP3, and MLKL. J Biol Chem 2013;288(43):31268–79.

[38] Ma Y, et al. *NF-kappaB protects macrophages from lipopolysaccharide-induced cell death: the role of caspase 8 and receptor-interacting protein.* J Biol Chem 2005;280(51):41827–34.

[39] McKenzie BA, Dixit VM, Power C. Fiery cell death: pyroptosis in the central nervous system. Trends in Neurosciences 2020;43(1):55–73.

[40] Lamkanfi M, Dixit VM. Inflammasomes and their roles in health and disease. Annual Review of Cell and Developmental Biology 2012;28(1):137–61.

[41] Rathinam VAK, Fitzgerald KA. Inflammasome complexes: emerging mechanisms and effector functions. Cell. 165(4): 792-800.

[42] Broz P, Pelegrín P, Shao F. The gasdermins, a protein family executing cell death and inflammation. Nat Rev Immunol 2019.

[43] Fink SL, Cookson BT. Caspase-1-dependent pore formation during pyroptosis leads to osmotic lysis of infected host macrophages. Cellular Microbiology 2006;8(11):1812–25.

[44] Kayagaki N, et al. Caspase-11 cleaves gasdermin D for non-canonical inflammasome signalling. Nature 2015;526:666.

[45] Liu X, et al. Inflammasome-activated gasdermin D causes pyroptosis by forming membrane pores. Nature 2016;535(7610):153–8.

[46] He Y, Hara H, Núñez G. Mechanism and regulation of NLRP3 inflammasome activation. Trends in Biochemical Sciences 2016;41(12):1012–21.

[47] Baker PJ, et al. NLRP3 inflammasome activation downstream of cytoplasmic LPS recognition by both caspase-4 and caspase-5. Eur J Immunol 2015;45(10):2918–26.

[48] Ahn BJ, et al. The N-terminal ectodomain of Ninjurin1 liberated by MMP9 has chemotactic activity. Biochem Biophys Res Commun 2012;428(4):438–44.
[49] Kayagaki N, et al. NINJ1 mediates plasma membrane rupture during lytic cell death. Nature 2021;591 (7848):131–6.
[50] Ahn BJ, et al. Ninjurin1 deficiency attenuates susceptibility of experimental autoimmune encephalomyelitis in mice. J Biol Chem 2014;289(6):3328–38.
[51] Degen M, et al. Structural basis of NINJ1-mediated plasma membrane rupture in cell death. Nature 2023;.
[52] Tan S, Schubert D, Maher P. Oxytosis: a novel form of programmed cell death. Curr Top Med Chem 2001;1(6):497–506.
[53] Dixon SJ, et al. Ferroptosis: an iron-dependent form of nonapoptotic cell death. Cell 2012;149(5):1060–72.
[54] Haber F, Weiss J. The catalytic decomposition of hydrogen peroxide by iron salts. Proc R Soc Lond - Math Phys Sci 1934;147(861):332–51.
[55] Walling C. Fenton's reagent revisited. Acc Chem Res 1975;8(4):125–31.
[56] Shah R, Shchepinov MS, Pratt DA. Resolving the role of lipoxygenases in the initiation and execution of ferroptosis. ACS Cent Sci 2018;4(3):387–96.
[57] Testa U, Pelosi E, Peschle C. The transferrin receptor. Crit Rev Oncog 1993;4(3):241–76.
[58] Feng H, et al. Transferrin receptor is a specific ferroptosis marker. Cell Rep 2020;30(10):3411–23 e7.
[59] Delaby C, et al. Subcellular localization of iron and heme metabolism related proteins at early stages of erythrophagocytosis. PLoS One 2012;7(7):e42199.
[60] White C, et al. HRG1 is essential for heme transport from the phagolysosome of macrophages during erythrophagocytosis. Cell Metab 2013;17(2):261–70.
[61] Simmons WR, et al. Normal iron homeostasis requires the transporter SLC48A1 for efficient heme-iron recycling in mammals. Front Genome Ed 2020;2:8.
[62] Campbell MR, et al. Novel hematopoietic target genes in the NRF2-mediated transcriptional pathway. Oxid Med Cell Longev 2013;120305 2013.
[63] Ursini F, et al. Purification from pig liver of a protein which protects liposomes and biomembranes from peroxidative degradation and exhibits glutathione peroxidase activity on phosphatidylcholine hydroperoxides. Biochim Biophys Acta 1982;710(2):197–211.
[64] Yang WS, et al. Regulation of ferroptotic cancer cell death by GPX4. Cell 2014;156(1-2):317–31.
[65] Ran Q, et al. Transgenic mice overexpressing glutathione peroxidase 4 are protected against oxidative stress-induced apoptosis. J Biol Chem 2004;279(53):55137–46.
[66] Esworthy RS, et al. Cloning and sequencing of the cDNA encoding a human testis phospholipid hydroperoxide glutathione peroxidase. Gene 1994;144(2):317–18.
[67] Bannai S. Exchange of cystine and glutamate across plasma membrane of human fibroblasts. J Biol Chem 1986;261(5):2256–63.
[68] Lee H, et al. Energy-stress-mediated AMPK activation inhibits ferroptosis. Nat Cell Biol 2020;22 (2):225–34.
[69] Dolma S, et al. Identification of genotype-selective antitumor agents using synthetic lethal chemical screening in engineered human tumor cells. Cancer Cell 2003;3(3):285–96.
[70] Chu B, et al. ALOX12 is required for p53-mediated tumour suppression through a distinct ferroptosis pathway. Nat Cell Biol 2019;21(5):579–91.
[71] Jiang X, Stockwell BR, Conrad M. Ferroptosis: mechanisms, biology and role in disease. Nat Rev Mol Cell Biol 2021;22(4):266–82.
[72] Lee JE, et al. H3K4 mono- and di-methyltransferase MLL4 is required for enhancer activation during cell differentiation. Elife 2013;2:e01503.
[73] Egolf S, et al. MLL4 mediates differentiation and tumor suppression through ferroptosis. Sci Adv 2021;7 (50):eabj9141.
[74] Warburg O. The metabolism of carcinoma cells. J Cancer Res 1925;9(1):148–63.
[75] Mills EL, et al. Succinate dehydrogenase supports metabolic repurposing of mitochondria to drive inflammatory macrophages. Cell 2016;167(2):457–70 e13.

[76] Bailey JD, et al. Nitric oxide modulates metabolic remodeling in inflammatory macrophages through TCA cycle regulation and itaconate accumulation. Cell Rep 2019;28(1):218–30 e7.
[77] Cheng SC, et al. mTOR- and HIF-1alpha-mediated aerobic glycolysis as metabolic basis for trained immunity. Science 2014;345(6204):1250684.
[78] Tannahill GM, et al. Succinate is an inflammatory signal that induces IL-1beta through HIF-1alpha. Nature 2013;496(7444):238–42.
[79] Michelucci A, et al. Immune-responsive gene 1 protein links metabolism to immunity by catalyzing itaconic acid production. Proc Natl Acad Sci U S A 2013;110(19):7820–5.
[80] Lee CG, et al. Cloning and analysis of gene regulation of a novel LPS-inducible cDNA. Immunogenetics 1995;41(5):263–70.
[81] Mills EL, et al. Itaconate is an anti-inflammatory metabolite that activates Nrf2 via alkylation of KEAP1. Nature 2018;556(7699):113–17.
[82] Bambouskova M, et al. Electrophilic properties of itaconate and derivatives regulate the IkappaBzeta-ATF3 inflammatory axis. Nature 2018;556(7702):501–4.
[83] Frezza C, et al. Haem oxygenase is synthetically lethal with the tumour suppressor fumarate hydratase. Nature 2011;477(7363):225–8.
[84] Yang M, et al. The succinated proteome of FH-mutant tumours. Metabolites 2014;4(3):640–54.
[85] Hooftman A, et al. Macrophage fumarate hydratase restrains mtRNA-mediated interferon production. Nature 2023.
[86] Hooftman A, et al. The immunomodulatory metabolite itaconate modifies NLRP3 and inhibits inflammasome activation. Cell Metab 2020;32(3):468–78 e7.
[87] Zecchini V, et al. Fumarate induces vesicular release of mtDNA to drive innate immunity. Nature 2023;615(7952):499–506.
[88] Grover SP, Mackman N. Tissue factor: an essential mediator of hemostasis and trigger of thrombosis. Arterioscler Thromb Vasc Biol 2018;38(4):709–25.
[89] Ryan TAJ, Preston RJS, O'Neill LAJ. Immunothrombosis and the molecular control of tissue factor by pyroptosis: prospects for new anticoagulants. Biochem J 2022;479(6):731–50.
[90] Ryan TAJ, et al. Dimethyl fumarate and 4-octyl itaconate are anticoagulants that suppress Tissue Factor in macrophages via inhibition of Type I Interferon. Nat Commun 2023;14(1):3513.
[91] Liu D, et al. Discovery of itaconate-mediated lysine acylation. J Am Chem Soc 2023;145(23):12673–81.
[92] Zhang D, et al. Metabolic regulation of gene expression by histone lactylation. Nature 2019;574(7779):575–80.
[93] Humphries F, et al. Succination inactivates gasdermin D and blocks pyroptosis. Science 2020;369(6511):1633–7.
[94] Balasubramanian A, et al. The palmitoylation of gasdermin D directs its membrane translocation and pore formation during pyroptosis. Sci Immunol 2024;9(94):eadn1452.
[95] Du G, et al. ROS-dependent S-palmitoylation activates cleaved and intact gasdermin D. Nature 2024;.
[96] Zhang N, et al. A palmitoylation-depalmitoylation relay spatiotemporally controls GSDMD activation in pyroptosis. Nat Cell Biol 2024;26(5):757–69.
[97] Blatnik M, et al. Inactivation of glyceraldehyde-3-phosphate dehydrogenase by fumarate in diabetes. Formation of S-(2-Succinyl)Cysteine, a Novel Chemical Modification of Protein and Possible Biomarker of Mitochondrial Stress 2008;57(1):41–9.
[98] Kato M, Sakai K, Endo A. Koningic acid (heptelidic acid) inhibition of glyceraldehyde-3-phosphate dehydrogenases from various sources. Biochim Biophys Acta 1992;1120(1):113–16.
[99] Zhang C, et al. Hereditary leiomyomatosis and renal cell cancer: recent insights into mechanisms and systemic treatment. Front Oncol 2021;11.
[100] Ashrafian H, et al. Fumarate is cardioprotective via activation of the Nrf2 antioxidant pathway. Cell Metabolism 2012;15(3):361–71.
[101] Zecchini V, et al. Fumarate induces vesicular release of mtDNA to drive innate immunity. Nature 2023;.

[102] Kornberg MD, et al. Dimethyl fumarate targets GAPDH and aerobic glycolysis to modulate immunity. Science 2018;360(6387):449–53.

[103] Hu H, et al. Dimethyl fumarate covalently modifies Cys673 of NLRP3 to exert anti-inflammatory effects. iScience 2024;27(4):109544.

[104] Schroeder A, et al. Targeting Thioredoxin-1 by dimethyl fumarate induces ripoptosome-mediated cell death. Sci Rep 2017;7:43168.

[105] Hayashi T, Ueno Y, Okamoto T. Oxidoreductive regulation of nuclear factor kappa B. Involvement of a cellular reducing catalyst thioredoxin. J Biol Chem 1993;268(15):11380–8.

[106] Micheau O, et al. NF-kappaB signals induce the expression of c-FLIP. Mol Cell Biol 2001;21(16):5299–305.

[107] Xie X, et al. Dimethyl fumarate induces necroptosis in colon cancer cells through GSH depletion/ROS increase/MAPKs activation pathway. Br J Pharmacol 2015;172(15):3929–43.

[108] Bambouskova M, et al. Itaconate confers tolerance to late NLRP3 inflammasome activation. Cell Rep 2021;34(10):108756.

[109] He Y, et al. NEK7 is an essential mediator of NLRP3 activation downstream of potassium efflux. Nature 2016;530(7590):354–7.

[110] Aksentijevich I, et al. The clinical continuum of cryopyrinopathies: novel CIAS1 mutations in North American patients and a new cryopyrin model. Arthritis Rheum 2007;56(4):1273–85.

[111] Booshehri LM, Hoffman HM. CAPS and NLRP3. J Clin Immunol 2019;39(3):277–86.

[112] Agostini L, et al. NALP3 forms an IL-1beta-processing inflammasome with increased activity in Muckle-Wells autoinflammatory disorder. Immunity 2004;20(3):319–25.

[113] Gross CJ, et al. K(+) efflux-independent NLRP3 inflammasome activation by small molecules targeting mitochondria. Immunity 2016;45(4):761–73.

[114] Martinon F, Burns K, Tschopp J. The inflammasome: a molecular platform triggering activation of inflammatory caspases and processing of proIL-beta. Mol Cell 2002;10(2):417–26.

[115] Sharif H, et al. Structural mechanism for NEK7-licensed activation of NLRP3 inflammasome. Nature 2019;570(7761):338–43.

[116] Kelley N, et al. The NLRP3 inflammasome: an overview of mechanisms of activation and regulation. Int J Mol Sci 2019;20(13).

[117] Weindel CG, et al. Mitochondrial ROS promotes susceptibility to infection via gasdermin D-mediated necroptosis. Cell 2022;185(17):3214–31 e23.

[118] Miao R, et al. Gasdermin D permeabilization of mitochondrial inner and outer membranes accelerates and enhances pyroptosis. Immunity 2023;56(11):2523–41 e8.

[119] Devant P, et al. Gasdermin D pore-forming activity is redox-sensitive. Cell Rep 2023;42(1):112008.

CHAPTER 5

Computational modeling of metabolism in oncology

Linda Fong[1], Meng Jin[1], Samir Kharbanda[1], Marc Creixell[1], Xiumin Wu[2], David Zhang[3], Juan Dubrot[4], Kathleen Yates[5], Robert Manguso[5], Benjamin Kauffman-Malaga[2], Sean Hackett[1] and Jonathan Powell[1]

[1]Calico Life Sciences, LLC, South San Francisco, CA, United States, [2]CA, United States, [3]Yale University, New Haven, CT, United States, [4]Clinica Universidad do Navarra, Madrid, Spain, [5]Broad Institute of MIT & Harvard, Cambridge, MA, United States

Introduction

Metabolism as a therapeutic avenue in oncology

Metabolic dysregulation is a critical and well-documented driver of cancer malignancy. Early observations that tumor cells could exploit glycolysis to fuel rapid cell division, known as the Warburg effect, have since motivated investigation into whether targeting metabolic dependencies might offer therapeutic benefit [1–3]. The exquisite flexibility of tumor cells to reprogram their metabolism has led to an explosion of biochemical and computational technologies aimed at profiling this molecular phenotype. Metabolomics and fluxomics have redefined our capabilities to measure biochemical difference (Box 5.1), while advances in single-cell measurements have revolutionized our understanding of tumor heterogeneity with unprecedented resolution. With the development of new technologies, efforts to generate metabolic resources for target discovery are on the rise; databases encompassing tumor cell line profiles [4] and unified genome-scale models [5] are now publicly available. This growing collection of data has made evident the central role that metabolism plays in integrating epigenomic, genomic, transcriptomic, proteomic, and extracellular/intercellular signals across vastly heterogeneous tumor, immune, and stromal cells to shape the tumor microenvironment [6]. We describe in this chapter how the characterization of metabolic networks, both experimentally and computationally, has been important for uncovering novel drug targets as well as elucidating the metabolic properties that govern therapeutic response [7].

> **BOX 5.1 Metabolome profiling strategies**
>
> As described previously [112,113], metabolome profiling aims to capture a comprehensive picture and can be performed in an untargeted or targeted fashion. In untargeted metabolomics, an unbiased approach provides the relative quantification of metabolites as measured by mass spectrometry. However, sample preparation, fragmentation, and downstream metabolite identification using available databases can deeply influence the metabolites recovered in each experiment. In contrast, targeted metabolomics rely on native and isotopically labeled analytes to more accurately quantify metabolites and enhance sensitivity. The opportunity to trace a labeled isotope through multiple substrates consequently enables researchers to compute flux based on uptake and secretion rates. Yet, targeted strategies often offer only partial coverage of the metabolome and therefore increase the chance of data misinterpretation. Although these techniques have been foundational in establishing our current understanding of cancer metabolism, they remain restricted to bulk-level measurements and therefore limited in their ability to uncover shifts in metabolite pathway utilization and to inform network analyses at the resolution of single cells.

Uncovering potential targets: altered metabolic programs in cancer cells

Considered to be a hallmark of tumorigenesis, oncogenic transformation requires the activation and reprogramming of key metabolic pathways to support cell growth and proliferation [8]. Downstream of receptor tyrosine kinases, oncogene-driven RAS, PI3K, MYC, and mTOR signaling have been consequently linked to alterations in glycolysis, TCA cycle, glutamine metabolism, fatty acid metabolism, and nucleotide synthesis [9–13]. Targeting differential demands on broadly utilized pathways, however, has been limited by small therapeutic windows due to off- and on-target effects on nonmalignant rapidly proliferating cells [14]. Given this, there has been deep interest in understanding selective metabolic vulnerabilities conferred by specific mutations. For example, in KEAP1-mutant lung adenocarcinoma, the constitutive induction of NRF2 signaling resulted in a selective dependency on increased glutaminolysis, which could be therapeutically exploited via glutaminase inhibition [15]. Perhaps the most notable success has been found in IDH1/2 mutant cancers, where targeted inhibition reduces the production of 2-hydroxyglutarate to enable differentiation in AML and to decrease stemness in glioma for clinical benefit [16,17].

In conjunction with these mutation-focused approaches, unbiased CRISPR screens have been implemented across a wide array of tumor models to identify metabolic vulnerabilities. Screens designed to examine the role of nutrient availability compared human plasma-like media (HPLM) conditions to high-glucose RPMI/DMEM conditions, uncovering cell-specific medium essential genes such as GPT2 and GLS [18]. In pancreatic cancer, CRISPR screens comparing in vitro and in vivo dependencies found most essential genes to be consistent, with two in vivo exceptions: heme synthesis limited tumor growth, while autophagic pathways were found to protect tumor cells from TNF-induced cell death [19]. In colorectal cancer, loss of CHSY1 led to succinate-mediated activation of PI3K/AKT/HIF1A, CD8 + T cell exhaustion, and PD-L1 upregulation [20]. Beyond libraries of metabolic genes, screens designed to search for tumor suppressor genes via proliferation have identified glycerolipid biosynthesis to be required for biomass generation in tumor cells [21].

CRISPR screens have also been used to expand our understanding of KEAP1-related metabolic changes. Zhao et al. performed combinatorial CRISPR-Cas9 screens to functionally evaluate a set of 51 genes and map differences in metabolic network topology [22]. The authors revealed that the KEAP1 mutation alters the relative importance of oxidative pentose phosphate pathway by modulating the redox gene expression as well as driving GSH synthesis and regeneration [22]. Larger scale drug-based modifier screens, comprising ~30,000 sgRNAs targeting ~3000 genes showed consistently altered GSH metabolism and further demonstrated that NADPH depletion by ATM inhibition drastically impaired the survival of KEAP1-deficient cells [23]. Taken together, the implementation of unbiased CRISPR screening has rapidly expanded our understanding of metabolic networks and unearthed tumor cell vulnerabilities that may serve as potential drug targets.

Emerging importance of metabolites as signals for immune cells and stromal cells

While targeting tumor cell metabolism may serve as a direct therapeutic strategy, we must also consider that tumor cells do not exist in isolation. The composition of the tumor microenvironment, often comprising diverse cell types, drastically influences the availability of nutrients, metabolites, and other factors that may constrain cellular function. Stealing key metabolites, such as glutamine, triple-negative breast cancer cells deprive tumor-infiltrating lymphocytes of much-needed amino acids, thereby impairing antitumor responses [24]. Nutrient partitioning between hubs of competing and cooperating cells, particularly within the harsh conditions of poorly vascularized tumors, can result in both spatial and functional heterogeneity to support the proliferation, evasion, and progression of disease [25,26]. Moreover, tumor cells not only affect the metabolism of neighboring cells by depleting levels of glucose, glutamine, and amino acids, and they also directly produce metabolites and high levels of lactic acid that dampen immune function, which has been shown on multiple occasions to restrict antitumor responses and adaptive T cell function [27–29]. This was recently demonstrated by Notarangelo et al. wherein the accumulation of D-2-hydroxyglutarate, produced by IDH1 mutant tumors, interacted directly with T cell lactate dehydrogenase, resulting in inhibited proliferation, cytokine production, and cytolytic function [30]. Thus it is necessary to understand how the myriad of cell types present in the tumor microenvironment interacts with and contributes to the overall metabolic profile. Most importantly, when developing therapeutic strategies, we must distinguish whether potential targets can sufficiently restrict tumor growth without impairing immune function within the tumor microenvironment.

To understand how metabolic activity can be exploited for productive versus nonproductive responses, we must first consider how different immune subsets utilize metabolites for context-dependent adaptation to support their differentiation and function. In many cases, perturbation-based screening efforts have been able to rapidly uncover several components essential for integrating nutrient signaling to activate immune cells.

CD8 T cells

T cells display tremendous flexibility in their ability to coopt bioenergetic pathways. As critical responders to both infection and cancer, they must fuel activation and differentiation programs following antigen stimulation. CD8 T cells are capable of consuming conventional fuels such as glucose and glutamine but can turn to other physiologic carbon sources to generate mitochondrial ATP when necessary. One such example of context-dependent utilization is lactate. Though tumor-derived lactate has been noted to drive immunosuppression by reducing anaplerosis via a succinate shunt [31], recent work has also shown that lactate can be preferentially oxidized, even in the presence of glucose, by CD8 T effector cells to drive T cell viability and IFNγ production [32]. Glutamate abundance has similarly been associated with improved CD8 T cell activation following αPD-1 therapy, with glutaminase inhibition significantly limiting activation and clonal T cell expansion [33]. Even alternative substrates, such as inosine, are capable of supporting T cell growth and function in the absence of glucose—by relieving tumor-imposed metabolic restrictions, inosine supplementation can be converted into central carbon metabolism precursors and consequently drive antitumor efficacy following immune checkpoint blockade [34]. Leone et al. found acetate could be utilized as a carbon source for the TCA cycle in the setting of glutamine blockade, through the upregulation of acyl-CoA synthetases ACSS1 and ACSS2 [35]. It is not only central carbon metabolism that drives T cell immunity, however, as alterations in methionine metabolism in T cells have been shown to reduce histone methylation and STAT5 expression, thereby limiting functional T cell signatures in colon cancer [36]. Similarly, serine deprivation diminishes the expansion of T cells in vivo, as the nonessential amino acid supplies components necessary for de novo nucleotide biosynthesis during proliferation [37]. Lastly, hypoxia has been shown to impair the mitochondrial dynamics of CD8 T cells and impede the proliferative capacity, function, and infiltration in multiple cancers [38–40]. These observations point to several metabolic programs that could be tuned or exploited to alter T cell function and, furthermore, suggest that systematic searches to characterize how nutrient competition can most effectively be addressed to aid in immune function would offer tremendous utility.

Toward that end, many CRISPR screens have uncovered metabolic factors that play a role in T cell function and fate. Between effector and memory T cell states, transporters Slc7a1 and Slc38a2 modulated mTOR signaling to promote an effector-like phenotype [41]. In the search for metabolic strategies that enabled homing to tissues and solid tumors, CRISPR screens revealed a reliance on nonsteroidal products of the mevalonate-cholesterol pathway, such as coenzyme Q, to drive induction of the transcription factor SREBP2 and enable tissue-resident T memory formation [42]. In the realm of adoptive cell therapy, genome-scale gain-of-function screens have also identified proline metabolism, particularly PRODH2 overexpression, as a target for enhancing CAR-T efficacy [43]. Importantly, the recent development of screening platforms designed to interrogate naïve and differentiated immune biology with greater editing penetrance, such as the X-CHIME series (combinatorial C-CHIME, inducible I-CHIME, lineage-based L-CHIME, and sequentially S-CHIME), will soon be able to more faithfully uncover in vivo metabolic dependencies [44].

CD4 T cells

The differentiation of CD4 T cell populations into effector or regulatory subsets is critical for providing help in the context of the antitumor response. While cytokines and transcription factors promoting Th1, Th2, and Th17 have been well-elucidated, literature characterizing the role of metabolic pathways—nutrients, growth factors, local oxygen levels, coactivation receptors, and metabolites—which are essential for differentiation and function is still emerging. Activation of CD4 cells into helper subsets is typically fueled by glycolytic metabolism and mTOR regulation. Consistent with this, metformin was shown to activate AMPK, reducing glycolysis in CD4 T cells and enhancing lipid oxidation by inhibiting the expression of mTOR, thus interfering with the differentiation and effector function of CD4 T cells [45,46]. Insufficiency of the glycolytic metabolite phosphoenolpyruvate (PEP), which is rate-limited by the enzyme *Enolase 1*, has also been shown to limit Ca^{2+}-NFAT-mediated T cell activation [28,47]. Not surprisingly, methionine has proven to be key nutrient in shaping epigenetic reprogramming of CD4 cells as well. Rapidly imported following activation of CD4 T helper (Th) cells, methionine was required to maintain S-adenosyl-methionine pools for histone H3K4 methylation and subsequent gene induction [48]. L-Arginine, another amino acid known to fuel CD4 T cells, has been shown to support viability and proliferation under nutrient-limiting conditions and can be obtained by CD4 populations following transfer from antigen-presenting cells [49]. Similar to CD8 findings, glutaminase (GLS) can drive differentiation toward Th1 phenotypes, increasing Tbet expression and altering chromatin accessibility to limit functions associated with Th17 cells.

In the tumor microenvironment, however, glucose is often depleted thereby inhibiting the differentiation of naïve CD4 T cells into pro-inflammatory effector phenotypes like Th1 and Th17. Short-chain fatty acids such as acetate (C2), propionate (C3), and butyrate (C4) have been shown to restrain CD4 T cell activation and the accumulation of memory T cells following CTLA-4 therapy [50]. As we look for therapeutic approaches to overcome newly defined CD4-mediated resistance and to drive CD4 effector functions and memory responses, CRISPR screens have yet again emerged as a valuable tool. Genome-wide CRISPR screens in Th2 cells have identified *PPARG* and *ABCD3*, two metabolic genes expressed in the peroxisome that regulate fatty acid uptake and glucose storage, as hits that enable effector transcription factor binding patterns, activation, and consequent differentiation [51]. In vivo screens in CD4 T cells found Socs1 to be an intrinsic checkpoint of Th1 differentiation; Socs1 deletion led to CD4 proliferation and the induction of metabolic genes, including the insulin growth factor regulator *HTRA1* and the metabolic checkpoint *NUAK1* thought to support the proliferative phenotype [52]. Screens identifying essential regulators CD4 T migration found the transcription factor Foxo1, a Myc-dependent metabolic regulator as a top-ranked hit [53,54]. It is evident from these series of CRISPR screens that the approach of engaging CD4-mediated help in the tumor environment may be an effective way to promote therapeutic responses in cancer treatment.

Regulatory T cells (T_{regs})

T regulatory cells can adapt to high lactate environments by suppressing glycolysis and enhancing oxidative phosphorylation through the expression of Foxp3 [55]. This reprogramming provides a metabolic advantage to these cells so that they can promote peripheral tolerance. In contrast to effector T cells, which utilize glycolytic and glutaminolytic pathways to support their survival, Foxp3 + T_{regs} and memory T cells rely on lipid oxidation [56,57]. Glutathione metabolism has also been shown to play a critical role in controlling ROS production in T_{regs} and restricting serine metabolism to enable the suppressive capacity of these cells. Loss of glutamate cysteine ligase (*Gclc*) led to enhanced antitumor responses and severe autoimmunity, through mechanisms such as restored serine metabolism, mTOR activation, and Foxp3 downregulation [58].

It is clear that systematically understanding the role of Foxp3, as a master regulator of the regulatory phenotype, would facilitate therapeutic approaches aimed at reprogramming T_{regs}. To ask this question, Cortez et al. developed a CRISPR-based pooled screening platform to interrogate 500 nuclear factors in primary mouse T_{regs} to identify gene regulatory networks that promoted or disrupted Foxp3 [59]. USP22 was found to be a positive regulator that stabilized Foxp3 expression, while Rnf20 was found to be a negative regulator, which when ablated, could rescue USP22 deficiency [59]. The BRD9-containing ncBAF complex was also found to be a regulator of Foxp3 in genome-wide CRISPR screens performed in primary mouse T_{regs}, with BRD9 loss enhancing antitumor immunity in the MC38 colorectal model [60]. Intriguingly, additional work has been done to determine whether tumor-infiltrating T_{regs} differ from peripheral T_{regs} and whether targeted master regulators of the former would serve as attractive immune-oncology targets. CRISPR-Cas9 screens performed in vivo using a chimeric hematopoietic stem cell transplant model found that *TRPS1* targeting inhibited tumor T_{reg} infiltration without depleting peripheral T_{regs} or inhibiting CD4 T conventional cells and provided cures in more than 50% of MCA205 fibrosarcoma tumors [61]. While early efforts in eliminating T$_{regs}$ often created unwanted autoimmune side effects, identifying preferential and selective regulators of the regulatory phenotype may be promising for future drug development efforts.

Natural killer cells

Natural killer (NK) cells and innate-like lymphocytes also have the potential to elicit highly potent antitumor activity, and novel checkpoint inhibitors against NKG2A are in development [62]. We can similarly rationalize that enhancing the cytolytic function of these innate defenders metabolically would drive immunotherapy response or even protect against oncogenesis. Many studies have shown that driving effector function in NK cells requires similar glycolytic pathway activation as in T cells [63,64]. NK cells increase glycolytic enzyme expression, glucose uptake, and flux through glycolysis to maintain an activated state [65], and if inhibited, interferon gamma production by the NK cell is impaired [66]. Different from other lymphocytes, however, NK cells are acutely regulated by amino acids, which control cMYC protein levels [67]. In unbiased efforts to identify drivers of NK function, CRISPR screens have identified that calcium regulators, such as *CALHM2*, impacted both in vitro and in vivo efficacy when perturbed in CAR-engineered NK [68,69]. Ongoing work examining oncometabolites, such as sodium succinate, has revealed that these environmental triggers negatively impact NK function and IFN-γ levels [70].

Tumor-associated macrophages and myeloid-derived suppressor cells

Tumor-associated macrophages (TAMs) and myeloid-derived suppressor cells (MDSCs) are commonly understood to mediate suppressive effects by consuming and releasing metabolites within the tumor microenvironment. The plasticity of MDSCs allows them to undergo metabolic reprogramming from glycolysis to fatty acid oxidation, particularly when lipid accumulation occurs in the tumor microenvironment [71]. MDSC development is also influenced by Notch-mediated lactate metabolism, promoting differentiation into a suppressive state rather than into mature macrophages [72]. Importantly, it has been shown that inhibiting glutamine metabolism in MDSCs can convert them to an inflammatory phenotype [73], reinforcing the concept that employing metabolic therapies may be beneficial in refractory cancer settings.

More recently, the role of these cells in manipulating metabolites for tumor resistance has come to light. Taken up by pancreatic cancer cells, TAMs released deoxycytidine which can mediate chemoresistance to gemcitabine via molecular competition. Validated in GEMMs, depletion of TAMs sensitized PDAC tumors to gemcitabine, while patients with low macrophage burden exhibit better response rates to gemcitabine treatment. Similarly, MDSCs were shown to secrete the metabolite dicarbonyl methylglyoxal, which, when transferred to T cells, paralyzed effector function [74]. Blocking mitochondrial complex I activity reversed the negative effect of this metabolite [74]. Targeting the immunosuppressive effects of myeloid cells has largely emerged in the form of cell-directed therapies, for example, *CSF1R* and *CD47* inhibiting or depleting biologics. However, these approaches have been tried with little to no success.

CRISPR screens have not only become a tool for identifying alternative approaches for remodeling and reprogramming myeloid cells but also generating resources of macrophage biology. In a pool-based metabolic CRISPR screen, *KEAP1* and *ACOD1* were found to be strong regulators of the pro-inflammatory myeloid state. ACOD1 depletion reduced levels of the immune-metabolite itaconate, which in turn allowed KEAP1 to sequester NRF2 from the nucleus and restrict its ability to induce an antiinflammatory program [75]. Other pooled screens have revealed that METTL3 serves as a positive regulator of the innate macrophage response and activation of TNFα by mediating RNA metabolism, and loss of METTL3 promoted TAM reprogramming and MC38 tumor growth in vivo [76]. Deeper investigation into whether genetic perturbations remodel the overall metabolite profile of the tumor microenvironment to promote TAM or MDSC activation will be needed.

While we continue to expand our understanding of tumor immunity [77], it is important to acknowledge the relevance of other tissue-resident stromal cells, such as fibroblasts, endothelial cells, and mesenchymal cells. The susceptibility of these cells to metabolite imbalances in the TME will vary from that of tumor cells, as different cell lineages express varying levels of salvage enzymes and solute transporters. In particular, it will be necessary to characterize how cancer-associated fibroblasts, a population of cells which can drive TME remodeling, oncogenesis, and resistance, mediate tissue-level metabolite availability to fuel tumor cell growth. For example, CAF-derived nucleosides have been shown to induce glucose consumption and a dependence on MYC, enabling PDAC tumor growth [78]. Insights into these mechanisms can lead to potential therapeutic targets.

It is to be expected that these cell−cell communication networks occur in both direct and indirect fashion—through receptor-ligand interactions as well as through cytokine or metabolite signaling. For this reason, many groups have sought to profile the tumor interstitial fluid (TIF) as a way of understanding this intermediary step. As mentioned previously, high levels of adenosine nucleosides present in the TIF facilitate immunosuppression. While tumor cells may be sensitive to dNTP imbalances and altered amino acid levels in the TIF, T cells are also impacted by alterations in intracellular uptake of adenosine and its ability to lead to DNA replication stress. For this reason, A2AR reinvigoration through the development of selective antagonists for A2A and A2B receptors is in development for enhancing immunotherapy as well as improving adoptive cell therapy [79]. Other potential targets were identified by Shifrut et al., who adapted their sgRNA lentiviral infection with Cas9 electroporation approach to identify genes that would render T cells resistant to adenosine-driven immunosuppression. In the presence of an adenosine receptor 2 (A2A) agonist (CGS-21680), loss of *ADORA2A* and *FAM105A* overcame adenosine suppression, driving proliferation and continued cytolytic function [80].

The functional role of metabolites following import or export from the TIF remains to be understood. Not to be overlooked, metabolic reprogramming can fuel epigenetic remodeling, enabling the addition or removal of histone marks to alter chromatin accessibility. Metabolite availability drives the epigenetic state of the cell by serving as signaling molecules or posttranslational modifications on DNA, thereby regulating gene expression, transcription, and translation. In fact, it has been shown that the uptake and consequent conversion of metabolites into palmitate and acetyl-CoA not only impact central carbon metabolism but also regulate the epigenome by priming cells for differentiation, cytokine production, and even survival in the tumor microenvironment [81,82]. Additionally, TCA metabolites such as α-ketoglutarate (αKG) are required for histone demethylase activity and can be inhibited by succinate, fumarate, or 2-hydroxyglutarate (2HG), demonstrating that distinct metabolic pathways regulate the abundance of metabolites and the flux of reactions required to maintain or reprogram the epigenome [83]. These efforts to elucidate the channels of continuous feedback between metabolite availability and intracellular metabolic enzymes, as sensors of ATP generation and the energetic state of the cell, may reveal impactful epigenetic modulators. We can then exploit these multicompartment metabolic networks to subsequently drive epigenetic remodeling and downstream effector programs, to improve immune cell function and promote therapeutic response, or to prevent lineage transitions that mediate tumor resistance.

Thus it is evident that advances in optimizing the metabolic state of key cytolytic immune cells and harnessing effector functions for tumor clearance present another direct avenue for drug discovery.

Computational models help provide a comprehensive and unifying picture

Much of the current metabolic understanding described above comes from reductionist biology approaches. CRISPR screens move our understanding in the direction of systems biology, but it may be necessary to consider that the entirety of the metabolic system is more than the sum of its parts. To this end, we turn to recent developments in computational models and linear programming representations that can capture and help elucidate metabolic programs and potential vulnerabilities of the tumor microenvironment.

In their simplest form, metabolic programs that support tumor growth can be viewed as a series of chemical reactions that dictate the molecular state. Through mathematical modeling at the genome-scale, we can computationally identify metabolites that serve as essential signaling molecules and metabolic enzymes that dictate cellular function in key cell types [5]. Computational metabolic analyses may also offer insight into cell–cell metabolite exchange, drug-resistance of tumor cells in certain tissue contexts, and even drug-based on-target effects versus side effects. Moreover, constraint-based metabolic models comprise the most widely used systems biology framework for interrogating metabolic states and can serve as helpful

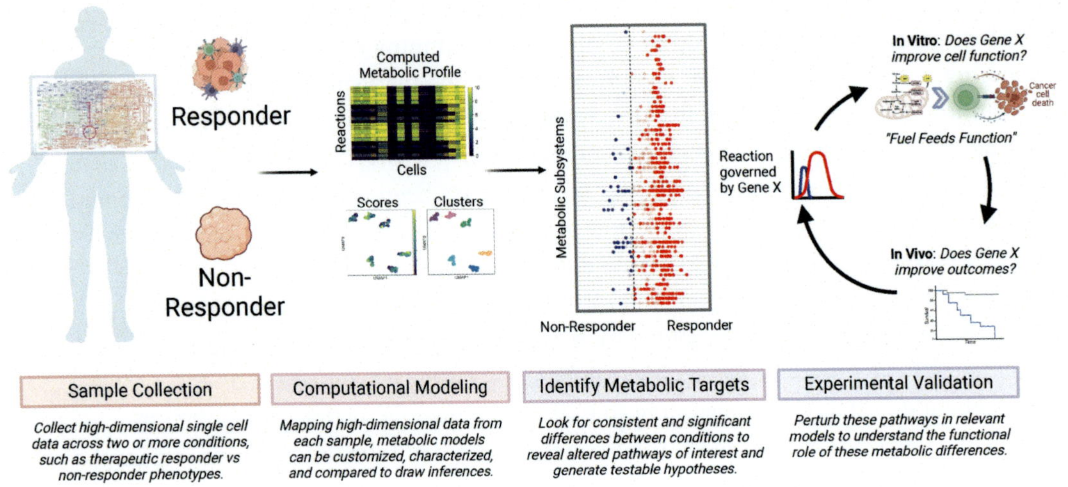

Figure 5.1: A framework for utilizing genome-scale metabolic models to identify metabolic programs that drive therapeutic response.
The comparison of responder versus nonresponder metabolic profiles can reveal bottlenecks and pathway remodeling upon treatment. The use of recently developed computational algorithms lends insight into metabolic differences at the single-cell level, which currently cannot be measured with traditional metabolomics approaches. Targeting differential pathways revealed by these analyses can generate testable hypotheses which, following in vitro and in vivo experimental validation, may lead to new therapeutic opportunities.

tools to computationally predict targetable reactions, metabolites, and enzymes that may perform well as metabolic therapies.

As we dive into the advancements and applications of genome-scale metabolic models, we will provide a framework of how scientists might leverage high-dimensional data to computationally derive metabolic profiles for single cells (Fig. 5.1), particularly in therapeutic settings where metabolic profiles may be difficult to obtain. Lastly, we highlight how the application of bulk- and single-cell computational algorithms has begun to uncover metabolic targets for drug discovery in the difficult-to-treat cancers. We conclude that we must harness the upcoming era of big data to improve our metabolic inferences and enable the study of which metabolites or enzymes govern key reactions in cancer and tumor immunity.

Development of genome-scale metabolic models and applications of constraint-based modeling in oncology

Constraint-based modeling utilizes genome-scale metabolic models

Constraint-based modeling and flux balance analysis aim to predict complete cellular reaction activities from large-scale gene expression and reaction stoichiometry information encoded in genome-scale metabolic models (GEMs) [84,85]. Under quasisteady state assumptions, metabolites within the system remain mass balanced, and reaction flux distributions can be solved by linear programming to optimize an objective function such as growth rate, biomass, or ATP production. Because we attribute biological importance to these objective functions, we can use these models to describe cellular behaviors. Additionally, we can incorporate prior knowledge of the system into these GEMs—stoichiometric, thermodynamic, and gene-association rules of the metabolic network are encoded on a per-model-organism basis.

Starting with generically defined GEMs, for example, HUMAN1 or Recon2, which have been extensively curated to generate consensus models of human metabolism [5], the Nielson group has recently developed an optimized approach called fast tINIT (ftINIT) to generate context-specific genome-scale models for 202 cell populations across 19 organs [86]. Running in two steps, reactions without gene associations are first omitted from the linear optimization problem, and then remaining reactions are selected based on fixed or individual gene expression thresholds. This custom collection of reactions is converted into a working metabolic model with the Gurobi solver. These models have revealed that several healthy tissues and their associated tumors had markedly different metabolic capabilities. Liver cancers show increased proline de novo synthesis relative to nontumor tissue; AML showed enhanced heme, DHA, glycine, and homocysteine de novo synthesis relative to Blood GTEx data [5]. Additional work examining metabolism across cell types in the tumor microenvironment of lung adenocarcinoma revealed that more than 1000 reactions were differentially on or off across the populations, consistent with metabolic network diversity. Moreover, tumor cells across several datasets were found to have altered fatty acid metabolism, acetyl-CoA metabolism, heme metabolism, and TCA metabolism [86].

As described above, tailoring GEMs provides insight into cellular and tissue differences between diseased and healthy states to generate hypotheses around metabolic mechanisms and potential therapeutic targets. However, it should be noted that unlike traditional metabolomics approaches (Box 5.1), constraint-based modeling does not produce true flux measurements. Rather, it estimates a solution space by imposing constraints on the range of potential flux values of model reactions [87]. Because FBA approaches rely on assumptions of optimal metabolic behaviors, such approaches may also oversimplify the complex programs of cancer cells. For example, objective functions that emphasize growth may overlook the importance of metabolite uptake and secretion within the tumor microenvironment and their abilities to metabolically influence surrounding cell types. Additionally, advances to improve reaction representation and metabolic subsystem classification in mammalian GEMs are still ongoing. Despite this, we strongly believe that the application of constraint-based modeling and GEMs can provide enormous value, particularly in contexts where bulk measurements prove insufficient such as cancer. Given the current limitations of making metabolomic measurements in single cells, these models serve as useful tools for probing tumor heterogeneity with respect to metabolic pathway utilization. Of course, the success of workflows which implement these computational approaches will require cross-validation. Efforts to compare the emergent properties of these models with CRISPR-edited essentialities are already promising [88]. Below, we provide a start-to-finish example of implementing and validating tumor-contextualized GEMs.

Validating constraint-based metabolic models for tumor cells in preclinical settings

To demonstrate the utility of our proposed framework (Fig. 5.1), we first provide an example of customizing constraint-based models with tumor cell transcriptomic data. Select syngeneic tumor models have been shown to be sensitive to glutamine modulation [35,89]. Specifically, treatment of MC38 colon carcinoma tumors with the glutamine antagonist DON (6-diazo-5-oxo-L-norleucine) has been shown to decrease tumor size and result in sustained therapeutic responses, while treatment of B16 melanoma tumors with DON showed little effect [35]. Taking bulk RNA sequencing data from both responsive MC38 tumors and nonresponsive B16 tumors, we contextualized the recently released Mouse-GEM model using fTINIT in the RAVEN Toolkit [90] and performed flux balance analysis (FBA) using the COBRApy package [91] (Fig. 5.2A). Following DON treatment, we identified that MC38 (DON-responsive) tumor cells failed to maintain flux through the TCA cycle, attenuating cell proliferation and survival. In contrast, B16 (DON-resistant) tumor cells showed positive fluxes for TCA reactions between AKGD/OGDH and MDH2 (Fig. 5.2B). This led us to hypothesize that differences in flux through the TCA cycle may enable resistance in the B16 model and that OGDH and MDH2 might serve as potential targets to sensitize the B16 model to DON therapy.

Additional validation by RNA sequencing demonstrated that DON treatment induced OGDH and MDH2 transcripts in a dose-dependent manner in B16 cells, but not in MC38 cells, providing further evidence that B16 cells could rewire this pathway to mediate resistance to DON (Fig. 5.2C and D). We next asked whether loss of OGDH or MDH2 could impact metabolic function sufficiently to alter tumor responsiveness to glutamine antagonism. Relative to B16 parental cells, we saw decreased OCR in OGDH and MDH2 knockout lines consistent with efficient gene editing (Fig. 5.2E and F). Upon implantation in vivo, we found that loss of flux through OGDH or MDH2 in combination with DON treatment delayed tumor growth and increased survival (Fig. 5.2G and H). Altogether, we were able to experimentally validate selectively active targets (OGDH and MDH2) derived from our computational analyses in responder (MC38 cells) and nonresponder (B16 cells) metabolic models.

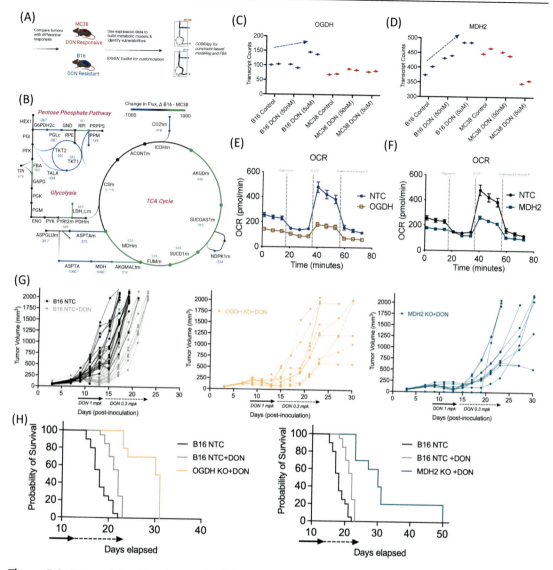

Figure 5.2: Target identification and validation following bulk RNA GEM customization and flux balance analyses in tumor cells.

(A) MC38 and B16 tumor cells were selected as responder versus nonresponder groups for metabolic modeling following glutamine antagonism. (B) Difference in FBA solutions between MC38 and B16 tumors following glutamine antagonism with DON. FBA changes in reaction flux are indicated by the colorbar. (C and D) Transcript counts for OGDH and MDH2 recovered from RNA sequencing validation in B16 and MC38 cell lines treated in vitro with increased doses of DON. (E and F) Seahorse OCR collected for NTC lines and OGDH or MDH2 KO lines used in validation studies. (G) In vivo validation shows decreased tumor growth when OGDH or MDH2 loss is combined with DON glutamine antagonism. (H) Kaplan–Meier curves capture survival benefits when OGDH or MDH2 loss is combined with DON glutamine antagonism. *NTC*, Nontargeting control; *GEMs*, genome-scale metabolic models.

Adapting constraint-based models for single-cell RNA sequencing (scRNA-seq) data

In oncology, capturing single-cell data modalities highlights the tremendous heterogeneity that exists within tumor cell populations and across tumor microenvironmental cell types, whilst enabling scientists to uncover mechanisms related to therapeutic response and resistance. Because the acquisition of single-cell metabolomic data in a high-throughput fashion remains a considerable challenge, the development of algorithms to infer metabolic fluxes from associated single-cell transcriptomic data has gained popularity (Table 5.1). These approaches apply constraint-based FBA on a per-cell basis, inferring the metabolic flux across all reactions of the metabolic network within a cell. Limits on reaction rates are computed on the basis of gene expression. scFBA determines a maximal theoretical flux of each reaction in the GEM and then applies flux constraints based on singe-cell RNA sequencing data [92]. Similarly, Compass computes a maximum flux per reaction but returns a solution with adjusted penalty scores that are inversely proportional to gene expression—reactions associated with a gene or transcript that has limited expression will be weighted with a higher penalty, while reactions associated with an abundant transcript may have a lower penalty and therefore a higher likelihood of occurrence [93]. METAflux takes a different approach, bootstrapping average gene expression in a cell group to define

Table 5.1: Single-cell algorithms applied to onco-metabolism or immunometabolism.

Algorithm	Application	Finding	References
scFBA	Extends flux balance analysis to scRNA-seq; Examined LUAD xenograft models and primary breast cancer samples.	Integrating scRNA-seq greatly reduces the space of feasible solutions that sustain metabolically-driven tumor growth, thereby restricting candidate drug targets.	Damiani et al. PLOS Computational Biology. 2019. Damiani et al. [92]
Compass	Extends flux balance analysis to scRNA-seq; Compared healthy Th17 and pathogenic Th17 in models of EAE (experimental autoimmune encephalomyelitis).	Inhibiting polyamine biosynthesis enzymes ODC1 and SAT1 alleviates autoimmune CNS inflammation.	Wagner et al. [93]
METAflux	Extends flux balance analysis to scRNA-seq; Applied to in vivo lymphoma model treated with CAR NK cells engineered to express IL15.	CAR NKs exhibit higher glycolysis and oxidative phosphorylation, competing with tumor cells for oxygen and glucose until relapse.	Huang et al. Nature Comm. 2023. Huang et al. [94]
scFEA	Graphical neural network infers the cell-wise fluxome; Assesses brain tumors, Alzheimer's, and spatial transcriptomics data.	In spatial tumor data, the ratio of pyruvate to lactate flux versus the ratio of pyruvate to TCA flux predicted regions of high hypoxia, consistent with high HIF1A gene expression.	Algahmdi et al. Genome Research. 2021. Alghamdi et al. [95]

the upper and lower bounds on reaction fluxes [94]. Additional inputs, such as metabolite concentration or nutrient profiles, can be added to further customize the model. Metabolic networks can then be interrogated across populations. Both Compass and METAflux provide nutrient uptake and secretion values, which can be interpreted to determine whether cell types are competing for a metabolite in the TME or acting cooperatively by secreting a metabolite that acts in a paracrine fashion. MERGE, a heuristic algorithm that uses a distance-based metric to infer the contribution of neighboring reactions to compute flux potential, optimizes the capture of tissue-relevant metabolic functions but has only been applied in the context of *C. elegans* metabolism [96].

In contrast to the GEM-based modeling approach, deep neural networks have been applied to infer nonlinear relationships between enzymes and metabolites. The algorithm scFEA encodes the GEM into a graphical neural network (GNN), with edges reflecting substrate and product relationships [95]. Trained on the single-cell RNA sequencing input data, the model aims to minimize flux imbalance; resulting pathways with high metabolite flux imbalances indicates metabolic stress [95]. FlowGAT combines FBA with a machine learning-based GNN trained on knockout-fitness scores. Different model architectures have helped to predict essential genes in *E. coli* thus far but require the central assumption that WT and perturbed strains hold the same fitness objective function [97].

Utilization of single-cell transcriptomic data for model customization

Single-cell metabolic modeling in immune cells

Given the technical difficulty of obtaining single-cell metabolomics measurements, the single-cell algorithms described (Table 5.1) are ideally suited to capture the metabolic heterogeneity of immune cells in the tumor microenvironments. To demonstrate the utility of these algorithms, we applied the Compass algorithm to reveal metabolic reactions with inferred differential activity in vivo following immunotherapy treatment. Single-cell RNA sequencing data was collected for CD45-enriched populations isolated from MC38 tumors (colon carcinoma) and KPC tumors (pancreatic cancer) following treatment with PD-1 or first-in-class small molecule immunotherapy ABBV-CLS-484 (484), an inhibitor against PTPN2/N1 [98]. MC38 is a well-documented PD-1-responsive model, while KPC is known to be a PD-1-refractory model, enabling interpretation by fitting into our comparative framework (Fig. 5.1). Although the microenvironment in each tumor is composed of diverse lymphocytic and myeloid populations, single-cell analyses allow us to effectively distinguish these populations through marker gene expression. Within each distinct population, information-sharing parameter lambda (λ) was set to 0.25 between cells to compensate for dropout in single-cell RNA sequencing data as recommended.

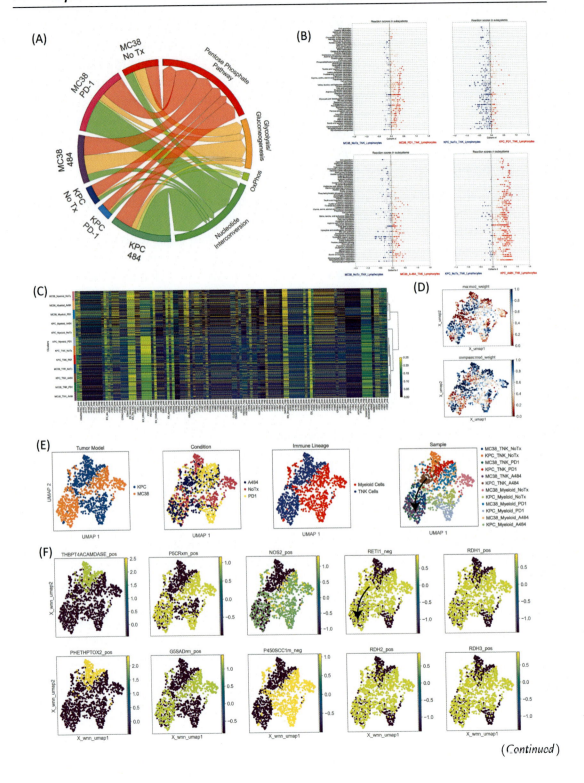

(Continued)

To visualize changes in lymphocyte metabolism for key subsystems such as pentose phosphate pathway, glycolysis, oxidative phosphorylation, and nucleotide interconversion, we tabulated reactions with significant positive flux as computed by Wilcoxon rank sum metrics in each of our conditions: untreated (No Tx), PD-1 treated (PD-1), and PTPN2/N1 treated (484) in MC38 and KPC tumors (Fig. 5.3A). Consistent with treatment response, we observe an increase in reactions with positive flux upon PD-1 or 484 treatment in MC38 relative to untreated conditions. PD-1 therapy in MC38 induces greater flux in several nucleotide interconversion reactions, as might be expected when lymphocytes undergo active proliferation following antigen stimulation. In contrast, KPC tumors treated with PD-1 showed few differences in their flux profiles for these subsystems when compared to untreated KPC tumors. We find through these analyses that PTPN2/N1 inhibition, which acts by unleashing the brakes on JAK/STAT signaling, can remodel central carbon metabolic pathways in KPC tumors, showing drastic increases in PPP and nucleotide interconversion on par with that observed in MC38 tumors.

Looking across all metabolic subsystems, we statistically computed differential reaction activity by estimated effect size with Cohen's distance [92,93] and plotted the median difference between these flux distributions for each reaction in the Recon2 GEM (Fig. 5.3B). We find that lymphocytes in MC38 tumors show increases in flux across multiple subsystems following PD-1 therapy, while lymphocytes in KPC tumors do not. We further find that PTPN2/N1 inhibition with 484 effectively induces metabolic remodeling in MC38 tumors like PD-1 treatment, with many subsystems exhibiting changes of similar magnitude. In KPC tumors, however, the metabolic differences induced by 484 are strikingly different. Again, we find that increased JAK/STAT signaling by 484 treatment elicits an overall metabolic rewiring of lymphocytes in a manner distinct from immune checkpoint blockade, correlating with its ability to overcome the limited efficacy of immunotherapy typically observed in this model. Hierarchical clustering of the reaction scores recovered by Compass highlights these similarities in metabolic state by grouping

Figure 5.3: Single-cell transcriptome-inferred metabolic activity computed with the Compass algorithm captures metabolic changes following immunotherapy.
(A) Chord diagram represents the proportion of reactions with significant inferred flux for each labeled metabolic subsystem in lymphocytes for each labeled condition. (B) Differential activity of metabolic reactions. Reactions (dots) are partitioned by Recon2 subsystems and colored by the sign of their Cohen's d statistic (effect size). (C) Hierarchical clustering of reaction score heatmap. (D) Modality weights assigned by WNN to integrate RNA and Compass scores. (E) UMAP visualization for tumor model, conditions, immune lineage, and samples for which Compass scores were computed. (F) UMAP visualization of reaction scores plotted for representative top differential reactions.

KPC tumors treated with 484 with treated lymphocytes from MC38-responsive tumors (Fig. 5.3C).

Utilizing the muon framework for multiomic data [99], we coembedded transcriptomic data with Compass-derived reaction scores, using a weighted nearest neighbors network analysis to integrate these layers and generate a UMAP visualization (Fig. 5.3D). We visualized conditions for both lymphoid and myeloid cells from our dataset, but for the purposes of this example, we will continue to focus on changes in lymphocyte metabolism. Within the UMAP representation, we found that lymphocytes from KPC untreated and KPC PD-1 treated conditions occupied a similar high-dimensional space (Fig. 5.3E). Furthermore, we found that KPC tumors treated with PTPN2/N1 inhibitor 484 mapped more closely to responsive and immune "hot" MC38 conditions (Fig. 5.3E).

By performing analyses analogs to differential gene expression, we utilized this single-cell data to identify differential reactions based on computed Compass scores. Among the most significantly different reactions, we found increased tetrahydrobiopterin (THBPT4ACAMDASE) and phenylalanine, tyrosine, and tryptophan (PHETHPTOX2) metabolism in KPC untreated and KPC PD-1 treated tumors (Fig. 5.3F). Increased arginine and proline metabolism (P5CRxm, G5SADrm, NOS2) was observed in MC38 tumor conditions, but not KPC (Fig. 5.3F). Myeloid cells showed high reaction scores for cholesterol metabolism reaction P450SCC1m, which was absent in lymphocytes. Lastly, we asked which metabolic changes drove KPC + PTPN2i-treated cells to cluster more closely to lymphocytes from MC38 tumors (Fig. 5.3F). We found changes in four significantly different reactions linked to retinoic acid metabolism (RET1, RDH1, RDH2, and RDH3), belonging to the vitamin A metabolism subsystem of Recon2 (Fig. 5.3F).

In this example, we can see how comparisons between inferred metabolic flux can be interpreted for hypothesis generation. Bolstered by reported literature, associations between tryptophan and cholesterol metabolism have previously been linked to immunotherapy resistance [100–105]. Recent findings also suggest that retinoic acid can potentiate immunotherapy response [106], playing a finely tuned role in T cell activation and tolerance [107]. Further investigation into the enzymes that regulate these differential reactions may lead to target discovery.

Applying metabolic models to clinical data

Clinical samples are not only difficult to acquire but also limited in nature, often not providing enough material for metabolic profiling via traditional assays like mass spectrometry. However, clinical samples are now more routinely undergoing single-cell RNA sequencing profiling to characterize changes in TME and in the periphery. Transcriptomic profiles of patient peripheral blood mononuclear cell (PBMC) populations or dissociated tumor cell populations can serve as direct inputs to the algorithms listed in Table 5.1, allowing researchers to ask whether the metabolic changes observed in preclinical models might direct clinical drug development and whether inferred metabolic profiles might prove useful as clinical biomarkers.

Comparing metabolic phenotypes of patients who exhibit clinical benefit (therapeutic response) versus those who progress (therapeutic nonresponders) may improve clinical trial success rates in addition to providing insight into resistance mechanisms (Fig. 5.1). Using our metabolic model example above (Fig. 5.3) along with other published findings, clinical researchers might hypothesize that vitamin A metabolites would potentiate interferon responses, sensitize tumors to checkpoint blockade, and improve patient outcomes. Thus we can see how identifying metabolic differences observed in vivo which hold true in patients may guide the design of prospective drug combinations entering the clinic. To this end, new clinical trials are pursuing this hypothesis, including six active clinical trials (NCT05482451, NCT05345002, NCT06371274, NCT04305041, NCT04303169, and NCT04305054) spanning multiple oncology indications such as melanoma, triple-negative breast cancer, pancreatic cancer, and recurrent IDH-mutant glioma. Future work will reveal whether metabolite-modulating approaches prove effective and their potential role in combination with more direct interferon-modulating therapies such as a PTPN2/N1 inhibitor (NCT06188975), due to their ability to influence and possibly amplify multiple pathways within tumor cells.

The use of these metabolic models may further serve to improve clinical biomarker signals. If metabolic changes directly reflect the mechanism of action of a given therapeutic, these approaches offer a straightforward measurement of pathway activity and provide added value as a pharmacodynamic readout in early phase clinical trials. However, because cancer cells rely on high metabolic activity to grow and proliferate, an alternative readout of these models may consist of evaluating the overall metabolic activity of profiled tumor cells. Tumor cells in patients with stable disease may exhibit less metabolic activity, while tumor cells of those with progressive disease may possess more significant reactions in subsystems correlated with biomass or resistance phenotypes. Thus capturing metabolic readouts through computational modeling may offer utility to clinical development strategies by providing earlier indicators of therapeutic response, as reflected by the overall metabolic activity of tumor cells.

Perspectives on the implementation of metabolic models in target discovery and clinical development

The tools that enable genome-scale metabolic interrogation have advanced alongside the rapid adoption of single-cell modalities. While it is evident that cellular metabolism plays a role in enabling or restricting response, not all metabolic phenotypes are straightforward and amenable to interpretation. Integrating the use of constraint-based models will help associate related metabolic subsystems and pathways to pinpoint a mechanistic, reaction-centric-based understanding. Moreover, these computational models will help reduce the search space for viable drug candidates to improve the success rates of drug development. Here, we not only highlight the implementation and validation of metabolic models, but we also demonstrate that different cell types present in the tumor microenvironment are governed by their own metabolic characteristics. Thus we conclude that the widespread use of single-cell algorithms will exponentially deepen our understanding of the metabolic heterogeneity present in the tumor microenvironment.

While we emphasize the development of algorithms that incorporate single-cell RNA sequencing data in their metabolic model customization, we recognize that other modalities may improve these models further. It remains an active area of research interest to develop methods capable of integrating -omic modalities beyond transcriptomics. For example, measurements of protein levels, which may differ from RNA levels, are often captured by antibody-based modalities like CITE-seq and flow cytometry. Proteomic-based mass spectrometry has been used in bulk settings to incorporate protein-level data into lower organism metabolic models, as demonstrated by GECKO [108], but such approaches need to be adapted to the single-cell level for higher organisms. As available CITE-seq panels have expanded from surface markers to accommodating intracellular proteins, these panels have become increasingly customizable—to the point of adding in antibodies for SLC transporters and other metabolic enzymes. As added flexibility in the conjugation of oligos to measuring metabolites becomes technically feasible, we will see further improvement of computations models due to the incorporation of "ground truth" readouts of metabolites to guide the model, rather than inferred activity from transcriptomic measurements.

Naturally, it is of deep interest to resolve single-cell metabolic differences spatially. The recently published single cell spatially resolved metabolic (scSpaMet) framework combines untargeted spatial metabolomics with targeted multiplex protein imaging to profile single immune and cancer cells for joint protein-metabolite profiling in immune and cancer cells across lung, tonsil, and endometrial tissues [109]. Hu et al. found that spatially resolving metabolic-protein relationships uncovered variation between cells in tumor versus stromal regions as well as elucidated localized hubs of metabolic competition [95]. Deep learning-based joint embeddings have also revealed unique metabolite-driven states in patient level tissues while trajectory inference shed light on metabolically driven differentiation [95]. Lastly, in resected primary and metastatic PDAC samples, the application of scFEA to evaluate local ecotypes revealed that while primary tumors exhibited reduced glycolysis, pentose phosphate pathway, and TCA flux, metastatic sites were enriched for these behaviors along with amino acid and glycan synthesis [110]. These profiles are not only suggestive of enhanced growth and biomass production in metastatic organs but may be critical considerations when designing therapeutic strategies for patients with diseases that span different anatomical locations.

Finally, with the advancement of large language models (LLM) as a method of generative AI, it may become possible to develop foundational models which utilize pretrained transformers to distill biological correlations between genes, proteins, and metabolites within a cell. The development of scGPT has already taken some of the first steps to build these AI-based models, enhancing pipeline tasks such as cell annotation, batch correction, gene-network inferences, and even perturbation predictions [111]. As the training of these foundational models expands to more cells, tissues, diseases, and organisms, we expect these models to be rapidly adopted into target discovery pipelines to improve the attrition rate of clinical drug development in cancer.

References

[1] DeBerardinis RJ, Chandel NS. We need to talk about the Warburg effect. Nat Metab 2020;2(2):127−9. Available from: https://doi.org/10.1038/s42255-020-0172-2, https://www.nature.com/natmetab/.

[2] Luengo A, Gui DY, Vander Heiden MG. Targeting metabolism for cancer therapy. Cell Chem Biol 2017;24(9):1161−80. Available from: https://doi.org/10.1016/j.chembiol.2017.08.028.

[3] Stine ZE, Schug ZT, Salvino JM, Dang CV. Targeting cancer metabolism in the era of precision oncology. Nat Rev Drug Discovery 2022;21(2):141−62. Available from: https://doi.org/10.1038/s41573-021-00339-6, https://www.nature.com/nrd/.

[4] Li H, Ning S, Ghandi M, Kryukov GV, Gopal S, Deik A, et al. The landscape of cancer cell line metabolism. Nat Med 2019;25(5):850−60. Available from: https://doi.org/10.1038/s41591-019-0404-8.

[5] Robinson JL, Kocabaş P, Wang H, Cholley PE, Cook D, Nilsson A, et al. An atlas of human metabolism. Sci Signal 2020;13(624). Available from: https://doi.org/10.1126/scisignal.aaz1482, https://stke.sciencemag.org/content/sigtrans/13/624/eaaz1482.full.pdf.

[6] Elia I, Haigis MC. Metabolites and the tumour microenvironment: from cellular mechanisms to systemic metabolism. Nat Metab 2021;3(1):21−32. Available from: https://doi.org/10.1038/s42255-020-00317-z, https://www.nature.com/natmetab/.

[7] Zaal EA, Berkers CR. The influence of metabolism on drug response in cancer. Front Oncol 2018;8. Available from: https://doi.org/10.3389/fonc.2018.00500, http://www.frontiersin.org/Oncology/about.

[8] Pavlova NN, Thompson CB. The emerging hallmarks of cancer metabolism. Cell Metab 2016;23(1):27−47. Available from: https://doi.org/10.1016/j.cmet.2015.12.006.

[9] Yuneva M, Zamboni N, Oefner P, Sachidanandam R, Lazebnik Y. Deficiency in glutamine but not glucose induces MYC-dependent apoptosis in human cells. J Cell Biol 2007;178(1):93−105. Available from: https://doi.org/10.1083/jcb.200703099, http://www.jcb.org/cgi/reprint/178/1/93.

[10] Yuneva MO, Fan TWM, Allen TD, Higashi RM, Ferraris DV, Tsukamoto T, et al. The metabolic profile of tumors depends on both the responsible genetic lesion and tissue type. Cell Metab 2012;15(2):157−70. Available from: https://doi.org/10.1016/j.cmet.2011.12.015.

[11] Liu GY, Sabatini DM. mTOR at the nexus of nutrition, growth, ageing and disease. Nat Rev Mol Cell Biol 2020;21(4):183−203. Available from: https://doi.org/10.1038/s41580-019-0199-y, http://www.nature.com/molcellbio.

[12] Mayers JR, Torrence ME, Danai LV, Papagiannakopoulos T, Davidson SM, Bauer MR, et al. Tissue of origin dictates branched-chain amino acid metabolism in mutant Kras-driven cancers. Science 2016;353(6304):1161−5. Available from: https://doi.org/10.1126/science.aaf5171, http://science.sciencemag.org/content/sci/353/6304/1161.full.pdf.

[13] Valvezan AJ, Turner M, Belaid A, Lam HC, Miller SK, McNamara MC, et al. mTORC1 couples nucleotide synthesis to nucleotide demand resulting in a targetable metabolic vulnerability. Cancer Cell 2017;32(5):624. Available from: https://doi.org/10.1016/j.ccell.2017.09.013, https://www.journals.elsevier.com/cancer-cell.

[14] Vander Heiden MG, DeBerardinis RJ. Understanding the intersections between metabolism and cancer biology. Cell 2017;168(4):657–69. Available from: https://doi.org/10.1016/j.cell.2016.12.039, https://www.sciencedirect.com/journal/cell.

[15] Romero R, Sayin VI, Davidson SM, Bauer MR, Singh SX, LeBoeuf SE, et al. Keap1 loss promotes Kras-driven lung cancer and results in dependence on glutaminolysis. Nat Med 2017;23(11):1362–8. Available from: https://doi.org/10.1038/nm.4407.

[16] Mellinghoff IK, Lu M, Wen PY, Taylor JW, Maher EA, Arrillaga-Romany I, et al. Vorasidenib and ivosidenib in IDH1-mutant low-grade glioma: a randomized, perioperative phase 1 trial. Nat Med 2023;29(3):615–22. Available from: https://doi.org/10.1038/s41591-022-02141-2, https://www.nature.com/nm/.

[17] Wang F, Travins J, DeLaBarre B, Penard-Lacronique V, Schalm S, Hansen E, et al. Targeted inhibition of mutant IDH2 in leukemia cells induces cellular differentiation. Science 2013;340(6132):622–6. Available from: https://doi.org/10.1126/science.1234769.

[18] Rossiter NJ, Huggler KS, Adelmann CH, Keys HR, Soens RW, Sabatini DM, et al. CRISPR screens in physiologic medium reveal conditionally essential genes in human cells. Cell Metab 2021;33(6):1248. Available from: https://doi.org/10.1016/j.cmet.2021.02.005, http://www.cellmetabolism.org/.

[19] Zhu XG, Chudnovskiy A, Baudrier L, Prizer B, Liu Y, Ostendorf BN, et al. Functional genomics in vivo reveal metabolic dependencies of pancreatic cancer cells. Cell Metab 2021;33(1):211. Available from: https://doi.org/10.1016/j.cmet.2020.10.017, http://www.cellmetabolism.org/.

[20] Sun G, Zhao S, Fan Z, Wang Y, Liu H, Cao H, et al. CHSY1 promotes CD8 + T cell exhaustion through activation of succinate metabolism pathway leading to colorectal cancer liver metastasis based on CRISPR/Cas9 screening. J Exp & Clin Cancer Res 2023;42(1). Available from: https://doi.org/10.1186/s13046-023-02803-0.

[21] Encarnación-Rosado J, Sohn ASW, Biancur DE, Lin EY, Osorio-Vasquez V, Rodrick T, et al. Targeting pancreatic cancer metabolic dependencies through glutamine antagonism. Nat Cancer 2024;5(1):85–99. Available from: https://doi.org/10.1038/s43018-023-00647-3.

[22] Zhao D, Badur MG, Luebeck J, Magaña JH, Birmingham A, Sasik R, et al. Combinatorial CRISPR-Cas9 metabolic screens reveal critical redox control points dependent on the KEAP1-NRF2 regulatory axis. Mol Cell 2018;69(4):699. Available from: https://doi.org/10.1016/j.molcel.2018.01.017.

[23] Li H, Liu Y, Xiao Y, Wilson CN, Bai HJ, Jones MD, et al. CRISPR metabolic screen identifies ATM and KEAP1 as targetable genetic vulnerabilities in solid tumors. Proc Natl Acad Sci 2023;120(6). Available from: https://doi.org/10.1073/pnas.2212072120.

[24] Edwards DN, Ngwa VM, Raybuck AL, Wang S, Hwang Y, Kim LC, et al. Selective glutamine metabolism inhibition in tumor cells improves antitumor T lymphocyte activity in triple-negative breast cancer. J Clin Investigation 2021;131(4). Available from: https://doi.org/10.1172/JCI140100, https://www.jci.org/articles/view/140100/pdf.

[25] Chang CH, Qiu J, O'Sullivan D, Buck MD, Noguchi T, Curtis JD, et al. Metabolic competition in the tumor microenvironment is a driver of cancer progression. Cell 2015;162(6):1229–41. Available from: https://doi.org/10.1016/j.cell.2015.08.016, https://www.sciencedirect.com/journal/cell.

[26] Arner EN, Rathmell JC. Metabolic programming and immune suppression in the tumor microenvironment. Cancer Cell 2023;41(3):421–33. Available from: https://doi.org/10.1016/j.ccell.2023.01.009, https://www.journals.elsevier.com/cancer-cell.

[27] Watson MLJ, Vignali PDA, Mullett SJ, Overacre-Delgoffe AE, Peralta RM, Grebinoski S, et al. Metabolic support of tumour-infiltrating regulatory T cells by lactic acid. Nature 2021;591(7851):645–51. Available from: https://doi.org/10.1038/s41586-020-03045-2.

[28] Ho PC, Bihuniak JD, MacIntyre AN, Staron M, Liu X, Amezquita R, et al. Phosphoenolpyruvate is a metabolic checkpoint of anti-tumor T cell responses. Cell 2015;162(6):1217–28. Available from: https://doi.org/10.1016/j.cell.2015.08.012, https://www.sciencedirect.com/journal/cell.

[29] Kim SK, Cho SW. The evasion mechanisms of cancer immunity and drug intervention in the tumor microenvironment. Front Pharmacology 2022;13. Available from: https://doi.org/10.3389/fphar.2022.868695, http://www.frontiersin.org/Pharmacology.

[30] Notarangelo G. Oncometabolite d-2HG alters T cell metabolism to impair CD8 + T cell function. Sci 2022;377:1519−29.

[31] Elia I, Rowe JH, Johnson S, Joshi S, Notarangelo G, Kurmi K, et al. Tumor cells dictate anti-tumor immune responses by altering pyruvate utilization and succinate signaling in CD8 + T cells. Cell Metab 2022;34(8):1137. Available from: https://doi.org/10.1016/j.cmet.2022.06.008.

[32] Kaymak I. Carbon source availability drives nutrient utilization in CD8 + T cells. Cell Metab 2022;34 (1296).

[33] Best SA, Gubser PM, Sethumadhavan S, Kersbergen A, Negrón Abril YL, Goldford J, et al. Glutaminase inhibition impairs CD8 T cell activation in STK11-/Lkb1-deficient lung cancer. Cell Metab 2022;34 (6):874. Available from: https://doi.org/10.1016/j.cmet.2022.04.003, http://www.cellmetabolism.org/.

[34] Wang T, Gnanaprakasam JNR, Chen X, Kang S, Xu X, Sun H, et al. Inosine is an alternative carbon source for CD8 + -T-cell function under glucose restriction. Nat Metab 2020;2(7):635−47. Available from: https://doi.org/10.1038/s42255-020-0219-4.

[35] Leone RD, Zhao L, Englert JM, Sun IM, Oh MH, Sun IH, et al. Glutamine blockade induces divergent metabolic programs to overcome tumor immune evasion. Science 2019;366(6468):1013−21. Available from: https://doi.org/10.1126/science.aav2588, https://science.sciencemag.org/content/366/6468/1013/tab-pdf.

[36] Bian Y, Li W, Kremer DM, Sajjakulnukit P, Li S, Crespo J, et al. Cancer SLC43A2 alters T cell methionine metabolism and histone methylation. Nature 2020;585(7824):277−82. Available from: https://doi.org/10.1038/s41586-020-2682-1.

[37] Ma EH, Bantug G, Griss T, Condotta S, Johnson RM, Samborska B, et al. Serine is an essential metabolite for effector T cell expansion. Cell Metab 2017;25(2):345−57. Available from: https://doi.org/10.1016/j.cmet.2016.12.011, http://www.cellmetabolism.org/.

[38] Liu Y-N, Yang J-F, Huang D-J, Ni H-H, Zhang C-X, Zhang L, et al. Hypoxia induces mitochondrial defect that promotes T cell exhaustion in tumor microenvironment through MYC-regulated pathways. Front Immunol 2020;11. Available from: https://doi.org/10.3389/fimmu.2020.01906.

[39] Bannoud N, Dalotto-Moreno T, Kindgard L, García PA, Blidner AG, Mariño KV, et al. Hypoxia supports differentiation of terminally exhausted CD8 T cells. Front Immunology 2021;12. Available from: https://doi.org/10.3389/fimmu.2021.660944.

[40] Scharping NE, Rivadeneira DB, Menk AV, Vignali PDA, Ford BR, Rittenhouse NL, et al. Mitochondrial stress induced by continuous stimulation under hypoxia rapidly drives T cell exhaustion. Nat Immunology 2021;22(2):205−15. Available from: https://doi.org/10.1038/s41590-020-00834-9, http://www.nature.com/ni.

[41] Huang H. In vivo CRISPR screening reveals nutrient signaling processes underpinning CD8 + T cell fate decisions. Cell. 184(1221).

[42] Reina-Campos M, Heeg M, Kennewick K, Mathews IT, Galletti G, Luna V, et al. Metabolic programs of T cell tissue residency empower tumour immunity. Nature 2023;621(7977):179−87. Available from: https://doi.org/10.1038/s41586-023-06483-w.

[43] Ye L, Park JJ, Peng L, Yang Q, Chow RD, Dong MB, et al. A genome-scale gain-of-function CRISPR screen in CD8 T cells identifies proline metabolism as a means to enhance CAR-T therapy. Cell Metab 2022;34(4):595. Available from: https://doi.org/10.1016/j.cmet.2022.02.009.

[44] LaFleur MW, Lemmen AM, Streeter ISL, Nguyen TH, Milling LE, Derosia NM, et al. X-CHIME enables combinatorial, inducible, lineage-specific and sequential knockout of genes in the immune system. Nat Immunology 2024;25(1):178−88. Available from: https://doi.org/10.1038/s41590-023-01689-6, https://www.nature.com/ni.

[45] Duan W. Metformin mitigates autoimmune insulitis by inhibiting Th1 and Th17 responses while promoting Treg production. Am J Transl Res 2019;11:2393−402.

[46] Liu S, Liao S, Liang L, Deng J, Zhou Y. The relationship between CD4 + T cell glycolysis and their functions. Trends Endocrinol Metab 2023;34(6):345−60. Available from: https://doi.org/10.1016/j.tem.2023.03.006, www.elsevier.com/locate/tem.

[47] Gemta LF, Siska PJ, Nelson ME, Gao X, Liu X, Locasale JW, et al. Impaired enolase 1 glycolytic activity restrains effector functions of tumor-infiltrating CD8 + T cells. Sci Immunology 2019;4(31). Available from: https://doi.org/10.1126/sciimmunol.aap9520, http://immunology.sciencemag.org/content/immunology/4/31/eaap9520.full.pdf.

[48] Roy DG, Chen J, Mamane V, Ma EH, Muhire BM, Sheldon RD, et al. Methionine metabolism shapes T helper cell responses through regulation of epigenetic reprogramming. Cell Metab 2020;31(2):250. Available from: https://doi.org/10.1016/j.cmet.2020.01.006, http://www.cellmetabolism.org/.

[49] Crowther RR, Schmidt SM, Lange SM, McKell MC, Robillard MC, Zhao J, et al. Cutting edge: L-arginine transfer from antigen-presenting cells sustains CD41 T cell viability and proliferation. J Immunology 2022;208(4):793−8. Available from: https://doi.org/10.4049/jimmunol.2100652, https://www.jimmunol.org/content/jimmunol/208/4/793.full.pdf.

[50] Coutzac C, Jouniaux J-M, Paci A, Schmidt J, Mallardo D, Seck A, et al. Systemic short chain fatty acids limit antitumor effect of CTLA-4 blockade in hosts with cancer. Nat Commun 2020;11(1). Available from: https://doi.org/10.1038/s41467-020-16079-x.

[51] Henriksson J, Chen X, Gomes T, Ullah U, Meyer KB, Miragaia R, et al. Genome-wide CRISPR screens in T helper cells reveal pervasive crosstalk between activation and differentiation. Cell 2019;176(4):882. Available from: https://doi.org/10.1016/j.cell.2018.11.044.

[52] Galy SD. In vivo genome-wide CRISPR screens identify SOCS1 as intrinsic checkpoint of CD4 + TH1 cell response. Sci Immunology 2021;6.

[53] Kendirli A, de la Rosa C, Lämmle KF, Eglseer K, Bauer IJ, Kavaka V, et al. A genome-wide in vivo CRISPR screen identifies essential regulators of T cell migration to the CNS in a multiple sclerosis model. Nat Neurosci 2023;26(10):1713−25. Available from: https://doi.org/10.1038/s41593-023-01432-2.

[54] Newton RH, Shrestha S, Sullivan JM, Yates KB, Compeer EB, Ron-Harel N, et al. Maintenance of CD4 T cell fitness through regulation of Foxo1. Nat Immunology 2018;19(8):838−48. Available from: https://doi.org/10.1038/s41590-018-0157-4, http://www.nature.com/ni.

[55] Angelin A, Gil-de-Gómez L, Dahiya S, Jiao J, Guo L, Levine MH, et al. Foxp3 reprograms T cell metabolism to function in low-glucose, high-lactate environments. Cell Metab 2017;25(6):1282. Available from: https://doi.org/10.1016/j.cmet.2016.12.018.

[56] Gerriets VA, Kishton RJ, Johnson MO, Cohen S, Siska PJ, Nichols AG, et al. Foxp3 and Toll-like receptor signaling balance T reg cell anabolic metabolism for suppression. Nat Immunology 2016;17(12):1459−66. Available from: https://doi.org/10.1038/ni.3577, http://www.nature.com/ni.

[57] Lim AR, Rathmell WK, Rathmell JC. The tumor microenvironment as a metabolic barrier to effector T cells and immunotherapy. elife Sci Publ Ltd, U S elife 2020;9:1−13. Available from: https://doi.org/10.7554/eLife.55185, https://elifesciences.org/articles/55185.

[58] Kurniawan H, Franchina DG, Guerra L, Bonetti L, Baguet LS, Grusdat M, et al. Glutathione restricts serine metabolism to preserve regulatory T cell function. Cell Metab 2020;31(5):920. Available from: https://doi.org/10.1016/j.cmet.2020.03.004.

[59] Cortez JT, Montauti E, Shifrut E, Gatchalian J, Zhang Y, Shaked O, et al. CRISPR screen in regulatory T cells reveals modulators of Foxp3. Nature 2020;582(7812):416−20. Available from: https://doi.org/10.1038/s41586-020-2246-4, http://www.nature.com/nature/index.html.

[60] Loo CS, Gatchalian J, Liang Y, Leblanc M, Xie M, Ho J, et al. A genome-wide crispr screen reveals a role for the non-canonical nucleosome-remodeling BAF complex in Foxp3 expression and regulatory T cell function. Immunity 2020;53(1):143. Available from: https://doi.org/10.1016/j.immuni.2020.06.011, https://www.immunity.com.

[61] Obradovic A, Ager C, Turunen M, Nirschl T, Khosravi-Maharlooei M, Iuga A, et al. Systematic elucidation and pharmacological targeting of tumor-infiltrating regulatory T cell master regulators. Cancer Cell 2023;41(5):933. Available from: https://doi.org/10.1016/j.ccell.2023.04.003.

[62] André P, Denis C, Soulas C, Bourbon-Caillet C, Lopez J, Arnoux T, et al. Anti-NKG2A mAb is a checkpoint inhibitor that promotes anti-tumor immunity by unleashing both T and NK cells. Cell 2018;175(7):1731. Available from: https://doi.org/10.1016/j.cell.2018.10.014.

[63] Wang Z, Guan D, Wang S, Chai LYA, Xu S, Lam K-P. Glycolysis and Oxidative phosphorylation play critical roles in natural killer cell receptor-mediated natural killer cell functions. Front Immunol 2020;11. Available from: https://doi.org/10.3389/fimmu.2020.00202.

[64] Sohn H, Cooper MA. Metabolic regulation of NK cell function: implications for immunotherapy. Immunometabolism 2023;5(1):e00020. Available from: https://doi.org/10.1097/in9.0000000000000020.

[65] Donnelly RP, Loftus RM, Keating SE, Liou KT, Biron CA, Gardiner CM, et al. MTORC1-dependent metabolic reprogramming is a prerequisite for NK cell effector function. J Immunology 2014;193 (9):4477–84. Available from: https://doi.org/10.4049/jimmunol.1401558, http://www.jimmunol.org/content/193/9/4477.full.pdf + html.

[66] O'Brien KL, Finlay DK. Immunometabolism and natural killer cell responses. Nat Rev Immunology 2019;19(5):282–90. Available from: https://doi.org/10.1038/s41577-019-0139-2, http://www.nature.com/nri/index.html.

[67] Loftus RM, Assmann N, Kedia-Mehta N, O'Brien KL, Garcia A, Gillespie C, et al. Amino acid-dependent cMyc expression is essential for NK cell metabolic and functional responses in mice. Nat Commun 2018;9(1). Available from: https://doi.org/10.1038/s41467-018-04719-2, http://www.nature.com/ncomms/index.html.

[68] Li YR, Lyu Z, Tian Y, Fang Y, Zhu Y, Chen Y, et al. Advancements in CRISPR screens for the development of cancer immunotherapy strategies. Mol Ther Oncolytics 2023;31. Available from: https://doi.org/10.1016/j.omto.2023.100733, https://www.journals.elsevier.com/molecular-therapy-oncolytics.

[69] Peng L. Perturbomics of tumor-infiltrating NK cells. bioRxiv. (2003).

[70] Sandro M, Xinyu W. Identification of the role of oncometabolites on natural killer cell in the tumor microenvironment by CRISPR screening. J ImmunoTherapy Cancer 2023;11.

[71] Yan D, Adeshakin AO, Xu M, Afolabi LO, Zhang G, Chen YH, et al. Lipid metabolic pathways confer the immunosuppressive function of myeloid-derived suppressor cells in tumor. Front Immunology 2019;10. Available from: https://doi.org/10.3389/fimmu.2019.01399.

[72] Zhao J-L, Ye Y-C, Gao C-C, Wang L, Ren K-X, Jiang R, et al. Notch-mediated lactate metabolism regulates MDSC development through the Hes1/MCT2/c-Jun axis. Cell Rep 2022;38(10):110451. Available from: https://doi.org/10.1016/j.celrep.2022.110451.

[73] Oh MH, Sun IH, Zhao L, Leone RD, Sun IM, Xu W, et al. Targeting glutamine metabolism enhances tumor-specific immunity by modulating suppressive myeloid cells. J Clin Investigation 2020;130(7):3865–84. Available from: https://doi.org/10.1172/JCI131859, https://www.jci.org/articles/view/131859/pdf.

[74] Baumann T, Dunkel A, Schmid C, Schmitt S, Hiltensperger M, Lohr K, et al. Regulatory myeloid cells paralyze T cells through cell–cell transfer of the metabolite methylglyoxal. Nat Immunology 2020;21 (5):555–66. Available from: https://doi.org/10.1038/s41590-020-0666-9.

[75] Wang X, Su S, Zhu Y, Cheng X, Cheng C, Chen L, et al. Metabolic Reprogramming via ACOD1 depletion enhances function of human induced pluripotent stem cell-derived CAR-macrophages in solid tumors. Nat Commun 2023;14(1). Available from: https://doi.org/10.1038/s41467-023-41470-9.

[76] Tong J, et al. Sci Adv 2021;7.

[77] Mellman I, Chen DS, Powles T, Turley SJ. The cancer-immunity cycle: indication, genotype, and immunotype. Immunity 2023;56(10):2188–205. Available from: https://doi.org/10.1016/j.immuni.2023.09.011, https://www.immunity.com.

[78] Yuan M, Tu B, Li H, Pang H, Zhang N, Fan M, et al. Cancer-associated fibroblasts employ NUFIP1-dependent autophagy to secrete nucleosides and support pancreatic tumor growth. Nat Cancer 2022;3 (8):945–60. Available from: https://doi.org/10.1038/s43018-022-00426-6.

[79] Sun C, Wang B, Hao S. Adenosine-A2A receptor pathway in cancer immunotherapy. Front Immunology 2022;13. Available from: https://doi.org/10.3389/fimmu.2022.837230.

[80] Shifrut E. Genome-wide CRISPR screens in primary human T cells reveal key regulators of immune function. Cell 1915;175.

[81] Arnold PK, Finley LWS. Regulation and function of the mammalian tricarboxylic acid cycle. J Biol Chem 2023;299(2). Available from: https://doi.org/10.1016/j.jbc.2022.102838, https://www.sciencedirect.com/journal/journal-of-biological-chemistry.

[82] Liu XZ, Rulina A, Choi MH, Pedersen L, Lepland J, Takle ST, et al. C/EBPB-dependent adaptation to palmitic acid promotes tumor formation in hormone receptor negative breast cancer. Nat Commun 2022;13(1). Available from: https://doi.org/10.1038/s41467-021-27734-2, http://www.nature.com/ncomms/index.html.

[83] Baksh SC, Finley LWS. Metabolic coordination of cell fate by α-ketoglutarate-dependent dioxygenases. Trends Cell Biol 2021;31(1):24−36. Available from: https://doi.org/10.1016/j.tcb.2020.09.010, https://www.elsevier.com/locate/tcb.

[84] Hrovatin K, Fischer DS, Theis FJ. Toward modeling metabolic state from single-cell transcriptomics. Mol Metab 2022;57. Available from: https://doi.org/10.1016/j.molmet.2021.101396, http://www.elsevier.com/wps/find/journaldescription.cws_home/728618/description.

[85] Orth JD, Thiele I, Palsson BO. What is flux balance analysis? Nat Biotechnol 2010;28(3):245−8. Available from: https://doi.org/10.1038/nbt.1614.

[86] Gustafsson J, Anton M, Roshanzamir F, Jörnsten R, Kerkhoven EJ, Robinson JL, et al. Generation and analysis of context-specific genome-scale metabolic models derived from single-cell RNA-Seq data. Proc Natl Acad Sci 2023;120(6). Available from: https://doi.org/10.1073/pnas.2217868120.

[87] Bordbar A, Monk JM, King ZA, Palsson BO. Constraint-based models predict metabolic and associated cellular functions. Nat Rev Genet 2014;15(2):107−20. Available from: https://doi.org/10.1038/nrg3643.

[88] Opdam S, Richelle A, Kellman B, Li S, Zielinski DC, Lewis NE. A systematic evaluation of methods for tailoring genome-scale metabolic models. Cell Syst 2017;4(3):318. Available from: https://doi.org/10.1016/j.cels.2017.01.010.

[89] Guo C, You Z, Shi H, Sun Y, Du X, Palacios G, et al. SLC38A2 and glutamine signalling in cDC1s dictate anti-tumour immunity. Nature 2023;620(7972):200−8. Available from: https://doi.org/10.1038/s41586-023-06299-8.

[90] Wang H, Marcišauskas S, Sánchez BJ, Domenzain I, Hermansson D, Agren R, et al. RAVEN 2.0: A versatile toolbox for metabolic network reconstruction and a case study on Streptomyces coelicolor. PLOS Computational Biol 2018;14(10):e1006541. Available from: https://doi.org/10.1371/journal.pcbi.1006541.

[91] Ebrahim A, Lerman JA, Palsson BO, Hyduke DR. COBRApy, COnstraints-Based Reconstruction and Analysis for Python. BMC Syst Biol 2013;7.

[92] Damiani C, Maspero D, Di Filippo M, Colombo R, Pescini D, Graudenzi A, et al. Integration of single-cell RNA-seq data into population models to characterize cancer metabolism. PLOS Computational Biol 2019;15(2):e1006733. Available from: https://doi.org/10.1371/journal.pcbi.1006733.

[93] Wagner A, Wang C, Fessler J, DeTomaso D, Avila-Pacheco J, Kaminski J, et al. Metabolic modeling of single Th17 cells reveals regulators of autoimmunity. Cell 2021;184(16):4168. Available from: https://doi.org/10.1016/j.cell.2021.05.045.

[94] Huang Y, Mohanty V, Dede M, Tsai K, Daher M, Li L, et al. Characterizing cancer metabolism from bulk and single-cell RNA-seq data using METAFlux. Nat Commun 2023;14(1). Available from: https://doi.org/10.1038/s41467-023-40457-w.

[95] Alghamdi N, Chang W, Dang P, Lu X, Wan C, Gampala S, et al. A graph neural network model to estimate cell-wise metabolic flux using single-cell RNA-seq data. Genome Res 2021;31(10):1867−84. Available from: https://doi.org/10.1101/gr.271205.120.

[96] Yilmaz LS, Li X, Nanda S, Fox B, Schroeder F, Walhout AJM. Modeling tissue-relevant Caenorhabditis elegans metabolism at network, pathway, reaction, and metabolite levels. Mol Syst Biol 2020;16(10). Available from: https://doi.org/10.15252/msb.20209649, https://onlinelibrary.wiley.com/journal/17444292.

[97] Hasibi R, Michoel T, Oyarzún DA. Integration of graph neural networks and genome-scale metabolic models for predicting gene essentiality. npj Syst Biol Appl 2024;10(1). Available from: https://doi.org/10.1038/s41540-024-00348-2, https://www.nature.com/npjsba/.

[98] Baumgartner CK, Ebrahimi-Nik H, Iracheta-Vellve A, Hamel KM, Olander KE, Davis TGR, et al. The PTPN2/PTPN1 inhibitor ABBV-CLS-484 unleashes potent anti-tumour immunity. Nature 2023;622(7984):850−62. Available from: https://doi.org/10.1038/s41586-023-06575-7, https://www.nature.com/nature/.

[99] Bredikhin D, Kats I, Stegle O. MUON: multimodal omics analysis framework. Genome Biol 2022;23(1). Available from: https://doi.org/10.1186/s13059-021-02577-8.
[100] Botticelli A, Mezi S, Pomati G, Cerbelli B, Cerbelli E, Roberto M, et al. Tryptophan catabolism as immune mechanism of primary resistance to anti-PD-1. Front Immunology 2020;11. Available from: https://doi.org/10.3389/fimmu.2020.01243.
[101] El-Kenawi A, Dominguez-Viqueira W, Liu M, Awasthi S, Abraham-Miranda J, Keske A, et al. Macrophage-derived cholesterol contributes to therapeutic resistance in prostate cancer. Cancer Res 2021;81(21):5477–90. Available from: https://doi.org/10.1158/0008-5472.can-20-4028.
[102] Goossens P, Rodriguez-Vita J, Etzerodt A, Masse M, Rastoin O, Gouirand V, et al. Membrane cholesterol efflux drives tumor-associated macrophage reprogramming and tumor progression. Cell Metab 2019;29(6):1376. Available from: https://doi.org/10.1016/j.cmet.2019.02.016.
[103] Li F, Zhao Z, Zhang Z, Zhang Y, Guan W. Tryptophan metabolism induced by TDO2 promotes prostatic cancer chemotherapy resistance in a AhR/c-Myc dependent manner. BMC Cancer 2021;21(1). Available from: https://doi.org/10.1186/s12885-021-08855-9.
[104] Opitz CA, Somarribas Patterson LF, Mohapatra SR, Dewi DL, Sadik A, Platten M, et al. The therapeutic potential of targeting tryptophan catabolism in cancer. Br J Cancer 2020;122(1):30–44. Available from: https://doi.org/10.1038/s41416-019-0664-6, http://www.nature.com/bjc/index.html.
[105] Sica A, Bleve A, Garassino MC. Membrane cholesterol regulates macrophage plasticity in cancer. Cell Metab 2019;29(6):1238–40. Available from: https://doi.org/10.1016/j.cmet.2019.05.011, http://www.cellmetabolism.org/.
[106] Tilsed CM, Casey TH, de Jong E, Bosco A, Zemek RM, Salmons J, et al. Retinoic acid induces an IFN-driven inflammatory tumour microenvironment, sensitizing to immune checkpoint therapy. Front Oncol 2022;12. Available from: https://doi.org/10.3389/fonc.2022.849793, http://www.frontiersin.org/Oncology/about.
[107] Larange A. A regulatory circuit controlled by extranuclear and nuclear retinoic acid receptor α determines T cell activation and function. Immunity 2010;56.
[108] Domenzain I, Sánchez B, Anton M, Kerkhoven EJ, Millán-Oropeza A, Henry C, et al. Reconstruction of a catalogue of genome-scale metabolic models with enzymatic constraints using GECKO 2.0. Nat Commun 2022;13(1). Available from: https://doi.org/10.1038/s41467-022-31421-1.
[109] Hu T, Allam M, Cai S, Henderson W, Yueh B, Garipcan A, et al. Single-cell spatial metabolomics with cell-type specific protein profiling for tissue systems biology. Nat Commun 2023;14(1). Available from: https://doi.org/10.1038/s41467-023-43917-5.
[110] Khaliq AM, Rajamohan M, Saeed O, Mansouri K, Adil A, Zhang C, et al. Spatial transcriptomic analysis of primary and metastatic pancreatic cancers highlights tumor microenvironmental heterogeneity. Nat Genet 2024. Available from: https://doi.org/10.1038/s41588-024-01914-4, https://www.nature.com/ng/.
[111] Cui H. Towards building a foundation model for single-cell multi-omics using generative AI. bioRxiv. (2004).
[112] Danzi F, Pacchiana R, Mafficini A, Scupoli MT, Scarpa A, Donadelli M, et al. To metabolomics and beyond: a technological portfolio to investigate cancer metabolism. Signal Transduct Target Ther 2023;8(1). Available from: https://doi.org/10.1038/s41392-023-01380-0.
[113] Antoniewicz MR. A guide to 13C metabolic flux analysis for the cancer biologist. Exp Mol Med 2018;50(4):1–13. Available from: https://doi.org/10.1038/s12276-018-0060-y.

CHAPTER 6

Immunometabolic contributions to the pathogenesis of cardiovascular disease

Emily Anne Day

Department of Physiology and Pharmacology, Schulich School of Medicine and Dentistry, The University of Western Ontario, London, ON, Canada

Introduction

Immune cells in cardiovascular disease

Cardiovascular diseases (CVDs) are the leading causes of morbidity and mortality worldwide. Cardiovascular disease is an umbrella term for a variety of conditions, including heart failure (HF), coronary artery disease (CAD) which is also referred to as coronary heart disease (CHD), cerebrovascular disease, peripheral artery disease (PAD), and aortic atherosclerosis. The development of cardiovascular disease involves both chronic low-grade inflammation and acute inflammation, particularly in cases of CAD, myocardial infarction (MI) and acute coronary syndrome. Chronic low-grade inflammation is a risk factor in CVD, contributing to unresolved inflammation and autoimmune responses in the arterial wall that can drive the progression of atherosclerosis as well as heart failure [1,2]. Chronic inflammation arises due to an inadequate resolution of the inflammatory process, which is often seen in individuals with metabolic risk factors such as obesity, diabetes, and hypertension. In acute coronary syndrome and MI, the blockage of blood flow or the rupture of plaques triggers acute inflammation, which can lead to long-term cardiac damage. Following reperfusion through coronary intervention with stents or thrombolysis, the degree of inflammatory resolution varies and holds prognostic significance for the progression of ischemic HF. Prolonged and severe inflammatory responses can result in adverse cardiac remodeling, eventually leading to HF.

Atherosclerosis is the process underlying most CVDs, characterized by the buildup of plaques within the arterial walls. Atherosclerotic cardiovascular disease (ASCVD) has evolved from being seen as a disease of passive cholesterol accumulation to a disease that is driven by chronic inflammation which initiates a plethora of biochemical and histologic phenomena that lead to atherosclerotic plaque formation narrowing the arteries and impeding blood flow and the triggering of plaque rupture events. In modern cardiology care, patients are treated with statins to reduce circulating LDLc which has been shown to reduce CVD events. However, among patients receiving statins, inflammation, assessed by high-sensitivity CRP, was a stronger predictor for risk of future cardiovascular events and death than cholesterol assessed by LDLc [2], which clearly highlights an important role for inflammation in CVD. Immune cells, particularly macrophages and T cells, are key contributors to the pathogenesis of CVD. Recent research has highlighted the significance of immune cell metabolism—specifically, the metabolites produced during cellular metabolic processes—in regulating immune cell function and influencing CVD outcomes. Metabolites such as lactate, succinate, and itaconate can act as signaling molecules, modulating immune cell activity, and altering the inflammatory environment within cardiovascular tissues. These metabolites not only reflect the metabolic state of immune cells but also actively contribute to the atherosclerotic processes by affecting plaque stability, endothelial function, and overall vascular health. Additionally, these metabolites can play a crucial role in the response to ischemia and reperfusion following MI and alter the cardiac remodeling worsening the progression of ischemic HF.

In this chapter, we will discuss the unique immunometabolic shifts occurring in CVD, with a particular focus on ASCVD, and discuss how they serve both protective and pathogenic roles and the implications for treating individuals with CVD.

Atherosclerotic plaque structure and environment

Atherosclerotic plaques develop within a unique microenvironment that is defined not only by the cellular and molecular interactions but also by distinct physical and metabolic conditions. The atherosclerotic plaque is a complex, heterogeneous structure composed of a fibrous cap, lipid core, and a variety of immune cells embedded within an extracellular matrix. The immunometabolic environment within the plaque is influenced by factors such as hypoxia, mechanical stress, and the availability of nutrients and oxygen, which collectively shape the disease's progression and stability.

The plaque's fibrous cap, primarily composed of collagen and smooth muscle cells, acts as a barrier separating the thrombogenic lipid core from the bloodstream. The integrity of this cap is critical for preventing plaque rupture, which can lead to acute cardiovascular events. Within the plaque, regions of hypoxia arise due to the imbalance between the increased metabolic demands of proliferating cells and the limited diffusion of oxygen from the lumen. Hypoxia-inducible factors (HIFs) become activated under these conditions, driving the expression of genes involved in angiogenesis, glycolysis, and inflammation, further influencing the behavior of immune cells.

The core of the plaque is often necrotic and characterized by a rich lipid environment with accumulated cholesterol crystals and cell debris. This necrotic core not only serves as a depot for lipids but also as a site of intense immune activity. The heterogeneity of the plaque environment also extends to its metabolic landscape. Variations in oxygen, pH, and nutrient availability create microdomains within the plaque that foster distinct immune cell phenotypes and functions. For example, regions of the plaque with lower oxygen levels favor the recruitment and activation of proinflammatory immune cells, while other areas may support a more reparative response. This metabolic heterogeneity is further influenced by the dynamic mechanical forces exerted by blood flow, which contribute to endothelial dysfunction and the focal nature of plaque development.

Immune cell metabolism

The metabolic pathways within immune cells are highly dynamic and adapt to the specific demands of immune activation, differentiation, and resolution of inflammation. Different immune cells, such as macrophages, T cells, and dendritic cells, rely on distinct metabolic pathways depending on their state of activation. For example, activated macrophages and effector T cells primarily utilize glycolysis to rapidly generate ATP and support the production of proinflammatory cytokines. In contrast, regulatory T cells and memory T cells rely more on oxidative phosphorylation to sustain their long-term, antiinflammatory functions. The metabolism of immune cells not only supports their energetic needs but also influences their function and fate. Metabolic intermediates and byproducts can serve as signaling molecules, regulating immune responses and shaping the overall immune landscape. As a result, immune cell metabolism plays a crucial role in both normal immune function and the pathogenesis of CVD. Almost every facet of immune cell metabolism can contribute to the pathogenesis of CVD. In the following sections, we will examine these metabolic pathways and their contributions to CVD across various immune cell types, highlighting their potential as therapeutic targets.

Metabolites in the pathogenesis of cardiovascular disease

Cholesterol and lipid metabolites

Low-density lipoproteins

Lipids are at the core of cardiovascular disease—low-density lipoproteins (LDL)—made by the liver play a central role in disease pathogenesis of CVD and particularly the development of plaques. Reduction in circulating LDLc is a key therapeutic strategy for the treatment of prevention of CVD and is targeted by several therapies, including statins, bempedoic acid, and PCSK9 inhibitors. Oxidized LDL (oxLDL) has been shown to be particularly atherogenic and is taken up by macrophages through scavenger receptors. The uptake of this oxLDL (and other modified LDL particles) results in the formation of foam cells—the main cell type of atherosclerotic plaques. These foam cells are proinflammatory and secrete cytokines to recruit more monocytes and macrophages to the plaque. Interestingly, the synthesis of fatty acids and cholesterol within macrophages can also be a key driver of atherosclerosis, evidenced by many genetic and small molecule modulators of lipogenesis (including AMPK activators, ACLY inhibitors, and FAS inhibition) having macrophage-specific effects on atherosclerosis [3–6]. In addition to macrophages, T cells have been shown to accumulate cholesterol to contribute to atherosclerosis, an effect which has been shown to be increased with age [7]. The accumulation of cholesterol promotes inflammation through changes to naïve T cell differentiation. Intracellular cholesterol in naïve T cells prevents their differentiation into Tregs and promotes their differentiation to Tfh cells [8]. In addition to cholesterol uptake and synthesis, the efflux of cholesterol by immune cells can also be an important contributor to atherosclerosis. Indeed, promotion of cholesterol efflux from macrophages has been shown to reduce atherosclerosis in animal models. Conversely, the blocking of cholesterol efflux in T cells has been shown to reduce atherosclerosis; however, this also results in T-cell apoptosis, which in turn reduced T-cell numbers in atherosclerotic plaques as well as aortic inflammation [9]. In addition to LDLc, lipoprotein(a) (LP(a)) has been shown to be a key driver of the inflammation seen in CVD. In patients with hyperlipoproteinemia(a), the content (absolute and relative) of nonclassical monocytes was higher [10]. **Lysophosphatidylcholine (LPC)** is also a major phospholipid component of oxidized low-density lipoproteins (OxLDL) and is implicated as a critical factor in the atherogenic activity of OxLDL.

Eicosanoids

In addition to lipoprotein particles and their components, several other lipid species contribute to immune cell activation and pathogenesis of cardiovascular disease, including eicosanoids such as **arachidonic acid (AA) and prostaglandins**. Eicosanoids are a class of molecules derived from 20 carbon ("eicosa" is Greek for 20) polyunsaturated fatty acids. **AA is a 20 carbon** omega-6 polyunsaturated fatty acid (PUFA) and the most abundant eicosanoid. Although eicosanoids are usually associated with proinflammatory responses [11], they are also known to play a key role in reducing inflammation by promoting the resolution of inflammation limiting immune cell infiltration, and initiating tissue repair mechanisms [12,13].

The three pathways responsible for the production of eicosanoids are recognized by the enzymes involved, such as cyclooxygenase-1 (COX-1), cyclooxygenase-2 (COX-2), lipoxygenases 5, 12, or 15 (5-LO, 12-LO, 15-LO), and cytochrome P450 (cyP450). Several studies have investigated the presence and activity of these enzymes in atherosclerosis. They found that COX-1 is expressed in normal arteries and in atherosclerotic lesions, while COX-2 is observed only in atherosclerotic plaques, mainly in macrophages [14]. COX-2 is also responsible for the production of PGE_2. PGE_2 has been viewed as one of the major mediators of inflammation; however, recent studies have demonstrated that PGE_2 can serve both pro- and antiinflammatory functions [15]. PGE_2 is an important negative regulator of neutrophil-mediated inflammation [16] and macrophage inflammation through inhibition of CCL5 [17]. In addition, to effects on macrophages, PGE_2 can also modulate platelet adhesion to ruptured plaques contributing to clot formation and thrombosis. Several PGE_2 receptor subtypes are present on platelets and have been shown to be involved in platelet aggregation [18]. However, the precise concentrations and pro- or antiaggregations effects of PGE_2 remain controversial [19]. In summary, COX-2 is highly expressed in plaque macrophages, resulting in PGE_2 production, but this seems to retain both protective and pathogenic roles in CVD.

Glucose metabolism and metabolites

Glucose and its metabolites play an especially important role in immune cells and the progression of CVD for two reasons. 1. High blood sugar (hyperglycemia) as seen in type 2 diabetes is a major risk factor for CVD. Adults with diabetes have 2–4 times increased cardiovascular risk compared with adults without diabetes, and the risk rises with worsening glycemic control. Further, diabetes has been associated with 75% increase in mortality rate in adults, and cardiovascular disease accounts for a large part of the excess mortality [20]. 2. **In response to inflammation, most immune cells dramatically shift their metabolism to favor glycolysis and down regulate Ox Phos.**

Advanced glycation end products

Hyperglycemia, glucose, and its metabolites can form advanced glycation end products (AGEs), which accumulate in the vasculature and contribute to endothelial dysfunction. The AGEs are a damage-associated molecular pattern (DAMP) which can be detected by their receptor (RAGE) on endothelial cells and macrophages, enhancing the recruitment of immune cells to sites of vascular injury and promoting atherosclerosis in diabetic mice [21]. Using bone marrow transplantation, hematopoietic RAGE signaling was shown to significantly contribute to diabetes-associated atherosclerosis [22]. Specifically in macrophages, AGE-RAGE interactions were shown to significantly attenuate cholesterol efflux to APOA1 and HDL and downregulated the cholesterol transporters Abca1 and Abcg1, at least in part through PPAR-γ-dependent regulation of these transporters [23] demonstrating an important role of these AGEs to regulate lipid metabolism and transport.

PKM2

In addition to glycation end products, glucose metabolism of lesion-residing macrophages is upregulated, such that atherosclerotic lesions can be visualized by positron emission tomography using 18F-fluorodeoxyglucose [24]. Macrophages and monocytes from individuals with CAD overuse glucose and upregulate several glycolytic genes, including PKM2 (pyruvate kinase muscle 2) [25]. PKM2 exists in tetramer or dimeric forms composed of the same monomers. When taking part in glycolysis, PKM2 is a tetramer. However, when in its dimeric form, PKM2 translocates to the nucleus where it can act as a coactivator for transcription factors implicated in the activation of the HIF1α (hypoxia-inducible factor-1α) and STAT3 (signal transducer and activator of transcription 3), which regulate proinflammatory genes [26]. Pharmacological inhibition of nuclear PKM2 translocation reduces lipopolysaccharides-induced proinflammatory cytokine secretion by macrophages and protects mice from lethal endotoxemia [26]. Consistent with PKM2 being proinflammatory, myeloid deletion of PKM2 reduced atherosclerosis through reduced inflammation and enhanced efferocytosis [27].

Lactate

Lactate is mainly generated through glycolysis in most tissues of the human body, with the highest level of production detected in muscles. In CVD it is difficult to ascertain the relative contribution of lactate from myocardium, cardiovascular tissue, smooth muscle, and immune cells; however, increased levels of lactate are associated with poor prognosis across CVDs [28–30]. Additionally, blood lactate levels have been associated with increased vascular wall thickness (a marker of atherosclerosis) [31]. Lactate, regardless of the source, can be recognized by lactate receptors on macrophages and leads to their antiinflammatory polarization [32]. Lactate promotes cardioprotective macrophage responses and preserves ventricular function after experimental MI [33] supporting a presumed role for efferocytotic-derived lactate in cardio protection after ischemic injury. However, lactate accumulation in the arterial wall has been shown to stabilize the hypoxia-inducible factor-1α (HIF1α), a transcription factor that drives the expression of proinflammatory genes in macrophages, suggesting a pro-atherosclerotic effect of lactate. While the role of lactate on different immune cell types has been extensively studied [34], further research is required in the context of CVD examining individual cell types.

HIF1α

HIF1α expression is increased in atherosclerotic plaques through PMK2 activity, lactate as well as hypoxic conditions in plaques. This increased HIF1α leads to the increase in glycolysis by upregulating the glucose transporter GLUT1. In addition, HIF1α induces the expression of key glycolytic enzymes HK2 and pyruvate dehydrogenase kinase 1 (PDK1), promoting glycolysis. Together, this results in a positive feedback loop which further enhances glycolysis, ROS production, and inflammation within atherosclerotic plaques. Furthermore, the importance of HIF1α in atherosclerosis was established by bone marrow-specific HIF1α deletion knockdown in $LDLR^{-/-}$ mice, resulting in reduced atherosclerotic plaque formation [35].

Pentose phosphate pathway

Another critical pathway in glucose metabolism is the pentose phosphate pathway (PPP), which branches from glycolysis at the level of glucose-6-phosphate. The PPP generates NADPH, a reducing agent required for the production of reactive oxygen species (ROS) in macrophages. While ROS are essential for pathogen defense, their overproduction in the context of atherosclerosis leads to oxidative stress, which can damage endothelial cells and contribute to the oxLDL, which is a key factor in foam cell formation and plaque development as described above. The NADPH oxidase family is a key source of reactive oxygen species (ROS) in the vasculature, primarily generating superoxide and hydrogen peroxide. These ROS are produced by endothelial cells, smooth muscle cells, fibroblasts, and infiltrating monocytes/macrophages. Several vascular NADPH oxidase isoforms, including Nox1, Nox2, Nox4, and Nox5, play significant roles in the development of human atherosclerosis [36,37]. Among these, the phagocytic NADPH oxidase isoform, Nox2, is particularly involved in the formation and progression of atherosclerotic lesions, predominantly through its activity in monocytes and macrophages [37–39]. Notably, the activity of Nox2 in blood phagocytes has been shown to positively correlate with carotid intima-media thickness (IMT) [40], a surrogate marker for atherosclerosis, as well as with plasma levels of matrix metalloproteinase-9 (MMP-9) [41], a marker of vascular remodeling, and an independent risk factor for atherothrombotic events, even in healthy individuals without clinical signs of atherosclerosis.

Amino acid metabolites

Arginine metabolism in immune cells

Arginine, a semiessential amino acid, is a substrate for several metabolic pathways in immune cells. Two key enzymes, nitric oxide synthase (NOS) and arginase, compete for arginine. NOS converts arginine into nitric oxide (NO) and citrulline. Endothelial cells produce NO through endothelial NOS (eNOS), while macrophages use inducible NOS (iNOS). NO is a signaling molecule with various physiological roles, including vasodilation, inhibition of platelet aggregation, and modulation of leukocyte adhesion. In the context of CVD, NO helps maintain vascular homeostasis by preventing endothelial dysfunction, reducing oxidative stress, and inhibiting inflammation [42]. It helps maintain vascular tone by relaxing smooth muscle cells, thereby preventing hypertension [43]—a major risk factor for CVD. NO also inhibits the adhesion of leukocytes to the endothelium [44], reducing inflammation and the formation of atherosclerotic plaques. In macrophages, iNOS is upregulated in response to inflammatory stimuli, and in this case, excessive NO production by iNOS can contribute to oxidative stress and tissue damage, exacerbating the inflammatory process in atherosclerotic lesions [45,46], and indeed, macrophage expression of iNOS is correlated with poor plaque stability in human coronary atherosclerotic plaque [47].

Arginase exists in two isoforms (Arginases I and II), which convert arginine into ornithine and urea. Ornithine can be further metabolized into polyamines and proline, contributing to cell proliferation and tissue repair. Arginase I is largely expressed by the liver, whereas Arginase II is found across several cell types. Importantly, increased activity and expression of arginase have been demonstrated in several pathological cardiovascular conditions, including hypertension, pulmonary arterial hypertension, atherosclerosis, myocardial ischemia, congestive heart failure, and vascular dysfunction [48]. This imbalance between arginase and NOS activity often occurs, leading to reduced NO production [48]. This shift can exacerbate endothelial dysfunction and promote atherosclerosis. Macrophages from Arg-II KO mice display reduced inflammatory cytokine production, and Arg-II KO mice have reduced atherosclerotic plaque formation with a decreased necrotic core, macrophage accumulation, and proinflammatory mediators in the plaque [49]. Together this data suggests that NO from macrophages is associated with acute inflammation but is largely protective from atherosclerosis, whereas macrophages display increased arginase activity in atherosclerosis, and this is associated with less stable more inflamed plaques.

Tryptophan metabolism and the kynurenine pathway

Tryptophan (Trp) is an essential amino acid with multiple roles in human physiology, including protein synthesis, serotonin production, and immune regulation. One of its significant metabolic pathways is the kynurenine pathway, which is increasingly recognized for its role in modulating immune responses. The kynurenine pathway is complex, generating several metabolites with diverse biological activities, including kynurenic, quinolinic, and anthranilic acids. This pathway has profound implications for cardiovascular health. The majority of tryptophan in the body is metabolized via the kynurenine pathway. This process is initiated by the enzymes indoleamine 2,3-dioxygenase (IDO) or tryptophan 2,3-dioxygenase (TDO), which convert tryptophan into N-formylkynurenine, subsequently leading to the production of kynurenine. IDO1, expressed in various immune cells like dendritic cells, macrophages, and certain endothelial cells, is a critical enzyme in this pathway. It is inducible by proinflammatory cytokines, particularly interferon-gamma (IFN-γ). The activation of IDO1 not only depletes tryptophan, suppressing the growth of pathogens and tumor cells, but also generates immunomodulatory kynurenine metabolites. IDO1 has been suggested to play a protective role in atherosclerosis due to its potential immunomodulatory effect [50]. IDO1 is expressed and upregulated in human and murine atherosclerosis where it colocalizes with macrophages [51,52]. Interestingly, in the murine systems, the absence of IDO1 was shown to protect against atherosclerosis [51]. In contrast, IDO1-mediated tryptophan depletion has antiinflammatory effects [53], and kynurenine dose-dependently decreases blood pressure in spontaneously hypertensive rats [54] which would suggest a potentially protective role of IDO1 in hypertension. The contrast of protective and pathogenic effects of IDO1 and kynurenine is likely due to its complex roles across several cell types. The depletion of tryptophan by IDO1 can suppress T-cell proliferation, promoting immune tolerance. Kynurenine promotes the differentiation of regulatory T cells (Tregs) [55], which should further promote immune tolerance. However, elevated levels of kynurenine and its metabolites have been observed in patients with CAD [56]. Studies have found that higher plasma kynurenine levels are associated with increased carotid intima-media thickness (CIMT) [57], a marker of atherosclerosis. Furthermore, in patients with heart failure, elevated kynurenine levels are correlated with worse outcomes [58]. However, these are observational correlations; therefore more research is required to understand the role of tryptophan, kynurenine, and IDO and their cell type-specific effects in CVD.

Glutamine

Glutamine is a critical amino acid in immune cell metabolism, serving as both a metabolic fuel and a precursor for biosynthetic processes. Immune cells, particularly those involved in inflammation such as macrophages and lymphocytes, have a high demand for glutamine to support their activation, proliferation, and function. Glutamine also contributes to the synthesis of glutathione (GSH), a key antioxidant that helps manage oxidative stress, which hypothetically would be protective in the context of atherosclerosis and CVD. However, circulating glutamine is associated with adverse events in patients with CAD [59]. Recent metabolomics studies have identified major changes in glutamine metabolism in macrophages upon exposure to M1- or M2-polarizing agents. Interestingly, both IL-4 and LPS-treated macrophages have been shown to increase their glutamine uptake, whereas IFN-γ + TNF-α-treated macrophages showed no change to glutamine uptake [60] and which of these inflammatory signals is more representative of what occurs in vivo is unclear. Treatment of macrophages with LPS results in a marked intracellular accumulation of succinate, which is derived from glutamine metabolism and acts as an endogenous danger signal and enhances the production of proinflammatory cytokines [61]. On the contrary, glutamine has been shown to be critical for the acquisition of the M2 polarization state and production of key antiinflammatory cytokines through its role in protein glycosylation [62]. To complicate matters further, macrophage supplementation with glutamine has been shown to increase lipid accumulation through increased lipid synthesis [63] suggesting a pro-atherogenic effect; however, the consequences of this supplementation on inflammatory cytokine production or polarization were not examined in detail. In addition to roles in atherosclerosis, glutamine is also important in its oxidative stress buffering capacity through synthesis of GSH and GSSG in response to myocardial infarction. This buffering of oxidative stress reduces ischemia reperfusion injury, although these effects are believed to largely be protective of the cardiomyocytes rather than immune cells [64]. Therefore the role of glutamine metabolism in CVD is nuanced and highly dependent on the precise inflammatory signals received, making it difficult to target therapeutically.

Homocysteine

Homocysteine (Hcy) is a sulfur-containing amino acid formed during the metabolism of methionine. Elevated levels of plasma Hcy result in a condition known as hyperhomocysteinemia (HHcy), which has long been suggested as an independent risk factor for atherosclerosis [65]. Hcy is associated with increased atherosclerosis through modulation of B-cells, T-cells, and macrophage metabolism. In macrophages, Hcy increases ROS production and MCP-1 expression to enhance atherosclerotic plaques [66]. In CD4 + T cells, Hcy enhances glucose metabolism and glycolysis, promotes interferon (IFN)-γ secretion and macrophage proinflammatory polarization, and ultimately accelerates atherosclerosis [67]. Furthermore, these T cells can release cytokines and cooperate with other immune cells, such as B cells and macrophages, to mediate HHcy-accelerated inflammation and atherosclerosis [68,69]. Several small molecules have been tested to treat HHcy-accelerated atherosclerosis and have shown promising effects through modulation of the T-cell phenotype associated with HHcy, which presents a novel therapeutic strategy for the treatment of CVD [67,69] and suggests that the effects of Hcy on atherosclerosis are a T cell rather than macrophage phenotype.

Tricarboxylic acid cycle intermediates

The mitochondrial **tricarboxylic acid (TCA) cyle**, also known as the citric acid cycle (CAC) or Krebs cycle, is crucial for ATP production. It serves as a central metabolic hub, linking various catabolic, anabolic, and anaplerotic reactions. Additionally, TCA-related metabolites play roles in diverse physiological processes, functioning as signaling molecules, epigenetic effectors, and modulators of immune and hypoxic responses. Interestingly, circulating levels of several TCA metabolites, including plasma 2-hydroxyglutarate, fumarate, and malate, were associated with increased cardiovascular risk [70]. Indeed, the disrupted TCA cycle is a hallmark of metabolism of inflammatory macrophages with increases in succinate, itaconate, and fumarate being reported [61,71,72].

Succinate

Succinate has been shown to accumulate in inflammatory macrophages through glutamine-dependent anaplerosis [61], although itaconate's inhibition of succinate dehydrogenase also contributes to these increases [73]. Succinate stabilizes HIF1α, which as described above promotes glycolysis and a proinflammatory state. Succinate acts as an inflammatory signal ligand, which can be transmitted through the receptor SUCNR1. SUCNR1 (also known as GPR91) is a G protein-coupled receptor responsible for succinate signaling and is widely expressed in systemic cell types. The effect of SUCNR1 activation in innate immune cells is environment dependent. For example, in human immature dendritic cells, SUCNR1 controls its chemotaxis in a succinate concentration-dependent manner [74]. However, the activation of SUCNR1 pathway seems to occur only in the acute phase of stimulation, since SUCNR1 is rapidly downregulated following the activation of dendritic cells. Interestingly, succinate has been shown to drive inflammation and cytokine release from macrophages; however, myeloid-specific deletion of SUCNR1 induced inflammation and worsened adipose tissue insulin resistance which highlights how succinate's inflammatory effects are likely not mediated through SUCNR1. Consistent with the inflammatory effects of succinate, succinate injections were shown to worsen atherosclerotic plaque formation in ApoE-/- mice [75] although whether these effects were specific to macrophages is unlikely.

In addition to effects on atherosclerosis, succinate accumulation is a metabolic signature of ischemia. During ischemia, the lack of blood flow results in the loss of ATP, lactate accumulation, and the buildup of metabolites, including those within the CAC, purine nucleotide degradation pathways, and those involved in fatty acid and amino acid metabolisms. However, this succinate is largely produced by the cardiac tissue itself rather than infiltrating immune cells and is therefore outside of the scope of this book chapter and has been reviewed elsewhere [76].

Itaconate

Itaconate is a myeloid-specific metabolite produced in response to inflammation through diversion from the TCA cycle by the enzyme Aconitase Decarboxylase 1 (ACOD1). This macrophage-specific enzyme (encoded by the gene *Irg1*) causes a large rewiring of metabolism. Itaconate has been proposed to work through three main mechanisms: 1. electrophilic modification of cysteine restudies [72,77], 2. inhibition of enzymes using structurally similar metabolites [73,78,79] and 3. breakdown into other metabolites mesaconate and citraconate [80,81]. Importantly, several cell-permeable derivatives have been made, including 4-octyl itaconate (4-OI), which has increased electrophilic properties and overlapping and unique mechanisms to itaconate [82]. Recently, two studies have shown that deletion of Irg1 exacerbates atherosclerosis [83,84]. Additionally, both studies also used 4-OI supplementation to limit the progression of atherosclerosis through the activation of Nrf2 and subsequent inhibition of inflammation [83,84]. Importantly, while both itaconate and 4-OI activate Nrf2, 4-OI is much more potent KEAP1 inhibitor and therefore Nrf2 activator than itaconate. Additionally, it is also likely that itaconate's regulation of hepatic lipid oxidation could also be contributing to the endogenous antiatherosclerotic effects of itaconate [85].

In addition to atherosclerosis, elevated levels of Irg1 and Nrf2 expression have also been shown to be associated with abdominal aortic aneurysm (AAA) lesions, although shRNA-mediated IRG1 knockdown exacerbated AAA growth and lesion inflammation [86], which suggests the increases in *Irg1* in human AAA are consequences not the cause of the lesions.

Short-chain fatty acids

Butyrate and propionate

Butyrate and propionate are short-chain fatty acids (SCFAs) produced primarily by the fermentation of dietary fibers by gut microbiota. These metabolites are not only key players in gut health but also have systemic effects, including significant roles in immune regulation. Largely seen as antiinflammatory molecules, experimental evidence suggests that these SCFAs are protective against CVD. These SCFAs have several distinct mechanisms of action, including binding of G Protein-Coupled Receptors (GPCRs), such as GPR41, GPR43, and GPR109A, on the surface of immune cells, inhibition of Histone Deacetylase (HDAC), to influence gene expression and cellular differentiation as well as promoting a general metabolic shift to an antiinflammatory phenotype [87].

Both butyrate and propionate have been shown to reduce atherosclerosis in experimental models by suppressing inflammation. For example, butyrate can inhibit the expression of vascular cell adhesion molecule-1 (VCAM-1) on endothelial cells [88], reducing the adhesion of monocytes and the subsequent formation of atherosclerotic plaques. Propionate has similar effects, promoting the differentiation of Tregs [89], which help maintain immune tolerance and reduce inflammation within atherosclerotic lesions. In addition, in a study of patients with coronary artery disease, lower circulating levels of butyrate and propionate were associated with increased systemic inflammation and greater atherosclerotic burden [90].

In addition to modulating atherosclerosis, SCFAs have also been associated with lower blood pressure and improved outcomes in heart failure. Propionate has been shown to lower blood pressure in animal models of hypertension. This effect is partly mediated by its action on immune cells within the vascular system [91]. In hypertensive mice, oral administration of propionate led to a significant reduction in blood pressure. This was accompanied by a decrease in inflammatory markers in the aorta and kidneys, highlighting the role of propionate in modulating immune-driven inflammation in hypertension [91]. Experimental studies in rodents have demonstrated that butyrate supplementation can attenuate cardiac hypertrophy and fibrosis in models of heart failure [92,93]. These beneficial effects are linked to butyrate's ability to reduce proinflammatory cytokine production and enhance the antiinflammatory activity of Tregs within the heart. Butyrate and propionate, as key metabolites produced by gut microbiota, have profound effects on immune cell function that influence cardiovascular health. Their ability to modulate inflammation, immune cell polarization, and endothelial function positions these SCFAs as important regulators in the pathogenesis of cardiovascular disease.

Conclusion

The intricate interplay between immune cell metabolism and CVD pathogenesis highlights the significant role of metabolic processes in shaping immune responses within the cardiovascular system. The metabolites generated through these pathways serve not only as energy sources but also as critical signaling molecules that modulate immune cell behavior and the inflammatory milieu. Understanding these immunometabolic processes opens up new avenues for therapeutic intervention. By targeting specific metabolic pathways or modulating key metabolites, it may be possible to attenuate the chronic inflammation that drives atherosclerosis, myocardial infarction, and other cardiovascular conditions. The therapeutic potential of such approaches is underscored by the success of interventions like statins and antiinflammatory agents, which already target related pathways with notable efficacy. However, the complexity of immunometabolism also presents challenges. The dual roles of certain metabolites, which can be either protective or pathogenic depending on context, necessitate a nuanced approach to therapeutic development. Future research must aim to unravel these complexities, with a focus on the context-specific effects of metabolic interventions and the potential for personalized medicine approaches in treating CVD. As spatial metabolomics from human samples advances, we will gain important insights into the context-dependent effects in real disease scenarios to address these questions. These insights will help understand the cellular, metabolic, and environmental heterogeneity in CVD, especially in the context of atherosclerosis and ischemia reperfusion injury.

In conclusion, the metabolic pathways within immune cells represent a productive ground for innovation in cardiovascular therapy. By continuing to explore and understand the dynamic interactions between metabolism and immunity, we can move closer to developing more effective strategies for preventing and treating cardiovascular diseases.

AI disclosure

During the preparation of this work, the author(s) used ChatGPT for editing and clarity. After using this tool/service, the author(s) reviewed and edited the content as needed and take(s) full responsibility for the content of the publication.

References

[1] Halade GV, Lee DH. Inflammation and resolution signaling in cardiac repair and heart failure. eBioMedicine 2022;79. Available from: https://doi.org/10.1016/j.ebiom.2022.103992, http://www.journals.elsevier.com/ebiomedicine/.

[2] Ridker PM, Bhatt DL, Pradhan AD, Glynn RJ, MacFadyen JG, Nissen SE. Inflammation and cholesterol as predictors of cardiovascular events among patients receiving statin therapy: a collaborative analysis of three randomised trials. Lancet 2023;401(10384):1293–301. Available from: https://doi.org/10.1016/S0140-6736(23)00215-5, http://www.journals.elsevier.com/the-lancet/.

[3] Day EA, Townsend LK, Rehal S, Batchuluun B, Wang D, Morrow MR, Lu R, Lundenberg L, Lu JH, Desjardins EM, Smith TKT, Raphenya AR, McArthur AG, Fullerton MD, Steinberg GR. Macrophage AMPK β1 activation by PF-06409577 reduces the inflammatory response, cholesterol synthesis, and atherosclerosis in mice. iScience 2023;26(11). Available from: https://doi.org/10.1016/j.isci.2023.108269, http://www.cell.com/iscience.

[4] Baardman J, Verberk SGS, van der Velden S, Gijbels MJJ, van Roomen CPPA, Sluimer JC, Broos JY, Griffith GR, Prange KHM, van Weeghel M, Lakbir S, Molenaar D, Meinster E, Neele AE, Kooij G, de Vries HE, Lutgens E, Wellen KE, de Winther MPJ, Van den Bossche J. Macrophage ATP citrate lyase deficiency stabilizes atherosclerotic plaques. Nat Commun 2020;11(1). Available from: https://doi.org/10.1038/s41467-020-20141-z, http://www.nature.com/ncomms/index.html.

[5] Schneider JG, Yang Z, Chakravarthy MV, Lodhi IJ, Wei X, Turk J, Semenkovich CF. Macrophage fatty-acid synthase deficiency decreases diet-induced atherosclerosis. J Biol Chem 2010;285(30):23398–409. Available from: https://doi.org/10.1074/jbc.M110.100321, http://www.jbc.org/content/285/30/23398.full.pdf+html, United.

[6] Day EA, Ford RJ, Smith BK, Houde VP, Stypa S, Rehal S, et al. Salsalate reduces atherosclerosis through AMPKβ1 in mice. Mol Metabol 2021;53:101321. Available from: https://doi.org/10.1016/j.molmet.2021.101321.

[7] Larbi A, Dupuis G, Khalil A, Douziech N, Fortin C, Fülöp T. Differential role of lipid rafts in the functions of CD4+ and CD8+ human T lymphocytes with aging. Cellular Signal 2006;18(7):1017–30. Available from: https://doi.org/10.1016/j.cellsig.2005.08.016.

[8] Gaddis DE, Padgett LE, Wu R, McSkimming C, Romines V, Taylor AM, McNamara CA, Kronenberg M, Crotty S, Thomas MJ, Sorci-Thomas MG, Hedrick CC. Apolipoprotein AI prevents regulatory to follicular helper T cell switching during atherosclerosis. Nat Commun 2018;9(1). Available from: https://doi.org/10.1038/s41467-018-03493-5, http://www.nature.com/ncomms/index.html.

[9] Bazioti V, La Rose AM, Maassen S, Bianchi F, de Boer R, Halmos B, Dabral D, Guilbaud E, Flohr-Svendsen A, Groenen AG, Marmolejo-Garza A, Koster MH, Kloosterhuis NJ, Havinga R, Pranger AT, Langelaar-Makkinje M, de Bruin A, van de Sluis B, Kohan AB, Yvan-Charvet L, van den Bogaart G, Westerterp M. T cell cholesterol efflux suppresses apoptosis and senescence and increases atherosclerosis in middle aged mice. Nat Commun 2022;13(1). Available from: https://doi.org/10.1038/s41467-022-31135-4.

[10] Afanasieva OI, Filatova AY, Arefieva TI, Klesareva EA, Tyurina AV, Radyukhina NV, Ezhov MV, Pokrovsky SN. The association of lipoprotein(a) and circulating monocyte subsets with severe coronary atherosclerosis. J Cardiovasc Dev Dis 2021;8(6). Available from: https://doi.org/10.3390/jcdd8060063, https://www.mdpi.com/2308-3425/8/6/63/pdf.

[11] Aoki T, Narumiya S. Prostaglandins and chronic inflammation. Trends Pharmacol Sci 2012;33(6):304–11. Available from: https://doi.org/10.1016/j.tips.2012.02.004.

[12] Pan WH, Hu X, Chen B, Xu QC, Mei HX. The effect and mechanism of lipoxin A4 on neutrophil function in LPS-induced lung injury. Inflammation 2022;45(5):1950–67. Available from: https://doi.org/10.1007/s10753-022-01666-5, http://www.wkap.nl/journalhome.htm/0360-3997.

[13] Serhan CN, Levy BD. Resolvins in inflammation: emergence of the pro-resolving superfamily of mediators. J Clin Invest 2018;128(7):2657–69. Available from: https://doi.org/10.1172/JCI97943, https://www.jci.org/articles/view/97943/pdf.

[14] Schonbeck U, Sukhova GK, Graber P, Coulter S, Libby P. Augmented expression of cyclooxygenase-2 in human atherosclerotic lesions. Am J Pathol 1999;155(4):1281–91. Available from: https://doi.org/10.1016/S0002-9440(10)65230-3, http://ajp.amjpathol.org/.

[15] Piper K, Garelnabi M. Eicosanoids: Atherosclerosis and cardiometabolic health. J Clin Translat Endocrinol 2020;19. Available from: https://doi.org/10.1016/j.jcte.2020.100216, http://www.journals.elsevier.com/journal-of-clinical-and-translational-endocrinology/.

[16] Frolov A, Yang L, Dong H, Hammock BD, Crofford LJ. Anti-inflammatory properties of prostaglandin E2: Deletion of microsomal prostaglandin E synthase-1 exacerbates non-immune inflammatory arthritis in mice. Prostaglandins Leukotrienes and Essential Fatty Acids 2013;89(5):351–8. Available from: https://doi.org/10.1016/j.plefa.2013.08.003.

[17] Qian X, Zhang J, Liu J. Tumor-secreted PGE2 Inhibits CCL5 Production in Activated Macrophages through cAMP/PKA Signaling Pathway. J Biol Chem 2011;286(3):2111–20. Available from: https://doi.org/10.1074/jbc.m110.154971.

[18] Philipose S, Konya V, Sreckovic I, Marsche G, Lippe IT, Peskar BA, Heinemann A, Schuligoi R. The prostaglandin E2 receptor EP4 is expressed by human platelets and potently inhibits platelet aggregation and thrombus formation. Arterioscl Thromb Vascul Biol 2010;30(12):2416−23. Available from: https://doi.org/10.1161/ATVBAHA.110.216374.

[19] Braune S, Küpper JH, Jung F. Effect of prostanoids on human platelet function: an overview. Int J Mol Sci 2020;21(23):1−20. Available from: https://doi.org/10.3390/ijms21239020, https://www.mdpi.com/1422-0067/21/23/9020/pdf.

[20] Dal Canto E, Ceriello A, Rydén L, Ferrini M, Hansen TB, Schnell O, Standl E, Beulens JWJ. Diabetes as a cardiovascular risk factor: An overview of global trends of macro and micro vascular complications. Eur J Prevent Cardiol 2019;26(2):25−32. Available from: https://doi.org/10.1177/2047487319878371, http://cpr.sagepub.com/content/by/year.

[21] Egaña-Gorroño L, López-Díez R, Yepuri G, Ramirez LS, Reverdatto S, Gugger PF, Shekhtman A, Ramasamy R, Schmidt AM. Receptor for advanced glycation end products (Rage) and mechanisms and therapeutic opportunities in diabetes and cardiovascular disease: Insights from human subjects and animal models. Front Cardiovasc Med 2020;7. Available from: https://doi.org/10.3389/fcvm.2020.00037, http://www.frontiersin.org/journals/cardiovascular-medicine.

[22] Koulis C, Kanellakis P, Pickering RJ, Tsorotes D, Murphy AJ, Gray SP, Thomas MC, Jandeleit-Dahm KAM, Cooper ME, Allen TJ. Role of bone-marrow- and non-bone-marrow-derived receptor for advanced glycation end-products (RAGE) in a mouse model of diabetes-associated atherosclerosis. Clin Sci 2014;127(7):485−97. Available from: https://doi.org/10.1042/cs20140045.

[23] Daffu G, Shen X, Senatus L, Thiagarajan D, Abedini A, Del Pozo CH, Rosario R, Song F, Friedman RA, Ramasamy R, Schmidt AM. RAGE suppresses ABCG1-mediated macrophage cholesterol efflux in diabetes. Diabetes 2015;64(12):4046−60. Available from: https://doi.org/10.2337/db15-0575, http://diabetes.diabetesjournals.org/content/64/12/4046.full.pdf+html.

[24] Rudd JHF, Warburton EA, Fryer TD, Jones HA, Clark JC, Antoun N, Johnström P, Davenport AP, Kirkpatrick PJ, Arch BN, Pickard JD, Weissberg PL. Imaging atherosclerotic plaque inflammation with [18 F]-fluorodeoxyglucose positron emission tomography. Circulation 2002;105(23):2708−11. Available from: https://doi.org/10.1161/01.cir.0000020548.60110.76.

[25] Shirai T, Nazarewicz RR, Wallis BB, Yanes RE, Watanabe R, Hilhorst M, Tian L, Harrison DG, Giacomini JC, Assimes TL, Goronzy JJ, Weyand CM. The glycolytic enzyme PKM2 bridges metabolic and inflammatory dysfunction in coronary artery disease. J Exp Med 2016;213(3):337−54. Available from: https://doi.org/10.1084/jem.20150900, http://jem.rupress.org/content/213/3/337.full.pdf.

[26] Palsson-Mcdermott EM, Curtis AM, Goel G, Lauterbach MAR, Sheedy FJ, Gleeson LE, Van Den Bosch MWM, Quinn SR, Domingo-Fernandez R, Johnson DGW, Jiang JK, Israelsen WJ, Keane J, Thomas C, Clish C, Vanden Heiden M, Xavier RJ, O'Neill LAJ. Pyruvate kinase M2 regulates hif-1α activity and il-1β induction and is a critical determinant of the warburg effect in LPS-activated macrophages. Metabolism 2015;21(1):65−80. Available from: https://doi.org/10.1016/j.cmet.2014.12.005, http://www.cellmetabolism.org/.

[27] Doddapattar P, Dev R, Ghatge M, Patel RB, Jain M, Dhanesha N, Lentz SR, Chauhan AK. Myeloid cell PKM2 deletion enhances efferocytosis and reduces atherosclerosis. Circul Res 2022;130(9):1289−305. Available from: https://doi.org/10.1161/CIRCRESAHA.121.320704, https://www.ovid.com/product-details.454.html.

[28] Vermeulen RP, Hoekstra M, Nijsten MWN, van der Horst IC, van Pelt LJ, Jessurun GA, Jaarsma T, Zijlstra F, van den Heuvel AF. Clinical correlates of arterial lactate levels in patients with ST-segment elevation myocardial infarction at admission: A descriptive study. Crit Care 2010;14(5). Available from: https://doi.org/10.1186/cc9253Netherlands, http://ccforum.com/content/14/5/R164.

[29] Biegus J, Zymliński R, Sokolski M, Jankowska EA, Banasiak W, Ponikowski P. Elevated lactate in acute heart failure patients with intracellular iron deficiency as an identifier of poor outcome. Kardiol Polska 2019;77(3):347−54. Available from: https://doi.org/10.5603/KP.a2019.0014, https://ojs.kardiologiapolska.pl/kp/article/view/KP.a2019.0014/10065.

[30] Zymliński R, Biegus J, Sokolski M, Siwołowski P, Nawrocka-Millward S, Todd J, Jankowska EA, Banasiak W, Cotter G, Cleland JG, Ponikowski P. Increased blood lactate is prevalent and identifies poor

[31] Shantha GPS, Wasserman B, Astor BC, Coresh J, Brancati F, Sharrett AR, Young JH. Association of blood lactate with carotid atherosclerosis: The Atherosclerosis Risk in Communities (ARIC) Carotid MRI Study. Atherosclerosis 2013;228(1):249–55. Available from: https://doi.org/10.1016/j.atherosclerosis.2013.02.014.

[32] Morioka S, Perry JSA, Raymond MH, Medina CB, Zhu Y, Zhao L, Serbulea V, Onengut-Gumuscu S, Leitinger N, Kucenas S, Rathmell JC, Makowski L, Ravichandran KS. Efferocytosis induces a novel SLC program to promote glucose uptake and lactate release. Nature 2018;563(7733):714–18. Available from: https://doi.org/10.1038/s41586-018-0735-5, http://www.nature.com/nature/index.html.

[33] Chen Y, Wu G, Li M, Hesse M, Ma Y, Chen W, Huang H, Liu Y, Xu W, Tang Y, Zheng H, Li C, Lin Z, Chen G, Liao W, Liao Y, Bin J, Chen Y. LDHA-mediated metabolic reprogramming promoted cardiomyocyte proliferation by alleviating ROS and inducing M2 macrophage polarization. Redox Biol 2022;56:102446. Available from: https://doi.org/10.1016/j.redox.2022.102446.

[34] Caslin HL, Abebayehu D, Pinette JA, Ryan JJ. Lactate is a metabolic mediator that shapes immune cell fate and function. Front Physiol 2021;12. Available from: https://doi.org/10.3389/fphys.2021.688485, http://www.frontiersin.org/Physiology/archive/.

[35] Aarup A, Pedersen TX, Junker N, Christoffersen C, Bartels ED, Madsen M, Nielsen CH, Nielsen LB. Hypoxia-inducible factor-1α expression in macrophages promotes development of atherosclerosis. Arterioscl Thromb Vasc Biol 2016;36(9):1782–90. Available from: https://doi.org/10.1161/ATVBAHA.116.307830, http://atvb.ahajournals.org/.

[36] Azumi H, Inoue N, Ohashi Y, Terashima M, Mori T, Fujita H, Awano K, Kobayashi K, Maeda K, Hata K, Shinke T, Kobayashi S, Hirata Ki, Kawashima S, Itabe H, Hayashi Y, Imajoh-Ohmi S, Itoh H, Yokoyama M. Superoxide generation in directional coronary atherectomy specimens of patients with angina pectoris: Important role of NAD(P)H oxidase. Arterioscl Thromb Vasc Biol 2002;22(11):1838–44. Available from: https://doi.org/10.1161/01.ATV.0000037101.40667.62.

[37] Sorescu D, Weiss D, Lassègue B, Clempus RE, Szöcs K, Sorescu GP, Valppu L, Quinn MT, Lambeth JD, Vega JD, Taylor WR, Griendling KK. Superoxide production and expression of Nox family proteins in human atherosclerosis. Circulation 2002;105(12):1429–35. Available from: https://doi.org/10.1161/01.CIR.0000012917.74432.66.

[38] Kalinina N, Agrotis A, Tararak E, Antropova Y, Kanellakis P, Ilyinskaya O, Quinn MT, Smirnov V, Bobik A. Cytochrome b558-dependent NAD(P)H oxidase-phox units in smooth muscle and macrophages of atherosclerotic lesions. Arterioscl Thromb Vasc Biol 2002;22(12):2037–43. Available from: https://doi.org/10.1161/01.ATV.0000040222.02255.0F.

[39] Madrigal-Matute J, Fernandez-Laso V, Sastre C, Llamas-Granda P, Egido J, Martin-Ventura JL, Zalba G, Blanco-Colio LM. TWEAK/Fn14 interaction promotes oxidative stress through NADPH oxidase activation in macrophages. Cardiovasc Res 2015;108(1):139–47. Available from: https://doi.org/10.1093/cvr/cvv204, http://cardiovascres.oxfordjournals.org/.

[40] Zalba G, Beloqui O, José GS, Moreno MU, Fortuño A. J. Díez, NADPH oxidase-dependent superoxide production is associated with carotid intima-media thickness in subjects free of clinical atherosclerotic disease. Arterioscl Thromb Vasc Biol 2005;25(7):1452–7. Available from: https://doi.org/10.1161/01.ATV.0000168411.72483.08.

[41] Zalba G, Fortuño A, Orbe J, San José G, Moreno MU, Belzunce M, Rodríguez JA, Beloqui O, Páramo JA, Díez J. Phagocytic NADPH oxidase-dependent superoxide production stimulates matrix metalloproteinase-9: Implications for human atherosclerosis. Arterioscl Thromb Vasc Biol 2007;27(3):587–93. Available from: https://doi.org/10.1161/01.ATV.0000256467.25384.c6.

[42] Cyr AR, Huckaby LV, Shiva SS, Zuckerbraun BS. Nitric oxide and endothelial dysfunction. Crit Care Clin 2020;36(2):307–21. Available from: https://doi.org/10.1016/j.ccc.2019.12.009, http://www.elsevier.com/inca/publications/store/6/2/3/1/3/2/index.htt.

[43] Chen K, Pittman RN, Popel AS. Nitric oxide in the vasculature: Where does it come from and where does it go? A quantitative perspective. Antioxidants Redox Signal 2008;10(7):1185–98. Available from: https://doi.org/10.1089/ars.2007.1959.
[44] D.N. Granger, E. Senchenkova, Leukocyte–Endothelial Cell Adhesion. (2010).
[45] Detmers PA, Hernandez M, Mudgett J, Hassing H, Burton C, Mundt S, Chun S, Fletcher D, Card DJ, Lisnock JM, Weikel R, Bergstrom JD, Shevell DE, Hermanowski-Vosatka A, Sparrow CP, Chao YS, Rader DJ, Wright SD, Pure E. Deficiency in inducible nitric oxide synthase results in reduced atherosclerosis in apolipoprotein E-deficient mice. J Immunol 2000;165(6):3430–5. Available from: https://doi.org/10.4049/jimmunol.165.6.3430, http://www.jimmunol.org/.
[46] Kuhlencordt PJ, Chen J, Han F, Astern J, Huang PL. Genetic deficiency of inducible nitric oxide synthase reduces atherosclerosis and lowers plasma lipid peroxides in apolipoprotein E-knockout mice. Circulation 2001;103(25):3099–104. Available from: https://doi.org/10.1161/01.CIR.103.25.3099, http://circ.ahajournals.org.
[47] Depre C, Havaux X, Renkin J, Vanoverschelde JLJ, Wijns W. Expression of inducible nitric oxide synthase in human coronary atherosclerotic plaque. Cardiovasc Res 1999;41(2):465–72. Available from: https://doi.org/10.1016/S0008-6363(98)00304-6.
[48] Pernow J, Jung C. Arginase as a potential target in the treatment of cardiovascular disease: Reversal of arginine steal? Cardiovasc Res 2013;98(3):334–43. Available from: https://doi.org/10.1093/cvr/cvt036.
[49] Ming X-F, Rajapakse AG, Yepuri G, Xiong Y, Carvas JM, Ruffieux J, Scerri I, Wu Z, Popp K, Li J, Sartori C, Scherrer U, Kwak BR, Montani J-P, Yang Z. Arginase II promotes macrophage inflammatory responses through mitochondrial reactive oxygen species, contributing to insulin resistance and atherogenesis. J Am Heart Assoc 2012;1(4). Available from: https://doi.org/10.1161/jaha.112.000992.
[50] Ramprasath T, Han YM, Zhang D, Yu CJ, Zou MH. Tryptophan catabolism and inflammation: a novel therapeutic target for aortic diseases. Front Immunol 2021;12. Available from: https://doi.org/10.3389/fimmu.2021.731701, https://www.frontiersin.org/journals/immunology#.
[51] Metghalchi S, Ponnuswamy P, Simon T, Haddad Y, Laurans L, Clément M, Dalloz M, Romain M, Esposito B, Koropoulis V, Lamas B, Paul J-L, Cottin Y, Kotti S, Bruneval P, Callebert J, den Ruijter H, Launay J-M, Danchin N, Sokol H, Tedgui A, Taleb S, Mallat Z. Indoleamine 2,3-dioxygenase fine-tunes immune homeostasis in atherosclerosis and colitis through repression of interleukin-10 production. Cell Metabol 2015;22(3):460–71. Available from: https://doi.org/10.1016/j.cmet.2015.07.004.
[52] Niinisalo P, Oksala N, Levula M, Pelto-Huikko M, Järvinen O, Salenius JP, Kytömäki L, Soini JT, Kähönen M, Laaksonen R, Hurme M, Lehtimäki T. Activation of indoleamine 2,3-dioxygenase-induced tryptophan degradation in advanced atherosclerotic plaques: Tampere Vascular Study. Ann Med 2010;42(1):55–63. Available from: https://doi.org/10.3109/07853890903321559.
[53] Seo SK, Kwon B. Immune regulation through tryptophan metabolism. Exp Mol Med 2023;55(7):1371–9. Available from: https://doi.org/10.1038/s12276-023-01028-7, https://www.nature.com/emm/.
[54] Wang Y, Liu H, McKenzie G, Witting PK, Stasch JP, Hahn M, Changsirivathanathamrong D, Wu BJ, Ball HJ, Thomas SR, et al. Kynurenine is a novel endothelium-derived relaxing factor produced during inflammation. Nat Med 2010;16:279. Available from: https://doi.org/10.1038/NM.2092.
[55] Stone TW, Williams RO. Modulation of T cells by tryptophan metabolites in the kynurenine pathway. Trends Pharm Sci 2023;44(7):442–56. Available from: https://doi.org/10.1016/j.tips.2023.04.006, http://www.elsevier.com/locate/tips.
[56] Gáspár R, Halmi D, Demján V, Berkecz R, Pipicz M, Csont T. Kynurenine Pathway metabolites as potential clinical biomarkers in coronary artery disease. Front Immunol 2022;12. Available from: https://doi.org/10.3389/fimmu.2021.768560, https://www.frontiersin.org/journals/immunology#.
[57] Hinderliter A, Padilla RL, Gillespie BW, Levin NW, Kotanko P, Kiser M, Finkelstein F, Rajagopalan S, Saran R. Association of carotid intima-media thickness with cardiovascular risk factors and patient outcomes in advanced chronic kidney disease: The RRI-CKD study. Clin Nephrol 2015;84(1):10–20. Available from: https://doi.org/10.5414/CN108494, http://www.dustri.com/index.php?id = 8&no_cache = 1&magId = 20&volId = 182&issueId = 13473.

[58] Lund A, Nordrehaug JE, Slettom G, Solvang SEH, Pedersen EKR, Midttun Ø, Ulvik A, Ueland PM, Nygard O, Giil LM. Plasma kynurenines and prognosis in patients with heart failure. PLoS ONE 2020;15(1). Available from: https://doi.org/10.1371/journal.pone.0227365, https://journals.plos.org/plosone/article/file?id = 10.1371/journal.pone.0227365&type = printable.

[59] Shah SH, Bain JR, Muehlbauer MJ, Stevens RD, Crosslin DR, Haynes C, Dungan J, Newby LK, Hauser ER, Ginsburg GS, Newgard CB, Kraus WE. Association of a peripheral blood metabolic profile with coronary artery disease and risk of subsequent cardiovascular events. Circul: Cardiovasc Genet 2010;3(2):207−14. Available from: https://doi.org/10.1161/CIRCGENETICS.109.852814.

[60] Tavakoli S, Downs K, Short JD, Nguyen HN, Lai Y, Jerabek PA, Goins B, Toczek J, Sadeghi MM, Asmis R. Characterization of macrophage polarization states using combined measurement of 2-deoxyglucose and glutamine accumulation: Implications for imaging of atherosclerosis. Arterioscl Thromb Vasc Biol 2017;37(10):1840−8. Available from: https://doi.org/10.1161/ATVBAHA.117.308848, http://atvb.ahajournals.org/.

[61] Tannahill GM, Curtis AM, Adamik J, Palsson-Mcdermott EM, McGettrick AF, Goel G, Frezza C, Bernard NJ, Kelly B, Foley NH, et al. Succinate is a danger signal that induces IL-1β via HIF-1α. Nature 2013;496:238. Available from: https://doi.org/10.1038/NATURE11986.

[62] Jha AK, Huang SCC, Sergushichev A, Lampropoulou V, Ivanova Y, Loginicheva E, Chmielewski K, Stewart KM, Ashall J, Everts B, Pearce EJ, Driggers EM, Artyomov MN. Network integration of parallel metabolic and transcriptional data reveals metabolic modules that regulate macrophage polarization. Immunity 2015;42(3):419−30. Available from: https://doi.org/10.1016/j.immuni.2015.02.005, www.immunity.com.

[63] Rom O, Grajeda-Iglesias C, Najjar M, Abu-Saleh N, Volkova N, Dar DE, Hayek T, Aviram M. Atherogenicity of amino acids in the lipid-laden macrophage model system in vitro and in atherosclerotic mice: a key role for triglyceride metabolism. J Nutr Biochem 2017;45:24−38. Available from: https://doi.org/10.1016/j.jnutbio.2017.02.023, http://www.elsevier.com/locate/jnutbio.

[64] Liu J., Marchase R.B., Chatham J.C.Glutamine-induced protection of isolated rat heart from ischemia/reperfusion injury is mediated via the hexosamine biosynthesis pathway and increased protein O-GlcNAc levels. J Mol Cell Cardiol 2007;42(1):177−185. Available from: https://doi.org/10.1016/j.yjmcc.2006.09.015.

[65] McCully KS. Homocysteine and vascular disease. Nat Med 1996;2(4):386−9. Available from: https://doi.org/10.1038/nm0496-386.

[66] Dai J, Li W, Chang L, Zhang Z, Tang C, Wang N, Zhu Y, Wang X. Role of redox factor-1 in hyperhomocysteinemia-accelerated atherosclerosis. Free Rad Biol Med 2006;41(10):1566−77. Available from: https://doi.org/10.1016/j.freeradbiomed.2006.08.020.

[67] Lü Sl, Dang Gh, Deng Jc, Liu Hy, Liu B, Yang J, Ma Xl, Miao Yt, Jiang Ct, Xu Qb, Wang X, Feng J. Shikonin attenuates hyperhomocysteinemia-induced CD4 + T cell inflammatory activation and atherosclerosis in ApoE − / − mice by metabolic suppression. Acta Pharm Sin 2020;41(1):47−55. Available from: https://doi.org/10.1038/s41401-019-0308-7, http://www.nature.com.

[68] Deng J, Lü S, Liu H, Liu B, Jiang C, Xu Q, Feng J, Wang X. Homocysteine activates B cells via regulating PKM2-dependent metabolic reprogramming. J Immunol 2017;198(1):170−83. Available from: https://doi.org/10.4049/jimmunol.1600613, http://www.jimmunol.org/content/198/1/170.full.pdf.

[69] Ma K, Lv S, Liu B, Liu Z, Luo Y, Kong W, Xu Q, Feng J, Wang X. CTLA4-IgG ameliorates homocysteine-accelerated atherosclerosis by inhibiting T-cell overactivation in apoE-/- mice. Cardiovasc Res 2013;97(2):349−59. Available from: https://doi.org/10.1093/cvr/cvs330.

[70] Santos JL, Ruiz-Canela M, Razquin C, Clish CB, Guasch-Ferré M, Babio N, Corella D, Gómez-Gracia E, Fiol M, Estruch R, Lapetra J, Fitó M, Aros F, Serra-Majem L, Liang L, Martínez MÁ, Toledo E, Salas-Salvadó J, Hu FB, Martínez-González MA. Circulating citric acid cycle metabolites and risk of cardiovascular disease in the PREDIMED study. Nutr Metabol Cardiovasc Dis 2023;33(4):835−43. Available from: https://doi.org/10.1016/j.numecd.2023.01.002, http://www.elsevier.com/wps/find/journaldescription.cws_home/704955/description#description.

[71] Hooftman A, Peace CG, Ryan DG, Day EA, Yang M, McGettrick AF, Yin M, Montano EN, Huo L, Toller-Kawahisa JE, Zecchini V, Ryan TAJ, Bolado-Carrancio A, Casey AM, Prag HA, Costa ASH, De

Los Santos G, Ishimori M, Wallace DJ, Venuturupalli S, Nikitopoulou E, Frizzell N, Johansson C, Von Kriegsheim A, Murphy MP, Jefferies C, Frezza C, O'Neill LAJ. Macrophage fumarate hydratase restrains mtRNA-mediated interferon production. Nature 2023;615(7952):490–8. Available from: https://doi.org/10.1038/s41586-023-05720-6, https://www.nature.com/nature/.

[72] Mills EL, Ryan DG, Prag HA, Dikovskaya D, Menon D, Zaslona Z, Jedrychowski MP, Costa ASH, Higgins M, Hams E, Szpyt J, Runtsch MC, King MS, McGouran JF, Fischer R, Kessler BM, McGettrick AF, Hughes MM, Carroll RG, Booty LM, Knatko EV, Meakin PJ, Ashford MLJ, Modis LK, Brunori G, Sévin DC, Fallon PG, Caldwell ST, Kunji ERS, Chouchani ET, Frezza C, Dinkova-Kostova AT, Hartley RC, Murphy MP, O'Neill LA. Itaconate is an anti-inflammatory metabolite that activates Nrf2 via alkylation of KEAP1. Nature 2018;556(7699):113–17. Available from: https://doi.org/10.1038/nature25986, http://www.nature.com/nature/index.html.

[73] Lampropoulou V, Sergushichev A, Bambouskova M, Nair S, Vincent EE, Loginicheva E, Cervantes-Barragan L, Ma X, Huang SCC, Griss T, Weinheimer CJ, Khader S, Randolph GJ, Pearce EJ, Jones RG, Diwan A, Diamond MS, Artyomov MN. Itaconate Links Inhibition of Succinate Dehydrogenase with Macrophage Metabolic Remodeling and Regulation of Inflammation. Cell Metab 2016;24(1):158–66. Available from: https://doi.org/10.1016/j.cmet.2016.06.004, http://www.cellmetabolism.org/.

[74] Saraiva AL, Veras FP, Peres RS, Talbot J, De Lima KA, Luiz JP, Carballido JM, Cunha TM, Cunha FQ, Ryffel B, Alves-Filho JC. Succinate receptor deficiency attenuates arthritis by reducing dendritic cell traffic and expansion of Th17 cells in the lymph nodes. FASEB J 2018;32(12):6550–8. Available from: https://doi.org/10.1096/fj.201800285, https://www.fasebj.org/doi/pdf/10.1096/fj.201800285.

[75] Xu J, Zheng Y, Zhao Y, Zhang Y, Li H, Zhang A, Wang X, Wang W, Hou Y, Wang J. Succinate/IL-1β Signaling Axis Promotes the Inflammatory Progression of Endothelial and Exacerbates Atherosclerosis. Front Immunol 2022;13. Available from: https://doi.org/10.3389/fimmu.2022.817572.

[76] Pell VR, Chouchani ET, Frezza C, Murphy MP, Krieg T. Succinate metabolism: A new therapeutic target for myocardial reperfusion injury. Cardiovasc Res 2016;111(2):134–41. Available from: https://doi.org/10.1093/cvr/cvw100, http://cardiovascres.oxfordjournals.org/.

[77] Bambouskova M, Gorvel L, Lampropoulou V, Sergushichev A, Loginicheva E, Johnson K, Korenfeld D, Mathyer ME, Kim H, Huang LH, Duncan D, Bregman H, Keskin A, Santeford A, Apte RS, Sehgal R, Johnson B, Amarasinghe GK, Soares MP, Satoh T, Akira S, Hai T, De Guzman Strong C, Auclair K, Roddy TP, Biller SA, Jovanovic M, Klechevsky E, Stewart KM, Randolph GJ, Artyomov MN. Electrophilic properties of itaconate and derivatives regulate the IκBζ-ATF3 inflammatory axis. Nature 2018;556(7702):501–4. Available from: https://doi.org/10.1038/s41586-018-0052-z, http://www.nature.com/nature/index.html.

[78] Chen LL, Morcelle C, Cheng ZL, Chen X, Xu Y, Gao Y, Song J, Li Z, Smith MD, Shi M, Zhu Y, Zhou N, Cheng M, He C, Liu K, Lu G, Zhang L, Zhang C, Zhang J, Sun Y, Qi T, Lyu Y, Ren ZZ, Tan XM, Yin J, Lan F, Liu Y, Yang H, Qian M, Duan C, Chang X, Zhou Y, Shen L, Baldwin AS, Guan KL, Xiong Y, Ye D. Itaconate inhibits TET DNA dioxygenases to dampen inflammatory responses. Nat Cell Biol 2022;24(3):353–63. Available from: https://doi.org/10.1038/s41556-022-00853-8, http://www.nature.com/ncb/index.html.

[79] O'Carroll S, et al. Itaconate drives mtRNA-mediated type I interferon production through inhibition of succinate dehydrogenase. Nature Metabolism 2024;. Available from: https://doi.org/10.1038/s42255-024-01204-7.

[80] He W, Henne A, Lauterbach M, Geißmar E, Nikolka F, Kho C, Heinz A, Dostert C, Grusdat M, Cordes T, Härm J, Goldmann O, Ewen A, Verschueren C, Blay-Cadanet J, Geffers R, Garritsen H, Kneiling M, Holm CK, Metallo CM, Medina E, Abdullah Z, Latz E, Brenner D, Hiller K. Mesaconate is synthesized from itaconate and exerts immunomodulatory effects in macrophages. Nat Metabol 2022;4(5):524–33. Available from: https://doi.org/10.1038/s42255-022-00565-1.

[81] Chen F, Elgaher WAM, Winterhoff M, Büssow K, Waqas FH, Graner E, et al. Citraconate inhibits ACOD1 (IRG1) catalysis, reduces interferon responses and oxidative stress, and modulates inflammation and cell metabolism. Nat Metabol 2022;4(5):534–46. Available from: https://doi.org/10.1038/s42255-022-00577-x.

[82] Day EA, O'Neill LAJ. Protein targeting by the itaconate family in immunity and inflammation. Biochem J 2022;479(24):2499−510. Available from: https://doi.org/10.1042/BCJ20220364, https://portlandpress.com/biochemj/article-pdf/479/24/2499/941401/bcj-2022-0364c.pdf.

[83] Cyr Y, Bozal FK, Barcia Durán JG, Newman AAC, Amadori L, Smyrnis P, Gourvest M, Das D, Gildea M, Kaur R, Zhang T, Wang KM, Von Itter R, Schlegel PM, Dupuis SD, Sanchez BF, Schmidt AM, Fisher EA, van Solingen C, Giannarelli C, Moore KJ. The IRG1-itaconate axis protects from cholesterol-induced inflammation and atherosclerosis. Proc Natl Acad Sci USA 2024;121(15). Available from: https://doi.org/10.1073/pnas.2400675121, https://www.pnas.org/doi/10.1073/pnas.2400675121.

[84] Song J, Zhang Y, Frieler RA, Andren A, Wood S, Tyrrell DJ, Sajjakulnukit P, Deng JC, Lyssiotis CA, Mortensen RM, Salmon M, Goldstein DR. Itaconate suppresses atherosclerosis by activating a Nrf2-dependent antiinflammatory response in macrophages in mice. J Clin Invest 2024;134(3). Available from: https://doi.org/10.1172/JCI173034, https://www.jci.org/articles/view/173034/pdf.

[85] Weiss JM, Palmieri EM, Gonzalez-Cotto M, Bettencourt IA, Megill EL, Snyder NW, McVicar DW. Itaconic acid underpins hepatocyte lipid metabolism in non-alcoholic fatty liver disease in male mice. Nat Metabol 2023;5(6):981−95. Available from: https://doi.org/10.1038/s42255-023-00801-2, https://www.nature.com/natmetab/.

[86] Song H, Xu T, Feng X, Lai Y, Yang Y, Zheng H, He X, Wei G, Liao W, Liao Y, Zhong L, Bin J. Itaconate prevents abdominal aortic aneurysm formation through inhibiting inflammation via activation of Nrf2. EBioMedicine 2020;57:102832. Available from: https://doi.org/10.1016/j.ebiom.2020.102832.

[87] Silva YP, Bernardi A, Frozza RL. The Role of Short-Chain Fatty Acids From Gut Microbiota in Gut-Brain Communication. Front Endocrinol 2020;11. Available from: https://doi.org/10.3389/fendo.2020.00025, https://www.frontiersin.org/journals/endocrinology#.

[88] Zapolska-Downar D, Siennicka A, Kaczmarczyk M, Kołodziej B, Naruszewicz M. Butyrate inhibits cytokine-induced VCAM-1 and ICAM-1 expression in cultured endothelial cells: The role of NF-κB and PPARα. J Nutr Biochem 2004;15(4):220−8. Available from: https://doi.org/10.1016/j.jnutbio.2003.11.008.

[89] Meyer F, Seibert FS, Nienen M, Welzel M, Beisser D, Bauer F, Rohn B, Westhoff TH, Stervbo U, Babel N. Propionate supplementation promotes the expansion of peripheral regulatory T-Cells in patients with end-stage renal disease. J Nephrol 2020;33(4):817−27. Available from: https://doi.org/10.1007/s40620-019-00694-z, http://www.springer.com/medicine/nephrology/journal/40620.

[90] Trøseid M, Andersen GØ, Broch K, Hov JR. The gut microbiome in coronary artery disease and heart failure: Current knowledge and future directions. EBioMedicine 2020;52. Available from: https://doi.org/10.1016/j.ebiom.2020.102649, http://www.journals.elsevier.com/ebiomedicine/.

[91] Bartolomaeus H, Balogh A, Yakoub M, Homann S, Markó L, Höges S, Tsvetkov D, Krannich A, Wundersitz S, Avery EG, Haase N, Kräker K, Hering L, Maase M, Kusche-Vihrog K, Grandoch M, Fielitz J, Kempa S, Gollasch M, Zhumadilov Z, Kozhakhmetov S, Kushugulova A, Eckardt KU, Dechend R, Rump LC, Forslund SK, Müller DN, Stegbauer J, Wilck N. Short-Chain Fatty Acid Propionate Protects from Hypertensive Cardiovascular Damage. Circulation 2019;139(11):1407−21. Available from: https://doi.org/10.1161/CIRCULATIONAHA.118.036652, http://circ.ahajournals.org.

[92] Jiang X, Huang X, Tong Y, Gao H. Butyrate improves cardiac function and sympathetic neural remodeling following myocardial infarction in rats. Can J Physiol Pharm 2020;98(6):391−9. Available from: https://doi.org/10.1139/cjpp-2019-0531, http://www.nrc.ca/cgi-bin/cisti/journals/rp/rp_desy_e?cjpp.

[93] Zhang L, Deng M, Lu A, Chen Y, Chen Y, Wu C, Tan Z, Boini KM, Yang T, Zhu Q, Wang L. Sodium butyrate attenuates angiotensin II-induced cardiac hypertrophy by inhibiting COX2/PGE2 pathway via a HDAC5/HDAC6-dependent mechanism. J Cell Mol Med 2019;23(12):8139−50. Available from: https://doi.org/10.1111/jcmm.14684, http://onlinelibrary.wiley.com/journal/10.1111/(ISSN)1582-4934.

CHAPTER 7

Damage-associated molecular patterns as metabolic regulators of innate immunity

Tristram A.J. Ryan, Ivan Zanoni and Marco Di Gioia

Harvard Medical School, and Division of Immunology, Division of Gastroenterology, Boston Children's Hospital, Boston, MA, United States

Introduction

Innate immune cells are strategically distributed throughout the body and respond rapidly to external threats, such as pathogen infections. Phagocytes, including macrophages, neutrophils, and dendritic cells, are equipped with a repertoire of specialized receptors known as pattern-recognition receptors (PRRs). These receptors recognize conserved structures associated with invading microorganisms, known as pathogen-associated molecular patterns (PAMPs), which trigger inflammatory responses aimed at eliminating the source of the infection and restoring tissue homeostasis. The functions of phagocytes in the context of inflammation are also influenced by endogenous molecules released from host cells during tissue damage or stress. These signals, known as damage-associated molecular patterns (DAMPs), include a wide range of molecules like nucleic acids, proteins, lipids, and metabolites. While these molecules typically do not trigger immune responses under normal conditions, they can undergo changes in their physical or chemical properties, as well as their cellular or tissue location and concentration, when tissue injury occurs. These alterations make DAMPs "visible" to PRRs, thus sustaining inflammation. While this inflammatory response can be beneficial by combatting an infection and/or initiating tissue homeostasis restoration, it may also contribute to the development of chronic inflammatory diseases.

DAMPs can originate from the permeabilization of cellular membranes, leading to the release of reactive molecules from dying or dead cells into the extracellular compartment, where they can act through paracrine mechanisms to reshape phagocyte responses. Additionally, DAMP formation can result from the loss of intracellular homeostasis due to metabolic alterations, such as mitochondrial dysfunction, where DAMPs can then influence the signaling and outcomes of PRR activation and cell death programs.

DAMPs control the final functions of activated phagocytes by directly influencing the PRR signaling cascade and orchestrating subcellular processes such as autophagy and caspase activation. In addition to these effects, an emerging DAMP-mediated mechanism influencing inflammation is the rewiring of phagocyte cellular metabolism. Indeed, phagocytes undergo metabolic shifts to mount an appropriate response, initiated by PAMP-PRR engagement, against a specific external cue [1]. This process is further modulated by the production of DAMPs, which control the extent and duration of the response, ultimately reshaping phagocyte behavior. This metabolic process adds a new layer of complexity to the study of immune responses, challenging our understanding of the behavior of phagocytes during both infectious and noninfectious diseases characterized by the presence of DAMPs. In this chapter, we will explore the effects of DAMPs on phagocyte metabolism and how they modulate the inflammatory functions initiated by PAMPs.

Intracellular metabolites function as damage-associated molecular patterns intrinsically modulating pathogen-associated molecular patterns-induced responses

After encountering PAMPs, phagocytes rapidly remodel their metabolism to support their functions. A primary example of this occurs upon recognition of the Gram-negative bacterial component lipopolysaccharide (LPS), one of the best characterized PAMPs. LPS is recognized by Toll-like receptor 4 (TLR4), which induces a global rewiring of major metabolic pathways to coordinate microbial killing processes, the production of proinflammatory mediators, and the maintenance of cell viability [2–7]. LPS-activated phagocytes increase glycolysis and the pentose phosphate pathway (PPP), providing ATP to fuel protein translation and generating metabolic intermediates like citrate. Citrate is converted to acetyl-coenzyme A (acetyl-CoA), which promotes histone acetylation, thereby enabling the transcription of proinflammatory genes through the enhancement of a permissive chromatin organization. Additionally, acetyl-CoA is used in the biosynthesis of fatty acids, which are necessary for the expansion of secretory structures, such as the endoplasmic reticulum and Golgi apparatus. These processes are essential for the production and secretion of proteins critical to phagocyte activation [3,5,8–11]. In addition to increased glucose utilization, mitochondria play a critical role in driving inflammation, rapidly altering their metabolism and structure to create a signaling hub that regulates and sustains the processes triggered by TLR4 engagement. Indeed, LPS-activated phagocytes exhibit a profound reorganization of mitochondrial metabolism driven by two primary mechanisms:

- Also known as the Krebs cycle or citric acid cycle, this metabolic pathway consists of eight consecutive enzymes that extract energy from proteins, fats, and carbohydrates to produce NADH and FADH$_2$. These molecules fuel the mitochondrial electron transport chain (ETC) to synthesize ATP via oxidative phosphorylation (OXPHOS). During LPS activation, the TCA cycle experiences two "breaks." The first occurs due to reduced expression and activity of isocitrate dehydrogenase (IDH), resulting from an autocrine response of type I interferon (IFN). This interruption redirects the TCA cycle flux towards citrate and cis-aconitate, supporting citrate accumulation that is necessary for controlling the functions previously described and favoring the production of itaconate, driven by a rapid induction of aconitate decarboxylase (*Acod1*), also known as immune responsive gene 1 (*Irg1*), which is virtually absent in resting cells but is strongly upregulated by LPS engagement. Itaconate accumulation triggers the second breakpoint in the TCA cycle by competitively inhibiting succinate dehydrogenase (SDH), also known as complex II of the ETC, limiting the reversible conversion of succinate to fumarate, and resulting in succinate accumulation. Succinate, in turn, regulates the activity of transcription factors, such as hypoxia-inducible factor 1-alpha (HIF-1α), which control the production of proinflammatory mediators.
- Depression of ETC activity: This occurs mainly due to the production of nitric oxide (NO) induced by LPS through *Nos2* upregulation [3,4,6,12]. NO inhibits cytochrome oxidase by competing with oxygen and irreversibly binding to ETC complexes. The resulting downregulation of OXPHOS forces the cells to rely on aerobic glycolysis for ATP production, thereby increasing glucose uptake. Furthermore, since the TCA cycle and OXPHOS are closely coupled, dysfunction in the latter supports the reprogramming of the TCA cycle, leading to the accumulation of key metabolites.

Mitochondrial metabolites accumulate via metabolic shifts and/or transcriptional reprogramming during infection or injury and are increasingly being recognized as critical signaling molecules that govern a plethora of responses in immune cells [13–15]. Thus metabolites act as "mitokines" to modulate immune cells both intracellularly and extracellularly, with receptors and transporters being identified for several mitochondrial metabolites, as we will discuss below. Functions of metabolites include regulation of gene transcription by metabolites via epigenetic modifications such as DNA methylation and histone modifications [16], protein-metabolite interactions [17], and induction of pro- or antiinflammatory responses [18], depending on the specific metabolite and the context. Based on the accumulating evidence, we propose that not only are metabolites key signaling molecules, but they are also, in fact, DAMPs which are necessary cogs in the immune machinery for generating a full and successful immune response.

Itaconate, succinate, and fumarate have emerged in the last decade as key signaling metabolites, or DAMPs, as we shall describe below.

Succinate

Succinate is a dicarboxylic acid and TCA cycle metabolite that is produced in mitochondria upon hydrolysis of succinyl-CoA by the enzyme succinyl-CoA synthetase. Succinate is an important TCA cycle intermediate that undergoes reversible oxidation to fumarate by SDH at complex II of the ETC, contributing to ATP production via OXPHOS. Succinate, however, also has multiple immunomodulatory properties, as we will describe below (Fig. 7.1).

In 2000 Baysal and colleagues provided the first evidence that mutations in *SDHD*—one of the genes that encodes for complex II of the ETC—are an underlying cause of hereditary paraganglioma (or more specifically phaeochromocytoma), a form of head and neck cancer [19]. This identification that SDH exerts a key role in tumor suppression, as well as OXPHOS, during homeostasis, directly linked mitochondria and the ETC to cancer. This finding initiated a wealth of research into the mechanisms underlying tumorigenesis initiated by mitochondrial dysfunction, and it was later identified that succinate—which accumulates upon SDH inhibition or mutation—is transported from the mitochondrion to the cytosol to inhibit hypoxia-inducible factor (HIF)-α prolyl hydroxylase enzymes (PHDs 1, 2, and 3), resulting in stabilization of the transcription factor HIF-1α [20]. HIF-1α then translocates to the nucleus, initiating transcriptional upregulation of genes governing processes such as glycolysis and angiogenesis.

This early evidence of succinate being released from mitochondria as a DAMP was assigned a direct immune function in 2013 when Tannahill and colleagues described succinate as being one of the most upregulated metabolites in LPS-activated—and therefore glycolytic—macrophages [3]. Succinate-mediated HIF-1α stabilization was shown to be responsible for the induction of the proinflammatory gene *Il1b*, a key mediator in many chronic inflammatory diseases [21], thus directly linking glycolysis and a TCA cycle metabolite with regulation of the innate immune response to inflammation. This was confirmed by showing that pretreatment of macrophages with 2-deoxyglucose (2-DG)—a glycolysis inhibitor—or a cell-permeable α-ketoglutarate (α-KG) derivative—which increases PHD activity—suppressed LPS-induced HIF-1α stabilization and subsequent *Il1b* mRNA induction. The source of succinate accumulation in this study was ascribed to glutamine anaplerosis—whereby glutamine-derived α-KG is converted to succinate in the TCA cycle resulting in an elevation in succinate—although we now know that the second breakpoint in the TCA cycle mediated by itaconate's inhibition of SDH likely plays a role.

Interestingly, inhibition of *Il1b* induction by α-KG, which is the succinate precursor in the TCA cycle, which is in contrast to succinate's effect on *Il1b*, was later elaborated on by Liu and colleagues [22] who identified that glutamine-derived α-KG governs alternative activation of macrophages, suppressing proinflammatory gene induction via epigenetic reprogramming of IL-4-activated macrophages and limiting activation of the transcription factor nuclear factor-

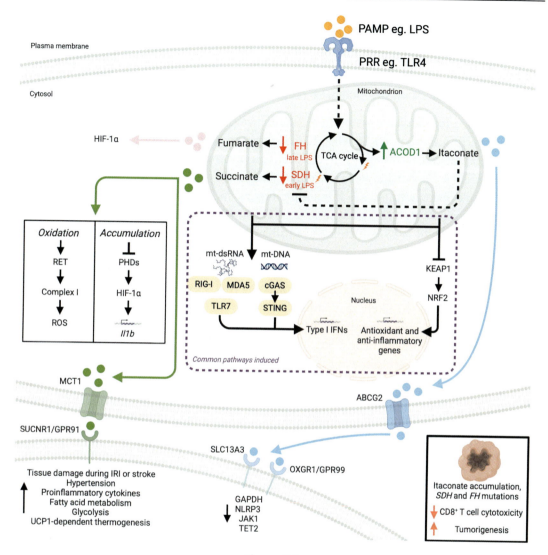

Figure 7.1

Immunomodulatory properties of the TCA cycle-derived metabolites itaconate, succinate, and fumarate. In LPS-activated macrophages, the metabolites itaconate, succinate, and fumarate accumulate to millimolar concentrations and signal as DAMPs to regulate a multitude of immune responses. These include targeting of GAPDH and NLRP3 by itaconate, stabilization of HIF-1α by fumarate, and elevation of complex I-dependent ROS via RET by succinate. All three metabolites share a common function in LPS-activated macrophages by amplifying LPS-induced type I IFN production via mt-nucleic acid release. All three metabolites also accumulate in cancers and are thought to be pro-tumorigenic. Collectively, an emerging consensus is that itaconate, succinate, and fumarate are critical cogs in the innate immune machinery that may have potential to be modulated for the treatment of human diseases. *DAMPs*, damage-associated molecular patterns; *LPS*, Lipopolysaccharide; *TCA*, tricarboxylic acid.

κB (NF-κB), which is commonly associated with upregulation of proinflammatory gene programs induced by LPS in classically activated macrophages. α-KG therefore restrains inflammation by suppressing HIF-1α stabilization and NF-κB activity, in contrast to succinate, with an elevated α-KG:succinate ratio being characteristic of an antiinflammatory macrophage, while a low α-KG:succinate ratio indicates proinflammatory macrophages.

Further evidence for succinate acting in a pathological role occurs in the context of ischemia-reperfusion injury (IRI), when blood supply to organs is transiently disrupted and the reoxygenation process damages tissue locally, as can occur during stroke or myocardial infarction. In 2014 Chouchani, Pell, and colleagues employed mouse models of IRI to identify that succinate accumulates in multiple organs due to a reversal of SDH. Re-oxidation of succinate by SDH leads to reverse electron transport (RET) at complex I of the ETC and production of ROS, which is responsible for the tissue damage during reperfusion [23]. Additionally, succinate may also accumulate during IRI via glutamine anaplerosis and a reduced α-KG:succinate ratio [24]. SDH inhibition was found to be protective against cardiac IRI in mice in these studies [23,24], meaning that succinate oxidation, rather than accumulation alone, is the likely mediator of succinate-induced pathology during IRI. Consistent with this, the competitive SDH inhibitor malonate, which limits succinate oxidation and therefore pathological ROS production at complex I, is protective when administered at reperfusion following IRI [25] or stroke [26] in mice. Notably, two-thirds of total succinate is released from ischemic hearts into the circulation within five minutes of reperfusion following ischemia [24]. This is consistent with reports that plasma succinate levels are elevated during conditions of stress such as hypoxia [27]—likely associated with HIF-1α stabilization and *Il1b* induction—and exercise [28].

This poses the question as to the extent of succinate's systemic signaling, acting as a DAMP released from mitochondria during inflammation. Succinate is released from cells in a monocarboxylated form via its transporter monocarboxylate transporter 1 (MCT1) as a result of a cytosolic acidification during conditions of stress such as exercise [29] or IRI [30]. Circulating or extracellular succinate signals through its G-protein-coupled receptor SUCNR1 (also called GPR91) to drive hypertension [31], induce proinflammatory cytokines [32], regulate vascular tone [33], fatty acid metabolism, glycolysis, and type I IFN signaling [34]. In contrast with these inflammatory roles associated with systemic succinate elevation, succinate has also been shown to protect against obesity in mice by driving brown adipocyte thermogenesis in an uncoupling protein 1 (UCP1)-dependent manner [35], as well as mediating an antiinflammatory genetic program in macrophages and in adipose tissue from lean humans but not obese humans [36].

This indicates that the effects of succinate are context-specific, and the kinetics of succinate accumulation, as well as the relative roles of succinate accumulation versus oxidation, need to be delineated in future studies. The emerging body of evidence also supports the concept that succinate accumulation is a conserved response mechanism during inflammation, with succinate being released from mitochondria and cells to act as a DAMP systemically to regulate further the host response.

Fumarate

Fumarate is another TCA cycle metabolite that has also been described to be an important modulator of the innate immune response. A direct substrate of succinate's reversible oxidation by SDH/complex II, fumarate is in turn reversibly hydrated to malate by the enzyme fumarate hydratase (FH). Notably, hydration of fumarate to malate can occur both in mitochondria and in the cytosol as FH is present in both cellular compartments [37] (Fig. 7.1).

As *SDH* mutations can drive tumorigenesis, mutations in *FH*—the gene that encodes for the enzyme that catalyzes the reversible hydration of fumarate to malate in the TCA cycle—can also cause cancers such as the hereditary cancer syndrome hereditary leiomyomatosis and renal cell carcinoma (HLRCC) [38], as well as gliomas and neuroblastomas [39]. Loss of function of *FH*, or *FH* deficiency, results in fumarate accumulation and cellular TCA cycle rewiring leading to increased glycolysis and pentose phosphate pathway activity [40]. FH deficiency leading to fumarate accumulation is associated with HIF stabilization during renal cancer via competitive inhibition of PHDs [41], which prevents HIF hydroxylation, in a manner similar to SDH inhibition and succinate-mediated HIF stabilization. Fumarate also competitively inhibits α-KG dioxygenases, such as the ten-eleven-translocation 5-methylcytosine (TET) dioxygenases involved in epigenetic regulation. This triggers induction of transcription factors associated with an epithelial-to-mesenchymal transition (EMT), characteristic of the initiation of metastasis that drives cancer progression [42]. This epigenetic modification mediated by fumarate likely contributes to its oncometabolic role in HLRCC.

Fumarate can posttranslationally modify proteins in a process termed succination by covalently reacting with cysteine residues of target proteins, forming *S*-(2-succinyl)cysteine (2SC) in an electrophilic Michael reaction [43]. Succination of proteins by fumarate, yielding 2SC, is strongly associated with *FH*-mutation-mediated HLRCC [44], making 2SC an important biomarker for the detection of FH inhibition or deficiency. Another primary example of succination is Kelch-like ECH-associated protein 1 (KEAP1). During homeostasis, KEAP1 acts as an important regulator of oxidative and electrophilic stress by binding and forming a complex with the antiinflammatory transcription factor nuclear factor-erythroid 2 p45-related factor 2 (NRF2), mediating NRF2 ubiquitination and degradation. Upon inflammation or mitochondrial stress, fumarate accumulation triggers succination of KEAP1, releasing NRF2 to induce transcription of antioxidant-associated genes [45,46] in concert with the transcription factor forkhead box protein A2 (FOXA2) [47]. In addition, fumarate has been shown to limit macrophage pyroptotic cell death—a programmed, proinflammatory, and lytic form of cell death that occurs in a caspase-dependent manner during inflammation—by succinating human Cys191 (mouse Cys192) in gasdermin D (GSDMD) [48]. This prevents oligomerization of GSDMD and subsequent lytic pore formation, protecting against cell death. These examples highlight the context-specific, protective, and pathological effects of fumarate-mediated succination of proteins.

Recently, a role for fumarate in the induction of the type I IFN response has been identified. In 2023 two laboratories reported that fumarate accumulation in bone marrow-derived macrophages and kidney epithelial cells, either as a result of LPS challenge or genetic *FH* loss, triggers mitochondrial membrane perturbations and the release of mitochondrial nucleic acids, namely, mitochondrial RNA (mtRNA) and DNA (mtDNA). Fumarate-mediated mtRNA release from the mitochondria into the cytosol was found to activate the RNA sensors RIG-I and MDA5, with a partial dependency on TLR7, inducing *Ifnb1* and the type I IFN response [49]. Fumarate was also found to trigger mtDNA release into the cytosol via mitochondrial-derived vesicles, which activated the cGAS-STING pathway, also inducing type I IFNs [50]. Interestingly, accumulation of fumarate after LPS challenge is multifaceted. At early timepoints (4-24 hours after LPS challenge), glutamine anaplerosis (which is also implicated in succinate accumulation at early timepoints) and an aspartate-argininosuccinate shunt from the mitochondria into the cytosol result in elevated cytosolic fumarate [49]. However, at later timepoints (24–48 hours after LPS challenge), prolonged LPS suppresses expression of *Fh* [49] by a currently unknown mechanism, mimicking the phenotype found in FH-deficient or FH-mutated tumors. Therefore while fumarate accumulation and export to the cytosol may be an important trigger, or indeed amplifier, of the finely tuned type I IFN response of the host to infections, metabolic alterations during conditions such as persistent bacterial or viral infections, or autoimmune conditions, may be a key contributor to exacerbated and prolonged type I IFN production, which is detrimental. Indeed, Hooftman and colleagues identified significantly suppressed expression of *FH* in PBMCs isolated from systemic lupus erythematosus (SLE) patients—an interferonopathy—compared with healthy controls [49]. This intriguing finding presents *FH* as a clinical biomarker for interferonopathies such as SLE, with impaired FH activity a newly identified target for the treatment and management of SLE.

Collectively, these studies highlight the role of fumarate acting as a DAMP within mitochondria during inflammation, triggering release of mtRNA or mtDNA as secondary DAMPs to modulate the type I IFN response. Further research in this area should unveil further regulation of the innate immune response by fumarate and indeed further consequences of impaired FH activity in the context of interferonopathies and associated autoimmune conditions.

Itaconate

Itaconate is another metabolite formed in the mitochondria and perhaps the best characterized TCA cycle-related metabolite in terms of regulation of the innate immune response to infection. Primarily produced in activated phagocytes such as macrophages, itaconate is not strictly a TCA cycle metabolite per se, as it is derived from the TCA cycle during the first breakpoint due to inhibition of IDH and simultaneous upregulation of *Acod1*, which is one of the most upregulated genes in activated macrophages. *Acod1* is upregulated by cytokines such as IFNs [51–54] and also via itaconate's inhibition of IDH2 [55], thus regulating its own synthesis. Collectively, this results in the synthesis of the unsaturated dicarboxylic acid itaconate from the decarboxylation of cis-aconitate [56].

Initially, itaconate was used primarily for industrial purposes such as the synthesis of polymers [57]. Itaconate was later identified in the 1970s as being antimicrobial via inhibition of isocitrate lyase, an enzyme in the glyoxylate shunt pathway which is critical for bacterial growth [58,59]. Furthermore, bacteria including *Mycobacterium tuberculosis* [60] and *Yersinia pestis* [61] carry genes encoding enzymes that degrade itaconate, highlighting its evolutionarily conserved antimicrobial properties.

As mentioned above, itaconate is the most upregulated metabolite in LPS-activated macrophages [4,62,63] and has recently emerged as a key immunometabolic player in macrophages—in addition to the newly characterized and related metabolites citraconate and mesaconate [64,65]—exerting various immunomodulatory effects (Fig. 7.1). An important finding in the rejuvenation of interest in itaconate came in 2016, with the description that itaconate inhibits SDH to elevate succinate levels during inflammation [66], with SDH inhibition alleviated in LPS-activated $Acod1^{-/-}$ macrophages due to their inability to synthesize itaconate [62]. Interestingly, it had previously been reported in 1949 that itaconate could inhibit SDH [67], but as itaconate lacked a characterized physiological role at the time, it was likely overlooked as a rather obscure, inconsequential metabolite. Itaconate may also inhibit IDH2, resulting in propagation of *Acod1* induction [55]. Thus itaconate directly links breakpoints 1 and 2 of the TCA cycle in activated macrophages. Intracellular abundance of itaconate has been shown to peak between 10 and 24 hours after LPS challenge, with itaconate secretion from macrophages peaking around 24 hours post challenge [62,68]. Therefore at early timepoints, itaconate's transient elevation and inhibition of SDH mediated by TCA cycle perturbations leads to HIF-1α stabilization, as described above. HIF-1α stabilization elevates expression of pyruvate dehydrogenase kinase 3 (*Pdk3*), which in turn reduces flux into acetyl-CoA and the TCA cycle at later timepoints (24-48 hours after LPS challenge) via inhibition of the pyruvate dehydrogenase complex [68]. This results in normalization of TCA cycle and reduced itaconate synthesis, alleviating itaconate's inhibition of SDH, thus repressing HIF-1α and restoring homeostasis [68]. Interestingly, there is also varying evidence that itaconate may suppress FH activity, in addition to its well-described role in inhibiting SDH. One study suggested that ACOD1/itaconate suppresses FH activity in human liver nonparenchymal cells activated with LPS for 6 hours [69], whilst another found elevated fumarate accumulation in $Acod1^{-/-}$ mouse bone marrow-derived macrophages activated with LPS for 24 hours [49]. This presents the intriguing hypothesis that itaconate may contribute to fumarate accumulation at early timepoints in LPS-activated cells in concert with the aspartate-argininosuccinate shunt, with the controlled reduction in itaconate at later timepoints (48 hours after LPS) making way for *Fh* suppression by LPS by an as-yet undefined mechanism. However, the different species and cell types used in these studies preclude to formally confirm the hypothesis of the dual inhibition of SDH and FH by itaconate, requiring further investigation. The differences in mouse and human biology are particularly pertinent with regard to itaconate as mouse ACOD1 has been reported to be approximately three-to-five-fold more active than human ACOD1 due to evolutionary substitution of isoleucine in mice with methionine in humans at position 154 in ACOD1 [70,71], which is important to note when drawing conclusions about itaconate biology elucidated in mice.

In the last decade, itaconate has been described as a potent antiinflammatory metabolite, with protective roles including activation of the antioxidant and antiinflammatory transcription factor NRF2 following LPS challenge [63], inhibition of GAPDH to suppress glycolysis [72], post-translational modification of NLRP3 and inhibition of inflammasome activation [73], as well as modification of JAK1 [74]. Itaconate also binds to TET2 at the same site as α-KG to suppress inflammation [75]. These studies, and many more documenting the antiinflammatory properties of itaconate, have been summarized in recent reviews [76,77].

Expanding on the repertoire of roles for endogenous itaconate, an itaconate transporter and receptor have both been recently described. Cytosolic itaconate was shown to be exported from human and mouse macrophages by ATP-binding cassette transporter G2 (ABCG2) [78], potentially mediating the elevation in extracellular itaconate during inflammation. Extracellular itaconate acts as a DAMP by signaling through the G-protein-coupled receptor oxoglutarate receptor 1 (OXGR1; also called GPR99) in mouse pulmonary epithelial cells [79]. This may be relevant in the context of *Staphylococcus aureus* pulmonary infection, where neutrophil-derived itaconate is released into the bronchoalveolar lavage fluid of mice to exert its immunomodulatory effects [80], potentially by signaling via OXGR1. Interestingly, a-KG has also been shown to signal through OXGR1 [31], highlighting the structural and physiological similarities between itaconate and α-KG. Itaconate can also be imported into hepatocytes via solute carrier family 13 member 3 (SLC13A3), also called Na^+/dicarboxylate cotransporter (NaDC3) [81]. Akin to OXGR1, receptors of the SLC13 family have previously been shown to mediate uptake of the related dicarboxylates succinate, fumarate, and α-KG [82], further emphasizing the similarities in receptors for structurally related metabolites. Whether ABCG2 as well as OXGR1 and SLC13A3 act as itaconate's transporter and receptors, respectively, in different cell types remains to be determined, but these studies describing a signaling axis for itaconate enhance the rationale for employing itaconate itself, rather than its derivatives (see below), in future experiments. This will help to elucidate the effects of itaconate in a more physiologically relevant and context-specific setup, where itaconate has been shown to exhibit both pro- and antiinflammatory effects. Indeed, despite the initial reports of itaconate's antiinflammatory effects, ACOD1/itaconate has been described as a putative target in cancer, with *ACOD1* expression and itaconate being upregulated in tumor-associated macrophages from mice in multiple models of cancer [83–85]. Itaconate is taken up by $CD8^+$ T cells in cancer, modifying their epigenome to suppress $CD8^+$ T cell cytotoxicity, resulting in tumor growth [84,86,87]. Itaconate has also recently been implicated in the pathogenesis of atherosclerosis [88]. Collectively, the body of research on the immunomodulatory metabolite itaconate continues to gain interest and grow, with exciting potential to harness itaconate's biochemical properties or indeed suppress its induction and accumulation when necessary to develop new clinical therapies based on this intriguing metabolite.

Metabolites and their derivatives: contrasting results in the context of type I interferons

It was originally thought that itaconate, like succinate and fumarate, was impermeable to immune cells in vitro when administered in its exogenous form. Therefore a number of cell-permeable itaconate derivatives were designed, most prominently 4-octyl itaconate (4-OI) and dimethyl itaconate (DI). Many of the early itaconate studies employed 4-OI and DI as proxies for endogenous itaconate, but we now know that these derivatives are much more highly electrophilic and cysteine reactive than endogenous itaconate, and a number of antiinflammatory properties assigned to itaconate are in retrospect more representative of 4-OI's and DI's innate electrophilicity. For example, 4-OI has been shown to exert its antiinflammatory effects by directly modifying cysteines of proteins such as NLRP3 [73], JAK1 [74], STING [89,90], and MAVS [91] in an alkylation reaction termed 2,3-dicarboxypropylation. These differing properties between itaconate and its derivatives may explain the contrasting reports in their effects, such as activation of NRF2, which has been reported for 4-OI [63] but is less clear for itaconate itself [92,93]. While alkylation of multiple proteins by 4-OI has been demonstrated, the evidence for itaconate modifying proteins is less clear-cut, although recent studies suggest that the transcription factor EB (TFEB) induces *Acod1* and itaconate in response to bacteria [94], with itaconate then alkylating TFEB to induce lysosomal biogenesis as a key mediator of itaconate's antibacterial properties [95]. Therefore further research into whether itaconate can modify similar targets to 4-OI on previously described 4-OI-target proteins, such as NLRP3 or STING, would yield interesting biology for the itaconate field.

Another difference between itaconate and its derivatives regards type I IFN signaling. 4-OI suppresses induction of type I IFNs [63,96,97], conferring protection in inflammatory models characterized by excess IFN production, such as IFN- and tissue factor-mediated coagulation [97]. However, the effects of itaconate on type I IFNs appear to be more nuanced. Itaconate itself elevates type I IFNs and interferon-stimulated genes in LPS-activated macrophages [98,99] via inhibition of SDH [100]. This triggers mtRNA release from mitochondria, which is detected by the cytosolic double-stranded RNA sensors RIG-I and MDA5, inducing type I IFNs [100]. Thus itaconate's induction of type I IFNs in LPS-activated macrophages occurs via a similar mechanism to fumarate [49]. In neurons, inhibition of SDH by itaconate has been implicated in induction of an antiviral state during infection with Zika virus [101]. Indeed, plasma itaconate levels are reported to be reduced in SARS-CoV-2-infected patients, which may be associated with a reduced IFN response, leading to increased viral susceptibility [102].

Contrastingly, in a model of influenza A virus (IAV) infection, itaconate has been shown to suppress STAT1 phosphorylation and subsequent type I IFN responses in human lung A549 cells [65,103]. Furthermore, Sohail and colleagues found that following IAV infection, $Acod1^{-/-}$ mice were more susceptible to pulmonary infection, weight loss, and mortality than their wild-type counterparts [103]. However, citraconate, a recently described endogenous ACOD1 inhibitor, also suppresses IAV-induced type I IFN responses [65], adding further complexity to the role of itaconate during viral infection. Collectively, this suggests that regulation of type I IFNs by itaconate differs by cell type and infection origin and requires further study to delineate these disparities and context-specific differences.

These contrasting effects are akin to the differential regulation of type I IFNs by succinate and fumarate and their related derivatives. SDH inhibition, which results in succinate accumulation, has been linked with induction of type I IFN signaling pathways [34] and an antiviral state [101], but its derivative diethyl succinate suppresses MAVS aggregation [104], which is required for type I IFN induction following detection of double-stranded RNA in the cytosol of immune cells. As a result, diethyl succinate inhibits type I IFNs in macrophages infected with vesicular stomatitis virus [104]. As discussed above, fumarate also elevates type I IFNs in LPS-activated macrophages via the release of mitochondrial nucleic acids [49,50], while the fumarate-based derivative, dimethyl fumarate (DMF), blocks type I IFNs [105]. DMF shares very similar structural and antiinflammatory properties with 4-OI, also driving NRF2 activation [106] and suppressing NLRP3 [48] and JAK1 activity [107], as well as pathological IFN- and tissue factor-driven coagulation [97]. In fact, DMF is clinically approved under the trade name Tecfidera™ for the treatment of psoriasis and multiple sclerosis, perhaps paving the way for similar TCA cycle-derived metabolite-inspired compounds such as 4-OI for assessment of their antiinflammatory potential in the clinic. Harnessing endogenous metabolic properties may in the future expand the arsenal of drugs in the clinic that exert their protective effects in-part via regulation of metabolism, such as the antidiabetic drug metformin which acts via activation of the master metabolic regulator AMP-activated protein kinase (AMPK) [108] and the appetite suppressor growth differentiation factor 15 (GDF15) [109,110] to mediate its beneficial effects on body weight and energy balance.

An ever-expanding array of immunomodulatory metabolites

In addition to the extensive immunomodulatory properties of the aforementioned succinate, fumarate, and itaconate, further metabolic regulators of immunity continue to be described. A recent prominent example is lactate. Formerly considered a waste product of aerobic glycolysis and Warburg metabolism, lactate exerts its immunomodulatory effects upon export from cells via the monocarboxylate transporter MCT4 [111]—which is upregulated in a HIF-1α-dependent manner [112]—and uptake via its receptor hydroxycarboxylic acid receptor 1 (HCAR1), formerly termed GPR81 [113,114]. Emerging evidence has identified lactate as an important regulator of glycolysis-mediated T cell proliferation [115], cell cycle [116], and post-translational modification of proteins [16]. Lactate can exert epigenetic modifications in immune cells, lactylating histones to reprogram gene transcription as a result of glycolysis induced during infection [117], which can result in the suppression of proinflammatory gene induction [118]. An example of this is lactylation of *Nos2* in proinflammatory macrophages, with the net effect being suppression of inducible nitric oxide synthase (iNOS)-mediated type I IFN production [119]. This lactate-mediated suppression of inflammation and return to homeostasis is an important checkpoint in immune cell activation, as chronic type I IFN exposure—such as those that may occur in interferonopathies such as SLE—limits lactate's ability to modify inflammatory mediators such as *Nos2*, amplifying and exacerbating type I IFN production [119]. Lactate can also sense and bind MAVS, inhibiting MAVS-induced type I IFNs [120,121], with the glycolysis inhibitor 2-DG restoring type I IFN production. Thus lactate has recently emerged as a critical regulator of type I IFN production. This is important as subcellular location of MAVS can dictate the specificity of IFN production, with peroxisomal MAVS guiding glycolysis toward pentose phosphate pathway-mediated type III IFN induction, whereas MAVS on mitochondria-associated endoplasmic reticulum membranes mediates hexosamine biosynthesis pathway-mediated type I IFN induction [122]. Therefore overarching regulation of type I IFN induction by lactate is another emerging example of a metabolite acting as a DAMP at a critical checkpoint to mediate innate immune activation.

Extracellular damage-associated molecular patterns as extrinsic regulators of pathogen-associated molecular pattern-initiated immunometabolism: the case of oxidized phospholipids

DAMPs, or their precursors, can be released by stressed cells into the extracellular environment, where they can also be modified to become active inflammation-modulating molecules. To date, several extracellular DAMPs have been identified in the context of infections or stress conditions, such as tumor progression. These molecules originate from cytosolic content, including macromolecules such as S100A8/A9, RNA, TCA metabolites (as mentioned earlier), and ATP, or from the nuclear space, such as high mobility group box 1 (HMGB1), histones, and genomic DNA [123,124]. Moreover, nonenzymatically modified lipids have emerged as a new class of extracellular DAMPs that may control the metabolism of phagocytes, as described for adipose tissue macrophages (ATM) in obese mice [125] and for circulating and tissue-resident monocytes/macrophages during atherosclerosis [126] or sepsis [127].

Lipids have a structural role in membranes and function as an energy source, but they are also well known for their capacity to modulate cellular signaling processes. To perform this last task, lipids are chemically and structurally modified obtaining a unique capacity to bind cellular targets and/or receptors. These modifications can occur through cell-controlled and programmed enzymatic pathways, as in the case of prostaglandins. Indeed, these mediators are products of the enzymatic oxidation of arachidonic acid, and their production results from the finely tuned expression and activation of a dedicated biosynthetic pathway [128]. In contrast, lipid oxidation can result from spontaneous and uncontrolled reactions triggered by the exposure of intracellular lipids to environmental oxygen concentrations or reactive oxygen species (ROS) produced during stress conditions. The nonenzymatically oxidization of phospholipids, which are part of cell membranes, lipid droplets, lung surfactants, and low-density lipoprotein (LDL) [4], originates DAMPs that contribute to the initiation and amplification of inflammation. In particular, the oxidative products derived from the phospholipid 1-palmitoyl-2-arachidonoyl-sn-glycero-3-phosphocholine (PAPC), collectively known as oxPAPC, are a prototype of nonenzymatically oxPLs. oxPAPC accumulates in oxidized LDL (oxLDL) [129,130], apoptotic cells, and microparticles released by activated or dying cells [131–133] and actively modulates cellular signaling processes that are associated with inflammatory diseases, including atherosclerosis [134], nonalcoholic steatohepatitis (NASH) [135], lung injury and viral infection [136], sepsis [127], leprosy [137], UV-irradiated skin [138], myocardial ischemia-reperfusion [139], and multiple sclerosis [140,141].

Increasing evidence suggests that oxPAPC reshapes the phagocytic responses induced by PAMPs (Fig. 7.2). Specifically, oxPAPC has been shown to modulate the phenotype of LPS-activated macrophages, altering the balance of their anti- and proinflammatory functions and supporting their persistence in local tissues. These effects are mediated by three interconnected mechanisms: (1) early inhibition of AKT, leading to the suppression of the antiinflammatory cytokine IL10 through epigenetic remodeling; (2) late and persistent reorganization of the mitochondrial metabolic reprogramming induced by LPS, resulting in a unique metabolic state that amplifies the production of proinflammatory cytokines; and (3) triggering an atypical inflammasome activation by directly interacting with caspase-11, inducing the active release of IL1β from long-lived phagocytes (Fig. 7.2).

oxPLs modulate early metabolic reprogramming and block antiinflammatory responses

AKT is a serine/threonine protein kinase that plays a key role in a plethora of cellular processes, including cell survival, proliferation, protein synthesis, migration, and metabolism. The activation of TLR4 by LPS results in the formation of a multiprotein signaling platform called the myddosome [142], which initiates molecular pathways that control the transcription of target genes and the rapid metabolic reprogramming of macrophages. This supramolecular organizing center (SMOC) is composed of the adaptors TIRAP/MAL and MyD88, and the

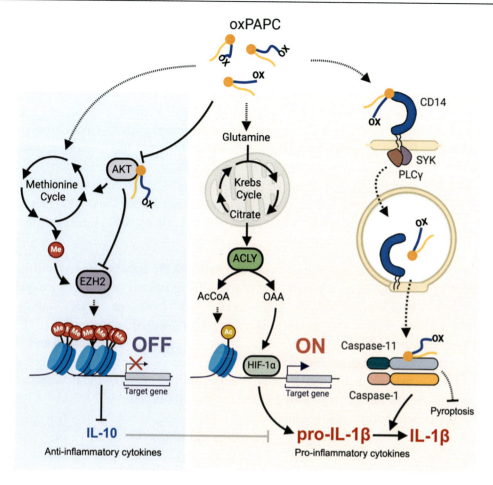

Figure 7.2

oxPAPC modulates phagocytic responses. In LPS-activated macrophages, oxPAPC sustains the activity of EZH2 through the potentiation of the methionine cycle and the direct inhibition of AKT. This results in the deposition of the histone modification H3K27me2/me3, which impairs the expression of the antiinflammatory cytokine IL10 (left). Moreover, oxPAPC reprograms the TCA cycle in a way that sustains ACLY activity, resulting in the production of AcCoA, which supports permissive histone acetylation and produces OAA that stabilizes HIF-1α, necessary for boosting the transcription of *Il1b*. Additionally, through CD14 internalization, oxPAPC directly binds caspase-11, inducing hyperinflammation through the release of bioactive IL-1β, while blocking pyroptosis (right). *LPS*, Lipopolysaccharide.

effector proteins IRAKs, TRAF6, and TBK1 [143]. The latter is responsible for AKT activation, which in turn controls the early increase in glucose utilization through the phosphorylation and mitochondrial translocation of the first enzyme of glycolysis, hexokinase 2 (HK2) [5]. This metabolic shift is the first step in the long-term metabolic changes that occur in phagocytes, helping the reprogramming of mitochondria and ultimately controlling epigenetic modifications and transcription, as described previously.

The concurrent recognition of LPS and oxPAPC leads to the suppression of the early glycolytic flux induced by AKT. A recent study has shown that oxPAPC directly inhibits AKT by binding to its catalytic domain. This was demonstrated using a biotinylated analog of oxPAPC in pull-down experiments and further confirmed by the suppressed activity of AKT in cell-free assays in the presence of oxPAPC [127]. AKT is modulated by the cellular redox state and by electrophilic molecules [144,145]. oxPAPC consists of electrophilic oxidized forms that are highly reactive to cysteine, such as 1-palmitoyl-2-(5,6-epoxyisoprostane E_2)-sn-glycero-3-phosphatidylcholine (PEIPC) [146]. These forms interact with reactive cysteine residues, as demonstrated for KEAP1, a cellular sensor for electrophiles that activates the antioxidative program initiated by NRF2 [147–149]. As described in the previous paragraph regarding succination and KEAP1, oxPAPC may similarly interact with cysteine residues in the catalytic domain of AKT, leading to the formation of an inactive AKT complex.

While the suppression of early glycolysis mediated by oxPAPC does not directly affect the transcription of LPS-target genes—likely due to oxPAPC inducing compensatory metabolic programs, as will be discussed in the following section—the inhibition of AKT activity also leads to the rewiring of other metabolic pathways, such as the methionine cycle [127]. The methionine cycle consists of a series of reactions that catabolize methionine and provide methyl groups for epigenetic modifications, such as DNA and histone methylation. S-adenosyl-homocysteine (SAH) and/or homocysteine, intermediates of the methionine cycle, were among the most upregulated metabolites in cells exposed to LPS and oxPAPC, or when AKT is pharmacologically inhibited [127]. Additionally, AKT controls the inhibitory phosphorylation at S21 [150] of the methyltransferase Enhancer of Zeste Homolog 2 (EZH2), which transfers methyl groups to H3K27, thereby suppressing the transcription of target genes. Thus through the suppression of AKT activity, oxPAPC leads to the activation of EZH2, which induces epigenetic modifications, such as H3K27me2/me3, a key modulator of gene silencing in mammals [151,152]. One of the affected target genes is *Il10*, a crucial autocrine and paracrine antiinflammatory mediator [153]. IL10 plays a key role in restraining the inflammatory responses of phagocytes, ensuring a controlled response and preventing the exacerbation of inflammation. By reducing IL10 production in macrophages, oxPAPC increases the production of proinflammatory cytokines and impairs the control of pathogenic infections. In murine models of sepsis and persistent viral lung infections, blocking oxPAPC accumulation has been shown to increase local and systemic IL10 levels, reshaping the inflammatory response and protecting the animals from death [127].

oxPLs modulate long-term metabolic processes and boost inflammatory responses

Prolonged exposure of LPS-activated macrophages to oxPAPC significantly alters the mitochondrial metabolic reprogramming induced by LPS, leading to a unique metabolic state that amplifies the production of proinflammatory cytokines [126]. While mitochondrial dysfunction occurs following TLR4 activation, as described above, the presence of oxPAPC not only preserves but enhances mitochondrial activity, maintaining the TCA cycle and OXPHOS. This enhancement is marked by a significant reduction in NO production, which preserves the integrity and function of ETC complexes. Additionally, the selective increase in IDH expression helps sustain an intact TCA cycle, facilitating the export of citrate to the cytosol, where ATP-citrate lyase (ACLY) converts it into acetyl-CoA and oxaloacetate (OAA). OAA inhibits PDHs as described above for succinate and fumarate [3,154], stabilizing HIF-1α, which significantly upregulates the transcription of IL1β. Notably, the acetyl-CoA generated during ACLY activation is employed by histone acetyltransferases (HATs) to transfer the acetyl group to conserved lysine on histone proteins [155], supporting a chromatin remodeling that facilitates the transcription of target genes [11,155,156]. In addition, oxPAPC treatment is sufficient to potently increase the mitochondrial potential ($\Delta\psi_m$) of macrophages [126], which is the gradient of the electric potential on the inner mitochondrial membrane generated by ETC proton pumps [157]. $\Delta\psi_m$ sustains the TCA cycle and OXPHOS and maintains a healthy mitochondria network, avoiding mitophagy and preserving mitochondrial mass [157]. Thus the conserved and increased mitochondrial fitness induced by oxPAPC, supported also by production of a redox-balancing response triggered by KEAP1-NRF2 activation [158], may prolong the lifespan of macrophages—as has been described in atherosclerotic lesions [159] and fibrosis [160]—and sustain their inflammatory signature. Notably, the novel metabolic configuration induced by oxPAPC relies strictly on the catabolism of glutamine rather than glycolysis. Glutamine is essential for sustaining the inflammatory phenotype of macrophages within atheromas, and inhibiting its utilization may improve outcomes in atherosclerotic mice [126].

oxPLs induce hyperinflammation

oxPAPC, in the presence of PAMPs, such as LPS, has the unique capacity to potently induce a form of inflammasome activation in phagocytes, which leads to the secretion of IL1β but prevents pyroptosis and favors cell survival [161,162]. This state, called "hyperactivation," is mediated by the ability of oxPAPC to directly bind caspase-11 and triggers an atypical inflammasome activation, culminating in active release of IL1β from long-living phagocytes [161]. This process is critical not only for establishing local and systemic inflammation but also for fostering a robust T cell response [161,163,164].

Extracellular oxPAPC can reach the cytosol through plasma membrane receptors such as CD36 and SR-BI [165]. Additionally, oxPAPC is carried by the TLR4 coreceptor CD14, which facilitates its internalization and triggers an endocytic process driven by phospholipase C gamma (PLCγ) and spleen tyrosine kinase (SYK). The mechanism by which oxPAPC exits the endosome and enters the cytosol remains unclear. It is possible that other lipid-specific receptors, like transmembrane protein 30A (TMEM30A) [166], play a role in this translocation. However, it is also plausible that oxPAPC may alter the plasma or endosomal membrane architecture, resulting in its translocation to the cytosol. Indeed, it has been shown that oxPAPC can insert itself into cellular membranes, altering the balance between liquid-ordered and liquid-disordered phases [167]. Furthermore, oxPAPC can be generated intracellularly in response to cellular stress. For instance, a study by Kerur and colleagues demonstrated that retinal pigmented epithelial cells produce oxPAPC in a model of age-related macular degeneration, contributing to their proinflammatory activity and the progression of the disease [168].

Caspase-11 is a cytosolic sensor for LPS, leading to the "noncanonical" activation of the NLRP3 inflammasome. This activation results in the proteolytic activation of caspase-1, which in turn promotes maturation of the proinflammatory cytokines, pro-IL1β and pro-IL18. Additionally, LPS-activated caspase-11 directly cleaves GSDMD, forming stable pores in the plasma membrane that induce pyroptosis and enable the secretion of mature cytokines.

In contrast to LPS, which binds to the CARD domain of caspase-11, promoting its interaction with NLRP3 and its proteolytic activity, cytosolic oxPAPC binds directly to the catalytic domain of caspase-11. This interaction induces caspase-11 oligomerization but does not activate its enzymatic activity. As a result, oxPAPC can drive the assembly of NLRP3 and the maturation of IL1b, while inhibiting the pyroptotic cell death program. The exact mechanism by which this cytokine is secreted from living cells remains unclear, though it is suggested that GSDMD pores still play a role in this process [169]. Indeed, it was hypothesized that hyperactive cells may engage a repair process involving the endosomal sorting complex required for transport (ESCRT) to address membrane damage and remove GSDMD pores as ectosomes [170]. Thus the rapid turnover of GSDMD pores facilitates IL1β secretion while preventing extensive damage to the plasma membrane, thus shielding the cell from pyroptosis. Moreover, as previously described with fumarate-induced succination, oxPAPC may lead to the accumulation of specific mitochondrial metabolites that can modify GSDMD activity. This modulation can help prevent excessive damage to the plasma membrane while maintaining sufficient pores to allow IL1β secretion.

In sum, these studies indicate that oxPLs are important immunomodulators and exert their context-dependent pro- or antiinflammatory effects via immunometabolic regulation. It will be intriguing in future studies to assess the full extent of their regulation of specific metabolites, or indeed if specific metabolites act as DAMPs to boost—or inhibit—the release of nonenzymatically modified lipids. This may lead to the development of a novel class of therapeutics specifically targeting oxidized phospholipid-mediated hyperinflammation during infections and inflammatory conditions such as atherosclerosis and sepsis.

Conclusion

Given the broad range of innate immune regulation by DAMPs such as mitochondrial metabolites and oxPLs, and the rapid rate at which new roles for these DAMPs are described, it is highly likely that we are only now at the precipice of understanding the true extent of the roles of DAMPs as regulators of immunometabolism and innate immunity. Herein, employing immunometabolites that accumulate in response to PAMPs as an example of intrinsic modulation of the immune system, as well as oxidized membrane phospholipids that accumulate during inflammation or injury as extrinsic modulators of the immune response, we have described how DAMPs are critical immunomodulatory signals and exert their immunoregulatory effects both in concert with, and by augmenting, activation of PAMP-PRR signaling, in addition to regulatory effects separate and distinct from PAMP-mediated responses. Importantly, and excitingly for the field, immunometabolism is emerging as a critical fulcrum in DAMP-mediated immune responses. This presents future studies exploring the role of intrinsic and extrinsic DAMPs as metabolic regulators of innate immunity as a highly relevant and topical niche with the potential for exciting discoveries ahead uncovering new biology. Ultimately, harnessing the innate immunomodulatory properties of DAMPs such as metabolites and oxPLs may yield new targets and therapeutics with clinical utility for the broad range of conditions associated with dysregulated immunometabolism and immune responses.

References

[1] Lachmandas E, Boutens L, Ratter JM, Hijmans A, Hooiveld GJ, Joosten LAB, et al. Microbial stimulation of different Toll-like receptor signalling pathways induces diverse metabolic programmes in human monocytes. Nat Microbiol 2016;2:1–10 Nature Publishing Group.

[2] Davies LC, Rice CM, Palmieri EM, Taylor PR, Kuhns DB, McVicar DW. Peritoneal tissue-resident macrophages are metabolically poised to engage microbes using tissue-niche fuels. Nat Commun 2017;8:2074 Nature Publishing Group.

[3] Tannahill GM, Curtis AM, Adamik J, Palsson-McDermott EM, McGettrick AF, Goel G, et al. Succinate is an inflammatory signal that induces IL-1β through HIF-1α. Nature 2013;496:238–42.

[4] Jha AK, Huang SC-C, Sergushichev A, Lampropoulou V, Ivanova Y, Loginicheva E, et al. Network integration of parallel metabolic and transcriptional data reveals metabolic modules that regulate macrophage polarization. Immunity 2015;42:419–30.

[5] Everts B, Amiel E, Huang SC-C, Smith AM, Chang C-H, Lam WY, et al. TLR-driven early glycolytic reprogramming via the kinases TBK1-IKKε supports the anabolic demands of dendritic cell activation. Nat Immunol 2014;15:323–32.

[6] Everts B, Amiel E, van der Windt GJW, Freitas TC, Chott R, Yarasheski KE, et al. Commitment to glycolysis sustains survival of NO-producing inflammatory dendritic cells. Blood 2012;120:1422–31.

[7] Krawczyk CM, Holowka T, Sun J, Blagih J, Amiel E, DeBerardinis RJ, et al. Toll-like receptor-induced changes in glycolytic metabolism regulate dendritic cell activation. Blood 2010;115:4742–9.

[8] Haschemi A, Kosma P, Gille L, Evans CR, Burant CF, Starkl P, et al. The sedoheptulose kinase CARKL directs macrophage polarization through control of glucose metabolism. Cell Metab 2012;15:813–26.

[9] Palsson-McDermott EM, Curtis AM, Goel G, Lauterbach MAR, Sheedy FJ, Gleeson LE, et al. Pyruvate kinase M2 regulates Hif-1α activity and IL-1β induction and is a critical determinant of the warburg effect in LPS-activated macrophages. Cell Metab 2015;21:65–80.

[10] Millet P, Vachharajani V, McPhail L, Yoza B, McCall CE. GAPDH Binding to TNF-α mRNA Contributes to Posttranscriptional Repression in Monocytes: A Novel Mechanism of Communication between Inflammation and Metabolism. J Immunol 2016;196:2541–51 American Association of Immunologists.

[11] Lauterbach MA, Hanke JE, Serefidou M, Mangan MSJ, Kolbe C-C, Hess T, et al. Toll-like receptor signaling rewires macrophage metabolism and promotes histone acetylation via ATP-citrate lyase. Immunity 2019;51:997–1011.e7.

[12] Bailey JD, Diotallevi M, Nicol T, McNeill E, Shaw A, Chuaiphichai S, et al. Nitric oxide modulates metabolic remodeling in inflammatory macrophages through TCA cycle regulation and itaconate accumulation. Cell Rep 2019;28:218–230.e7.

[13] Martínez-Reyes I, Chandel NS. Mitochondrial TCA cycle metabolites control physiology and disease. Nat Commun 2020;11:102.

[14] Baker SA, Rutter J. Metabolites as signalling molecules. Nat Rev Mol Cell Biol 2023;24:355–74.

[15] Marques E, Kramer R, Ryan DG. Multifaceted mitochondria in innate immunity. NPJ Metab Health Dis 2024;2:6.

[16] Diskin C, Ryan Ta J, O'Neill La J. Modification of Proteins by Metabolites in Immunity. Immunity 2021;54:19–31.

[17] Hicks KG, Cluntun AA, Schubert HL, Hackett SR, Berg JA, Leonard PG, et al. Protein-metabolite interactomics of carbohydrate metabolism reveal regulation of lactate dehydrogenase. Science 2023;379:996–1003.

[18] Zasłona Z, O'Neill LAJ. Cytokine-like roles for metabolites in immunity. Mol Cell 2020;78:814–23.

[19] Baysal BE, Ferrell RE, Willett-Brozick JE, Lawrence EC, Myssiorek D, Bosch A, et al. Mutations in SDHD, a mitochondrial complex II gene, in hereditary paraganglioma. Science 2000;287:848–51.

[20] Selak MA, Armour SM, MacKenzie ED, Boulahbel H, Watson DG, Mansfield KD, et al. Succinate links TCA cycle dysfunction to oncogenesis by inhibiting HIF-alpha prolyl hydroxylase. Cancer Cell 2005;7:77–85.

[21] Dinarello CA. Interleukin-1 in the pathogenesis and treatment of inflammatory diseases. Blood 2011;117:3720–32.

[22] Liu P-S, Wang H, Li X, Chao T, Teav T, Christen S, et al. α-ketoglutarate orchestrates macrophage activation through metabolic and epigenetic reprogramming. Nat Immunol 2017;18:985–94.

[23] Chouchani ET, Pell VR, Gaude E, Aksentijević D, Sundier SY, Robb EL, et al. Ischaemic accumulation of succinate controls reperfusion injury through mitochondrial ROS. Nature 2014;515:431–5.

[24] Zhang J, Wang YT, Miller JH, Day MM, Munger JC, Brookes PS. Accumulation of Succinate in Cardiac Ischemia Primarily Occurs via Canonical Krebs Cycle Activity. Cell Rep 2018;23:2617–28.

[25] Prag HA, Aksentijevic D, Dannhorn A, Giles AV, Mulvey JF, Sauchanka O, et al. Ischemia-Selective Cardioprotection by Malonate for Ischemia/Reperfusion Injury. Circ Res 2022;131:528–41.

[26] Mottahedin A, Prag HA, Dannhorn A, Mair R, Schmidt C, Yang M, et al. Targeting succinate metabolism to decrease brain injury upon mechanical thrombectomy treatment of ischemic stroke. Redox Biol 2023;59:102600.

[27] Hochachka PW, Owen TG, Allen JF, Whittow GC. Multiple end products of anaerobiosis in diving vertebrates. Comp Biochem Physiol B 1975;50:17–22.

[28] Hochachka PW, Dressendorfer RH. Succinate accumulation in man during exercise. Eur J Appl Physiol 1976;35:235–42.

[29] Reddy A, Bozi LHM, Yaghi OK, Mills EL, Xiao H, Nicholson HE, et al. pH-Gated Succinate Secretion Regulates Muscle Remodeling in Response to Exercise. Cell 2020;183:62–75.e17.

[30] Prag HA, Gruszczyk AV, Huang MM, Beach TE, Young T, Tronci L, et al. Mechanism of succinate efflux upon reperfusion of the ischaemic heart. Cardiovasc Res 2021;117:1188–201.

[31] He W, Miao FJ-P, Lin DC-H, Schwandner RT, Wang Z, Gao J, et al. Citric acid cycle intermediates as ligands for orphan G-protein-coupled receptors. Nature 2004;429:188–93.

[32] Rubic T, Lametschwandtner G, Jost S, Hinteregger S, Kund J, Carballido-Perrig N, et al. Triggering the succinate receptor GPR91 on dendritic cells enhances immunity. Nat Immunol 2008;9:1261–9.

[33] Leite LN, Gonzaga NA, Simplicio JA, do Vale GT, Carballido JM, Alves-Filho JC, et al. Pharmacological characterization of the mechanisms underlying the vascular effects of succinate. Eur J Pharmacol 2016;789:334–43.

[34] Mills EL, Kelly B, Logan A, Costa ASH, Varma M, Bryant CE, et al. Succinate dehydrogenase supports metabolic repurposing of mitochondria to drive inflammatory macrophages. Cell 2016;167:457–470.e13.

[35] Mills EL, Pierce KA, Jedrychowski MP, Garrity R, Winther S, Vidoni S, et al. Accumulation of succinate controls activation of adipose tissue thermogenesis. Nature 2018;560:102–6.

[36] Keiran N, Ceperuelo-Mallafré V, Calvo E, Hernández-Alvarez MI, Ejarque M, Núñez-Roa C, et al. SUCNR1 controls an anti-inflammatory program in macrophages to regulate the metabolic response to obesity. Nat Immunol 2019;20:581–92.

[37] Sass E, Blachinsky E, Karniely S, Pines O. Mitochondrial and cytosolic isoforms of yeast fumarase are derivatives of a single translation product and have identical amino termini. J Biol Chem 2001;276:46111–17.

[38] Tomlinson IPM, Alam NA, Rowan AJ, Barclay E, Jaeger EEM, Kelsell D, et al. Germline mutations in FH predispose to dominantly inherited uterine fibroids, skin leiomyomata and papillary renal cell cancer. Nat Genet 2002;30:406–10.

[39] Zhang J, Walsh MF, Wu G, Edmonson MN, Gruber TA, Easton J, et al. Germline mutations in predisposition genes in pediatric cancer. N Engl J Med 2015;373:2336–46.

[40] Valcarcel-Jimenez L, Frezza C. Fumarate hydratase (FH) and cancer: a paradigm of oncometabolism. Br J Cancer 2023;129:1546–57.

[41] Isaacs JS, Jung YJ, Mole DR, Lee S, Torres-Cabala C, Chung Y-L, et al. HIF overexpression correlates with biallelic loss of fumarate hydratase in renal cancer: novel role of fumarate in regulation of HIF stability. Cancer Cell 2005;8:143–53.

[42] Sciacovelli M, Gonçalves E, Johnson TI, Zecchini VR, da Costa ASH, Gaude E, et al. Fumarate is an epigenetic modifier that elicits epithelial-to-mesenchymal transition. Nature 2016;537:544–7.

[43] Alderson NL, Wang Y, Blatnik M, Frizzell N, Walla MD, Lyons TJ, et al. S-(2-Succinyl)cysteine: a novel chemical modification of tissue proteins by a Krebs cycle intermediate. Arch Biochem Biophys 2006;450:1–8.

[44] Bardella C, El-Bahrawy M, Frizzell N, Adam J, Ternette N, Hatipoglu E, et al. Aberrant succination of proteins in fumarate hydratase-deficient mice and HLRCC patients is a robust biomarker of mutation status. J Pathol 2011;225:4–11.

[45] Ooi A, Wong J-C, Petillo D, Roossien D, Perrier-Trudova V, Whitten D, et al. An antioxidant response phenotype shared between hereditary and sporadic type 2 papillary renal cell carcinoma. Cancer Cell 2011;20:511–23.

[46] Adam J, Hatipoglu E, O'Flaherty L, Ternette N, Sahgal N, Lockstone H, et al. Renal cyst formation in Fh1-deficient mice is independent of the Hif/Phd pathway: roles for fumarate in KEAP1 succination and Nrf2 signaling. Cancer Cell 2011;20:524–37.

[47] Rogerson C, Sciacovelli M, Maddalena LA, Pouikli A, Segarra-Mondejar M, Valcarcel-Jimenez L, et al. FOXA2 controls the anti-oxidant response in FH-deficient cells. Cell Rep 2023;42:112751.

[48] Humphries F, Shmuel-Galia L, Ketelut-Carneiro N, Li S, Wang B, Nemmara VV, et al. Succination inactivates gasdermin D and blocks pyroptosis. Science 2020;369:1633–7.

[49] Hooftman A, Peace CG, Ryan DG, Day EA, Yang M, McGettrick AF, et al. Macrophage fumarate hydratase restrains mtRNA-mediated interferon production. Nature 2023;615:490–8.

[50] Zecchini V, Paupe V, Herranz-Montoya I, Janssen J, Wortel IMN, Morris JL, et al. Fumarate induces vesicular release of mtDNA to drive innate immunity. Nature 2023;615:499–506.

[51] Degrandi D, Hoffmann R, Beuter-Gunia C, Pfeffer K. The proinflammatory cytokine-induced IRG1 protein associates with mitochondria. J Interferon Cytokine Res J Int Soc Interferon Cytokine Res 2009;29:55–67.

[52] de Weerd NA, Vivian JP, Nguyen TK, Mangan NE, Gould JA, Braniff S-J, et al. Structural basis of a unique interferon-β signaling axis mediated via the receptor IFNAR1. Nat Immunol 2013;14:901–7.

[53] Naujoks J, Tabeling C, Dill BD, Hoffmann C, Brown AS, Kunze M, et al. IFNs modify the proteome of legionella-containing vacuoles and restrict infection Via IRG1-derived itaconic acid. PLoS Pathog 2016;12:e1005408.

[54] De Souza DP, Achuthan A, Lee MK, Binger KJ, Lee M-C, Davidson S, et al. Autocrine IFN-I inhibits isocitrate dehydrogenase in the TCA cycle of LPS-stimulated macrophages. J Clin Invest 2019;129:4239–44.

[55] Heinz A, Nonnenmacher Y, Henne A, Khalil M-A, Bejkollari K, Dostert C, et al. Itaconate controls its own synthesis via feedback-inhibition of reverse TCA cycle activity at IDH2. Biochim Biophys Acta Mol Basis Dis 2022;1868:166530.

[56] Michelucci A, Cordes T, Ghelfi J, Pailot A, Reiling N, Goldmann O, et al. Immune-responsive gene 1 protein links metabolism to immunity by catalyzing itaconic acid production. Proc Natl Acad Sci U S A 2013;110:7820–5.

[57] Hooftman A, O'Neill LAJ. The immunomodulatory potential of the metabolite itaconate. Trends Immunol 2019;40:687–98.

[58] Williams JO, Roche TE, McFadden BA. Mechanism of action of isocitrate lyase from Pseudomonas indigofera. Biochemistry 1971;10:1384–90.

[59] Rittenhouse JW, McFadden BA. Inhibition of isocitrate lyase from Pseudomonas indigofera by itaconate. Arch Biochem Biophys 1974;163:79–86.

[60] Wang H, Fedorov AA, Fedorov EV, Hunt DM, Rodgers A, Douglas HL, et al. An essential bifunctional enzyme in Mycobacterium tuberculosis for itaconate dissimilation and leucine catabolism. Proc Natl Acad Sci U S A 2019;116:15907–13.

[61] Sasikaran J, Ziemski M, Zadora PK, Fleig A, Berg IA. Bacterial itaconate degradation promotes pathogenicity. Nat Chem Biol 2014;10:371–7.

[62] Lampropoulou V, Sergushichev A, Bambouskova M, Nair S, Vincent EE, Loginicheva E, et al. Itaconate links inhibition of succinate dehydrogenase with macrophage metabolic remodeling and regulation of inflammation. Cell Metab 2016;24:158–66.

[63] Mills EL, Ryan DG, Prag HA, Dikovskaya D, Menon D, Zaslona Z, et al. Itaconate is an anti-inflammatory metabolite that activates Nrf2 via alkylation of KEAP1. Nature 2018;556:113–17.

[64] He W, Henne A, Lauterbach M, Geißmar E, Nikolka F, Kho C, et al. Mesaconate is synthesized from itaconate and exerts immunomodulatory effects in macrophages. Nat Metab 2022;4:524–33.

[65] Chen F, Elgaher Wa M, Winterhoff M, Büssow K, Waqas FH, Graner E, et al. Citraconate inhibits ACOD1 (IRG1) catalysis, reduces interferon responses and oxidative stress, and modulates inflammation and cell metabolism. Nat Metab 2022;4:534–46.

[66] Cordes T, Wallace M, Michelucci A, Divakaruni AS, Sapcariu SC, Sousa C, et al. Immunoresponsive gene 1 and itaconate inhibit succinate dehydrogenase to modulate intracellular succinate levels. J Biol Chem 2016;291:14274–84.

[67] Ackermann WW, Potter VR. Enzyme inhibition in relation to chemotherapy. Proc Soc Exp Biol Med Soc Exp Biol Med N Y N 1949;72:1–9.

[68] Seim GL, Britt EC, John SV, Yeo FJ, Johnson AR, Eisenstein RS, et al. Two-stage metabolic remodelling in macrophages in response to lipopolysaccharide and interferon-γ stimulation. Nat Metab 2019;1:731–42.

[69] Azzimato V, Chen P, Barreby E, Morgantini C, Levi L, Vankova A, et al. Hepatic miR-144 drives fumarase activity preventing NRF2 activation during obesity. Gastroenterology 2021;161:1982–1997.e11.

[70] Chen F, Lukat P, Iqbal AA, Saile K, Kaever V, van den Heuvel J, et al. Crystal structure of cis-aconitate decarboxylase reveals the impact of naturally occurring human mutations on itaconate synthesis. Proc Natl Acad Sci U S A 2019;116:20644–54.

[71] Chen F, Yalcin I, Zhao M, Chen C, Blankenfeldt W, Pessler F, et al. Amino acid positions near the active site determine the reduced activity of human ACOD1 compared to murine ACOD1. Sci Rep 2023;13:10360.

[72] Liao S-T, Han C, Xu D-Q, Fu X-W, Wang J-S, Kong L-Y. 4-Octyl itaconate inhibits aerobic glycolysis by targeting GAPDH to exert anti-inflammatory effects. Nat Commun 2019;10:5091.
[73] Hooftman A, Angiari S, Hester S, Corcoran SE, Runtsch MC, Ling C, et al. The Immunomodulatory Metabolite Itaconate Modifies NLRP3 and Inhibits Inflammasome Activation. Cell Metab 2020;32:468–478.e7.
[74] Runtsch MC, Angiari S, Hooftman A, Wadhwa R, Zhang Y, Zheng Y, et al. Itaconate and itaconate derivatives target JAK1 to suppress alternative activation of macrophages. Cell Metab 2022;34:487–501.e8.
[75] Chen L-L, Morcelle C, Cheng Z-L, Chen X, Xu Y, Gao Y, et al. Itaconate inhibits TET DNA dioxygenases to dampen inflammatory responses. Nat Cell Biol 2022;24:353–63.
[76] Peace CG, O'Neill LA. The role of itaconate in host defense and inflammation. J Clin Invest 2022;132:e148548.
[77] Day EA, O'Neill LAJ. Protein targeting by the itaconate family in immunity and inflammation. Biochem J 2022;479:2499–510.
[78] Chen C, Zhang Z, Liu C, Sun P, Liu P, Li X. ABCG2 is an itaconate exporter that limits antibacterial innate immunity by alleviating TFEB-dependent lysosomal biogenesis. Cell Metab 2024;36:498–510.e11.
[79] Zeng Y-R, Song J-B, Wang D, Huang Z-X, Zhang C, Sun Y-P, et al. The immunometabolite itaconate stimulates OXGR1 to promote mucociliary clearance during the pulmonary innate immune response. J Clin Invest 2023;133:e160463.
[80] Tomlinson KL, Riquelme SA, Baskota SU, Drikic M, Monk IR, Stinear TP, et al. Staphylococcus aureus stimulates neutrophil itaconate production that suppresses the oxidative burst. Cell Rep 2023;42:112064.
[81] Chen C, Liu C, Sun P, Zhang Z, Wang Z, Liu P, et al. Itaconate uptake via SLC13A3 improves hepatic antibacterial innate immunity. Dev Cell 2024; S1534-5807(24)00448-9.
[82] Pajor AM. Sodium-coupled dicarboxylate and citrate transporters from the SLC13 family. Pflug Arch 2014;466:119–30.
[83] Weiss JM, Davies LC, Karwan M, Ileva L, Ozaki MK, Cheng RY, et al. Itaconic acid mediates crosstalk between macrophage metabolism and peritoneal tumors. J Clin Invest 2018;128:3794–805.
[84] Chen Y-J, Li G-N, Li X-J, Wei L-X, Fu M-J, Cheng Z-L, et al. Targeting IRG1 reverses the immunosuppressive function of tumor-associated macrophages and enhances cancer immunotherapy. Sci Adv 2023;9:eadg0654.
[85] Wang X, Su S, Zhu Y, Cheng X, Cheng C, Chen L, et al. Metabolic Reprogramming via ACOD1 depletion enhances function of human induced pluripotent stem cell-derived CAR-macrophages in solid tumors. Nat Commun 2023;14:5778.
[86] Zhao H, Teng D, Yang L, Xu X, Chen J, Jiang T, et al. Myeloid-derived itaconate suppresses cytotoxic CD8 + T cells and promotes tumour growth. Nat Metab 2022;4:1660–73.
[87] Gu X, Wei H, Suo C, Shen S, Zhu C, Chen L, et al. Itaconate promotes hepatocellular carcinoma progression by epigenetic induction of CD8 + T-cell exhaustion. Nat Commun 2023;14:8154.
[88] Harber, Neele KJ, van Roomen AE, Gijbels CP, Beckers L MJ, Toom, et al. Targeting the ACOD1-itaconate axis stabilizes atherosclerotic plaques. Redox Biol 2024;70:103054.
[89] Li W, Li Y, Kang J, Jiang H, Gong W, Chen L, et al. 4-octyl itaconate as a metabolite derivative inhibits inflammation via alkylation of STING. Cell Rep 2023;42:112145.
[90] Su C, Cheng T, Huang J, Zhang T, Yin H. 4-Octyl itaconate restricts STING activation by blocking its palmitoylation. Cell Rep 2023;42:113040.
[91] Kurmasheva N, Said A, Wong B, Kinderman P, Han X, Rahimic AHF, et al. Octyl itaconate enhances VSVΔ51 oncolytic virotherapy by multitarget inhibition of antiviral and inflammatory pathways. Nat Commun 2024;15:4096.
[92] Bambouskova M, Gorvel L, Lampropoulou V, Sergushichev A, Loginicheva E, Johnson K, et al. Electrophilic properties of itaconate and derivatives regulate the IκBζ-ATF3 inflammatory axis. Nature 2018;556:501–4.
[93] Sun KA, Li Y, Meliton AY, Woods PS, Kimmig LM, Cetin-Atalay R, et al. Endogenous itaconate is not required for particulate matter-induced NRF2 expression or inflammatory response. eLife 2020;9:e54877.

[94] Schuster E-M, Epple MW, Glaser KM, Mihlan M, Lucht K, Zimmermann JA, et al. TFEB induces mitochondrial itaconate synthesis to suppress bacterial growth in macrophages. Nat Metab 2022;4:856−66.

[95] Zhang Z, Chen C, Yang F, Zeng Y-X, Sun P, Liu P, et al. Itaconate is a lysosomal inducer that promotes antibacterial innate immunity. Mol Cell 2022;82:2844−2857.e10.

[96] Olagnier D, Brandtoft AM, Gunderstofte C, Villadsen NL, Krapp C, Thielke AL, et al. Nrf2 negatively regulates STING indicating a link between antiviral sensing and metabolic reprogramming. Nat Commun 2018;9:3506.

[97] Ryan TAJ, Hooftman A, Rehill AM, Johansen MD, Brien ECO, Toller-Kawahisa JE, et al. Dimethyl fumarate and 4-octyl itaconate are anticoagulants that suppress Tissue Factor in macrophages via inhibition of Type I Interferon. Nat Commun 2023;14:3513.

[98] Swain A, Bambouskova M, Kim H, Andhey PS, Duncan D, Auclair K, et al. Comparative evaluation of itaconate and its derivatives reveals divergent inflammasome and type I interferon regulation in macrophages. Nat Metab 2020;2:594−602.

[99] Waqas SF-U-H, Sohail A, Nguyen AHH, Usman A, Ludwig T, Wegner A, et al. ISG15 deficiency features a complex cellular phenotype that responds to treatment with itaconate and derivatives. Clin Transl Med 2022;12:e931.

[100] O'Carroll SM, Peace CG, Toller-Kawahisa JE, Min Y, Hooftman A, Charki S, et al. Itaconate drives mtRNA-mediated type I interferon production through inhibition of succinate dehydrogenase. Nat Metab 2024.

[101] Daniels BP, Kofman SB, Smith JR, Norris GT, Snyder AG, Kolb JP, et al. The Nucleotide Sensor ZBP1 and Kinase RIPK3 Induce the Enzyme IRG1 to Promote an Antiviral Metabolic State in Neurons. Immunity 2019;50:64−76.e4.

[102] Song J-W, Lam SM, Fan X, Cao W-J, Wang S-Y, Tian H, et al. Omics-driven systems interrogation of metabolic dysregulation in COVID-19 pathogenesis. Cell Metab 2020;32:188−202.e5.

[103] Sohail A, Iqbal AA, Sahini N, Chen F, Tantawy M, Waqas SFH, et al. Itaconate and derivatives reduce interferon responses and inflammation in influenza A virus infection. PLoS Pathog 2022;18:e1010219.

[104] Xiao Y, Chen X, Wang Z, Quan J, Zhao X, Tang H, et al. Succinate Is a natural suppressor of antiviral immune response by targeting MAVS. Front Immunol 2022;13:816378.

[105] Zaro BW, Vinogradova EV, Lazar DC, Blewett MM, Suciu RM, Takaya J, et al. Dimethyl fumarate disrupts human innate immune signaling by targeting the IRAK4-MyD88 complex. J Immunol Baltim Md 1950 2019;202:2737−46.

[106] Linker RA, Lee D-H, Ryan S, van Dam AM, Conrad R, Bista P, et al. Fumaric acid esters exert neuroprotective effects in neuroinflammation via activation of the Nrf2 antioxidant pathway. Brain J Neurol 2011;134:678−92.

[107] Schmitt A, Xu W, Bucher P, Grimm M, Konantz M, Horn H, et al. Dimethyl fumarate induces ferroptosis and impairs NF-κB/STAT3 signaling in DLBCL. Blood 2021;138:871−84.

[108] Zhou G, Myers R, Li Y, Chen Y, Shen X, Fenyk-Melody J, et al. Role of AMP-activated protein kinase in mechanism of metformin action. J Clin Invest 2001;108:1167−74.

[109] Day EA, Ford RJ, Smith BK, Mohammadi-Shemirani P, Morrow MR, Gutgesell RM, et al. Metformin-induced increases in GDF15 are important for suppressing appetite and promoting weight loss. Nat Metab 2019;1:1202−8.

[110] Coll AP, Chen M, Taskar P, Rimmington D, Patel S, Tadross JA, et al. GDF15 mediates the effects of metformin on body weight and energy balance. Nature 2020;578:444−8.

[111] Sonveaux P, Végran F, Schroeder T, Wergin MC, Verrax J, Rabbani ZN, et al. Targeting lactate-fueled respiration selectively kills hypoxic tumor cells in mice. J Clin Invest 2008;118:3930−42.

[112] Ullah MS, Davies AJ, Halestrap AP. The plasma membrane lactate transporter MCT4, but not MCT1, is up-regulated by hypoxia through a HIF-1alpha-dependent mechanism. J Biol Chem 2006;281:9030−7.

[113] Cai T-Q, Ren N, Jin L, Cheng K, Kash S, Chen R, et al. Role of GPR81 in lactate-mediated reduction of adipose lipolysis. Biochem Biophys Res Commun 2008;377:987−91.

[114] Ahmed K, Tunaru S, Tang C, Müller M, Gille A, Sassmann A, et al. An autocrine lactate loop mediates insulin-dependent inhibition of lipolysis through GPR81. Cell Metab 2010;11:311−19.

[115] Quinn WJ, Jiao J, TeSlaa T, Stadanlick J, Wang Z, Wang L, et al. Lactate limits T cell proliferation via the NAD(H) redox state. Cell Rep 2020;33:108500.

[116] Liu W, Wang Y, Bozi LHM, Fischer PD, Jedrychowski MP, Xiao H, et al. Lactate regulates cell cycle by remodelling the anaphase promoting complex. Nature 2023;616:790–7.

[117] Zhang D, Tang Z, Huang H, Zhou G, Cui C, Weng Y, et al. Metabolic regulation of gene expression by histone lactylation. Nature 2019;574:575–80.

[118] Shi W, Cassmann TJ, Bhagwate AV, Hitosugi T, Ip WKE. Lactic acid induces transcriptional repression of macrophage inflammatory response via histone acetylation. Cell Rep 2024;43:113746.

[119] Reynolds MB, Klein B, McFadden MJ, Judge NK, Navarrete HE, Michmerhuizen BC, et al. Type I interferon governs immunometabolic checkpoints that coordinate inflammation during Staphylococcal infection. Cell Rep 2024;43:114607.

[120] Zhang W, Wang G, Xu Z-G, Tu H, Hu F, Dai J, et al. Lactate is a natural suppressor of RLR signaling by targeting MAVS. Cell 2019;178:176–189.e15.

[121] Zhou L, He R, Fang P, Li M, Yu H, Wang Q, et al. Hepatitis B virus rigs the cellular metabolome to avoid innate immune recognition. Nat Commun 2021;12:98.

[122] He Q-Q, Huang Y, Nie L, Ren S, Xu G, Deng F, et al. MAVS integrates glucose metabolism and RIG-I-like receptor signaling. Nat Commun 2023;14:5343.

[123] Ma M, Jiang W, Zhou R. DAMPs and DAMP-sensing receptors in inflammation and diseases. Immunity 2024;57:752–71.

[124] Huang Y, Jiang W, Zhou R. DAMP sensing and sterile inflammation: intracellular, intercellular and inter-organ pathways. Nat Rev Immunol 2024.

[125] Serbulea V, Upchurch CM, Schappe MS, Voigt P, DeWeese DE, Desai BN, et al. Macrophage phenotype and bioenergetics are controlled by oxidized phospholipids identified in lean and obese adipose tissue. Proc Natl Acad Sci U S A 2018;115:E6254–63.

[126] Di Gioia M, Spreafico R, Springstead JR, Mendelson MM, Joehanes R, Levy D, et al. Endogenous oxidized phospholipids reprogram cellular metabolism and boost hyperinflammation. Nat Immunol 2020;21:42–53.

[127] Di Gioia M, Poli V, Tan PJ, Spreafico R, Chu A, Cuenca AG, et al. Host-derived oxidized phospholipids initiate effector-triggered immunity fostering lethality upon microbial encounter. BioRxiv Prepr Serv Biol 2023; 2023.11.21.568047.

[128] Furuyashiki T, Narumiya S. Stress responses: the contribution of prostaglandin E2 and its receptors. Nat Rev Endocrinol 2011;7:163–75 Nature Publishing Group.

[129] Watson AD, Leitinger N, Navab M, Faull KF, Hörkkö S, Witztum JL, et al. Structural identification by mass spectrometry of oxidized phospholipids in minimally oxidized low density lipoprotein that induce monocyte/endothelial interactions and evidence for their presence in vivo. J Biol Chem 1997;272:13597–607.

[130] Navab M, Ananthramaiah GM, Reddy ST, Lenten BJV, Ansell BJ, Fonarow GC, et al. Thematic review series: The Pathogenesis of Atherosclerosis The oxidation hypothesis of atherogenesis: the role of oxidized phospholipids and HDL. J Lipid Res 2004;45:993–1007.

[131] Tsiantoulas D, Perkmann T, Afonyushkin T, Mangold A, Prohaska TA, Papac-Milicevic N, et al. Circulating microparticles carry oxidation-specific epitopes and are recognized by natural IgM antibodies. J Lipid Res 2015;56:440–8.

[132] Yang M, Du Q, Goswami J, Varley PR, Chen B, Wang R, et al. Interferon regulatory factor 1–Rab27a regulated extracellular vesicles promote liver ischemia/reperfusion injury. Hepatology 2018;67:1056–70.

[133] Binder CJ, Papac-Milicevic N, Witztum JL. Innate sensing of oxidation-specific epitopes in health and disease. Nat Rev Immunol 2016;16:485–97.

[134] Que X, Hung M-Y, Yeang C, Gonen A, Prohaska TA, Sun X, et al. Oxidized phospholipids are proinflammatory and proatherogenic in hypercholesterolaemic mice. Nature 2018;558:301–6.

[135] Sun X, Seidman JS, Zhao P, Troutman TD, Spann NJ, Que X, et al. Neutralization of oxidized phospholipids ameliorates non-alcoholic steatohepatitis. Cell Metab 2020;31:189–206.e8.

[136] Imai Y, Kuba K, Neely GG, Yaghubian-Malhami R, Perkmann T, van Loo G, et al. Identification of oxidative stress and Toll-like receptor 4 signaling as a key pathway of acute lung injury. Cell 2008;133:235—49.

[137] Cruz D, Watson AD, Miller CS, Montoya D, Ochoa M-T, Sieling PA, et al. Host-derived oxidized phospholipids and HDL regulate innate immunity in human leprosy. J Clin Invest 2008;118:2917—28.

[138] Gruber F, Oskolkova O, Leitner A, Mildner M, Mlitz V, Lengauer B, et al. Photooxidation generates biologically active phospholipids that induce heme oxygenase-1 in skin cells. J Biol Chem 2007;282:16934—41.

[139] Nakanishi H, Iida Y, Shimizu T, Taguchi R. Analysis of oxidized phosphatidylcholines as markers for oxidative stress, using multiple reaction monitoring with theoretically expanded data sets with reversed-phase liquid chromatography/tandem mass spectrometry. J Chromatogr B Anal Technol Biomed Life Sci 2009;877:1366—74.

[140] Kanter JL, Narayana S, Ho PP, Catz I, Warren KG, Sobel RA, et al. Lipid microarrays identify key mediators of autoimmune brain inflammation. Nat Med 2006;12:138—43.

[141] Qin J, Goswami R, Balabanov R, Dawson G. Oxidized phosphatidylcholine is a marker for neuroinflammation in multiple sclerosis brain. J Neurosci Res 2007;85:977—84.

[142] Fisch D, Zhang T, Sun H, Ma W, Tan Y, Gygi SP, et al. Molecular definition of the endogenous Toll-like receptor signalling pathways. Nature 2024;631:635—44.

[143] Fitzgerald KA, Kagan JC. Toll-like receptors and the control of immunity. Cell 2020;180:1044—66.

[144] Su Z, Burchfield JG, Yang P, Humphrey SJ, Yang G, Francis D, et al. Global redox proteome and phosphoproteome analysis reveals redox switch in Akt. Nat Commun 2019;10:5486.

[145] Long MJC, Parvez S, Zhao Y, Surya SL, Wang Y, Zhang S, et al. Akt3 is a privileged first responder in isozyme-specific electrophile response. Nat Chem Biol., 13. Nature Publishing Group; 2017. p. 333—8.

[146] Springstead JR, Gugiu BG, Lee S, Cha S, Watson AD, Berliner JA. Evidence for the importance of OxPAPC interaction with cysteines in regulating endothelial cell function. J Lipid Res 2012;53:1304—15.

[147] Jyrkkänen H-K, Kansanen E, Inkala M, Kivelä AM, Hurttila H, Heinonen SE, et al. Nrf2 regulates antioxidant gene expression evoked by oxidized phospholipids in endothelial cells and murine arteries in vivo. Circ Res 2008;103:e1—9.

[148] Bretscher P, Egger J, Shamshiev A, Trötzmüller M, Köfeler H, Carreira EM, et al. Phospholipid oxidation generates potent anti-inflammatory lipid mediators that mimic structurally related pro-resolving eicosanoids by activating Nrf2. EMBO Mol Med 2015;7:593—607 Springer Nature.

[149] Muri J, Feng Q, Wolleb H, Shamshiev A, Ebner C, Tortola L, et al. Cyclopentenone prostaglandins and structurally related oxidized lipid species instigate and share distinct pro- and anti-inflammatory pathways. Cell Rep 2020;30:4399—4417.e7.

[150] Cha T-L, Zhou BP, Xia W, Wu Y, Yang C-C, Chen C-T, et al. Akt-mediated phosphorylation of EZH2 suppresses methylation of lysine 27 in histone H3. Science 2005;310:306—10.

[151] Sankar A, Mohammad F, Sundaramurthy AK, Wang H, Lerdrup M, Tatar T, et al. Histone editing elucidates the functional roles of H3K27 methylation and acetylation in mammals. Nat Genet 2022;54:754—60.

[152] Scacchetti A, Bonasio R. Histone gene editing probes functions of H3K27 modifications in mammals. Nat Genet 2022;54:746—7.

[153] Moore KW, de Waal Malefyt R, Coffman RL. O'Garra A. Interleukin-10 and the interleukin-10 receptor. Annu Rev Immunol 2001;19:683—765.

[154] Fong G-H, Takeda K. Role and regulation of prolyl hydroxylase domain proteins. Cell Death Differ 2008;15:635—41 Nature Publishing Group.

[155] Wellen KE, Hatzivassiliou G, Sachdeva UM, Bui TV, Cross JR, Thompson CB. ATP-citrate lyase links cellular metabolism to histone acetylation. Science 2009;324:1076—80 American Association for the Advancement of Science.

[156] Covarrubias A.J., Aksoylar H.I., Yu J., Snyder N.W., Worth A.J., Iyer S.S. Akt-mTORC1 signaling regulates Acly to integrate metabolic input to control of macrophage activation. In: Wallach D., editor. eLife. eLife Sciences Publications, Ltd; 2016. p. e11612. 5.

[157] Zorova LD, Popkov VA, Plotnikov EY, Silachev DN, Pevzner IB, Jankauskas SS, et al. Mitochondrial membrane potential. Anal Biochem 2018;552:50–9.

[158] Serbulea V, Upchurch CM, Ahern KW, Bories G, Voigt P, DeWeese DE, et al. Macrophages sensing oxidized DAMPs reprogram their metabolism to support redox homeostasis and inflammation through a TLR2-Syk-ceramide dependent mechanism. Mol Metab 2017;7:23–34.

[159] Robbins CS, Hilgendorf I, Weber GF, Theurl I, Iwamoto Y, Figueiredo J-L, et al. Local proliferation dominates lesional macrophage accumulation in atherosclerosis. Nat Med 2013;19:1166–72.

[160] Monocyte-derived alveolar macrophages drive lung fibrosis and persist in the lung over the life span | Journal of Experimental Medicine | Rockefeller University Press [Internet]. [cited 2020 Aug 31]. Available from: https://rupress-org.ezp-prod1.hul.harvard.edu/jem/article/214/8/2387/42522/Monocyte-derived-alveolar-macrophages-drive-lung.

[161] Zanoni I, Tan Y, Di Gioia M, Broggi A, Ruan J, Shi J, et al. An endogenous caspase-11 ligand elicits interleukin-1 release from living dendritic cells. Science 2016;352:1232–6.

[162] Zanoni I, Tan Y, Di Gioia M, Springstead JR, Kagan JC. By capturing inflammatory lipids released from dying cells, the receptor CD14 induces inflammasome-dependent phagocyte hyperactivation. Immunity 2017;47:697–709.e3.

[163] Zhivaki D, Borriello F, Chow OA, Doran B, Fleming I, Theisen DJ, et al. Inflammasomes within hyperactive murine dendritic cells stimulate long-lived T cell-mediated anti-tumor immunity. Cell Rep 2020;33:108381.

[164] Zhivaki D, Kennedy SN, Park J, Boriello F, Devant P, Cao A, et al. Correction of age-associated defects in dendritic cells enables CD4 + T cells to eradicate tumors. Cell, 187. Elsevier; 2024. p. 3888–903. e18.

[165] Podrez EA, Poliakov E, Shen Z, Zhang R, Deng Y, Sun M, et al. Identification of a novel family of oxidized phospholipids that serve as ligands for the macrophage scavenger receptor CD36. J Biol Chem 2002;277:38503–16.

[166] Chen R, Brady E, McIntyre TM. Human TMEM30a Promotes Uptake of Anti-tumor and Bioactive Choline Phospholipids into Mammalian Cells. J Immunol Baltim Md 1950 2011;186:3215–25.

[167] Cavazos AT, Pennington ER, Dadoo S, Gowdy KM, Wassall SR, Shaikh SR. OxPAPC stabilizes liquid-ordered domains in biomimetic membranes. Biophys J 2023;122:1130–9.

[168] Kerur N, Fukuda S, Banerjee D, Kim Y, Fu D, Apicella I, et al. cGAS drives noncanonical-inflammasome activation in age-related macular degeneration. Nat Med 2018;24:50–61 Nature Publishing Group.

[169] Evavold CL, Ruan J, Tan Y, Xia S, Wu H, Kagan JC. The Pore-Forming Protein Gasdermin D Regulates Interleukin-1 Secretion from Living Macrophages. Immunity 2018;48:35–44.e6.

[170] Rühl S, Shkarina K, Demarco B, Heilig R, Santos JC, Broz P. ESCRT-dependent membrane repair negatively regulates pyroptosis downstream of GSDMD activation. Science 2018;362:956–60.

CHAPTER 8

Adaptive immunity and metabolism

Katherine C. Verbist, Piyush Sharma, Helen Beere and Douglas R. Green
Department of Immunology, St. Jude Children's Research Hospital, Memphis, TN, United States

Introduction

The adaptive immune response is characterized by lymphocytes and their functions. Several inherent properties of lymphocytes dictate their demand for energy and consequent metabolic states: (1) They are long-lived, as naïve and memory cells persist in a host for many decades; (2) they have enormous proliferative capacity, as effector T cells or germinal center B cells produce millions of daughter cells; (3) they differentiate into effector cells producing large numbers of cytotoxic granules, cytokines, or antibodies; (4) they are highly mobile; and (5) they must glean nutrients from very different tissue microenvironments.

Despite a great deal of speculation about the high energetic costs of an adaptive immune response, this has not been rigorously assessed in any system. One study in congenic mice using an antigen that induces a rapid antibody response (Keyhole Lipid Hemocyanin in saline) showed some enhancing effect on oxygen consumption [1]; however, this was not tested in animals incapable of mounting an adaptive immune response (e.g., RAG- or IgM-deficient animals). Other studies in a variety of outbred animals of different species showed conflicting results [2,3].

Based on the known adenosine triphosphate (ATP) requirements, we can broadly estimate the energetic costs of T- and B-cell proliferation. The major cost is the replication and maintenance of the lymphocyte cellular proteome of about 4×10^8 proteins with an average length of 300–400 amino acids, requiring about 8×10^{11} ATP. If we factor in the synthesis of lipids and nucleic acids, the cost for a single division of a lymphocyte is about 10^{12} ATP [4]. The most rapidly dividing cell in the human body is an activated $CD8^+$ T cell, which divides every 4–6 hours [5] and thus requires about 2×10^8 ATP per second. Activated $CD4^+$ T cells and B cells divide more slowly but still rapidly compared to other cells in the body. Since activated lymphocytes have additional demands beyond division, as outlined above, let's increase our estimate to 3×10^8 ATP per second (probably an overestimate). Generic cells in the human body generate about 10^8 ATP per second [4]. While we know that the many thousands of activated lymphocytes that function in an adaptive immune response increase their metabolism to meet the increased demand for ATP and the material for biomass, it is nevertheless unlikely that this represents a major drain on the metabolic resources of the body overall. (Innate responses, including fever, may cause such a drain, but here we are only considering the costs of the adaptive immune response.)

In this chapter, we consider how the adaptive immune response is metabolically fueled and how different immune cells participating in such responses rewire their metabolism to meet the demands of responding to a foreign antigen.

Metabolism of the antigen-presenting cells

Most of the adaptive immune response comprises the actions of lymphocytes, but the initiation of this response is governed by dendritic cells (DCs), myeloid antigen-presenting cells that provide stimulation in the form of cognate antigen, costimulation, and cytokine signals to specific T cells. They can also produce the state known as immunological tolerance, a subsequent inability of the adaptive immune system to respond to a specific antigen. It is now appreciated that the metabolic state of the antigen-presenting cells helps shape the subsequent T cell response. Activated DCs are highly glycolytic and adopt this metabolic pathway when initiating T-cell responses [6]. The switch to glycolysis in response to an activating signal (lipopolysaccharide) was found to be dependent on phosphoinositide-3-kinase (PI3K) and AKT and antagonized by adenosine monophosphate (AMP)-activated protein kinase (AMPK). Inhibition of glycolysis prevented DC activation and antigen presentation to T cells [7]. Similar studies have also implicated Hypoxia-Induced Factor-1 (HIF-1) in the switch to glycolysis in activated DCs [8].

In contrast, DCs that induce immune tolerance, similar to immature DCs, are characterized by oxidative phosphorylation (OXPHOS) [9,10]. The tolerogenic properties of DCs have been linked to increased fatty-acid oxidation (FAO) [11]. Human monocyte-derived DCs, treated with dexamethasone and vitamin D_3 to induce tolerogenic DCs, induced unresponsiveness in allogeneic T cells, and this was partially reversed by inhibition of FAO [10].

Metabolism of $CD8^+$ T cells

Naïve T cell metabolism

Naïve T cells are long-lasting, metabolically quiescent cells, maintained in a homeostatic state by signals induced by tonic T cell receptor (TCR) signaling, sphingosine 1-phosphate (S1P), and IL-7, which, in combination with AKT signaling, regulate glucose receptor Glut1 expression to maintain glucose uptake. Glucose is subsequently metabolized into pyruvate, fueling the TCA cycle and mitochondrial OXPHOS to fulfill the ATP demand

[12,13]. Studies have further shown that mitochondrial complex III or IV deficiency leads to a decreased number of naïve T cells, suggesting a role for the electron transport chain (ETC) in naïve T cell maturation and survival [14,15]. IL-7 signaling is critical for naïve T cell maintenance, as studies have demonstrated that loss of function mutation in IL-7R severely compromises the survival of naïve T cells [16]. IL-7 expression is maintained by forkhead box protein O1 (FOXO1), and the recruitment of IL-7R into lipid rafts sustains IL7 signaling [17,18]. S1P, which supports naïve T cell survival and is important for T cell migration, facilitates OXPHOS by suppressing mitophagy [19]. Fatty acids contribute to energy production via mitochondrial-dependent FAO. Both short-chain and long-chain fatty acids (SCFAs and LCFAs) act as substrates for FAO, while SCFA can freely diffuse into the mitochondrial matrix, and the transport of LCFA is regulated by Carnitine Palmitoyltransferase-1 (Cpt1) [20]. FAO catabolizes acyl-CoA, generating acetyl-CoA, which is shuttled into the TCA cycle and further oxidized to generate ATP [21]. Acetyl-CoA also promotes lipid and cholesterol synthesis via the mevalonate pathway. Collectively, naïve T cells maintain a minimal metabolic state, which is primarily sustained by the energy generated from OXPHOS and FAO.

T cell activation

Upon cognate antigen recognition, naïve T cells undergo rapid transformation, which is visually observed as a rapid increase in cellular mass and number. T cell receptor (TCR) stimulation combined with CD28 costimulation facilitates the PI3K-AKT axis, which, in combination with nuclear factor of activated T cells (NFAT), upregulates GLUT1 and ASCT2 transporters. This upregulation ensures glucose and glutamine uptake, the two major metabolic contributors to T cell activation, prioritizing anabolism over catabolism. Glutamine plays a significant role in the quiescence exit of naïve T cells, and its catabolism by glutaminolysis aids in biosynthesis and generates glutathione, thereby counteracting reactive oxygen species (ROS). Glutaminolysis is also coupled with the biosynthesis of polyamines, where ornithine (precursor of polyamines) is generated from glutamine [22] as well as arginine [23]. It further facilitates T cell proliferation by promoting leucine uptake via LAT1-CD98 and subsequently activates mammalian target of rapamycin complex I (mTORC1) [24]. Next, the transcription factor Myc is expressed in an mTORC1-dependent manner and regulates the expression of GLUT1 and glutaminase I (GLS1), supporting T cell proliferation by promoting both glucose and glutamine metabolism [25]. Although Myc regulates glutamine uptake and catabolism, glutamine is shown to be required for sustained Myc expression, where glutamine starvation significantly dampens Myc expression and consequently T cell proliferation [21]. Studies indicate that Myc is frequently asymmetrically sorted upon division mediated by the TORC1-eIF4F complex, which influences the differentiation of effector or memory T cells [26,27]. The mTOR-Myc axis is important in initiating and maintaining the activation-induced proteomic and metabolomic flux necessary to sustain the proliferative demand.

Mitochondrial metabolism dynamics in T cell activation

Mitochondria are key organelles in T cell activation. Metabolic intermediates from both glucose and glutamine catabolism enter the TCA cycle in the mitochondria, subsequently regulating OXPHOS, NADPH, and glycolysis for energy production. Upon activation, glutaminolysis results in conversion of glutamine to glutamate, which further feeds into generation of α-ketoglutarate (α-KG). α-KG is then metabolized via the TCA cycle to generate citrate and pyruvate, supporting glycolysis [21]. While not mitochondrial, the pentose phosphate pathway (PPP) is crucial for NADPH and ribose-5-phosphate (for nucleotide synthesis) generation. The PPP is fueled via the glucose catabolic pathway at glucose-6-phosphate, which is catalyzed by glucose-6-phosphate dehydrogenase (G6PD) to generate NADPH [28]. To further support OXPHOS, mitochondrial biogenesis is upregulated via mTORC1-dependent remodeling of the mitochondrial proteome. The balance between glycolysis and OXPHOS is crucial during T cell activation. Mitochondrial pyruvate carrier (MPC) transports pyruvate into mitochondria, effectively reducing its availability in the cytoplasm, leading to the generation of acetyl-CoA, promoting the TCA and OXPHOS. Inhibition of MPC favors glycolysis [29]. Another mitochondrial metabolite that is crucial for optimal activation is ROS, which must be regulated as excess ROS can lead to cellular oxidative damage. Mitochondrial ROS induction is coupled with increased transcription of glutamate-cysteine ligase catalytic subunit (GCLC), which is the rate-limiting enzyme of glutathione (GSH) biosynthesis [30]. GSH is utilized by glutathione peroxidase 4 (GPX4) to combat lipid hydroperoxides generated by oxidant ROS species H_2O_2, to prevent ferroptosis [31]. Additionally, GCLC ablation has been shown to be associated with defective TCR-induced Myc expression and T cell activation, via dampening aerobic glycolysis and glutaminolysis and reduced NFAT signaling [32].

Ca^{2+}-mediated NFAT signaling is crucial for initial T cell activation. Studies indicate that the glycolytic metabolite phosphoenolpyruvate (PEP) inhibits sarco/endoplasmic reticulum Ca^{2+}-ATPase (SERCA) activity, thereby sustaining TCR-mediated NFAT signaling [33].

T cells have also been shown to utilize lactate dehydrogenase A (LDHA), which converts pyruvate to lactate, sustaining NAD^+/NADH ratios [34]. Studies have further demonstrated that T cells can utilize lactate as a source of pyruvate to fuel the TCA cycle [35].

Although T cells can scavenge nucleotides [36], they can also produce them *de novo*. Mitochondrial function is necessary for pyrimidine synthesis, as one step in this process occurs in the mitochondrial intermembrane space and is dependent on ubiquinone generated by the Q cycle in the ETC. Another important pathway is the one-carbon (1 C) pathway, which supports mitochondrial NADPH generation and nucleotide synthesis. The 1 C pathway is initiated by donating one carbon to tetrahydro-folate (THF) through the conversion of serine into glycine in a reversible reaction via serine hydroxyl-methyltransferase 1 or 2 (SHMT1/2), generating 5,10-methylene-THF (5,10-me-THF), used in the production of purines [37].

Fatty-acid metabolism in activated T cells

T cell activation involves accumulation of metabolites associated with fatty-acid synthesis (FAS), with a concomitant decrease in FAO pathway metabolites. This metabolic shift from FAO to FAS is dependent on the mTORC1-Myc axis [38], and studies have shown that deletion of Raptor, an mTORC1 scaffolding protein, led to compromised de novo lipid synthesis [39]. Mechanistically, mTORC1 induces sterol regulatory element-binding proteins 1 and 2 (SREBP1/2), which subsequently bind to the promoter region of key genes involved in lipid synthesis, including genes encoding acetyl-CoA carboxylase (*Acaca*), fatty-acid synthesis (*Fasn*), and hydroxymethylglutaryl-CoA reductase (*Hmgcr*, encoding the rate-limiting enzyme of cholesterol synthesis). Cell-specific deletion of *Srebp* or *Acc1* has been shown to significantly decrease T cell proliferation and differentiation [40].

Amino acid metabolism in activated T cells

In addition to protein generation, amino acids are critical for the biosynthesis of nucleotides, polyamines, and antioxidants (GSH). Upon activation, naïve T cells induce mTORC-Myc-mediated upregulation of multiple solute transporters, for example, the glutamine-specific transporters Slc32a1 and Slc32a2, the L-amino acid transporter Slc7a5, and the antiporter Slc7a11, among others, enabling influx of amino acids necessary for optimal activation. Arginine is converted to ornithine and citrulline, further aiding in the generation of polyamines and GSH. Studies have demonstrated that arginine deprivation induces T cell proliferation arrest via General Control Nonderepressible-2 (GCN2), highlighting the crucial role of arginine in T cell proliferation following activation [41]. However, another study found that Gcn2-deficient CD8[+] T cells fail to proliferate in response to presented antigen under in vitro or in vivo conditions of limiting amounts of arginine, asparagine, lysine, tryptophan, or leucine [42].

Leucine, a large neutral amino acid, is important in mTORC1 activation and is primarily transported by Slc7a5 and Slc3a2 [43,44]. Methionine is an essential amino acid required for protein synthesis as well as cellular methylome maintenance through the generation of methyl-donor S-adenosyl methionine (SAM). It can be transported by several solute transporters, with Slc7a5 being the essential one [45]. Asparagine is a nonessential amino acid, transported by alanine, serine, and cysteine transporter 2 (ASCT2) and utilized for protein synthesis and post-translational modifications. T cells, upon activation, upregulate asparagine synthetase (ASNS) in an mTOR-Myc-dependent manner, which generates asparagine and glutamate from glutamine and aspartate. Studies reveal that extracellular availability of asparagine is inversely related to ASNS levels [46]. Furthermore, direct binding of asparagine to Src-family tyrosine kinase Lck strengthens phosphorylation at Tyr394, enhancing TCR signaling [47]. Collectively, amino acid metabolism is important during T cell activation, aiding in proteome and epigenome maintenance and proliferation.

Effector and memory CD8+ T cells

Effector T cells (Teff) are cytolytic cells that eliminate infected or malignant cells and exhibit a short lifespan, whereas memory T cells (Tmem) are long-lived, antigen-specific cells that undergo a rapid proliferative response upon antigen recognition and can differentiate into Teff to mediate recall responses.

Upon activation, T cells maintain their effector function primarily through glycolysis, while still executing OXPHOS [25,48]. Similarly to the activation state, fully differentiated Teff cells utilize both glucose and glutamine to meet their ATP requirements and to maintain redox balance, while directing lipids and amino acids toward biomass generation and proliferation. Although most of the metabolic state of Teff cells resembles that observed during T cell activation, certain pathways warrant emphasis due to their importance in Teff maintenance and function. Glycolytic metabolism directly correlates with Teff function, as studies have demonstrated that mTORC1 inhibition decreases glycolysis and effector function. A reduction in glucose availability diminishes glucose-derived pyruvate, attenuates acetyl-CoA generation with a subsequent decrease in protein and histone acetylation, and diverts glyceraldehyde 3-phosphate dehydrogenase (GAPDH) activity as a glycolytic enzyme towards binding to the 3'UTR of IFN-γ, limiting its synthesis [49]. Along with generation of acetyl-CoA, the mitochondrial ETC is critical for Teff function, where complex III regulates ROS production for NFAT signaling and interleukin-2 (IL-2) production [15]. Despite heavily relying on glycolysis, Teff cells still regulate OXPHOS. This is further regulated by cytochrome oxidase (COX), and deletion of COX (Cox10) led to decreased OXPHOS and increased T cell apoptosis after activation [14].

FAS is a hallmark of Teff cells. The mTORC1-mediated induction of the SREBP pathway is crucial for maintaining Teff cells, and deletion of SREBP cleavage activating protein (SCAP) resulted in significantly impaired Teff differentiation. This effect was also attributed to inhibition of the glycolytic switch in SCAP-deficient cells. Moreover, exogenous cholesterol was able to rescue SCAP-deficient T cells, reinforcing the role of lipid synthesis in Teff differentiation and function [40].

As with activated T cells, glutamine, serine, and arginine are important for the maintenance and proliferation of Teff cells. Arginine supplementation promotes both serine biosynthesis and OXPHOS, which enhances T cell survival but attenuates effector responses [23]. Conversely, limiting methionine availability can disrupt Teff function through reduction in H3K79me2 methylation and decreased STAT5 function [50].

Tmem can be further delineated into T effector memory (Tem, $CD44^{hi}$ $CD62L^{lo}$ $CCR7^{lo}$), T central memory (Tcm, $CD44^{hi}$ $CD62L^{hi}$ $CCR7^{hi}$), and T resident memory (Trm, $CD103^{+}CD69^{+}$). As Tmem are long-lived, they exhibit a metabolic state similar to that of naïve T cells, characterized by increased mitochondrial OXPHOS over glycolysis. While

Teff rely on FAS, Tmem transition to FAO. Tmem possess increased mitochondrial mass comprised of densely packed cristae, increasing the efficiency of the ETC and further increasing mitochondrial spare respiratory capacity. This phenomenon is associated with increased expression of CPT1a, a rate-limiting protein for FAO [51,52]. Studies emphasize the role of AMPK signaling in upregulation of FAO in Tmem, and mice lacking tumor necrosis factor (TNF) receptor factor 6 (TRAF6) failed to upregulate FAO, leading to a defect in Tmem generation, which was subsequently rescued by the AMPK agonist metformin [53]. T cells can fuel their FAO via multiple mechanisms: by increasing aquaporin 9 (AQP9)-mediated glycerol uptake to promote triacylglyceride (TAG) synthesis [54], liposomal lipolysis of glucose-mediated de novo synthesized fatty acids [55], and uptake of extracellular free fatty acid, which is specifically critical for skin Trm, mediated by fatty acid binding protein 4 and 5 (FABP4, 5) [56].

The microenvironment plays a crucial role in Tmem survival, such as in adipose tissue, where T cells exhibit elevated FAO, specifically in white adipose tissue (WAT) [57]. Despite the fact that Tmem prefer OXPHOS, there have been conflicting reports regarding whether glycolysis inhibits Tmem generation. One study indicates that inhibition of glycolysis by 2-deoxyglucose (2-DG) treatment promotes Tmem generation [58], whereas another study concludes that despite elevated glycolysis achieved by deletion of the E3 ligase von Hippel-Lindau (VHL) under normoxia, Tmem generation remains unaffected [59]. These studies suggest that Tmem are metabolically adaptable and capable of adjusting to different metabolic environments to ensure their longevity.

T cell exhaustion

T cell exhaustion is a consequence of persistent antigen stimulation and/or an impaired microenvironment, such as hypoxia or elevated ROS levels [60]. This state is characterized by diminished functionality and proliferation of T cells upon antigen re-exposure. Exhausted T cells can be further categorized into T progenitor exhausted (Tpex) and T terminal exhausted (Tex) subsets. Tpex cells retain the capacity for proliferation and effector function and are known to be responsive to immune checkpoint-blockade therapy, whereas Tex cells are nonresponsive and exhibit severely compromised effector function. Tpex cells exhibit catabolic metabolism with mitochondrial FAO and OXPHOS, which enables them to generate sufficient ATP to sustain proliferation and cytokine production. Conversely, Tex cells demonstrate reduced GLUT1 expression, leading to decreased glucose uptake and diminished expression of peroxisome proliferator-activated receptor γ coactivator-1α (PGC-1α). This results in reduced mitochondrial biomass and membrane potential, culminating in insufficient OXPHOS and ATP generation [61,62]. Tex cells also exhibit elevated levels of ROS, which has been attributed to mitochondrial fission. This excess of mitochondrial ROS is hypothesized to activate NFAT in a persistent manner, which has been demonstrated to promote Tex cell development [15]. Despite our current understanding of exhausted T cell generation, the precise mechanisms by which metabolism affects and promotes exhaustion remain incompletely elucidated.

Metabolism of CD4$^+$ T cells

Similar to CD8$^+$ T cells, CD4$^+$ T cells (sometimes referred to as "T helper cells") undergo dynamic metabolic changes closely coupled to their differentiation status. Like most resting, healthy cells without the need to spare nutrient-derived carbons for biomolecule production, naïve CD4$^+$ T cells rely primarily on OXPHOS as an energy source but shift into aerobic glycolysis upon activation [63,64]. This metabolic process is fueled by increased glycolysis, glutaminolysis, and OXPHOS, and involves FAS, as discussed above for CD8$^+$ T cells. More distinctly than their cytotoxic counterparts, CD4$^+$ T cell activation is highly informed by cytokine signaling, which leads them to differentiate into defined Teff subsets (Th1, Th2, Th9, Th17, Tfh, or induced regulatory T cells (Treg)). Th1 cells participate in cell-mediated immunity; Th2 in humoral immunity; Th9 in helminth infections, allergic reactions, and autoimmunity; Tfh in germinal center reactions; and Th17 in mucosal immunity and inflammation, while Treg limit inappropriate or excessive immune responses by suppressing Teff cells [65]. Just as each of these phenotypically distinct Teff subsets plays its own role in immunity, each is associated with different metabolic demands and programs [66].

Metabolism of CD4$^+$ Treg cells

Forkhead box p3 (Foxp3)-expressing Tregs are critical for immune regulation and may be generated during CD4$^+$ T cell development in the thymus (natural Treg) or during CD4$^+$ T cell differentiation in the periphery (iTreg) [67]. In either case, Treg do not share the same metabolic requirements as other Teff. First, Treg do not depend on glucose to the same extent as other Teff. They express low levels of Glut1 and exhibit lower levels of glycolysis [68]. Foxp3 increases the expression of ETC protein complexes and decreases glycolysis by directly suppressing c-Myc expression through binding to its TATA box [69]. Instead, a high rate of lipid oxidation and the ability of Treg to persist when glycolysis is inhibited suggest that Treg utilize lipid catabolism for energy [70,71]. Tregs have lipidomes distinct from other Teff and can link glycolysis to FAS, using glucose or lactate as fuels for FAS [72]. Glucose metabolism can be greatly impaired by knockout of the transcription factor *Estrogen-Related Receptor alpha* (*ERRα*), and this inhibits T cell differentiation both in vitro and in vivo, but Treg are selectively rescued by the addition of exogenous fatty acids [73]. TGFβ/Smad signaling pathways drive FAO [74] by activating peroxisome proliferator-activated receptor (PPAR) signaling pathways [75]. PPAR signaling promotes the expression of CD36 and CPT1A, two key proteins involved in fatty-acid uptake and oxidation, which leads to enhanced generation of acetyl-CoA and subsequent biogenesis of uridine diphospho-*N*-acetylglucosamine (UDP-GlcNAc). This molecule acts as a sugar-nucleotide donor substrate to promote N-linked glycosylation [76] and facilitates cell surface retention of type II TGF-β receptor (TβRII) and IL-2 receptor α (IL-2Rα), which perpetuate the feed-forward loop that leads to Foxp3 induction and subsequent Treg differentiation [75,77,78].

Treg are characterized by greater mitochondrial mass and greater OXPHOS capacity than other Teff [79]. In line with this, ablation of the metabolic sensor *Liver Kinase B1* (*Lkb1*) impaired Treg cell survival and function by decreasing mitochondrial mass, compromising OXPHOS, and inhibiting the subsequent generation of ATP [80]. Accordingly, disruptions to the ETC result in impaired Treg differentiation. Specifically, inhibition of complex I promotes upregulation and mitochondrial localization of Notch1 with disruptions to Treg function without affecting Foxp3 expression [81–83]. Blocking complex III, on the other hand, downregulates Foxp3 expression and leads to a proinflammatory phenotype in Treg cells [84]. ETC complex III supports Treg function, as loss of this complex promotes the generation of 2-hydroxyglutarate and succinate, which in turn inhibits ten-eleven translocation (TET) family DNA demethylases and suppresses expression of genes associated with Treg function (including *Nrp1*, *Pdcd1*, *Nt5e*, *Tigit*, and *Flg2*) [84,85]. Ablation of *cytochrome oxidase* (*Cox*), specifically *Cox10* in the ETC complex IV, led to increased Treg cell apoptosis and impaired function in vivo [86]. Conversely, blocking complex V, which couples ATP synthesis through the energy accumulated in the proton gradient across the inner membrane, promotes Foxp3 induction and the generation of induced Treg under conditions for the generation of Th17 cells (see below) [87].

Moreover, while amino acids are essential for Teff activation, Tregs seem to be less dependent on them. For example, activation of naive $CD4^+$ T cells under conditions of glutamine deprivation resulted in skewing towards the Treg phenotype [88,89]. Under conditions of enhanced glutaminolysis, there is an accumulation of 2-hydroxyglutarate (2-HG) the direct product of error-prone dehydrogenase activity on the substrate α-KG, which results in hypermethylation of the Foxp3 gene locus, inhibited Foxp3 transcription, and induction of Th17 cell differentiation instead [90]. Similarly, deprivation of tryptophan metabolites promotes Treg expansion [91]. Treg differentiation, however, is correlated with expression of the amino acid transporter Slc3a2, which is primarily responsible for the uptake of branched-chain amino acids [92], and Treg proliferation and activation is induced by treatment with these amino acids in vitro [93]. Sphinganine, an intermediate metabolite in sphingolipid synthesis, was also found to support Treg differentiation and immune suppression through interaction with the transcription factor c-Fos, which further enhances the transcription of Foxp3 [94]. It remains unclear how other specific amino acids may modulate Treg differentiation, proliferation, and function.

Consistent with the hypothesis that amino acid metabolism may be overall less important for Treg than other Teff, inhibition of mTORC1 via rapamycin promotes FAO and the generation of Treg at the expense of Teff differentiation [95]. In vitro, naive T cells lacking mTOR expression spontaneously develop into Treg after TCR stimulation even in the absence of exogenous TGFβ [96]. Complimentary studies in which the mTOR pathway is made constitutively active by *Tuberous sclerosis complex* (*Tsc1*) deletion promoted glycolysis and impaired the formation of Treg cells [97]. Upstream of mTORC1, the AMP-activated kinase (AMPK) can phosphorylate Tsc2, which in turn inhibits mTORC1 activity [98] and promotes catabolic processes [99]. Tregs have high levels of phospho-AMPK, and treatment with metformin, an indirect activator of AMPK, induces the generation of Treg in a model of allergic asthma [71]. Activation of AMPK may also contribute to Treg cell differentiation through phosphorylation-mediated inhibition of acetyl-CoA carboxylase and enhancement of mitochondrial FAO [100]. Activation of AMPK by the pharmaceutical agonist 5-aminoimidazole-4-carboxamide ribonucleotide (AICAR) enhanced fatty-acid uptake and promoted Treg cell differentiation, which could be reversed by etomoxir, an inhibitor of FAO, suggesting that the induction of Treg cell AMPK activation is mediated by FAO metabolism [101].

Still, the role of mTOR in Tregs is more complex than initially appreciated, since Foxp3cre-Raptor$^{fl/fl}$ mice (which lack mTORC1 in Treg) develop general autoimmune responses, indicating that Tregs fail to function [102]. In Foxp3cre-Raptor$^{fl/fl}$, Rictor$^{fl/fl}$ mice (lacking both mTORC1 and mTORC2 in Treg), there is an amelioration of this inflammatory phenotype. In the same study, in Foxp3cre-Rictor$^{fl/fl}$ mice (lacking mTORC2 in Treg), Treg appear to retain their function. Overall, these data would suggest that mTORC2 is dispensable for Treg function, but inhibition of this complex is required for Treg development. Indeed, transient inhibition of mTOR is necessary for Treg proliferation [103], which may lead to difficulty culturing these cells in nutrient-replete media wherein mTOR activation is likely continuous. In vivo, nutrient availability varies, and consequently, the metabolic state of Treg and their development and function are likely altered by their environment [103].

Targeting Treg metabolism

Tregs exhibit metabolic adaptions that allow them to function in low-glucose, high-lactate environments. Such metabolic adaptations are essential for Treg function in inflamed tissues but also confer upon them a survival advantage in tumors where their presence is maladaptive to the organism [69]. In these high-lactate environments, lactate dehydrogenase (LDH) favors the conversion of lactate into pyruvate while using NAD + as a cofactor, which would lead Teff to a redox imbalance, and glycolysis would be prevented (as would further Teff differentiation). In Treg, however, OXPHOS is promoted, allowing the generation of NAD$^+$ by oxidation in the TCA cycle [69], giving them a survival advantage. Although metabolism in anti-cancer immunity is discussed in detail elsewhere in this volume, this highlights the potential power of exploiting the unique metabolic features of Treg in treating cancers.

Metabolism of CD4$^+$ Th1 T cells

Th1 cells mainly secrete interferon gamma (IFNγ), which allows these cells to eliminate intracellular pathogens and activate the phagocytic activity of macrophages. The master transcriptional regulator of Th1 differentiation is *T-box transcription factor (T-bet)*, and many of the downstream targets of T-bet result in aerobic glycolysis [34,49]. The importance of aerobic glycolysis in T cell activation is debated, yet in the differentiation of CD4$^+$ T cells into Th1 cells, there is a clear example of the need for this particular pathway, as the glycolytic enzyme GAPDH, in the absence of substrate, interferes with the translation of IFNγ, a primary effector molecule of Th1 cells [49]. It is possible, then, that GAPDH and other glycolytic enzymes could function as metabolic checkpoints by linking T cell effector function to glucose availability, and in this way, T cells could use it indirectly to sense the environment, ensuring that activation is only achieved in the presence of abundant glucose. Another study proposed that to maintain aerobic glycolysis and further support Th1 differentiation, LDHA confers epigenetic control over the *Ifnγ* locus, and hence its expression in these effector T cells is a major prerequisite [104]. The ramping up of glycolysis upon TCR triggering in Th1 cells is also necessary to deliver glucose to the PPP for generation of biosynthetic precursor molecules needed for growth and proinflammatory cytokines [105].

Along with glycolysis, Th1 cells also rely upon glutaminolysis for their growth and proliferation. In Th1 polarizing conditions, CD4$^+$ T cells that lack a glutamine supply generate Foxp3$^+$ Treg [106], and this effect can be prevented by a cell-permeable α-ketoglutarate analogue (dimethyl-2-oxoglutarate), as α-ketoglutarate has been shown to enhance T-bet expression [88]. Apart from glutamine, other branched-chain amino acids (such as valine, leucine, and isoleucine) and aromatic amino acids (such as phenylalanine, tyrosine, and tryptophan) are required for in vitro differentiation into Th1 cells [44]. Therefore the expression of the amino acid transporter CD98 is necessary for in vitro Th1 differentiation [44].

Finally, complex II of the ETC is known to play roles in Th1 differentiation. While inhibiting Complex II promotes the proliferation of Th1 cells, genetic removal of the Complex II subunit succinate dehydrogenase complex leads to a compromised capacity for IFNγ production with elevated H3K9 and K27 acetylation. Thus Complex II counteracts Th cell differentiation by negatively regulating both proliferation and histone acetylation [107].

Targeting Th1 metabolism

Overactivation of Th1 cells underlies several inflammatory diseases, among them Rheumatoid Arthritis (RA) [108]. $CD4^+$ T cells participating in RA appear to utilize glucose differently than healthy T cell controls [108]. They fail to upregulate the key glycolytic enzyme 6-Phosphofructo-2-Kinase/Fructose-2,6-Bisphosphatase 3 (PFKFB3) and further shift glucose toward the PPP. Glucose-6-phosphate dehydrogenase (G6PD) acts as a gatekeeper to the PPP and is upregulated in $CD4^+$ T cells from patients [109,110]. Thus in RA patients, the balance in expression of PFKFB3 and G6PD is shifted toward G6PD, a phenomenon that correlates with disease severity and suggests that G6PD might be a druggable target in RA [109,111]. Furthermore, mitochondrial insufficiency in these T cells (perhaps from accumulation of damaged mitochondrial DNA (mtDNA)) prevents FAS and promotes deposition of cytoplasmic lipid droplets that are utilized in expansion and mobilization of the cell membrane for tissue invasion [108,112,113].

Treatment with leflunomide, an inhibitor of dihydroorotate dehydrogenase (DHODH), has been implemented for several autoimmune diseases, including RA and psoriatic arthritis. DHODH is a mitochondrial enzyme involved in pyrimidine synthesis, which accepts electrons from ubiquinone. Inhibition of DHODH by leflunomide might therefore interfere with OXPHOS in activated T cells via functional inhibition of complex III of the ETC, consequently inducing a shift from Th1 to Th2 subpopulations [114,115]. Finally, since the function of Th1 cells depends so heavily on the production of inflammatory cytokines and mediators, it is aided by nutrient-replete environments, which are sensed by the mTOR complex. The mTORC1 complex directly phosphorylates T-bet and leads to T-bet-dependent IFNγ production, and indeed, inhibition of mTORC1 activation leads to the suppression of Th1 differentiation [116]. Likewise, metformin, a mild Complex I inhibitor, impairs Th1 differentiation [117].

Metabolism of $CD4^+$ Th2 cells

Th2 cells are involved in combatting infections caused by extracellular parasites and secrete IL-4, IL-5, and IL-13, cytokines important for aiding IgE class switching and degranulation of basophils and eosinophils. IL-4-induced signal transducer and activator of transcription 6 (STAT6) drives the expression of GATA-binding protein (GATA3), the master regulator of Th2 cells [118,119]. All Th subsets are glycolytic, but, Th2 cells appear to be the most glycolytic subset (among Th1, Th2, Th17, and Treg) and show the highest expression of Glut1 [71,120]. Likewise, all Th lineages (except Treg) depend on mTOR, but mTORC2, rather than mTORC1, seems to be more important for Th2 cells. Blocking glutaminase 1 (GLS1), the enzyme that converts glutamine to glutamate in T cell mitochondria, was found to promote Th2 cell differentiation by inactivating the mTORC1 pathway [89]. T cells specifically lacking mTORC1 activity (due to deletion of the upstream molecule Rheb) cannot develop into Th1 and Th17 cells, while Th2 differentiation is normal [96]. Instead, deletion of Rictor, a scaffolding protein essential for mTORC2, restrains Th2 development [121]. Moreover, activation of mTORC2 downstream targets Ras homolog gene family member A (RhoA) and serum/glucocorticoid-regulated kinase 1 (SGK1) play important roles in Th2 differentiation. RhoA initiates Th2 differentiation and allergic airway inflammation by regulating IL-4 receptor mRNA expression [122] but is not required for Th2 maintenance [123]. SGK1 promotes Th2 commitment and inhibits the degradation of JunB [124], another transcription factor that controls the Th2 cytokine program [125].

Extracellular metabolites have also been reported to influence Th2 differentiation and functions. Lactate secreted by B cells (especially in aging) may skew $CD4^+$ T cells away from a Th2 phenotype and towards more proinflammatory subsets such as Th1 and Th17 [126]. ATP and an enzyme involved in tryptophan metabolism, indoamine 2,3-dioxygenase (IDO) potentiate [127,128], whereas glutamine suppresses [129], Th2 differentiation. Short-chain fatty acids have also been studied, but contradictory results have been obtained, so more investigation is needed as to how these might influence Th2 cells [130–132].

Targeting Th2 metabolism

Like Th1 cells, Th2 cells can be pathogenic upon entry into tissues wherein they can cause damage. In the lungs, the transcription factor nuclear factor erythroid 2-related factor 2 (Nrf2) upregulates glycolysis and OXPHOS in Th2 cells and regulates their polyfunctionality, making this a possible therapeutic target during allergic inflammation [133]. Itaconate has also been used to attenuate Th2 responses in the lungs of house dustmite-challenged mice, presumably because itaconate can act as a competitive inhibitor of succinate dehydrogenase (complex II of the ETC) [134]. Th2 cells in other tissues display heightened levels of lipid metabolism, such as in metabolic signatures from Th2 cells in the airways of mice challenged with dustmite antigens compared to those in lymph nodes, and inhibitors of lipid metabolism resulted in a reduction of associated pathologies [120]. This reliance on lipid metabolism may be regulated by PPARγ [135–138] as PPARγ expression is induced by IL-4R and STAT6 activation in other cell types [139–141]. Targeting PPARγ has been shown to reduce immunity toward the nematode *Heligmosomoides polygyrus*, which depends on Th2 function, and improve pathology in Th2-driven airway inflammation models [136,138].

Metabolism of $CD4^+$ Th9 T cells

In 2008 Veldhoen and Dardalhon reported that TGFβ and IL-4 induced the generation of $Foxp3^-$ T cells that mainly secreted IL-9 and IL-10 and were designated as a novel subset of the $CD4^+$ Th cells called Th9 cells [142,143]. Th9 cells are important in the defense against solid tumors [144−146] and helminth infections [147] and are also implicated in various autoimmune disorders [148,149]. The transcriptional driver of Th9 cells is *PU.1* (also known as *Spi-1 proto-oncogene* (*SPI1*)) [142,150]. Although it was shown that inhibiting mitogen-activated protein kinase kinase kinase 7 (MAP3K7), also known as TAK1 in naïve $CD4^+$ T cells with 5z-7-oxozeaenol almost completely blocked Th9 differentiation [151], little else is currently known about metabolic features unique to this subset of Th cells.

Metabolism of $CD4^+$ Th17 T cells

$CD4^+$ T cells activated in the presence of IL-6 and TGFβ express the transcription factor *retinoic-acid-receptor-related orphan nuclear receptor gamma* (*RORγt*, also called *RORC*) and consequently produce IL17 and other inflammatory cytokines, including IL-22, GM-CSF, TNF, IL-9, and IL-21 [152]. Studies so far confirm the PI3K/AKT/mTOR signaling pathway as a prerequisite for Th17 differentiation. A study using mice with a T cell-specific deletion of Raptor (essential for mTORC1 activity) showed that mTORC1 was required for Th17, but not Th1 development [153]. It was suggested that mTORC1 activity may support Th17 development through S6 Kinase (S6K) 2, which binds RORγt and facilitates its nuclear localization [153]. Likewise, activation of S6K1 (a homolog of S6K2 also downstream of mTORC1) was implicated exclusively in Th17 cells [154]. Higher mTOR activity from impaired AMPK signaling (deletion of AMPK regulator LKB1 or AMPK target TSC1) predisposes $CD4^+$ T cells to differentiate into Th17 cells [70,101] and lower mTOR signaling from AMPK activation impairs Th17 differentiation [155,156].

A transcription factor that serves as a major metabolic hub for Th17 differentiation is hypoxia-inducible factor 1-alpha (Hif-1α). Although HIF-1α is rapidly induced upon activation in all T cells, it seems to be dispensable for the initiation of metabolic changes in most T cells [25], but Th17 differentiation is uniquely impaired by the loss of this pathway [70,157]. Hif-1α expression is at least in part regulated by pyruvate dehydrogenase (PDH) activity, as abolishing its activity leads to diminished acetyl-CoA production, reduced Hif-1α expression, and ultimately suppressed *IL17A* and *IL17F* mRNA expression [158]. Hif-1α expression is also reduced following inhibition of methylenetetrahydrofolate dehydrogenase (MTHFD2), an essential mitochondrial folate enzyme, and ablating this enzyme in naïve $CD4^+$ T cells reduced Th17 differentiation [159].

Like their proinflammatory counterparts, Th1 cells, glutamine metabolism is also a strong regulator of Th17 differentiation, likely through epigenetic regulation. The aberrant activation of GLS-dependent glutaminolysis triggers H3K9Ac and H3K27Ac epigenetic modifications within the *IL17 A* gene promoter, which further enhances the chromatin accessibility of *RORγt* [160]. Inhibition of GLS enhanced global H3K27 trimethylation in Th1 cells, while that in Th17 cells decreased, and cytokine production and proliferation are similarly reduced and increased in Th17 and Th1 cells, respectively [89]. The metabolite of mitochondrial glutaminolysis, αKG, participates in this glutaminolysis-mediated epigenetic remodeling by regulating histone and DNA methylation levels as a substrate for dioxygenases, including histone demethylases and TET family hydroxylases [161]. It has been reported that Th17 cells produce the most αKG among Th cells, suggesting a strong correlation between Th17 polarization and glutaminolysis [89]. Metabolites downstream of αKG such as 2-HG also promote Th17 cell differentiation by inhibiting Tet-methylcytosine dioxygenase 1−3, resulting in methylation and suppression of *FOXP3* transcription to promote *IL17A/IL-17F* expression [90]. 2-HG can also regulate KDM5-specific H3K4me3 modifications in the promoter and CNS2 enhancer of the *IL17 A* gene locus and facilitate the differentiation of Th17 cells directly [162].

Glutaminolysis also provides essential precursors for GSH production, and this is an important antioxidant in T cells [163]. By blocking glutaminolysis-mediated GSH generation in naïve T cells, the redox balance shifts toward an oxidative state, which subsequently restricts Th17 cell differentiation [164]. Analysis of the downstream pathway revealed that treatment with a GLS inhibitor inhibits GSH production, leading to increased ROS levels that suppress the expression of RORγt [162].

Where Treg can utilize extracellular fatty acids, other T cell lineages rely on de novo FAS, and this pathway may be especially important for Th17 cells. Acetyl-CoA carboxylase (ACC1) (required for FAS) inhibition has the strongest impact on Th17 development [165,166]. When cells synthesize lipids from glucose, the final glycolytic product, pyruvate, moves into the mitochondria to form acetyl-CoA and then citrate, which then moves into the cytosol and gets converted back to acetyl-CoA, which fuels FAS. Cytosolic acetyl-CoA can also be catalyzed in the mevalonate−cholesterol synthetic pathway. Inhibition of 3-hydroxy-3-methylglutaryl CoA reductase (HMGCR), a rate-limiting enzyme in the mevalonate−cholesterol pathway, has been reported to impair Th17 differentiation [167,168]. Consistently, intermediates of cholesterol metabolism, such as desmosterol or the endogenous cholesterol-derivative oxysterol, can act as RORγt agonists and enhance Th17 differentiation [169].

Finally, the ETC may serve as an important regulator of Th17 differentiation. Inhibition of complex I with the compound rotenone blocks de novo aspartate and N-carbamoyl-L-aspartate synthesis and interferes with the cellular $NAD^+/NADH$ balance and results in altered localization of Notch1 and RORγt in the nucleus and impairs IL17-dependent Th17 differentiation [81]. Similarly, inhibition of complex V leads to diminished proliferation of Th17 cells and reduced RORγt expression and IL17 production [87].

Targeting Th17 metabolism

Th17 cells have garnered significant attention due to their role in the pathology of several autoimmune diseases such as multiple sclerosis (MS), psoriasis, Crohn's disease, systemic lupus erythematosus (SLE), and ulcerative colitis [170]. As it appears that the PI3K−AKT−mTORC1 pathway and LKB1−AMPK pathway may serve as connecting pathways between environmental cues and T cell commitment to Th17 cells, many of the proteins in these pathways may be therapeutic targets in Th17-mediated diseases. Chemical inhibition of mTORC1 with arctigenin, a substance isolated from the fruit *Arctium lappa*, impaired Th17 induction (as well as Th1 cells) [171], and metformin treatment impairs Th17 differentiation [117,172].

Upstream of mTORC1, the dependency of TH17s on glutaminolysis may also represent a viable therapeutic target. Diminishing glutaminolysis in lupus-prone murine models through either GLS1 deletion or inhibition results in fewer Th17 cells and a concomitant reduction in disease activity [173]. Glutaminolysis has been shown to promote experimental autoimmune encephalomyelitis (EAE), an established animal model of MS [174,175], and studies in this model suggest that interrupting CD4$^+$ T cell glutaminolysis impaired mTORC1 activation, limited Th1 and Th17 cell expansion, and suppressed immune cell infiltrates in the central nervous system [32,176]. Like its effect on EAE, blocking glutamine metabolism in a chronic inflammatory liver disease ameliorated disease progression by inhibiting the differentiation and function of Th1 and Th17 cells [177].

Further targeting of Th17 metabolism has been explored in EAE, where Th17 cells are known to be especially detrimental. In this model, deletion of Hif-1α in Th17 cells leads to delayed development of disease [178], and mice are protected from this disease with treatment with ACC1-specific inhibitors [169]. The supplementation of propionic acid restored the Th17/Treg balance in EAE, leading to the amelioration of inflammation [179]. Mechanistically, supplementation with propionic acid specifically upregulated expression of peroxisomal carnitine O-octanoyltransferase (Crot), leading to the promotion of FAO and the generation of acetyl-CoA, skewing activated T cells away from Th17 development and toward Treg [180]. The obstruction of the ETC-mediated ATP production with oligomycin during Th17 differentiation reduced frequencies of these cells and downregulated the expression of genes associated with the pathogenicity of Th17 cells, including *Il17a*, *Tgfb3*, *Il23r*, *Stat4*, and *Gpr65* and led to a substantial delay in the onset of EAE and concomitant reduction in severity [87]. T cell-specific deletion of spermine N1-acetyltransferase 1 (SAT1, a rate-limiting enzyme of polyamine recycling) also significantly delays the onset and severity of EAE [181,182], as does restriction of methionine [159], implying that one-carbon metabolism might be an especially attractive target in Th17 cells.

Metabolism of CD4$^+$ Tfh cells

Tfh cells are found primarily within B cell follicles of secondary lymphoid tissues and are critical to the generation of T-dependent antibody responses [183]. *Bcl6*, the transcriptional regulator of Tfh differentiation, is antagonistic to Blimp-1, an important regulator of Th2 differentiation; thus these two lineages tend to be mutually exclusive [184]. While this mutual antagonism between subsets is almost certain to lead to important metabolic differences between these two Th subsets, unfortunately to date not much research in this area has yet been pursued.

Targeting Tfh metabolism

Tfh cells may be particularly important in the pathogenesis of SLE, yet the findings on the role of their metabolism in SLE patients are conflicting. Through a combination of RNA-seq and metabolomics, specific anabolic programs characterized by enhanced glutamate metabolism were identified in Tfh cells from patients with SLE [185]. However, the inhibition of glutamine metabolism by the glutamine analog 6-diazo-5-oxo-L-norleucine (DON) had no effect on Tfh polarization [186]. A potential explanation is that dysfunctional mitophagy in Tfh cells, rather than glutamate metabolism per se, is the more important factor. Enhanced glutamate metabolism upon T cell activation may lead to dysfunctional mitophagy, unrestrained production of ROS, and promote the expansion of Tfh cells [187,188]. It is also known that pathways downstream of transaldolase deficiency induce mitophagy dysfunction, promote mTORC1 activation, and increase complex I expression [189,190], and mTORC1-dependent mitophagy dysfunction has been proposed to be a key factor contributing to the generation of autoantibodies and exacerbation of SLE pathogenesis [191,192].

Metabolism of humoral immunity

Throughout their lifetime, B cells must rapidly switch from periods of quiescence to those of intense growth and proliferation as well as undergoing dramatic changes in differentiation state. To accommodate these distinct changes, the metabolic status of the cells must alternate accordingly to fulfill the demands of altered B cell function and activity [193–198]. The metabolic requirements to sustain B cells at each stage within the developmental trajectory from their early development in the bone marrow and transition to the spleen where they emerge as long-lived memory B cells and antibody-secreting plasma cells are discussed herein.

The bone marrow provides the appropriate environment in which pro-B cells develop and are marked by rearrangement of the immunoglobulin heavy chain locus and assembly of the pre-B cell receptor. Resulting pre-B cells undergo a proliferative burst before rearrangement of the immunoglobulin light chain locus. At this point the immature B cells, expressing the B cell receptor (BCR) undergo negative selection to establish central tolerance. Those that survive exit the bone marrow compartment and transition through a developmental process to generate mature follicular (Fo) or innate like marginal zone (MZ) B cells. Following infection or immunization, antigen-activated B cells undergo responses within the germinal centers in a T cell-dependent manner or at extrafollicular (EF) sites independently of T cell help [199]. The EF sites within secondary lymphoid organs provide the niche in which activated B cells undergo rapid proliferation and differentiation into low affinity antibody-secreting plasmablasts. Alternatively, in the context of appropriate antigen stimulation and T cell-mediated help, formation of the germinal center reaction is initiated. Germinal centers provide the developmental niche in which B cells undergo the processes of activation-induced cytidine deaminase (AID)-driven somatic hypermutation, class-switch recombination (CSR), selection, and clonal expansion to generate a population of plasma cells (PCs) able to secrete high-affinity antibodies [200–202]. The germinal center is characterized by two distinct zones, the dark compartment, in which rapid proliferation and somatic hypermutation of the germinal center B cells takes place, and the light zone that is recognized as the region in which the B cells are relatively quiescent and interact with follicular dendritic cells and follicular helper T cells and undergo clonal selection. From this complex series of events, PCs and long-lived memory B cells emerge that respond to antigenic rechallenge and maintain the secretion of high-affinity antibodies.

B cell development

B cell development is marked by periods of intense proliferative activity punctuated by metabolic quiescence during which the critical Ig rearrangement events occur [193]. Proliferation of pro- and pre-B cells is fueled by an increase in glucose uptake, HIF-1α-mediated glycolysis, and marked by mitochondrial ROS production [203–206]. The reliance of B cell development on HIF-1α-mediated glycolysis is critical for the transition of pro-B cells to pre-B cells but dispensable for the progression of pre-B cells to IgM$^+$ immature B cells [205]. Pro-/pre-B cells also increase their oxygen consumption rate and utilize glucose and fatty acids for OXPHOS [207]. Conditional deletion of the mTORC1 regulator, *Raptor,* induced a block in B cell development at the early pre-B cell stage, with a corresponding decrease in both OXPHOS and glycolysis, consistent with an essential role for mTOR-mediated regulation of metabolism during B cell development [208]. Corroboration of these observations using an mTOR hypomorph mutant showed a block at the large pre-B to small pre-B stage and corresponding decrease in mature B cells [209]. In addition, deletion of *Rictor,* to specifically disrupt the mTORC2 complex, showed an accumulation of pro-B, pre-B, and immature B cells [210]. Furthermore, a block at the large pre-B cell stage identified a metabolic checkpoint mediated by Folliculin Interacting Protein-1 (FNIP3), the ablation of which led to metabolic insufficiency and dysregulation of AMPK-mediated inhibition of mTOR signaling and increased sensitivity to apoptosis induced by nutrient or IL-7 deprivation [211]. The transcription factors Paired box gene 5 (PAX5) and IKAROS family zinc finger 1 (IKZF1), critical for early B cell development, also act as metabolic checkpoints by sustaining AMPK activity to enforce a state of energy restriction in pre-B cells [212]. Pre-BCR-mediated regulation of the inner mitochondrial membrane protein, Swiprosin-2/EFhd1, during the pro- to pre-B cell transition was also shown to coordinate metabolic events to ensure normal B cell development [213].

Following a period of clonal expansion, the pre-B cell returns to a state of metabolic inactivity, upon which further VJ recombination takes place to generate the BCR. The immature B cell then migrates to the spleen and differentiates to generate mature resting Fo and MZ B cells that maintain minimal metabolic activity via FAO [214]. The acquisition of metabolic quiescence, characterized by increased extracellular adenosine salvage, a decrease in protein synthesis and mTORC1 signaling also appears critical for transitional to Fo B cell maturation [215]. Furthermore, a role for mTORC2 signaling in peripheral B cell development was characterized by an increase in transitional B cells and disruption of MZ and Fo B cell maturation [216]. *Tsc1* ablation in B cells, characterized by hyperactivation of mTORC1, led to a depletion of Fo B cells and a complete loss of the MZ population [217,218]. Distinct metabolic features of MZ and Fo B cells are further exemplified by their differing GSH-based redox dependencies [219]. Abrogation of GSH synthesis by the deletion of *Gclc* resulted in a loss of MZ B cells, suggesting that their persistence is dependent upon GSH. Although numbers of *Gclc*-deficient Fo B cells were unaffected, they displayed upregulation of mTORC1, enhanced glucose uptake, and a glycolytic phenotype, metabolic properties ordinarily associated with WT MZ B cells. Furthermore, disruption of redox homeostasis in Fo B cells led to elevated ROS, a block in the ETC, and significantly impaired mitochondrial respiration [219]. GPX4, which helps to maintain redox homeostasis by utilizing glutathione to prevent lipid peroxidation and ferroptotic cell death, is critical for the development and activities of MZ B cells but dispensable for the generation of functional Fo B cells [220].

B cell activation

Naive B cells remain metabolically quiescent until they encounter antigen, upon which they undergo a rapid program of growth and proliferation, and dramatic changes in metabolic programming is observed. The quiescent metabolic state is maintained by one of several checkpoint molecules, including tumor necrosis factor receptor-associated factor 3 (TRAF-3) [221], glycogen synthase kinase 3 (GSK-3) [222] and the miRNA Let-7 [223] that function to limit nutrient uptake. Inactive splenic B cells maintain their low metabolic activity by FAO to generate ATP [214]. Activation of B cells either via the BCR or Toll-like receptor (TLR) stimulation leads to a rapid increase in GLUT1-mediated glucose import [214,222,224,225] and elevated aerobic glycolysis followed by a progressive shift toward glucose oxidation via the PPP and mitochondrial TCA cycle [224,225]. These events occur independently of HIF-1a but require c-*Myc* [214] and PI3K/AKT signaling events [224,226]. Utilization of glucose for de novo lipogenesis via an ATP-citrate lyase-dependent pathway was shown to be critical for proliferation, survival, and differentiation of splenic B cells activated by lipopolysaccharide (LPS) [227]. Stimulation of naïve B cells with CD40L and IL-4 confirmed an enhanced glucose uptake and flux through the glycolytic pathway [214,224,225], but failure to accumulate glycolytic intermediates was consistent with glucose utilization by alternative metabolic pathways, including lipid synthesis and the PPP to generate ribose-5-phosphate for nucleotides. The increase in OXPHOS occurred independently of glucose, and robust uptake of glutamine fueled induction of the TCA cycle. Significantly, in this study, glucose restriction only minimally limited B cell activation, differentiation, and proliferation [228]. The metabolic changes following stimulation via the BCR must be sustained by T_H cell interactions or TLR signaling. In the absence of these secondary signals, mediated in part by PKCB [229], perturbation of calcium homeostasis, loss of glycolytic capacity, and mitochondrial dysfunction trigger eventual cell death [230].

Germinal center reaction

The germinal center is characterized by two distinct zones—the light zone in which B cells present antigen to Tfh cells and a dark zone in which B cells undergo clonal expansion and somatic hypermutation. Multiple rounds of migration between these two zones ultimately generate clones with higher affinity BCRs. Distinct differences in the microenvironment of these two regions [231] and in the metabolic demands of the B cells in them are reflected by the use of differential metabolic resources. Glycolysis is the preferred pathway of energy production in the light zone, characterized by robust expression of glycolytic genes and glucose uptake [232]. In contrast, dark zone B cells are marked by transcriptional profiles associated with OXPHOS and FAO with disruption of the ETC by the deletion of cytochrome oxidase, impairing clonal expansion and positive selection [232].

PCs are terminally differentiated B cells that utilize their metabolic resources predominantly to constitutively secrete antibodies, and whose longevity determines the durability of humoral immunity. The transition from a metabolically quiescent naïve B cell to a mature antibody-secreting PC depends on energetically costly proliferation and differentiation events. PCs can be characterized as short-lived antibody-secreting plasmablasts and plasma cells (SLPCs) that arise from the EF region of the lymphoid tissue and long-lived plasma cells (LLPCs) that undergo affinity maturation within the germinal centers [233]. Comparative metabolic analysis demonstrated that in contrast to SLPCs, their long-lived counterparts exhibited an elevated maximal respiratory capacity, enhanced glucose uptake and glycolysis-mediated generation of pyruvate [234,235]. In vivo ablation of mitochondrial pyruvate carrier 2 (Mpc2), a critical component of the mitochondrial pyruvate carrier, led to a decrease in LLPC frequency and accompanying loss of antigen-specific antibodies [234]. Glucose utilization was thought to be primarily diverted toward glycosylation of antibodies,

Disruption of *Slc2a1* (encoding Glut1) that encodes for the major glucose transporter on lymphocytes, in the B cells of mature mice with an intact preimmune repertoire, confirmed significantly elevated glucose uptake into PCs in addition to showing impairment of GLUT1-deficient B cell number early in an activation response with a requirement of glucose for proliferation and differentiation to the PC functional phenotype [236]. Evaluation of the metabolic fate of glucose in activated B cells by flux analysis revealed both glycolytic and mitochondrial utilization and diversion into the PPP and regulation of ROS in the development of PCs and antibody production [236]. Glutamine uptake was shown to contribute to the TCA cycle via anapleurosis via succinate oxidation as well as for generation of aspartate and glutamate for use in PC antibody production [235]. In contrast to previous observations [214], B cell development was unaffected by the deletion of GLUT1 in mature B2 cells, but a reduction in germinal center B cells and PCs was observed, indicating a critical role for glucose uptake in mature B cells for the development of PCs and antibody secretion. Increases in mitochondrial mass and transcription of genes associated with glycolysis, the TCA cycle, and hexosamine synthesis in GLUT1-deficient B cells failed to compensate for the lack in glucose availability [237].

Disruption of mtDNA in BCR- and LPS-activated B cells, using a B cell-specific dominant negative mutant of the mitochondrial DNA helicase Twinkle (TWNK), perturbed the generation and assembly of mitochondrially encoded ETC complexes, reduced OXPHOS, and disrupted the TCA cycle while the levels of glycolysis increased. While B cell development was normal under these conditions, germinal center formation, CSR, and maturation of PCs as well as both T cell-dependent and -independent events were impaired, indicating that mtDNA homeostasis in B cells is critical to maintain the metabolic requirements for an effective humoral immune response. Corroborating observations [238,239] show a progressive LPS-induced expression of electron transport and TCA components and a corresponding incremental increase in OXPHOS during the transition of naïve B cells to active plasmablasts [239]. An inverse relationship between OXPHOS and glycolysis usage was observed, with activated B cells showing a metabolic reliance on both pathways, while plasmablasts exclusively utilized OXPHOS in a BLIMP-1-dependent manner. The distinction between the metabolic requirements of activated B cells and germinal center responses is further illustrated by the deletion of LDHA at various points during B cell development. LDHA catalyzes the conversion of pyruvate to lactate and drives aerobic glycolysis. While naïve B cells were essentially unaffected by the ablation of LDHA and underwent an LPS-induced extrafollicular B cell response, their ability to form GCs and generate antibody responses was severely impacted [240].

In contrast to the reported requirement of glucose to facilitate the development of germinal center B cells (GCBCs) to mature antibody-producing PCs [236,237], GCBCs were shown to rely only minimally on glycolysis for their energy needs and to instead utilize FAO as their preferential energy source [241]. Ex vivo GCBCs showed their preference for oxidation of both endogenous and exogenous fatty acids to drive OXPHOS as their energy source with very limited input from glucose uptake and glycolysis. Consistent with this, inhibition of Cpt1-mediated fatty-acid import into mitochondria partially reduced oxygen consumption rate (OCR). Selective inhibition of fatty-acid import into peroxisomes further demonstrated that GCBCs conduct both mitochondrial and peroxisomal FAO. Interestingly, even under conditions of complete inhibition of FAO, glucose uptake was not engaged, suggesting an active repression of glycolysis. BCL-6, a critical transcription factor for GCBCs, has been shown to suppress glycolysis in T cells [242].

The mTOR complex, a key regulator of growth and proliferation in response to signals, including nutrients, growth factors, energy levels, and oxygen [243], plays a critical role at multiple points in the activation and differentiation of B cells (also see above) [244]. mTOR hypomorphic mutant mice were found defective in GC formation and antibody production after immunization that was reflected by a reduced expression of AID and lower levels of somatic hypermutation and CSR [209]. Impaired GC formation and an altered antibody repertoire after treatment with rapamycin before influenza infection helped to define a specific role for TORC1 [245]. Accordingly, inducible deletion of *Raptor* in mature B cells confirmed disruption of GC establishment and reduced differentiation of antibody-producing PCs [246]. Collectively, the mTOR signaling pathway clearly plays a critical role in the homeostasis and functional differentiation of B cells.

References

[1] Demas GE, Chefer V, Talan MI, Nelson RJ. Metabolic costs of mounting an antigen-stimulated immune response in adult and aged C57BL/6J mice. Am J Physiol 1997;273:R1631–7. Available from: https://doi.org/10.1152/ajpregu.1997.273.5.R1631.

[2] Segerstrom SC. Stress, energy, and immunity: an ecological view. Curr Dir Psychol Sci 2007;16:326–30. Available from: https://doi.org/10.1111/j.1467-8721.2007.00522.x.

[3] Buttemer WA, O'Dwyer TW, Astheimer LB, Klasing KC, Hoye BJ. No evidence of metabolic costs following adaptive immune activation or reactivation in house sparrows. Biol Lett 2022;1820220036. Available from: https://doi.org/10.1098/rsbl.2022.0036.

[4] Flamholz A, Phillips R, Milo R. The quantified cell. Mol Biol Cell 2014;25:3497–500. Available from: https://doi.org/10.1091/mbc.E14-09-1347.

[5] Yoon H, Kim TS, Braciale TJ. The cell cycle time of CD8 + T cells responding in vivo is controlled by the type of antigenic stimulus. PLoS One 2010;5:e15423. Available from: https://doi.org/10.1371/journal.pone.0015423.

[6] Patente TA, Pelgrom LR, Everts B. Dendritic cells are what they eat: how their metabolism shapes T helper cell polarization. Curr Opin Immunol 2019;58:16–23. Available from: https://doi.org/10.1016/j.coi.2019.02.003.

[7] Krawczyk CM, et al. Toll-like receptor-induced changes in glycolytic metabolism regulate dendritic cell activation. Blood 2010;115:4742–9. Available from: https://doi.org/10.1182/blood-2009-10-249540.

[8] Jantsch J, et al. Hypoxia and hypoxia-inducible factor-1 alpha modulate lipopolysaccharide-induced dendritic cell activation and function. J Immunol 2008;180:4697–705. Available from: https://doi.org/10.4049/jimmunol.180.7.4697.

[9] O'Neill LA, Pearce EJ. Immunometabolism governs dendritic cell and macrophage function. J Exp Med 2016;213:15−23. Available from: https://doi.org/10.1084/jem.20151570.

[10] Malinarich F, et al. High mitochondrial respiration and glycolytic capacity represent a metabolic phenotype of human tolerogenic dendritic cells. J Immunol 2015;194:5174−86. Available from: https://doi.org/10.4049/jimmunol.1303316.

[11] Osorio F, Fuentes C, Lopez MN, Salazar-Onfray F, Gonzalez FE. Role of Dendritic Cells in the Induction of Lymphocyte Tolerance. Front Immunol 2015;6:535. Available from: https://doi.org/10.3389/fimmu.2015.00535.

[12] Macintyre AN, et al. The glucose transporter Glut1 is selectively essential for CD4 T cell activation and effector function. Cell Metab 2014;20:61−72. Available from: https://doi.org/10.1016/j.cmet.2014.05.004.

[13] Rathmell JC, Vander Heiden MG, Harris MH, Frauwirth KA, Thompson CB. In the absence of extrinsic signals, nutrient utilization by lymphocytes is insufficient to maintain either cell size or viability. Mol Cell 2000;6:683−92. Available from: https://doi.org/10.1016/s1097-2765(00)00066-6.

[14] Tarasenko TN, et al. Cytochrome c oxidase activity is a metabolic checkpoint that regulates cell fate decisions during T cell activation and differentiation. Cell Metab 2017;25:1254−68. Available from: https://doi.org/10.1016/j.cmet.2017.05.007 e1257.

[15] Sena LA, et al. Mitochondria are required for antigen-specific T cell activation through reactive oxygen species signaling. Immunity 2013;38:225−36. Available from: https://doi.org/10.1016/j.immuni.2012.10.020.

[16] Jacobs SR, Michalek RD, Rathmell JC. IL-7 is essential for homeostatic control of T cell metabolism in vivo. J Immunol 2010;184:3461−9. Available from: https://doi.org/10.4049/jimmunol.0902593.

[17] Carrette F, Surh CD. IL-7 signaling and CD127 receptor regulation in the control of T cell homeostasis. Semin Immunol 2012;24:209−17. Available from: https://doi.org/10.1016/j.smim.2012.04.010.

[18] Kerdiles YM, et al. Foxo1 links homing and survival of naive T cells by regulating L-selectin, CCR7 and interleukin 7 receptor. Nat Immunol 2009;10:176−84. Available from: https://doi.org/10.1038/ni.1689.

[19] Mendoza A, et al. Lymphatic endothelial S1P promotes mitochondrial function and survival in naive T cells. Nature 2017;546:158−61. Available from: https://doi.org/10.1038/nature22352.

[20] Geltink RIK, Kyle RL, Pearce EL. Unraveling the complex interplay between T cell metabolism and function. Annu Rev Immunol 2018;36:461−88. Available from: https://doi.org/10.1146/annurev-immunol-042617-053019.

[21] Wang R, Green DR. Metabolic reprogramming and metabolic dependency in T cells. Immunol Rev 2012;249:14−26. Available from: https://doi.org/10.1111/j.1600-065X.2012.01155.x.

[22] Wu G, Haynes TE, Li H, Meininger CJ. Glutamine metabolism in endothelial cells: ornithine synthesis from glutamine via pyrroline-5-carboxylate synthase. Comp Biochem Physiol A Mol Integr Physiol 2000;126:115−23. Available from: https://doi.org/10.1016/s1095-6433(00)00196-3.

[23] Geiger R, et al. L-arginine modulates T cell metabolism and enhances survival and anti-tumor activity. Cell 2016;167:829−42. Available from: https://doi.org/10.1016/j.cell.2016.09.031 e813.

[24] Kwon NH, Fox PL, Kim S. Aminoacyl-tRNA synthetases as therapeutic targets. Nat Rev Drug Discov 2019;18:629−50. Available from: https://doi.org/10.1038/s41573-019-0026-3.

[25] Wang R, et al. The transcription factor Myc controls metabolic reprogramming upon T lymphocyte activation. Immunity 2011;35:871−82. Available from: https://doi.org/10.1016/j.immuni.2011.09.021.

[26] Verbist KC, et al. Metabolic maintenance of cell asymmetry following division in activated T lymphocytes. Nature 2016;532:389−93. Available from: https://doi.org/10.1038/nature17442.

[27] Liedmann S, et al. Localization of a TORC1-eIF4F translation complex during CD8(+) T cell activation drives divergent cell fate. Mol Cell 2022;82:2401−14. Available from: https://doi.org/10.1016/j.molcel.2022.04.016 e2409.

[28] Morre DJ, Rodriguez-Aguilera JC, Navas P, Morre DM. Redox modulation of the response of NADH oxidase activity of rat liver plasma membranes to cyclic AMP plus ATP. Mol Cell Biochem 1997;173:71−7. Available from: https://doi.org/10.1023/a:1006880419063.

[29] Bricker DK, et al. A mitochondrial pyruvate carrier required for pyruvate uptake in yeast, Drosophila, and humans. Science 2012;337:96−100. Available from: https://doi.org/10.1126/science.1218099.

[30] Klein Geltink RI, O'Sullivan D, Pearce EL. Caught in the cROSsfire: GSH Controls T Cell Metabolic Reprogramming. Immunity 2017;46:525−7. Available from: https://doi.org/10.1016/j.immuni.2017.03.022.

[31] Matsushita M, et al. T cell lipid peroxidation induces ferroptosis and prevents immunity to infection. J Exp Med 2015;212:555−68. Available from: https://doi.org/10.1084/jem.20140857.

[32] Mak TW, et al. Glutathione primes T cell metabolism for inflammation. Immunity 2017;46:675−89. Available from: https://doi.org/10.1016/j.immuni.2017.03.019.

[33] Ho PC, et al. Phosphoenolpyruvate is a metabolic checkpoint of anti-tumor T cell responses. Cell 2015;162:1217−28. Available from: https://doi.org/10.1016/j.cell.2015.08.012.

[34] Peng M, et al. Aerobic glycolysis promotes T helper 1 cell differentiation through an epigenetic mechanism. Science 2016;354:481−4. Available from: https://doi.org/10.1126/science.aaf6284.

[35] Kaymak I, et al. Carbon source availability drives nutrient utilization in CD8(+) T cells. Cell Metab 2022;34:1298−311. Available from: https://doi.org/10.1016/j.cmet.2022.07.012 e1296.

[36] Imanishi T, et al. Nucleic acid sensing by T cells initiates Th2 cell differentiation. Nat Commun 2014;5:3566. Available from: https://doi.org/10.1038/ncomms4566.

[37] Kurniawan H, Kobayashi T, Brenner D. The emerging role of one-carbon metabolism in T cells. Curr Opin Biotechnol 2021;68:193−201. Available from: https://doi.org/10.1016/j.copbio.2020.12.001.

[38] Powell JD, Pollizzi KN, Heikamp EB, Horton MR. Regulation of immune responses by mTOR. Annu Rev Immunol 2012;30:39−68. Available from: https://doi.org/10.1146/annurev-immunol-020711-075024.

[39] Yang K, et al. T cell exit from quiescence and differentiation into Th2 cells depend on Raptor-mTORC1-mediated metabolic reprogramming. Immunity 2013;39:1043−56. Available from: https://doi.org/10.1016/j.immuni.2013.09.015.

[40] Kidani Y, et al. Sterol regulatory element-binding proteins are essential for the metabolic programming of effector T cells and adaptive immunity. Nat Immunol 2013;14:489−99. Available from: https://doi.org/10.1038/ni.2570.

[41] Rodriguez PC, Quiceno DG, Ochoa AC. L-arginine availability regulates T-lymphocyte cell-cycle progression. Blood 2007;109:1568−73. Available from: https://doi.org/10.1182/blood-2006-06-031856.

[42] Van de Velde LA, et al. Stress Kinase GCN2 Controls the Proliferative Fitness and Trafficking of Cytotoxic T Cells Independent of Environmental Amino Acid Sensing. Cell Rep 2016;17:2247−58. Available from: https://doi.org/10.1016/j.celrep.2016.10.079.

[43] Hayashi K, Jutabha P, Endou H, Sagara H, Anzai N. LAT1 is a critical transporter of essential amino acids for immune reactions in activated human T cells. J Immunol 2013;191:4080−5. Available from: https://doi.org/10.4049/jimmunol.1300923.

[44] Sinclair LV, et al. Control of amino-acid transport by antigen receptors coordinates the metabolic reprogramming essential for T cell differentiation. Nat Immunol 2013;14:500−8. Available from: https://doi.org/10.1038/ni.2556.

[45] Sinclair LV, et al. Antigen receptor control of methionine metabolism in T cells. Elife 2019;8. Available from: https://doi.org/10.7554/eLife.44210.

[46] Hope HC, et al. Coordination of asparagine uptake and asparagine synthetase expression modulates CD8 + T cell activation. JCI Insight 2021;6. Available from: https://doi.org/10.1172/jci.insight.137761.

[47] Wu J, et al. Asparagine enhances LCK signalling to potentiate CD8(+) T-cell activation and anti-tumour responses. Nat Cell Biol 2021;23:75−86. Available from: https://doi.org/10.1038/s41556-020-00615-4.

[48] Frauwirth KA, et al. The CD28 signaling pathway regulates glucose metabolism. Immunity 2002;16:769−77. Available from: https://doi.org/10.1016/s1074-7613(02)00323-0.

[49] Chang CH, et al. Posttranscriptional control of T cell effector function by aerobic glycolysis. Cell 2013;153:1239−51. Available from: https://doi.org/10.1016/j.cell.2013.05.016.

[50] Bian Y, et al. Cancer SLC43A2 alters T cell methionine metabolism and histone methylation. Nature 2020;585:277−82. Available from: https://doi.org/10.1038/s41586-020-2682-1.

[51] van der Windt GJ, et al. Mitochondrial respiratory capacity is a critical regulator of CD8 + T cell memory development. Immunity 2012;36:68–78. Available from: https://doi.org/10.1016/j.immuni.2011.12.007.

[52] Klein Geltink RI, et al. Mitochondrial Priming by CD28. Cell 2017;171:385–97. Available from: https://doi.org/10.1016/j.cell.2017.08.018 e311.

[53] Pearce EL, et al. Enhancing CD8 T-cell memory by modulating fatty acid metabolism. Nature 2009;460:103–7. Available from: https://doi.org/10.1038/nature08097.

[54] Cui G, et al. IL-7-induced glycerol transport and TAG synthesis promotes memory CD8 + T cell longevity. Cell 2015;161:750–61. Available from: https://doi.org/10.1016/j.cell.2015.03.021.

[55] O'Sullivan D, et al. Memory CD8(+) T cells use cell-intrinsic lipolysis to support the metabolic programming necessary for development. Immunity 2014;41:75–88. Available from: https://doi.org/10.1016/j.immuni.2014.06.005.

[56] Pan Y, et al. Survival of tissue-resident memory T cells requires exogenous lipid uptake and metabolism. Nature 2017;543:252–6. Available from: https://doi.org/10.1038/nature21379.

[57] Han SJ, et al. White adipose tissue is a reservoir for memory T cells and promotes protective memory responses to infection. Immunity 2017;47:1154–68. Available from: https://doi.org/10.1016/j.immuni.2017.11.009 e1156.

[58] Sukumar M, et al. Inhibiting glycolytic metabolism enhances CD8 + T cell memory and antitumor function. J Clin Invest 2013;123:4479–88. Available from: https://doi.org/10.1172/JCI69589.

[59] Phan AT, et al. Constitutive glycolytic metabolism supports CD8(+) T cell effector memory differentiation during viral infection. Immunity 2016;45:1024–37. Available from: https://doi.org/10.1016/j.immuni.2016.10.017.

[60] Scharping NE, et al. Mitochondrial stress induced by continuous stimulation under hypoxia rapidly drives T cell exhaustion. Nat Immunol 2021;22:205–15. Available from: https://doi.org/10.1038/s41590-020-00834-9.

[61] Schurich A, et al. Distinct metabolic requirements of exhausted and functional virus-specific CD8 T cells in the same host. Cell Rep 2016;16:1243–52. Available from: https://doi.org/10.1016/j.celrep.2016.06.078.

[62] Vardhana SA, et al. Impaired mitochondrial oxidative phosphorylation limits the self-renewal of T cells exposed to persistent antigen. Nat Immunol 2020;21:1022–33. Available from: https://doi.org/10.1038/s41590-020-0725-2.

[63] Gerriets VA, Rathmell JC. Metabolic pathways in T cell fate and function. Trends Immunol 2012;33:168–73. Available from: https://doi.org/10.1016/j.it.2012.01.010.

[64] van der Windt GJ, Pearce EL. Metabolic switching and fuel choice during T-cell differentiation and memory development. Immunol Rev 2012;249:27–42. Available from: https://doi.org/10.1111/j.1600-065X.2012.01150.x.

[65] Saravia J, Chapman NM, Chi H. Helper T cell differentiation. Cell Mol Immunol 2019;16:634–43. Available from: https://doi.org/10.1038/s41423-019-0220-6.

[66] Balyan R, Gautam N, Gascoigne NRJ. The ups and downs of metabolism during the lifespan of a T cell. Int J Mol Sci 2020;21. Available from: https://doi.org/10.3390/ijms21217972.

[67] Schmitt EG, Williams CB. Generation and function of induced regulatory T cells. Front Immunol 2013;4:152. Available from: https://doi.org/10.3389/fimmu.2013.00152.

[68] Wieman HL, Wofford JA, Rathmell JC. Cytokine stimulation promotes glucose uptake via phosphatidylinositol-3 kinase/Akt regulation of Glut1 activity and trafficking. Mol Biol Cell 2007;18:1437–46. Available from: https://doi.org/10.1091/mbc.e06-07-0593.

[69] Angelin A, et al. Foxp3 reprograms T cell metabolism to function in low-glucose, high-lactate environments. Cell Metab 2017;25:1282–93. Available from: https://doi.org/10.1016/j.cmet.2016.12.018 e1287.

[70] Shi LZ, et al. HIF1alpha-dependent glycolytic pathway orchestrates a metabolic checkpoint for the differentiation of TH17 and Treg cells. J Exp Med 2011;208:1367–76. Available from: https://doi.org/10.1084/jem.20110278.

[71] Michalek RD, et al. Cutting edge: distinct glycolytic and lipid oxidative metabolic programs are essential for effector and regulatory CD4 + T cell subsets. J Immunol 2011;186:3299–303. Available from: https://doi.org/10.4049/jimmunol.1003613.

[72] de Kivit S, et al. Immune suppression by human thymus-derived effector Tregs relies on glucose/lactate-fueled fatty acid synthesis. Cell Rep 2024;43114681. Available from: https://doi.org/10.1016/j.celrep.2024.114681.

[73] Michalek RD, et al. Estrogen-related receptor-alpha is a metabolic regulator of effector T-cell activation and differentiation. Proc Natl Acad Sci U S A 2011;108:18348–53. Available from: https://doi.org/10.1073/pnas.1108856108.

[74] Fang Y, et al. Mitochondrial fusion induced by transforming growth factor-beta1 serves as a switch that governs the metabolic reprogramming during differentiation of regulatory T cells. Redox Biol 2023;62102709. Available from: https://doi.org/10.1016/j.redox.2023.102709.

[75] Miao Y, et al. The activation of PPARgamma enhances Treg responses through up-regulating CD36/CPT1-mediated fatty acid oxidation and subsequent N-glycan branching of TbetaRII/IL-2Ralpha. Cell Commun Signal 2022;20:48. Available from: https://doi.org/10.1186/s12964-022-00849-9.

[76] Araujo L, Khim P, Mkhikian H, Mortales CL, Demetriou M. Glycolysis and glutaminolysis cooperatively control T cell function by limiting metabolite supply to N-glycosylation. Elife 2017;6. Available from: https://doi.org/10.7554/eLife.21330.

[77] Zhang B, et al. Proximity-enabled covalent binding of IL-2 to IL-2Ralpha selectively activates regulatory T cells and suppresses autoimmunity. Signal Transduct Target Ther 2023;8:28. Available from: https://doi.org/10.1038/s41392-022-01208-3.

[78] Ansa-Addo EA, et al. Membrane-organizing protein moesin controls Treg differentiation and antitumor immunity via TGF-beta signaling. J Clin Invest 2017;127:1321–37. Available from: https://doi.org/10.1172/JCI89281.

[79] Shi H, Chi H. Metabolic control of Treg cell stability, plasticity, and tissue-specific heterogeneity. Front Immunol 2019;10:2716. Available from: https://doi.org/10.3389/fimmu.2019.02716.

[80] He N, et al. Metabolic control of regulatory T cell (Treg) survival and function by Lkb1. Proc Natl Acad Sci U S A 2017;114:12542–7. Available from: https://doi.org/10.1073/pnas.1715363114.

[81] Ozay EI, et al. Rotenone treatment reveals a role for electron transport complex I in the subcellular localization of key transcriptional regulators during T helper cell differentiation. Front Immunol 2018;9:1284. Available from: https://doi.org/10.3389/fimmu.2018.01284.

[82] Beier UH, et al. Essential role of mitochondrial energy metabolism in Foxp3(+) T-regulatory cell function and allograft survival. FASEB J 2015;29:2315–26. Available from: https://doi.org/10.1096/fj.14-268409.

[83] Marcel N, Sarin A. Notch1 regulated autophagy controls survival and suppressor activity of activated murine T-regulatory cells. Elife 2016;5. Available from: https://doi.org/10.7554/eLife.14023.

[84] Corte-Real BF, et al. Sodium perturbs mitochondrial respiration and induces dysfunctional Tregs. Cell Metab 2023;35:299–315. Available from: https://doi.org/10.1016/j.cmet.2023.01.009 e298.

[85] Weinberg SE, et al. Mitochondrial complex III is essential for suppressive function of regulatory T cells. Nature 2019;565:495–9. Available from: https://doi.org/10.1038/s41586-018-0846-z.

[86] Saravia J, et al. Homeostasis and transitional activation of regulatory T cells require c-Myc. Sci Adv 2020;6eaaw6443. Available from: https://doi.org/10.1126/sciadv.aaw6443.

[87] Shin B, et al. Mitochondrial oxidative phosphorylation regulates the fate decision between pathogenic Th17 and regulatory T cells. Cell Rep 2020;30:1898–909. Available from: https://doi.org/10.1016/j.celrep.2020.01.022 e1894.

[88] Klysz D, et al. Glutamine-dependent alpha-ketoglutarate production regulates the balance between T helper 1 cell and regulatory T cell generation. Sci Signal 2015;8:ra97. Available from: https://doi.org/10.1126/scisignal.aab2610.

[89] Johnson MO, et al. Distinct Regulation of Th17 and Th1 Cell Differentiation by Glutaminase-Dependent Metabolism. Cell 2018;175:1780–95. Available from: https://doi.org/10.1016/j.cell 2018.10.001 e1719.

[90] Xu T, et al. Metabolic control of T(H)17 and induced T(reg) cell balance by an epigenetic mechanism. Nature 2017;548:228–33. Available from: https://doi.org/10.1038/nature23475.

[91] Rankin LC, et al. Dietary tryptophan deficiency promotes gut RORgammat(+) Treg cells at the expense of Gata3(+) Treg cells and alters commensal microbiota metabolism. Cell Rep 2023;42112135. Available from: https://doi.org/10.1016/j.celrep.2023.112135.

[92] Geng J, et al. CD98-induced CD147 signaling stabilizes the Foxp3 protein to maintain tissue homeostasis. Cell Mol Immunol 2021;18:2618–31. Available from: https://doi.org/10.1038/s41423-021-00785-7.

[93] Ikeda K, et al. Slc3a2 Mediates Branched-Chain Amino-Acid-Dependent Maintenance of Regulatory T Cells. Cell Rep 2017;21:1824–38. Available from: https://doi.org/10.1016/j.celrep.2017.10.082.

[94] Ma S, et al. Serine enrichment in tumors promotes regulatory T cell accumulation through sphinganine-mediated regulation of c-Fos. Sci Immunol 2024;9:eadg8817. Available from: https://doi.org/10.1126/sciimmunol.adg8817.

[95] Battaglia M, Stabilini A, Roncarolo MG. Rapamycin selectively expands CD4 + CD25 + FoxP3 + regulatory T cells. Blood 2005;105:4743–8. Available from: https://doi.org/10.1182/blood-2004-10-3932.

[96] Delgoffe GM, et al. The kinase mTOR regulates the differentiation of helper T cells through the selective activation of signaling by mTORC1 and mTORC2. Nat Immunol 2011;12:295–303. Available from: https://doi.org/10.1038/ni.2005.

[97] Haxhinasto S, Mathis D, Benoist C. The AKT-mTOR axis regulates de novo differentiation of CD4 + Foxp3 + cells. J Exp Med 2008;205:565–74. Available from: https://doi.org/10.1084/jem.20071477.

[98] Inoki K, Zhu T, Guan KL. TSC2 mediates cellular energy response to control cell growth and survival. Cell 2003;115:577–90. Available from: https://doi.org/10.1016/s0092-8674(03)00929-2.

[99] Mihaylova MM, Shaw RJ. The AMPK signalling pathway coordinates cell growth, autophagy and metabolism. Nat Cell Biol 2011;13:1016–23. Available from: https://doi.org/10.1038/ncb2329.

[100] Houten SM, Violante S, Ventura FV, Wanders RJ. The biochemistry and physiology of mitochondrial fatty acid beta-oxidation and its genetic disorders. Annu Rev Physiol 2016;78:23–44. Available from: https://doi.org/10.1146/annurev-physiol-021115-105045.

[101] Gualdoni GA, et al. The AMP analog AICAR modulates the Treg/Th17 axis through enhancement of fatty acid oxidation. FASEB J 2016;30:3800–9. Available from: https://doi.org/10.1096/fj.201600522R.

[102] Zeng H, et al. mTORC1 couples immune signals and metabolic programming to establish T(reg)-cell function. Nature 2013;499:485–90. Available from: https://doi.org/10.1038/nature12297.

[103] Procaccini C, et al. An oscillatory switch in mTOR kinase activity sets regulatory T cell responsiveness. Immunity 2010;33:929–41. Available from: https://doi.org/10.1016/j.immuni.2010.11.024.

[104] Dai M, et al. LDHA as a regulator of T cell fate and its mechanisms in disease. Biomed Pharmacother 2023;158114164. Available from: https://doi.org/10.1016/j.biopha.2022.114164.

[105] Wu B, Goronzy JJ, Weyand CM. Metabolic fitness of T cells in autoimmune disease. Immunometabolism 2020;2. Available from: https://doi.org/10.20900/immunometab20200017.

[106] Metzler B, Gfeller P, Guinet E. Restricting glutamine or glutamine-dependent purine and pyrimidine syntheses promotes human T cells with high FOXP3 expression and regulatory properties. J Immunol 2016;196:3618–30. Available from: https://doi.org/10.4049/jimmunol.1501756.

[107] Bailis W, et al. Distinct modes of mitochondrial metabolism uncouple T cell differentiation and function. Nature 2019;571:403–7. Available from: https://doi.org/10.1038/s41586-019-1311-3.

[108] Weyand CM, Goronzy JJ. The immunology of rheumatoid arthritis. Nat Immunol 2021;22:10–18. Available from: https://doi.org/10.1038/s41590-020-00816-x.

[109] Yang Z, et al. Restoring oxidant signaling suppresses proarthritogenic T cell effector functions in rheumatoid arthritis. Sci Transl Med 2016;8. Available from: https://doi.org/10.1126/scitranslmed.aad7151 331ra338.

[110] Abboud G, et al. Inhibition of glycolysis reduces disease severity in an autoimmune model of rheumatoid arthritis. Front Immunol 2018;9:1973. Available from: https://doi.org/10.3389/fimmu.2018.01973.

[111] Weyand CM, Goronzy JJ. A mitochondrial checkpoint in autoimmune disease. Cell Metab 2018;28:185–6. Available from: https://doi.org/10.1016/j.cmet.2018.07.014.

[112] Shao L, et al. Deficiency of the DNA repair enzyme ATM in rheumatoid arthritis. J Exp Med 2009;206:1435−49. Available from: https://doi.org/10.1084/jem.20082251.

[113] Li Y, et al. The DNA repair nuclease MRE11A functions as a mitochondrial protector and prevents T cell pyroptosis and tissue inflammation. Cell Metab 2019;30:477−92. Available from: https://doi.org/10.1016/j.cmet.2019.06.016 e476.

[114] Klotz L, et al. Teriflunomide treatment for multiple sclerosis modulates T cell mitochondrial respiration with affinity-dependent effects. Sci Transl Med 2019;11. Available from: https://doi.org/10.1126/scitranslmed.aao5563.

[115] Fragoso YD, Brooks JB. Leflunomide and teriflunomide: altering the metabolism of pyrimidines for the treatment of autoimmune diseases. Expert Rev Clin Pharmacol 2015;8:315−20. Available from: https://doi.org/10.1586/17512433.2015.1019343.

[116] Chornoguz O, et al. mTORC1 promotes T-bet phosphorylation to regulate Th1 differentiation. J Immunol 2017;198:3939−48. Available from: https://doi.org/10.4049/jimmunol.1601078.

[117] Zhao D, et al. Metformin decreases IL-22 secretion to suppress tumor growth in an orthotopic mouse model of hepatocellular carcinoma. Int J Cancer 2015;136:2556−65. Available from: https://doi.org/10.1002/ijc.29305.

[118] Glimcher LH, Murphy KM. Lineage commitment in the immune system: the T helper lymphocyte grows up. Genes Dev 2000;14:1693−711.

[119] Kaplan MH, Schindler U, Smiley ST, Grusby MJ. Stat6 is required for mediating responses to IL-4 and for development of Th2 cells. Immunity 1996;4:313−19. Available from: https://doi.org/10.1016/s1074-7613(00)80439-2.

[120] Tibbitt CA, et al. Single-cell RNA sequencing of the T helper cell response to house dust mites defines a distinct gene expression signature in airway Th2 cells. Immunity 2019;51:169−84. Available from: https://doi.org/10.1016/j.immuni.2019.05.014 e165.

[121] Lee K, et al. Mammalian target of rapamycin protein complex 2 regulates differentiation of Th1 and Th2 cell subsets via distinct signaling pathways. Immunity 2010;32:743−53. Available from: https://doi.org/10.1016/j.immuni.2010.06.002.

[122] Yang JQ, et al. RhoA orchestrates glycolysis for TH2 cell differentiation and allergic airway inflammation. J Allergy Clin Immunol 2016;137:231−45. Available from: https://doi.org/10.1016/j.jaci.2015.05.004 e234.

[123] Rodriguez A, Ezquerro S, Mendez-Gimenez L, Becerril S, Fruhbeck G. Revisiting the adipocyte: a model for integration of cytokine signaling in the regulation of energy metabolism. Am J Physiol Endocrinol Metab 2015;309:E691−714. Available from: https://doi.org/10.1152/ajpendo.00297.2015.

[124] Heikamp EB, et al. The AGC kinase SGK1 regulates TH1 and TH2 differentiation downstream of the mTORC2 complex. Nat Immunol 2014;15:457−64. Available from: https://doi.org/10.1038/ni.2867.

[125] Li B, Tournier C, Davis RJ, Flavell RA. Regulation of IL-4 expression by the transcription factor JunB during T helper cell differentiation. EMBO J 1999;18:420−32. Available from: https://doi.org/10.1093/emboj/18.2.420.

[126] Romero M, et al. Immunometabolic effects of lactate on humoral immunity in healthy individuals of different ages. Nat Commun 2024;15:7515. Available from: https://doi.org/10.1038/s41467-024-51207-x.

[127] Clark DA, et al. Reduced uterine indoleamine 2,3-dioxygenase versus increased Th1/Th2 cytokine ratios as a basis for occult and clinical pregnancy failure in mice and humans. Am J Reprod Immunol 2005;54:203−16. Available from: https://doi.org/10.1111/j.1600-0897.2005.00299.x.

[128] Xu H, Zhang GX, Ciric B, Rostami A. IDO: a double-edged sword for T(H)1/T(H)2 regulation. Immunol Lett 2008;121:1−6. Available from: https://doi.org/10.1016/j.imlet.2008.08.008.

[129] Chang WK, Yang KD, Shaio MF. Effect of glutamine on Th1 and Th2 cytokine responses of human peripheral blood mononuclear cells. Clin Immunol 1999;93:294−301. Available from: https://doi.org/10.1006/clim.1999.4788.

[130] Wen T, Rothenberg ME. Cell-by-cell deciphering of T cells in allergic inflammation. J Allergy Clin Immunol 2019;144:1143−8. Available from: https://doi.org/10.1016/j.jaci.2019.10.001.

[131] Trompette A, et al. Gut microbiota metabolism of dietary fiber influences allergic airway disease and hematopoiesis. Nat Med 2014;20:159–66. Available from: https://doi.org/10.1038/nm.3444.

[132] Thio CL, Chi PY, Lai AC, Chang YJ. Regulation of type 2 innate lymphoid cell-dependent airway hyperreactivity by butyrate. J Allergy Clin Immunol 2018;142:1867–83. Available from: https://doi.org/10.1016/j.jaci.2018.02.032 e1812.

[133] Choi G, et al. NRF2 is a spatiotemporal metabolic hub essential for the polyfunctionality of Th2 cells. Proc Natl Acad Sci U S A 2024;121. Available from: https://doi.org/10.1073/pnas.2319994121 e2319994121.

[134] Li Y, et al. Itaconate suppresses house dust mite-induced allergic airways disease and Th2 cell differentiation. Mucosal Immunol 2024;. Available from: https://doi.org/10.1016/j.mucimm.2024.08.001.

[135] Robinette ML, et al. Transcriptional programs define molecular characteristics of innate lymphoid cell classes and subsets. Nat Immunol 2015;16:306–17. Available from: https://doi.org/10.1038/ni.3094.

[136] Nobs SP, et al. PPARgamma in dendritic cells and T cells drives pathogenic type-2 effector responses in lung inflammation. J Exp Med 2017;214:3015–35. Available from: https://doi.org/10.1084/jem.20162069.

[137] Lefterova MI, Haakonsson AK, Lazar MA, Mandrup S. PPARgamma and the global map of adipogenesis and beyond. Trends Endocrinol Metab 2014;25:293–302. Available from: https://doi.org/10.1016/j.tem.2014.04.001.

[138] Chen T, et al. PPAR-gamma promotes type 2 immune responses in allergy and nematode infection. Sci Immunol 2017;2. Available from: https://doi.org/10.1126/sciimmunol.aal5196.

[139] Szanto A, et al. STAT6 transcription factor is a facilitator of the nuclear receptor PPARgamma-regulated gene expression in macrophages and dendritic cells. Immunity 2010;33:699–712. Available from: https://doi.org/10.1016/j.immuni.2010.11.009.

[140] Odegaard JI, et al. Macrophage-specific PPARgamma controls alternative activation and improves insulin resistance. Nature 2007;447:1116–20. Available from: https://doi.org/10.1038/nature05894.

[141] Daniel B, et al. The Nuclear receptor PPARgamma controls progressive macrophage polarization as a ligand-insensitive epigenomic ratchet of transcriptional memory. Immunity 2018;49:615–26. Available from: https://doi.org/10.1016/j.immuni.2018.09.005 e616.

[142] Dardalhon V, et al. IL-4 inhibits TGF-beta-induced Foxp3 + T cells and, together with TGF-beta, generates IL-9 + IL-10 + Foxp3(-) effector T cells. Nat Immunol 2008;9:1347–55. Available from: https://doi.org/10.1038/ni.1677.

[143] Veldhoen M, et al. Transforming growth factor-beta 'reprograms' the differentiation of T helper 2 cells and promotes an interleukin 9-producing subset. Nat Immunol 2008;9:1341–6. Available from: https://doi.org/10.1038/ni.1659.

[144] Lu Y, et al. Th9 cells promote antitumor immune responses in vivo. J Clin Invest 2012;122:4160–71. Available from: https://doi.org/10.1172/JCI65459.

[145] Purwar R, et al. Robust tumor immunity to melanoma mediated by interleukin-9-producing T cells. Nat Med 2012;18:1248–53. Available from: https://doi.org/10.1038/nm.2856.

[146] Lu Y, et al. Tumor-specific IL-9-producing CD8 + Tc9 cells are superior effector than type-I cytotoxic Tc1 cells for adoptive immunotherapy of cancers. Proc Natl Acad Sci U S A 2014;111:2265–70. Available from: https://doi.org/10.1073/pnas.1317431111.

[147] Zielinski CE, et al. Dissecting the human immunologic memory for pathogens. Immunol Rev 2011;240:40–51. Available from: https://doi.org/10.1111/j.1600-065X.2010.01000.x.

[148] Raphael I, Nalawade S, Eagar TN, Forsthuber TG. T cell subsets and their signature cytokines in autoimmune and inflammatory diseases. Cytokine 2015;74:5–17. Available from: https://doi.org/10.1016/j.cyto.2014.09.011.

[149] Deng Y, et al. Th9 cells and IL-9 in autoimmune disorders: Pathogenesis and therapeutic potentials. Hum Immunol 2017;78:120–8. Available from: https://doi.org/10.1016/j.humimm.2016.12.010.

[150] Schmitt E, Klein M, Bopp T. Th9 cells, new players in adaptive immunity. Trends Immunol 2014;35:61–8. Available from: https://doi.org/10.1016/j.it.2013.10.004.

[151] Nakatsukasa H, et al. The DNA-binding inhibitor Id3 regulates IL-9 production in CD4(+) T cells. Nat Immunol 2015;16:1077−84. Available from: https://doi.org/10.1038/ni.3252.

[152] Sandquist I, Kolls J. Update on regulation and effector functions of Th17 cells. F1000Res 2018;7:205. Available from: https://doi.org/10.12688/f1000research.13020.1.

[153] Kurebayashi Y, et al. PI3K-Akt-mTORC1-S6K1/2 axis controls Th17 differentiation by regulating Gfi1 expression and nuclear translocation of RORgamma. Cell Rep 2012;1:360−73. Available from: https://doi.org/10.1016/j.celrep.2012.02.007.

[154] Sasaki CY, et al. p((7)(0)S(6)K(1)) in the TORC1 pathway is essential for the differentiation of Th17 Cells, but not Th1, Th2, or Treg cells in mice. Eur J Immunol 2016;46:212−22. Available from: https://doi.org/10.1002/eji.201445422.

[155] Andrzejewski S, Gravel SP, Pollak M, St-Pierre J. Metformin directly acts on mitochondria to alter cellular bioenergetics. Cancer Metab 2014;2:12. Available from: https://doi.org/10.1186/2049-3002-2-12.

[156] Wheaton WW, et al. Metformin inhibits mitochondrial complex I of cancer cells to reduce tumorigenesis. Elife 2014;3e02242. Available from: https://doi.org/10.7554/eLife.02242.

[157] Dang EV, et al. Control of T(H)17/T(reg) balance by hypoxia-inducible factor 1. Cell 2011;146:772−84. Available from: https://doi.org/10.1016/j.cell.2011.07.033.

[158] Soriano-Baguet L, et al. Pyruvate dehydrogenase fuels a critical citrate pool that is essential for Th17 cell effector functions. Cell Rep 2023;42112153. Available from: https://doi.org/10.1016/j.celrep.2023.112153.

[159] Sugiura A, et al. MTHFD2 is a metabolic checkpoint controlling effector and regulatory T cell fate and function. Immunity 2022;55:65−81. Available from: https://doi.org/10.1016/j.immuni.2021.10.011 e69.

[160] Xia X, et al. GLS1-mediated glutaminolysis unbridled by MALT1 protease promotes psoriasis pathogenesis. J Clin Invest 2020;130:5180−96. Available from: https://doi.org/10.1172/JCI129269.

[161] Xiao M, et al. Inhibition of alpha-KG-dependent histone and DNA demethylases by fumarate and succinate that are accumulated in mutations of FH and SDH tumor suppressors. Genes Dev 2012;26:1326−38. Available from: https://doi.org/10.1101/gad.191056.112.

[162] Miao Y, et al. The role of GLS1-mediated glutaminolysis/2-HG/H3K4me3 and GSH/ROS signals in Th17 responses counteracted by PPARgamma agonists. Theranostics 2021;11:4531−48. Available from: https://doi.org/10.7150/thno.54803.

[163] Muri J, Kopf M. Redox regulation of immunometabolism. Nat Rev Immunol 2021;21:363−81. Available from: https://doi.org/10.1038/s41577-020-00478-8.

[164] Lian G, et al. Glutathione de novo synthesis but not recycling process coordinates with glutamine catabolism to control redox homeostasis and directs murine T cell differentiation. Elife 2018;7. Available from: https://doi.org/10.7554/eLife.36158.

[165] Berod L, et al. De novo fatty acid synthesis controls the fate between regulatory T and T helper 17 cells. Nat Med 2014;20:1327−33. Available from: https://doi.org/10.1038/nm.3704.

[166] Endo Y, et al. Obesity drives Th17 cell differentiation by inducing the lipid metabolic kinase, ACC1. Cell Rep 2015;12:1042−55. Available from: https://doi.org/10.1016/j.celrep.2015.07.014.

[167] Timilshina M, et al. Activation of mevalonate pathway via LKB1 Is essential for stability of T(reg) cells. Cell Rep 2019;27:2948−61. Available from: https://doi.org/10.1016/j.celrep.2019.05.020 e2947.

[168] Forero-Pena DA, Gutierrez FR. Statins as modulators of regulatory T-cell biology. Mediators Inflamm 2013;2013167086. Available from: https://doi.org/10.1155/2013/167086.

[169] Hu X, et al. Sterol metabolism controls T(H)17 differentiation by generating endogenous RORgamma agonists. Nat Chem Biol 2015;11:141−7. Available from: https://doi.org/10.1038/nchembio.1714.

[170] Zambrano-Zaragoza JF, Romo-Martinez EJ, Duran-Avelar Mde J, Garcia-Magallanes N, Vibanco-Perez N. Th17 cells in autoimmune and infectious diseases. Int J Inflam 2014;2014651503. Available from: https://doi.org/10.1155/2014/651503.

[171] Wu X, et al. Arctigenin exerts anti-colitis efficacy through inhibiting the differentiation of Th1 and Th17 cells via an mTORC1-dependent pathway. Biochem Pharmacol 2015;96:323−36. Available from: https://doi.org/10.1016/j.bcp.2015.06.008.

[172] Kang KY, et al. Metformin downregulates Th17 cells differentiation and attenuates murine autoimmune arthritis. Int Immunopharmacol 2013;16:85−92. Available from: https://doi.org/10.1016/j.intimp.2013.03.020.

[173] Kono M, et al. Glutaminase 1 inhibition reduces glycolysis and ameliorates lupus-like disease in MRL/lpr mice and experimental autoimmune encephalomyelitis. Arthritis Rheumatol 2019;71:1869−78. Available from: https://doi.org/10.1002/art.41019.

[174] Andersen JV, Westi EW, Neal ES, Aldana BI, Borges K. beta-Hydroxybutyrate and medium-chain fatty acids are metabolized by different cell types in mouse cerebral cortex slices. Neurochem Res 2023;48:54−61. Available from: https://doi.org/10.1007/s11064-022-03726-6.

[175] Dabrowska-Bouta B, Struzynska L, Sidoryk-Wegrzynowicz M, Sulkowski G. Memantine improves the disturbed glutamine and gamma-amino butyric acid homeostasis in the brain of rats subjected to experimental autoimmune encephalomyelitis. Int J Mol Sci 2023;24. Available from: https://doi.org/10.3390/ijms241713149.

[176] Nakaya M, et al. Inflammatory T cell responses rely on amino acid transporter ASCT2 facilitation of glutamine uptake and mTORC1 kinase activation. Immunity 2014;40:692−705. Available from: https://doi.org/10.1016/j.immuni.2014.04.007.

[177] Yu Q, et al. Targeting glutamine metabolism ameliorates autoimmune hepatitis via inhibiting T cell activation and differentiation. Front Immunol 2022;13880262. Available from: https://doi.org/10.3389/fimmu.2022.880262.

[178] Nutsch K, Hsieh C. When T cells run out of breath: the HIF-1alpha story. Cell 2011;146:673−4. Available from: https://doi.org/10.1016/j.cell.2011.08.018.

[179] Haase S, et al. Propionic acid rescues high-fat diet enhanced immunopathology in autoimmunity via effects on Th17 responses. Front Immunol 2021;12701626. Available from: https://doi.org/10.3389/fimmu.2021.701626.

[180] Duscha A, et al. Propionic acid shapes the multiple sclerosis disease course by an immunomodulatory mechanism. Cell 2020;180:1067−80. Available from: https://doi.org/10.1016/j.cell.2020.02.035 e1016.

[181] Damasceno LEA, et al. PKM2 promotes Th17 cell differentiation and autoimmune inflammation by fine-tuning STAT3 activation. J Exp Med 2020;217. Available from: https://doi.org/10.1084/jem.20190613.

[182] Wagner A, et al. Metabolic modeling of single Th17 cells reveals regulators of autoimmunity. Cell 2021;184:4168−85. Available from: https://doi.org/10.1016/j.cell.2021.05.045 e4121.

[183] Wellford SA, Schwartzberg PL. Help me help you: emerging concepts in T follicular helper cell differentiation, identity, and function. Curr Opin Immunol 2024;87:102421. Available from: https://doi.org/10.1016/j.coi.2024.102421.

[184] Cruz-Morales E, Hart AP, Fossett GM, Laufer TM. Helios(+) and RORgammat(+) Treg populations are differentially regulated by MHCII, CD28, and ICOS to shape the intestinal Treg pool. Mucosal Immunol 2023;16:264−74. Available from: https://doi.org/10.1016/j.mucimm.2023.02.007.

[185] Gong M, et al. Transcriptional and metabolic programs promote the expansion of follicular helper T cells in lupus-prone mice. iScience 2023;26106774. Available from: https://doi.org/10.1016/j.isci.2023.106774.

[186] Zou X, et al. Metabolic regulation of follicular helper T cell differentiation in a mouse model of lupus. Immunol Lett 2022;247:13−21. Available from: https://doi.org/10.1016/j.imlet.2022.03.008.

[187] Oaks Z, Winans T, Huang N, Banki K, Perl A. Activation of the mechanistic target of rapamycin in SLE: explosion of evidence in the last five years. Curr Rheumatol Rep 2016;18:73. Available from: https://doi.org/10.1007/s11926-016-0622-8.

[188] Laniak OT, Winans T, Patel A, Park J, Perl A. Redox pathogenesis in rheumatic diseases. ACR Open Rheumatol 2024;6:334−46. Available from: https://doi.org/10.1002/acr2.11668.

[189] Winans T, et al. mTOR-dependent loss of PON1 secretion and antiphospholipid autoantibody production underlie autoimmunity-mediated cirrhosis in transaldolase deficiency. J Autoimmun 2023;140103112. Available from: https://doi.org/10.1016/j.jaut.2023.103112.

[190] Oaks Z, et al. Cytosolic aldose metabolism contributes to progression from cirrhosis to hepatocarcinogenesis. Nat Metab 2023;5:41–60. Available from: https://doi.org/10.1038/s42255-022-00711-9.

[191] Oaks Z, et al. Mitochondrial dysfunction in the liver and antiphospholipid antibody production precede disease onset and respond to rapamycin in lupus-prone mice. Arthritis Rheumatol 2016;68:2728–39. Available from: https://doi.org/10.1002/art.39791.

[192] Caza TN, et al. HRES-1/Rab4-mediated depletion of Drp1 impairs mitochondrial homeostasis and represents a target for treatment in SLE. Ann Rheum Dis 2014;73:1888–97. Available from: https://doi.org/10.1136/annrheumdis-2013-203794.

[193] Akkaya M, Pierce SK. From zero to sixty and back to zero again: the metabolic life of B cells. Curr Opin Immunol 2019;57:1–7. Available from: https://doi.org/10.1016/j.coi.2018.09.019.

[194] Boothby M, Rickert RC. Metabolic regulation of the immune humoral response. Immunity 2017;46:743–55. Available from: https://doi.org/10.1016/j.immuni.2017.04.009.

[195] Boothby MR, Brookens SK, Raybuck AL, Cho SH. Supplying the trip to antibody production-nutrients, signaling, and the programming of cellular metabolism in the mature B lineage. Cell Mol Immunol 2022;19:352–69. Available from: https://doi.org/10.1038/s41423-021-00782-w.

[196] Jellusova J. Cross-talk between signal transduction and metabolism in B cells. Immunol Lett 2018;201:1–13. Available from: https://doi.org/10.1016/j.imlet.2018.11.003.

[197] Jellusova J. Metabolic control of B cell immune responses. Curr Opin Immunol 2020;63:21–8. Available from: https://doi.org/10.1016/j.coi.2019.11.002.

[198] Jellusova J, Rickert RC. A brake for B cell proliferation: appropriate responses to metabolic stress are crucial to maintain B cell viability and prevent malignant outgrowth. Bioessays 2017;39. Available from: https://doi.org/10.1002/bies.201700079.

[199] Elsner RA, Shlomchik MJ. Germinal center and extrafollicular B cell responses in vaccination, immunity, and autoimmunity. Immunity 2020;53:1136–50. Available from: https://doi.org/10.1016/j.immuni.2020.11.006.

[200] Victora GD, Nussenzweig MC. Germinal centers. Annu Rev Immunol 2012;30:429–57. Available from: https://doi.org/10.1146/annurev-immunol-020711-075032.

[201] Shlomchik MJ, Weisel F. Germinal center selection and the development of memory B and plasma cells. Immunol Rev 2012;247:52–63. Available from: https://doi.org/10.1111/j.1600-065X.2012.01124.x.

[202] Shlomchik MJ, Luo W, Weisel F. Linking signaling and selection in the germinal center. Immunol Rev 2019;288:49–63. Available from: https://doi.org/10.1111/imr.12744.

[203] Rolink AG, Winkler T, Melchers F, Andersson J. Precursor B cell receptor-dependent B cell proliferation and differentiation does not require the bone marrow or fetal liver environment. J Exp Med 2000;191:23–32. Available from: https://doi.org/10.1084/jem.191.1.23.

[204] Zouali M. Transcriptional and metabolic pre-B cell receptor-mediated checkpoints: implications for autoimmune diseases. Mol Immunol 2014;62:315–20. Available from: https://doi.org/10.1016/j.molimm.2014.01.009.

[205] Kojima H, et al. Differentiation stage-specific requirement in hypoxia-inducible factor-1alpha-regulated glycolytic pathway during murine B cell development in bone marrow. J Immunol 2010;184:154–63. Available from: https://doi.org/10.4049/jimmunol.0800167.

[206] Clark MR, Mandal M, Ochiai K, Singh H. Orchestrating B cell lymphopoiesis through interplay of IL-7 receptor and pre-B cell receptor signalling. Nat Rev Immunol 2014;14:69–80. Available from: https://doi.org/10.1038/nri3570.

[207] Urbanczyk S, et al. Regulation of energy metabolism during early B lymphocyte development. Int J Mol Sci 2018;19. Available from: https://doi.org/10.3390/ijms19082192.

[208] Iwata TN, et al. Conditional disruption of raptor reveals an essential role for mTORC1 in B cell development, survival, and metabolism. J Immunol 2016;197:2250–60. Available from: https://doi.org/10.4049/jimmunol.1600492.

[209] Zhang S, et al. B cell-specific deficiencies in mTOR limit humoral immune responses. J Immunol 2013;191:1692–703. Available from: https://doi.org/10.4049/jimmunol.1201767.

[210] Zhang Y, et al. Rictor is required for early B cell development in bone marrow. PLoS One 2014;9: e103970. Available from: https://doi.org/10.1371/journal.pone.0103970.

[211] Park H, et al. Disruption of Fnip1 reveals a metabolic checkpoint controlling B lymphocyte development. Immunity 2012;36:769–81. Available from: https://doi.org/10.1016/j.immuni.2012.02.019.

[212] Chan LN, et al. Metabolic gatekeeper function of B-lymphoid transcription factors. Nature 2017;542:479–83. Available from: https://doi.org/10.1038/nature21076.

[213] Stein M, et al. A defined metabolic state in pre B cells governs B-cell development and is counterbalanced by Swiprosin-2/EFhd1. Cell Death Differ 2017;24:1239–52. Available from: https://doi.org/10.1038/cdd.2017.52.

[214] Caro-Maldonado A, et al. Metabolic reprogramming is required for antibody production that is suppressed in anergic but exaggerated in chronically BAFF-exposed B cells. J Immunol 2014;192:3626–36. Available from: https://doi.org/10.4049/jimmunol.1302062.

[215] Farmer JR, et al. Induction of metabolic quiescence defines the transitional to follicular B cell switch. Sci Signal 2019;12. Available from: https://doi.org/10.1126/scisignal.aaw5573.

[216] Lee K, et al. Requirement for Rictor in homeostasis and function of mature B lymphoid cells. Blood 2013;122:2369–79. Available from: https://doi.org/10.1182/blood-2013-01-477505.

[217] Benhamron S, Tirosh B. Direct activation of mTOR in B lymphocytes confers impairment in B-cell maturation andloss of marginal zone B cells. Eur J Immunol 2011;41:2390–6. Available from: https://doi.org/10.1002/eji.201041336.

[218] Ci X, et al. TSC1 promotes B cell maturation but is dispensable for germinal center formation. PLoS One 2015;10:e0127527. Available from: https://doi.org/10.1371/journal.pone.0127527.

[219] Franchina DG, et al. Glutathione-dependent redox balance characterizes the distinct metabolic properties of follicular and marginal zone B cells. Nat Commun 2022;13:1789. Available from: https://doi.org/10.1038/s41467-022-29426-x.

[220] Muri J, Thut H, Bornkamm GW, Kopf M. B1 and marginal zone B cells but not follicular B2 cells require Gpx4 to prevent lipid peroxidation and ferroptosis. Cell Rep 2019;29:2731–44. Available from: https://doi.org/10.1016/j.celrep.2019.10.070 e2734.

[221] Mambetsariev N, Lin WW, Wallis AM, Stunz LL, Bishop GA. TRAF3 deficiency promotes metabolic reprogramming in B cells. Sci Rep 2016;6:35349. Available from: https://doi.org/10.1038/srep35349.

[222] Jellusova J, et al. Gsk3 is a metabolic checkpoint regulator in B cells. Nat Immunol 2017;18:303–12. Available from: https://doi.org/10.1038/ni.3664.

[223] Jiang S, Yan W, Wang SE, Baltimore D. Let-7 suppresses B cell activation through restricting the availability of necessary nutrients. Cell Metab 2018;27:393–403. Available from: https://doi.org/10.1016/j.cmet.2017.12.007 e394.

[224] Doughty CA, et al. Antigen receptor-mediated changes in glucose metabolism in B lymphocytes: role of phosphatidylinositol 3-kinase signaling in the glycolytic control of growth. Blood 2006;107:4458–65. Available from: https://doi.org/10.1182/blood-2005-12-4788.

[225] Dufort FJ, et al. Cutting edge: IL-4-mediated protection of primary B lymphocytes from apoptosis via Stat6-dependent regulation of glycolytic metabolism. J Immunol 2007;179:4953–7. Available from: https://doi.org/10.4049/jimmunol.179.8.4953.

[226] Patke A, Mecklenbrauker I, Erdjument-Bromage H, Tempst P, Tarakhovsky A. BAFF controls B cell metabolic fitness through a PKC beta- and Akt-dependent mechanism. J Exp Med 2006;203:2551–62. Available from: https://doi.org/10.1084/jem.20060990.

[227] Dufort FJ, et al. Glucose-dependent de novo lipogenesis in B lymphocytes: a requirement for atp-citrate lyase in lipopolysaccharide-induced differentiation. J Biol Chem 2014;289:7011–24. Available from: https://doi.org/10.1074/jbc.M114.551051.

[228] Waters LR, Ahsan FM, Wolf DM, Shirihai O, Teitell MA. Initial B Cell Activation Induces Metabolic Reprogramming and Mitochondrial Remodeling. iScience 2018;5:99–109. Available from: https://doi.org/10.1016/j.isci.2018.07.005.

[229] Tsui C, et al. Protein kinase C-beta dictates B cell fate by regulating mitochondrial remodeling, metabolic reprogramming, and heme biosynthesis. Immunity 2018;48:1144–59. Available from: https://doi.org/10.1016/j.immuni.2018.04.031 e1145.

[230] Akkaya M, et al. Second signals rescue B cells from activation-induced mitochondrial dysfunction and death. Nat Immunol 2018;19:871–84. Available from: https://doi.org/10.1038/s41590-018-0156-5.

[231] Cho SH, et al. Germinal centre hypoxia and regulation of antibody qualities by a hypoxia response system. Nature 2016;537:234–8. Available from: https://doi.org/10.1038/nature19334.

[232] Chen D, et al. Coupled analysis of transcriptome and BCR mutations reveals role of OXPHOS in affinity maturation. Nat Immunol 2021;22:904–13. Available from: https://doi.org/10.1038/s41590-021-00936-y.

[233] Lam WY, Bhattacharya D. Metabolic links between plasma cell survival, secretion, and stress. Trends Immunol 2018;39:19–27. Available from: https://doi.org/10.1016/j.it.2017.08.007.

[234] Lam WY, et al. Mitochondrial pyruvate import promotes long-term survival of antibody-secreting plasma cells. Immunity 2016;45:60–73. Available from: https://doi.org/10.1016/j.immuni.2016.06.011.

[235] Lam WY, et al. Metabolic and transcriptional modules independently diversify plasma cell lifespan and function. Cell Rep 2018;24:2479–92. Available from: https://doi.org/10.1016/j.celrep.2018.07.084 e2476.

[236] Brookens SK, et al. Plasma cell differentiation, antibody quality, and initial germinal center B cell population depend on glucose influx rate. J Immunol 2024;212:43–56. Available from: https://doi.org/10.4049/jimmunol.2200756.

[237] Bierling TEH, et al. GLUT1-mediated glucose import in B cells is critical for anaplerotic balance and humoral immunity. Cell Rep 2024;43113739. Available from: https://doi.org/10.1016/j.celrep.2024.113739.

[238] Barwick BG, Scharer CD, Bally APR, Boss JM. Plasma cell differentiation is coupled to division-dependent DNA hypomethylation and gene regulation. Nat Immunol 2016;17:1216–25. Available from: https://doi.org/10.1038/ni.3519.

[239] Price MJ, Patterson DG, Scharer CD, Boss JM. Progressive upregulation of oxidative metabolism facilitates plasmablast differentiation to a T-independent antigen. Cell Rep 2018;23:3152–9. Available from: https://doi.org/10.1016/j.celrep.2018.05.053.

[240] Sharma R, et al. Distinct metabolic requirements regulate B cell activation and germinal center responses. Nat Immunol 2023;24:1358–69. Available from: https://doi.org/10.1038/s41590-023-01540-y.

[241] Weisel FJ, et al. Germinal center B cells selectively oxidize fatty acids for energy while conducting minimal glycolysis. Nat Immunol 2020;21:331–42. Available from: https://doi.org/10.1038/s41590-020-0598-4.

[242] Oestreich KJ, et al. Bcl-6 directly represses the gene program of the glycolysis pathway. Nat Immunol 2014;15:957–64. Available from: https://doi.org/10.1038/ni.2985.

[243] Saxton RA, Sabatini DM. mTOR signaling in growth, metabolism, and disease. Cell 2017;169:361–71. Available from: https://doi.org/10.1016/j.cell.2017.03.035.

[244] Iwata TN, Ramirez-Komo JA, Park H, Iritani BM. Control of B lymphocyte development and functions by the mTOR signaling pathways. Cytokine Growth Factor Rev 2017;35:47–62. Available from: https://doi.org/10.1016/j.cytogfr.2017.04.005.

[245] Keating R, et al. The kinase mTOR modulates the antibody response to provide cross-protective immunity to lethal infection with influenza virus. Nat Immunol 2013;14:1266–76. Available from: https://doi.org/10.1038/ni.2741.

[246] Jones DD, et al. mTOR has distinct functions in generating versus sustaining humoral immunity. J Clin Invest 2016;126:4250–61. Available from: https://doi.org/10.1172/JCI86504.

CHAPTER 9

Regulation of cytokine secretion by immunometabolites

Alexander Hooftman
Swiss Federal Institute of Technology Lausanne (EPFL), Global Health Institute, Lausanne, Switzerland

A summary of the cytokines mentioned in this chapter and their regulation by immunometabolites is given in Table 9.1. These effects will be discussed in more detail in subsequent sections.

IL-1β

IL-1β, part of the IL-1 family of cytokines, was first cloned by Charles Dinarello and colleagues in 1977 [1]. It is a proinflammatory, fever-inducing (pyrogenic) cytokine, produced predominantly by innate immune cells, which exists as a larger (31 kDa) intracellular pro-form and a smaller (17 kDa) secreted active form. The existence of these two forms of IL-1β requires that the release of active, cleaved IL-1β is a two-step process. While pro-IL-1β transcription is induced by PRR ligation and NF-κB signaling (signal 1), its subsequent processing and release is executed by caspase-1, a protein that forms part of an intracellular multiprotein complex named the inflammasome [2]. The fact that multiple levels of regulation exist for IL-1β has facilitated the development of novel therapeutics targeting various stages of IL-1β transcription, release, and signaling. The inflammasome in particular has been the subject of intense research, as its hyperactivation has been implicated in numerous inflammatory disorders [3].

While its multiple layers of regulation make IL-1β an attractive therapeutic target, it also makes it susceptible to endogenous regulation by immunometabolites, as summarized in Fig. 9.1. Succinate, one of the earliest examples of a signaling immunometabolite, can regulate IL-1β release through several mechanisms. The LPS-induced accumulation of succinate leads to stabilization of the IL-1β-promoting transcription factor HIF-1α [4]; [5]. This effect is dependent on succinate's role as an inhibitor of the PHD enzymes [6], which can therefore be overcome by treatment with the PHD substrate metabolite α-KG. The induction of IL-1β may also be dependent on the activity of SDH, which can generate high

Table 9.1: Regulation of cytokine secretion by immunometabolites.

Cytokine	Metabolite	Increase/Decrease	Cell type impacted	Target
IL-1β	L-2-HG	Increase	Macrophage	HIF-1α
	D-2-HG	Decrease	Macrophage	N/A
	Fumarate	Decrease	Macrophage	GAPDH, GSDMD
	Itaconate	Decrease	Macrophage	SDH, NRF2, GAPDH, ALDOA, NLRP3, GSDMD
	KYNA	Decrease	Macrophage	GPR35
	Succinate	Increase	Macrophage	HIF-1α, GPR91
TNF-α	Fumarate	Increase	Monocyte/macrophage	KDM5, c-Fos
	Lactoylglutathione	Increase	Macrophage	Histone lactoylation
IL-6	Fumarate	Increase	Monocyte	KDM5
	Itaconate	Decrease	Macrophage	ATF3, TET2
	KYNA	Increase	Cancer cell	AHR
	Lactoylglutathione	Increase	Macrophage	Histone lactoylation
Type I IFN	Cholesterol	Decrease	Macrophage	STING
	Itaconate	Increase	Macrophage	SDH
	Lactate	Decrease	Liver epithelial cells	MAVS
	Fumarate	Increase	Kidney epithelial cells	cGAS-STING
IFN-γ/IL-2	D-2-HG	Decrease	T cell	LDH
	L-2-HG	Increase	T cell	HIF-1α
	L-arginine	Increase	T cell	BAZ1B, PSIP1, TSN
	Fumarate	Decrease	T cell	ZAP70
	Itaconate	Decrease	T cell	Reduced aspartate, serine, glycine
	Lactate	Decrease	T cell, NK cell	NFAT
	Methionine	Increase	T cell	Histone methylation
	Methylglyoxal	Decrease	T cell	N/A
IL-17	2-HG	Decrease	T cell	FOXP3
	Itaconate	Decrease	T cell	RORγt

levels of mitochondrial ROS through reverse electron transport (RET), also leading to HIF-1α stabilization [7]. Alternatively, the role of succinate in promoting IL-1β release may be mediated by paracrine signaling through activation of GPR91 [8]; [9].

The accumulation of succinate in inflammatory macrophages is inextricably linked to the accumulation of a more recently defined immunometabolite, itaconate. Itaconate, as an inhibitor of SDH [10]; [11], can contribute to the accumulation of succinate by blocking its conversion to fumarate. While some of the aforementioned effects resulting from succinate accumulation may therefore be indirectly attributable to itaconate, itaconate can regulate IL-1β release by various means in addition to its role as an SDH inhibitor. In contrast to

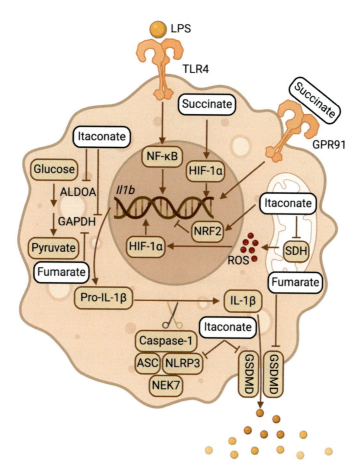

Figure 9.1: Regulation of IL-1β release by immunometabolites.
Succinate promotes expression of *Il1b* through activation of HIF-1α or ligation of cell-surface GPR91. Itaconate suppresses SDH activity, thereby reducing ROS generation, HIF-1α activation, and *Il1b* induction. It can also activate NRF2, driving transcriptional suppression of *Il1b*, or inactivate the glycolytic enzymes ALDOA and GAPDH, thereby suppressing the glycolytic shift and associated *Il1b* induction. Itaconate may also inhibit the processing of pro-IL-1β into mature IL-1β by inactivating the inflammasome proteins NLRP3 or GSDMD. The inactivation of GAPDH and GSDMD is a property that is shared with fumarate. *Created with Biorender.com.*

succinate, itaconate possesses a reactive carbon–carbon double bond which renders it an electrophile, allowing it to modify and inactivate target proteins. Inactivation of one such protein, KEAP1, liberates the antiinflammatory transcription factor NRF2 [12], which suppresses IL-1β transcription, either by promoting an antioxidant transcriptional response or by suppressing RNA Pol II recruitment to the IL-1β promoter [13]. The metabolic shift away from oxidative metabolism toward glycolysis is a hallmark of signal 1 and is required to support the transcriptional upregulation of pro-IL-1β. The activities of glycolytic enzymes such as GAPDH and aldolase A (ALDOA) are necessary for this shift to occur yet also possess cysteines that may be modified by electrophiles such as itaconate. Indeed, modification of specific cysteines in GAPDH [14] and ALDOA [15] by itaconate blocks the activity of these enzymes, resulting in a reduced glycolytic shift and reduced IL-1β expression. The nature of itaconate as an electrophile also has consequences for inflammasome activation, the second signal required for mature IL-1β release. The NLRP3 inflammasome, the best characterized and most widely studied of the inflammasomes, is composed of several proteins that are susceptible to modification by electrophiles such as itaconate. Modification of NLRP3 [16], as well as the pyroptosis executioner gasdermin D [17], has been demonstrated, resulting in reduced IL-1β release and pyroptosis. Conversely, macrophages that lack IRG1 and the capacity to synthesize endogenous itaconate exhibit heightened inflammasome activation and IL-1β release [17]; [16].

The modification of gasdermin D is a property that is shared by fumarate, a structurally similar metabolite that functions as an intermediate in the Krebs cycle. Again, both exogenous delivery of a fumarate derivative and the endogenous augmentation of fumarate levels using an inhibitor of fumarate hydratase blocked NLRP3 inflammasome activation and IL-1β release in macrophages [18]. This is not the only immunomodulatory mechanism shared by fumarate and itaconate, as fumarate has been shown to exert similar inhibition of GAPDH activity, glycolysis, and pro-IL-1β induction [19]. While the mechanisms of inhibition are broadly conserved between itaconate and fumarate, the respective papers did find that the modified cysteines were not conserved between the two metabolites, with itaconate modifying C77 on gasdermin D [17] and C22 on GAPDH [14], while fumarate was found to modify C192 on gasdermin D [18] and C150 on GAPDH [19].

The tryptophan catabolic pathway, which generates the metabolites kynurenine (L-KYN) and kynurenic acid (KYNA), has also been implicated in the regulation of NLRP3. These findings were framed in the context of a social stress-exacerbated colitis model, where chronic social defeat stress (CSDS) in mice worsened colonic inflammation. This phenomenon mimics the scenario in humans, as psychological stress is known to increase susceptibility to and relapse of colitis. In mice, this was found to be dependent on the colonic accumulation of KYNA, which activated GPR35 to drive autophagic degradation of NLRP3 in macrophages [20]. Since NLRP3 inflammasome activation is protective in colitis models [21], reduced NLRP3 levels led to an increased susceptibility to colonic injury.

2-Hydroxyglutarate (2-HG) is a dicarboxylic acid that is structurally similar to α-KG. 2-HG exists as two enantiomeric forms that exert markedly contrasting effects on inflammatory macrophages. Both enantiomers accumulate upon LPS stimulation of TLR4, with D-2-HG being the predominant enantiomer under these conditions [22]; [23]. While L-2-HG was found to support the glycolytic shift, HIF-1α stabilization, and associated IL-1β expression [23], D-2-HG was found to suppress IL-1β release along with multiple other inflammatory cytokines through an as yet unidentified mechanism which is independent of PHDs and HIF-1α [22]. The divergent effects of L-2-HG and D-2-HG highlight the sensitivity and specificity which exists in the metabolic regulation of cytokine responses.

TNF-α and IL-6

TNF-α and IL-6 are proinflammatory cytokines that contribute important roles to the innate immune response. Their roles are highly multifunctional and are reviewed elsewhere [24]; [25]. As an indication of their importance, the targeting of IL-6 and TNF-α has yielded several effective therapies for the treatment of autoimmune diseases, including siltuximab (anti-IL-6), tocilizumab (anti-IL-6R), infliximab (anti-TNF), and etanercept (soluble TNF receptor).

Cytokine expression in activated immune cells is supported by epigenetic changes, in addition to conventional signaling events that occur immediately downstream of ligand binding to PRRs. Epigenetic remodeling also plays an important role in models of trained immunity, whereby cells exhibit heightened cytokine responses to successive exposures to the same PAMP [26]. These epigenetic changes are believed to be supported by the glycolytic shift and, more specifically, an accumulation of fumarate [27]; [28]. By reducing the activity of the histone demethylase KDM5, fumarate can promote levels of the activating histone mark H3K4me3 at the promoters of TNF and IL-6, thereby increasing TNF-α and IL-6 release upon LPS restimulation [27]. As well as indirectly affecting the epigenetic landscape through modulation of epigenetic writers and erasers such as KDM5, specific immunometabolites may also directly modify histones. Examples of this are histone lactylation by lactate, which promotes homeostatic gene expression in M1 macrophages [29], and histone lactoylation by lactoylglutathione, which promotes TNF-a and IL-6 release from M1 macrophages [30].

A role for fumarate in boosting conventional TNF-α release has also been described, involving the antiinflammatory cytokine IL-10. Fumarate was found to suppress activity of c-Fos, a member of the AP-1 transcription factor complex, leading to a reduction in IL-10 release, which, given its role as an immunosuppressive cytokine that restrains the production of TNF-α, led to a concomitant increase in TNF-α release [31].

An important distinction exists in the regulation of TNF-α and IL-6, as TNF-α is generally considered to be a primary response gene following LPS stimulation, while IL-6 is a secondary response gene. The basis of this distinction is that TNF-α upregulation occurs directly downstream of LPS signaling and is driven by class I transcription factors such as NF-κB, while the upregulation of IL-6 occurs later and requires the expression of additional class II transcription factors [32]. IκBζ is an example of a class II transcription factor which regulates LPS-induced IL-6 production [33], the activation of which may be inhibited by electrophiles, such as itaconate, in a mechanism dependent on ATF3 [34]. While endogenous itaconate, a weak electrophile, exhibited modest inhibition of IκBζ and IL-6 release, treatment of macrophages with more electrophilic itaconate derivatives caused more profound inhibition [34]. The same compounds did not affect LPS-induced TNF-α release, indicating that itaconate selectively inhibits secondary, but not primary, transcriptional responses to LPS. An alternative mechanism was later proposed for the itaconate-mediated suppression of IL-6 involving the DNA dioxygenase TET2, the activity of which is suppressed by itaconate treatment, leading to reduced expression of *Nfkbiz* (the gene encoding IκBζ) and reduced expression of IL-6 and other secondary transcriptional genes [35]. Thus DNA modifications as well as histone modifications may be remodeled by immunometabolites.

The upregulation and release of IL-6 by inflammatory stimuli can be augmented by activation of the aryl hydrocarbon receptor (AHR) [36], a transcription factor which can be activated by the binding of a wide variety of exogenous and endogenous ligands. AHR activation was initially associated with the transcriptional upregulation of genes involved in xenobiotic metabolism, but its range of targets was later expanded to also include immunoregulatory effects, including the induction of IL-6. KYNA was discovered to be a potent endogenous ligand of AHR in cancer cells, linking tryptophan metabolism to xenobiotic metabolism [37]. The relationship between AHR and tryptophan metabolism appears to be bidirectional, as AHR activation can drive tryptophan catabolism in dendritic cells through the upregulation of the catabolic enzyme indoleamine 2,3-dioxygenase (IDO). Accumulation of the resulting product L-KYN in dendritic cells skewed T cell differentiation away from Th17 cells towards T_{reg} cells [38].

Type I interferons

Type I IFNs are a family of proinflammatory cytokines that play a major role in antiviral immunity. In humans, 13 functional IFN genes exist as part of the type I IFN family, encoding IFN-α and IFN-β among other type I IFN proteins. All type I IFNs signal through the IFN-α receptor (IFNAR), subsequently driving JAK/STAT signaling and culminating in the transcriptional activation of interferon-stimulated genes (ISGs), which have a wide range of antiviral functions. On the one hand, type I IFNs are critical for antiviral defense, yet their aberrant release contributes to the pathogenesis of certain autoimmune diseases including both heterogenous diseases, such as systemic lupus erythematosus (SLE), and monogenic diseases driven by activating mutations in signaling adaptor proteins, such as STING-associated vasculopathy with onset in infancy (SAVI). The upregulation and release of type I IFNs can be initiated by cell surface PRR sensing of extracellular pathogens, as well as the sensing of host-derived danger signals by intracellular PRRs. cGAS, RIG-I, and MDA5 are intracellular sensors of nucleic acids, which may be derived from host mitochondria, ensuring a means by which metabolic health can be communicated as an inflammatory readout. We will now outline the main mechanisms by which type I IFN is regulated by specific immunometabolites. These are also displayed in Fig. 9.2.

Numerous triggers have been described for the release of mitochondrial nucleic acids, most of which are associated with mitochondrial dysfunction and impaired mitophagy. While these mechanisms are comprehensively reviewed elsewhere [39], we will highlight some recent studies implicating specific metabolic signaling events in the generation of mitochondrial nucleic acids. Excessive cholesterol accumulation in macrophages, as a result of altered lipid metabolism, can lead to a suppression in mitochondrial respiration and the release of mitochondrial DNA into the cytosol, which subsequently drives AIM2 inflammasome activation [40]. Cholesterol synthesis was also shown to regulate interferon signaling, as suppressing the cholesterol biosynthesis pathway could spontaneously drive cGAS-STING-dependent type I IFN expression [41]. There is also evidence that perturbation of central carbon metabolic pathways can lead to the release of mitochondrial nucleic acids. Fumarate hydratase (FH), the enzyme that converts fumarate to malate in the Krebs cycle, is suppressed in activated macrophages. This process, coupled with increased bioenergetic stress and mitochondrial membrane potential, results in the release of immunostimulatory mitochondrial RNA (mtRNA) from these dysfunctional mitochondria. Extramitochondrial RNA resulting from FH loss subsequently drives a RIG-I/MDA5-dependent IFN response. Suppressed *FH* expression was also reported in cells isolated from the whole blood of SLE patients, indicating that the loss of FH may contribute to the IFN signature observed in these patients [31]. A separate publication found that the loss of FH in kidney epithelial cells drives the fumarate-dependent release of mtDNA-containing mitochondria-derived vesicles, leading to a cGAS-STING-dependent IFN response. Tumor tissue samples isolated from patients with *FH*-deficient renal cancer, termed hereditary leiomyomatosis and renal cell carcinoma (HLRCC), were found to exhibit increased expression of interferon-stimulated genes (ISGs) [42]. These two papers provide fascinating evidence of the importance of FH loss in the context of autoimmune disease and cancer, respectively, and the role of fumarate as a signaling immunometabolite that may boost type I IFN responses.

The evidence concerning the role of itaconate in regulating IFN responses is slightly less clear-cut. Initial studies, which used the itaconate derivative 4-octyl itaconate (4-OI) as a tool compound to model the effects of itaconate, found 4-OI to suppress type I IFN responses [12]; [43]. Various mechanisms have been proposed for this effect, including NRF2 activation [44] and the suppression of STING [45]; [46]. These effects were not fully verified in $Irg1^{-/-}$ macrophages, and it has been reported that unmodified itaconate in fact exerts the opposite effect by increasing the release of IFN-β from LPS-stimulated macrophages [47]. This was recently shown to be dependent on the inhibition of SDH and

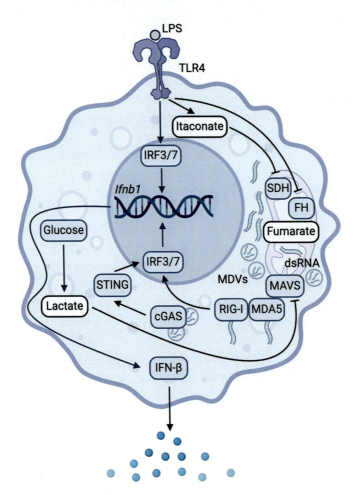

Figure 9.2: Regulation of type I IFN release by immunometabolites.
LPS signaling through TLR4 drives FH suppression and fumarate accumulation, leading to the release of mitochondrial dsRNA and mitochondrial DNA enclosed within MDVs, which, respectively, bind and activate the RIG-I/MDA5 and cGAS-STING signaling pathways, culminating in the transcriptional upregulation of *Ifnb1*. The release of mitochondrial dsRNA may also be triggered by the LPS-driven accumulation of itaconate, which does so by inhibiting SDH. Lactate, derived from glycolysis, binds and inactivates MAVS, thereby suppressing RIG-I/MDA5-driven *Ifnb1* induction. Itaconate can augment LPS-induced *Ifnb1* induction through an as yet unidentified mechanism. *dsRNA*, Double-stranded RNA; *FH*, fumarate hydratase; *IFN*, type I Iinterferon; *MDVs*, mitochondria-derived vesicles. *Created with Biorender.com.*

resultant release of mtRNA [48], similar to the phenotype observed upon FH inhibition. The discrepancy between the study of unmodified itaconate and the use of itaconate derivatives such as 4-OI perhaps owes itself to a difference in ability to modify cysteine residues, which is heightened for derivatives such as 4-OI (Hooftman & O'Neill, 2019).

In contrast to what is observed during early-phase (4 hours) TCA cycle rewiring following LPS stimulation, where an accumulation of specific TCA cycle intermediates can be observed coupled with an increase in glycolysis, the activation of the RIG-I-like receptors (RLRs) by transfection with poly (I:C) in HEK293 cells leads to an initial downregulation of glucose metabolism [49]. It is thought that the suppression of glycolysis licenses RLR activation by restricting the accumulation of the glycolytic end-product lactate. Lactate was found to interact with the RLR signaling adaptor protein MAVS, inhibiting its oligomerization and mitochondrial localization, where it usually interacts with RIG-I [49]. MAVS activity has been implicated in SLE, where an oligomerization-deficient mutant of MAVS is associated with milder disease activity [50]. Therefore the discovery that MAVS is susceptible to metabolic regulation might inform the design of novel therapeutics for this disease.

T cell cytokines

The majority of studies investigating the immunometabolic regulation of T cells have framed their findings in the context of the tumor microenvironment. In general, immunometabolites in this compartment can be derived from three possible cell types: from T cells themselves, from cancer cells, or from myeloid cells.

T cell-derived metabolites

Activated T cells have a large appetite for the amino acid L-arginine, which is rapidly metabolized to support their survival and various antitumor functions, including the release of the cytokine IFN-γ [51]. However, the availability of arginine in the tumor microenvironment may be limited by competition from tumor cells, which also consume large amounts of arginine, as well as the expression of arginases by tumor-infiltrating dendritic cells and macrophages [52]; [53]. The amino acid methionine is similarly limited in the tumor microenvironment, where it is consumed by tumor cells expressing high levels of the methionine transporter SLC43A2. This limits the amount of methionine available for T cell consumption, where it fuels the epigenetic changes required to support T cell survival and cytokine release [54]; [55].

The two enantiomers of 2-HG, previously described herein for their contrasting effects on macrophage cytokine release, also exhibit differing roles in the context of cancer. L-2-HG (also known as S-2-HG) predominantly accumulates in $CD8^+$ T cells [56], while D-2-HG (also known as *R*-2-HG) accumulates in cancer cells exhibiting mutations in IDH1/2 [57] (see subsequent section). As in macrophages, the accumulation of L-2-HG following T cell receptor (TCR) triggering in T cells is associated with a hypoxic response and the activation of HIF-1α, resulting in epigenetic changes that support T cell activation, including the release of the T cell activation cytokine IL-2 [56]. The accumulation of 2-HG may also be important in regulating T cell fate determination between T_H17 and induced T_{reg} cells. Using a pharmacological inhibitor called aminooxyacetic acid (AOA) to suppress GOT1 activity and 2-HG accumulation, the authors could link 2-HG accumulation to hypermethylation and increased expression of the *Foxp3* locus. This resulted in a balance shift away from T_H17 toward iT_{reg} differentiation [58]. However, these findings were disputed by a separate publication that used a genetic model of GOT1 depletion [59].

Tumor cell—derived metabolites

Mutations in key metabolic enzymes, such as IDH1/2, FH, and SDH, are associated with particular subsets of cancers, providing clinical evidence of how tumor cell metabolism can be rewired to support malignancy. The metabolites that arise from these mutations, so-called oncometabolites, can exert both intra- and intercellular roles in the tumor microenvironment. Mutation of IDH1 occurs in more than 70% of glioma cases, while many of the remaining cases have mutations in IDH2 [60]. The accumulation of D-2-HG, which reaches concentrations of up to ∼30 mM in the tumor microenvironment as a result of these mutations, drives the epigenetic changes that characterize the glioma phenotype [61]; [62]. Its extracellular accumulation means that it can also be taken up by $CD8^+$ T cells in the tumor microenvironment, where it inhibits effector functions, including the release of IFN-γ, in a mechanism dependent on inactivation of lactate dehydrogenase [63].

It is well-established that cancer cells rewire their glucose metabolism towards aerobic glycolysis in a metabolic switch termed the "Warburg Effect" [64]. The Warburg Effect creates a tumor microenvironment which is hypoxic, low-glucose, and high-lactate, an environment which impacts upon the functionality of the various infiltrating immune cell subsets. Lactate functions as an oncometabolite in this environment. It polarizes macrophages toward a tumor-associated M2 phenotype [65], inhibits NK cell function, supports the generation of myeloid-derived suppressor cells (MDSCs) [66], suppresses $CD8^+$ T cell activation and cytokine release [67], and supports survival and PD-1 expression on regulatory T cells (T_{reg} cells) [68]; [69].

Heterozygous germline mutations in FH predispose to HLRCC, and the loss of heterozygosity over time can lead to the development of a range of cancers which fall under this collective name, including a highly aggressive renal cell carcinoma. The loss of FH leads to a buildup of the oncometabolite fumarate. Fumarate, due to its structural similarity to α-KG, competitively inhibits the α-KG-dependent PHD enzymes [70], which hydroxylate the HIFs. Inhibition of the PHDs leads to stabilization of HIF-1α, which initiates a pro-tumorigenic transcriptional program in tumor cells. Fumarate can also function intercellularly, as its uptake from the tumor microenvironment can suppress $CD8^+$ T cell activation, TNF-α release, and IFN-γ release. This occurs through modification and inactivation of ZAP70, a kinase which functions in TCR signaling [71].

Myeloid cell–derived metabolites

The production of D-2-HG, lactate, and fumarate from tumor cells highlights the role that metabolites can play as oncogenic signaling molecules. Myeloid cells can also alter the metabolic makeup of the microenvironment through the secretion of immunometabolites, including itaconate and methylglyoxal.

Given the extent of its upregulation in activated myeloid cells, the release of itaconate into the tumor microenvironment by MDSCs is not entirely surprising. While $CD8^+$ T cells do not synthesize endogenous itaconate, they do take up secreted itaconate from the surrounding environment. The uptake of itaconate by $CD8^+$ T cells is thought to suppress their activation and the release of proinflammatory cytokines, including IFN-γ, TNF-α, and IL-2, thereby impairing their antitumor activity [72]. The recent characterisation of SLC13A3 as the transporter of itaconate has led to further discoveries concerning the role of itaconate in impairing antitumor immunity. SLC13A3 transports itaconate into tumor cells, where it protects these cells against an inflammatory form of cell death termed ferroptosis [73]. Itaconate was also shown to modify and stabilise PD-L1 expression on tumor cells, thereby also impairing antitumor immune responses [74]. These studies have highlighted SLC13A3 as a potential target for cancer immunotherapy. Itaconate was also shown to modulate T cell function in the context of autoimmunity, where it inhibited the differentiation of Th17 cells and the associated production of IL-17A. This was coupled with an increase in T_{reg} cell differentiation [75]. Therefore the role of itaconate as an immunometabolite is no longer confined to innate immune cells.

In contrast to the extracellular transfer of itaconate from MDSCs to T cells, the dicarbonyl radical methylglyoxal is transferred through direct cell-cell contact. Human MDSCs were found to be metabolically suppressed when compared to conventional monocytes and were able to transfer this metabolic paralysis to $CD8^+$ T cells through the cell–cell transfer of methylglyoxal. Neutralization of the glycation activity of methylglyoxal, in conjunction with checkpoint inhibition, was able to restore $CD8^+$ T cell function, in the form of IFN-γ and TNF-α production, thereby rescuing antitumor immunity. This work provides a first report of the emerging role of methylglyoxal as an immunometabolite [76].

Concluding remarks

The various ways in which immunometabolites regulate cytokine expression and release that have been described here will soon be added to, particularly with the use of more complex model systems, such as coculture and in vivo disease models, to capture novel metabolic signaling pathways. Some of the more intriguing recent findings describe roles for metabolites in intercellular communication, including the presence of fumarate, itaconate, and lactate, among others, in the tumor microenvironment, where they may be taken up by cancer cells or invading T cells. These reports also highlight the potential of delivering exogenous metabolites into diseased tissue as a means of treatment, which, given the various cytokine-remodeling effects that we have described here, might one day prove to be of great therapeutic benefit.

References

[1] Dinarello CA, Renfer L, Wolff SM. Human leukocytic pyrogen: Purification and development of a radioimmunoassay. Proceedings of the National Academy of Sciences of the United States of America 1977;74(10):4624–7. Available from: https://doi.org/10.1073/pnas.74.10.4624.

[2] Martinon F, Burns K, Tschopp J. The inflammasome: A molecular platform triggering activation of inflammatory caspases and processing of proIL-beta. Molecular Cell 2002;10(2):417–26. Available from: https://doi.org/10.1016/s1097-2765(02)00599-3.

[3] Mangan MSJ, Olhava EJ, Roush WR, Seidel HM, Glick GD, Latz E. Targeting the NLRP3 inflammasome in inflammatory diseases. Nature Reviews Drug Discovery 2018;17(8):588–606. Available from: https://doi.org/10.1038/nrd.2018.97.

[4] Palsson-McDermott EM, Curtis AM, Goel G, Lauterbach MAR, Sheedy FJ, Gleeson LE, van den Bosch MWM, Quinn SR, Domingo-Fernandez R, Johnston DGW, Jiang J, Israelsen WJ, Keane J, Thomas C, Clish C, Vander Heiden M, Xavier RJ, O'Neill LAJ. Pyruvate Kinase M2 Regulates Hif-1α Activity and IL-1β Induction and Is a Critical Determinant of the Warburg Effect in LPS-Activated Macrophages. Cell Metabolism 2015;21(1):65–80. Available from: https://doi.org/10.1016/j.cmet.2014.12.005.

[5] Tannahill GM, Curtis AM, Adamik J, Palsson-McDermott EM, McGettrick AF, Goel G, Frezza C, Bernard NJ, Kelly B, Foley NH, Zheng L, Gardet A, Tong Z, Jany SS, Corr SC, Haneklaus M, Caffrey BE, Pierce K, Walmsley S, et al. Succinate is an inflammatory signal that induces IL-1β through HIF-1α. Nature 2013;496(7444):238–42. Available from: https://doi.org/10.1038/nature11986.

[6] Selak MA, Armour SM, MacKenzie ED, Boulahbel H, Watson DG, Mansfield KD, Pan Y, Simon MC, Thompson CB, Gottlieb E. Succinate links TCA cycle dysfunction to oncogenesis by inhibiting HIF-α prolyl hydroxylase. Cancer Cell 2005;7(1):77–85. Available from: https://doi.org/10.1016/j.ccr.2004.11.022.

[7] Mills EL, Kelly B, Logan A, Costa ASH, Varma M, Bryant CE, Tourlomousis P, Däbritz JHM, Gottlieb E, Latorre I, Corr SC, McManus G, Ryan D, Jacobs HT, Szibor M, Xavier RJ, Braun T, Frezza C, Murphy MP, O'Neill LA. Succinate Dehydrogenase Supports Metabolic Repurposing of Mitochondria to Drive Inflammatory Macrophages. Cell 2016;167(2):457–470.e13. Available from: https://doi.org/10.1016/j.cell.2016.08.064.

[8] Littlewood-Evans A, Sarret S, Apfel V, Loesle P, Dawson J, Zhang J, Muller A, Tigani B, Kneuer R, Patel S, Valeaux S, Gommermann N, Rubic-Schneider T, Junt T, Carballido JM. GPR91 senses extracellular succinate released from inflammatory macrophages and exacerbates rheumatoid arthritis. Journal of Experimental Medicine 2016;213(9):1655–62. Available from: https://doi.org/10.1084/jem.20160061.

[9] Rubic T, Lametschwandtner G, Jost S, Hinteregger S, Kund J, Carballido-Perrig N, Schwärzler C, Junt T, Voshol H, Meingassner JG, Mao X, Werner G, Rot A, Carballido JM. Triggering the succinate receptor GPR91 on dendritic cells enhances immunity. Nature Immunology 2008;9(11):1261−9. Available from: https://doi.org/10.1038/ni.1657.

[10] Cordes T, Wallace M, Michelucci A, Divakaruni AS, Sapcariu SC, Sousa C, Koseki H, Cabrales P, Murphy AN, Hiller K, Metallo CM. Immunoresponsive Gene 1 and Itaconate Inhibit Succinate Dehydrogenase to Modulate Intracellular Succinate Levels. Journal of Biological Chemistry 2016;291 (27):14274−84. Available from: https://doi.org/10.1074/jbc.M115.685792.

[11] Lampropoulou V, Sergushichev A, Bambouskova M, Nair S, Vincent EE, Loginicheva E, Cervantes-Barragan L, Ma X, Huang SC-C, Griss T, Weinheimer CJ, Khader S, Randolph GJ, Pearce EJ, Jones RG, Diwan A, Diamond MS, Artyomov MN. Itaconate Links Inhibition of Succinate Dehydrogenase with Macrophage Metabolic Remodeling and Regulation of Inflammation. Cell Metabolism 2016;24 (1):158−66. Available from: https://doi.org/10.1016/j.cmet.2016.06.004.

[12] Mills EL, Ryan DG, Prag HA, Dikovskaya D, Menon D, Zaslona Z, Jedrychowski MP, Costa ASH, Higgins M, Hams E, Szpyt J, Runtsch MC, King MS, McGouran JF, Fischer R, Kessler BM, McGettrick AF, Hughes MM, Carroll RG, et al. Itaconate is an anti-inflammatory metabolite that activates Nrf2 via alkylation of KEAP1. Nature 2018;556(7699):113−17. Available from: https://doi.org/10.1038/nature25986.

[13] Kobayashi EH, Suzuki T, Funayama R, Nagashima T, Hayashi M, Sekine H, Tanaka N, Moriguchi T, Motohashi H, Nakayama K, Yamamoto M. Nrf2 suppresses macrophage inflammatory response by blocking proinflammatory cytokine transcription. Nature Communications 2016;7(1):11624. Available from: https://doi.org/10.1038/ncomms11624.

[14] Liao S-T, Han C, Xu D-Q, Fu X-W, Wang J-S, Kong L-Y. 4-Octyl itaconate inhibits aerobic glycolysis by targeting GAPDH to exert anti-inflammatory effects. Nature Communications 2019;10(1):5091. Available from: https://doi.org/10.1038/s41467-019-13078-5.

[15] Qin W, Qin K, Zhang Y, Jia W, Chen Y, Cheng B, Peng L, Chen N, Liu Y, Zhou W, Wang Y-L, Chen X, Wang C. S-glycosylation-based cysteine profiling reveals regulation of glycolysis by itaconate. Nature Chemical Biology 2019;15(10):983−91. Available from: https://doi.org/10.1038/s41589-019-0323-5.

[16] Hooftman A, Angiari S, Hester S, Corcoran SE, Runtsch MC, Ling C, Ruzek MC, Slivka PF, McGettrick AF, Banahan K, Hughes MM, Irvine AD, Fischer R, O'Neill LAJ. The Immunomodulatory Metabolite Itaconate Modifies NLRP3 and Inhibits Inflammasome Activation. Cell Metabolism 2020;32(3):468−478. e7. Available from: https://doi.org/10.1016/j.cmet.2020.07.016.

[17] Bambouskova M, Potuckova L, Paulenda T, Kerndl M, Mogilenko DA, Lizotte K, Swain A, Hayes S, Sheldon RD, Kim H, Kapadnis U, Ellis AE, Isaguirre C, Burdess S, Laha A, Amarasinghe GK, Chubukov V, Roddy TP, Diamond MS, et al. Itaconate confers tolerance to late NLRP3 inflammasome activation. Cell Reports 2021;34(10):108756. Available from: https://doi.org/10.1016/j.celrep.2021.108756.

[18] Humphries F, Shmuel-Galia L, Ketelut-Carneiro N, Li S, Wang B, Nemmara VV, Wilson R, Jiang Z, Khalighinejad F, Muneeruddin K, Shaffer SA, Dutta R, Ionete C, Pesiridis S, Yang S, Thompson PR, Fitzgerald KA. Succination inactivates gasdermin D and blocks pyroptosis. Science 2020;369 (6511):1633−7. Available from: https://doi.org/10.1126/science.abb9818.

[19] Kornberg MD, Bhargava P, Kim PM, Putluri V, Snowman AM, Putluri N, Calabresi PA, Snyder SH. Dimethyl fumarate targets GAPDH and aerobic glycolysis to modulate immunity. Science 2018;360 (6387):449−53. Available from: https://doi.org/10.1126/science.aan4665.

[20] Zheng X, Hu M, Zang X, Fan Q, Liu Y, Che Y, Guan X, Hou Y, Wang G, Hao H. Kynurenic acid/ GPR35 axis restricts NLRP3 inflammasome activation and exacerbates colitis in mice with social stress. Brain, Behavior, and Immunity 2019;79:244−55. Available from: https://doi.org/10.1016/j.bbi.2019.02.009.

[21] Villani A-C, Lemire M, Fortin G, Louis E, Silverberg MS, Collette C, Baba N, Libioulle C, Belaiche J, Bitton A, Gaudet D, Cohen A, Langelier D, Fortin PR, Wither JE, Sarfati M, Rutgeerts P, Rioux JD, Vermeire S, et al. Common variants in the NLRP3 region contribute to Crohn's disease susceptibility. Nature Genetics 2009;41(1):71−6. Available from: https://doi.org/10.1038/ng.285.

[22] de Goede KE, Harber KJ, Gorki FS, Verberk SGS, Groh LA, Keuning ED, Struys EA, van Weeghel M, Haschemi A, de Winther MPJ, van Dierendonck XAMH, Van den Bossche J. D-2-Hydroxyglutarate is an anti-inflammatory immunometabolite that accumulates in macrophages after TLR4 activation. Biochimica et Biophysica Acta (BBA) - Molecular Basis of Disease 2022;1868(9):166427. Available from: https://doi.org/10.1016/j.bbadis.2022.166427.

[23] Williams NC, Ryan DG, Costa ASH, Mills EL, Jedrychowski MP, Cloonan SM, Frezza C, O'Neill LA. Signaling metabolite L-2-hydroxyglutarate activates the transcription factor HIF-1α in lipopolysaccharide-activated macrophages. Journal of Biological Chemistry 2022;298(2):101501. Available from: https://doi.org/10.1016/j.jbc.2021.101501.

[24] Choy EH, De Benedetti F, Takeuchi T, Hashizume M, John MR, Kishimoto T. Translating IL-6 biology into effective treatments. Nature Reviews Rheumatology 2020;16(6):335−45. Available from: https://doi.org/10.1038/s41584-020-0419-z.

[25] van Loo G, Bertrand MJM. Death by TNF: a road to inflammation. Nature Reviews Immunology 2023;23(5):289−303. Available from: https://doi.org/10.1038/s41577-022-00792-3.

[26] Netea MG, Domínguez-Andrés J, Barreiro LB, Chavakis T, Divangahi M, Fuchs E, Joosten LAB, van der Meer JWM, Mhlanga MM, Mulder WJM, Riksen NP, Schlitzer A, Schultze JL, Stabell Benn C, Sun JC, Xavier RJ, Latz E. Defining trained immunity and its role in health and disease. Nature Reviews Immunology 2020;20(6):375−88. Available from: https://doi.org/10.1038/s41577-020-0285-6.

[27] Arts RJW, Novakovic B, ter Horst R, Carvalho A, Bekkering S, Lachmandas E, Rodrigues F, Silvestre R, Cheng S-C, Wang S-Y, Habibi E, Gonçalves LG, Mesquita I, Cunha C, van Laarhoven A, van de Veerdonk FL, Williams DL, van der Meer JWM, Logie C, et al. Glutaminolysis and Fumarate Accumulation Integrate Immunometabolic and Epigenetic Programs in Trained Immunity. Cell Metabolism 2016;24(6):807−19. Available from: https://doi.org/10.1016/j.cmet.2016.10.008.

[28] Cheng S-C, Quintin J, Cramer RA, Shepardson KM, Saeed S, Kumar V, Giamarellos-Bourboulis EJ, Martens JHA, Rao NA, Aghajanirefah A, Manjeri GR, Li Y, Ifrim DC, Arts RJW, van der Veer BMJW, Deen PMT, Logie C, O'Neill LA, Willems P, et al. mTOR- and HIF-1α−mediated aerobic glycolysis as metabolic basis for trained immunity. Science 2014;345(6204):1250684. Available from: https://doi.org/10.1126/science.1250684.

[29] Zhang D, Tang Z, Huang H, Zhou G, Cui C, Weng Y, Liu W, Kim S, Lee S, Perez-Neut M, Ding J, Czyz D, Hu R, Ye Z, He M, Zheng YG, Shuman HA, Dai L, Ren B, et al. Metabolic regulation of gene expression by histone lactylation. Nature 2019;574(7779):575−80. Available from: https://doi.org/10.1038/s41586-019-1678-1.

[30] Trujillo MN, Jennings EQ, Hoffman EA, Zhang H, Phoebe AM, Mastin GE, Kitamura N, Reisz JA, Megill E, Kantner D, Marcinkiewicz MM, Twardy SM, Lebario F, Chapman E, McCullough RL, D'Alessandro A, Snyder NW, Cusanovich DA, Galligan JJ. Lactoylglutathione promotes inflammatory signaling in macrophages through histone lactoylation. Molecular Metabolism 2024;81101888. Available from: https://doi.org/10.1016/j.molmet.2024.101888.

[31] Hooftman A, Peace CG, Ryan DG, Day EA, Yang M, McGettrick AF, Yin M, Montano EN, Huo L, Toller-Kawahisa JE, Zecchini V, Ryan TAJ, Bolado-Carrancio A, Casey AM, Prag HA, Costa ASH, De Los Santos G, Ishimori M, Wallace DJ, et al. Macrophage fumarate hydratase restrains mtRNA-mediated interferon production. Nature 2023;615(7952):490−8. Available from: https://doi.org/10.1038/s41586-023-05720-6.

[32] Medzhitov R, Horng T. Transcriptional control of the inflammatory response. Nature Reviews Immunology 2009;9(10):692−703. Available from: https://doi.org/10.1038/nri2634.

[33] Yamamoto M, Yamazaki S, Uematsu S, Sato S, Hemmi H, Hoshino K, Kaisho T, Kuwata H, Takeuchi O, Takeshige K, Saitoh T, Yamaoka S, Yamamoto N, Yamamoto S, Muta T, Takeda K, Akira S. Regulation of Toll/IL-1-receptor-mediated gene expression by the inducible nuclear protein IκBζ. Nature 2004;430(6996):218−22. Available from: https://doi.org/10.1038/nature02738.

[34] Bambouskova M, Gorvel L, Lampropoulou V, Sergushichev A, Loginicheva E, Johnson K, Korenfeld D, Mathyer ME, Kim H, Huang L-H, Duncan D, Bregman H, Keskin A, Santeford A, Apte RS, Sehgal R,

Johnson B, Amarasinghe GK, Soares MP, et al. Electrophilic properties of itaconate and derivatives regulate the IκBζ–ATF3 inflammatory axis. Nature 2018;556(7702):501–4. Available from: https://doi.org/10.1038/s41586-018-0052-z.

[35] Chen L-L, Morcelle C, Cheng Z-L, Chen X, Xu Y, Gao Y, Song J, Li Z, Smith MD, Shi M, Zhu Y, Zhou N, Cheng M, He C, Liu K, Lu G, Zhang L, Zhang C, Zhang J, et al. Itaconate inhibits TET DNA dioxygenases to dampen inflammatory responses. Nature Cell Biology 2022;24(3):353–63. Available from: https://doi.org/10.1038/s41556-022-00853-8.

[36] Hollingshead BD, Beischlag TV, DiNatale BC, Ramadoss P, Perdew GH. Inflammatory Signaling and Aryl Hydrocarbon Receptor Mediate Synergistic Induction of Interleukin 6 in MCF-7 Cells. Cancer Research 2008;68(10):3609–17. Available from: https://doi.org/10.1158/0008-5472.CAN-07-6168.

[37] DiNatale BC, Murray IA, Schroeder JC, Flaveny CA, Lahoti TS, Laurenzana EM, Omiecinski CJ, Perdew GH. Kynurenic Acid Is a Potent Endogenous Aryl Hydrocarbon Receptor Ligand that Synergistically Induces Interleukin-6 in the Presence of Inflammatory Signaling. Toxicological Sciences 2010;115(1):89–97. Available from: https://doi.org/10.1093/toxsci/kfq024.

[38] Nguyen NT, Kimura A, Nakahama T, Chinen I, Masuda K, Nohara K, Fujii-Kuriyama Y, Kishimoto T. Aryl hydrocarbon receptor negatively regulates dendritic cell immunogenicity via a kynurenine-dependent mechanism. Proceedings of the National Academy of Sciences 2010;107(46):19961–6. Available from: https://doi.org/10.1073/pnas.1014465107.

[39] Newman LE, Shadel GS. Mitochondrial DNA Release in Innate Immune Signaling. Annual Review of Biochemistry 2023;Vol. 92:299–332. Available from: https://doi.org/10.1146/annurev-biochem-032620-104401 Annual Reviews.

[40] Dang EV, McDonald JG, Russell DW, Cyster JG. Oxysterol Restraint of Cholesterol Synthesis Prevents AIM2 Inflammasome Activation. Cell 2017;171(5):1057–1071.e11. Available from: https://doi.org/10.1016/j.cell.2017.09.029.

[41] York AG, Williams KJ, Argus JP, Zhou QD, Brar G, Vergnes L, Gray EE, Zhen A, Wu NC, Yamada DH, Cunningham CR, Tarling EJ, Wilks MQ, Casero D, Gray DH, Yu AK, Wang ES, Brooks DG, Sun R, et al. Limiting Cholesterol Biosynthetic Flux Spontaneously Engages Type I IFN Signaling. Cell 2015;163(7):1716–29. Available from: https://doi.org/10.1016/j.cell.2015.11.045.

[42] Zecchini V, Paupe V, Herranz-Montoya I, Janssen J, Wortel IMN, Morris JL, Ferguson A, Chowdury SR, Segarra-Mondejar M, Costa ASH, Pereira GC, Tronci L, Young T, Nikitopoulou E, Yang M, Bihary D, Caicci F, Nagashima S, Speed A, et al. Fumarate induces vesicular release of mtDNA to drive innate immunity. Nature 2023;615(7952):499–506. Available from: https://doi.org/10.1038/s41586-023-05770-w.

[43] Olagnier D, Brandtoft AM, Gunderstofte C, Villadsen NL, Krapp C, Thielke AL, Laustsen A, Peri S, Hansen AL, Bonefeld L, Thyrsted J, Bruun V, Iversen MB, Lin L, Artegoitia VM, Su C, Yang L, Lin R, Balachandran S, et al. Nrf2 negatively regulates STING indicating a link between antiviral sensing and metabolic reprogramming. Nature Communications 2018;9(1):3506. Available from: https://doi.org/10.1038/s41467-018-05861-7.

[44] Ryan DG, Knatko EV, Casey AM, Hukelmann JL, Dayalan Naidu S, Brenes AJ, Ekkunagul T, Baker C, Higgins M, Tronci L, Nikitopolou E, Honda T, Hartley RC, O'Neill LAJ, Frezza C, Lamond AI, Abramov AY, Arthur JSC, Cantrell DA, et al. Nrf2 activation reprograms macrophage intermediary metabolism and suppresses the type I interferon response. iScience 2022;25(2):103827. Available from: https://doi.org/10.1016/j.isci.2022.103827.

[45] Li W, Li Y, Kang J, Jiang H, Gong W, Chen L, Wu C, Liu M, Wu X, Zhao Y, Ren J. 4-octyl itaconate as a metabolite derivative inhibits inflammation via alkylation of STING. Cell Reports 2023;42(3):112145. Available from: https://doi.org/10.1016/j.celrep.2023.112145.

[46] Su C, Cheng T, Huang J, Zhang T, Yin H. 4-Octyl itaconate restricts STING activation by blocking its palmitoylation. Cell Reports 2023;42(9):113040. Available from: https://doi.org/10.1016/j.celrep.2023.113040.

[47] Swain A, Bambouskova M, Kim H, Andhey PS, Duncan D, Auclair K, Chubukov V, Simons DM, Roddy TP, Stewart KM, Artyomov MN. Comparative evaluation of itaconate and its derivatives reveals

divergent inflammasome and type I interferon regulation in macrophages. Nature Metabolism 2020;2 (7):594–602. Available from: https://doi.org/10.1038/s42255-020-0210-0.

[48] O'Carroll SM, Peace CG, Toller-Kawahisa JE, Min Y, Hooftman A, Charki S, Kehoe L, O'Sullivan MJ, Zoller A, Mcgettrick AF, Zotta A, Day EA, Simarro M, Armstrong N, Annes JP, O'Neill LAJ. Itaconate drives mtRNA-mediated type I interferon production through inhibition of succinate dehydrogenase. Nature Metabolism 2024;6(11):2060–9. Available from: https://doi.org/10.1038/s42255-024-01145-1.

[49] Zhang W, Wang G, Xu Z-G, Tu H, Hu F, Dai J, Chang Y, Chen Y, Lu Y, Zeng H, Cai Z, Han F, Xu C, Jin G, Sun L, Pan B-S, Lai S-W, Hsu C-C, Xu J, et al. Lactate Is a Natural Suppressor of RLR Signaling by Targeting MAVS. Cell 2019;178(1):176–189.e15. Available from: https://doi.org/10.1016/j.cell.2019.05.003.

[50] Buskiewicz IA, Montgomery T, Yasewicz EC, Huber SA, Murphy MP, Hartley RC, Kelly R, Crow MK, Perl A, Budd RC, Koenig A. Reactive oxygen species induce virus-independent MAVS oligomerization in systemic lupus erythematosus. Science Signaling 2016;9(456). Available from: https://doi.org/10.1126/scisignal.aaf1933 ra115.

[51] Geiger R, Rieckmann JC, Wolf T, Basso C, Feng Y, Fuhrer T, Kogadeeva M, Picotti P, Meissner F, Mann M, Zamboni N, Sallusto F, Lanzavecchia A. L-Arginine Modulates T Cell Metabolism and Enhances Survival and Anti-tumor Activity. Cell 2016;167(3):829–842.e13. Available from: https://doi.org/10.1016/j.cell.2016.09.031.

[52] Norian LA, Rodriguez PC, O'Mara LA, Zabaleta J, Ochoa AC, Cella M, Allen PM. Tumor-Infiltrating Regulatory Dendritic Cells Inhibit CD8+ T Cell Function via l-Arginine Metabolism. Cancer Research 2009;69(7):3086–94. Available from: https://doi.org/10.1158/0008-5472.CAN-08-2826.

[53] Rodriguez PC, Quiceno DG, Zabaleta J, Ortiz B, Zea AH, Piazuelo MB, Delgado A, Correa P, Brayer J, Sotomayor EM, Antonia S, Ochoa JB, Ochoa AC. Arginase I Production in the Tumor Microenvironment by Mature Myeloid Cells Inhibits T-Cell Receptor Expression and Antigen-Specific T-Cell Responses. Cancer Research 2004;64(16):5839–49. Available from: https://doi.org/10.1158/0008-5472.CAN-04-0465.

[54] Bian Y, Li W, Kremer DM, Sajjakulnukit P, Li S, Crespo J, Nwosu ZC, Zhang L, Czerwonka A, Pawłowska A, Xia H, Li J, Liao P, Yu J, Vatan L, Szeliga W, Wei S, Grove S, Liu JR, et al. Cancer SLC43A2 alters T cell methionine metabolism and histone methylation. Nature 2020;585(7824):277–82. Available from: https://doi.org/10.1038/s41586-020-2682-1.

[55] Roy DG, Chen J, Mamane V, Ma EH, Muhire BM, Sheldon RD, Shorstova T, Koning R, Johnson RM, Esaulova E, Williams KS, Hayes S, Steadman M, Samborska B, Swain A, Daigneault A, Chubukov V, Roddy TP, Foulkes W, et al. Methionine Metabolism Shapes T Helper Cell Responses through Regulation of Epigenetic Reprogramming. Cell Metab 2020;31(2):250–266.e9. Available from: https://doi.org/10.1016/j.cmet.2020.01.006 PubMed.

[56] Tyrakis PA, Palazon A, Macias D, Lee Kian L, Phan Anthony T, Veliça P, You J, Chia GS, Sim J, Doedens A, Abelanet A, Evans CE, Griffiths JR, Poellinger L, Goldrath AW, Johnson RS. S-2-hydroxyglutarate regulates CD8+ T-lymphocyte fate. Nature 2016;540(7632):236–41. Available from: https://doi.org/10.1038/nature20165.

[57] Dang L, White DW, Gross S, Bennett BD, Bittinger MA, Driggers EM, Fantin VR, Jang HG, Jin S, Keenan MC, Marks KM, Prins RM, Ward PS, Yen KE, Liau LM, Rabinowitz JD, Cantley LC, Thompson CB, Vander Heiden MG, Su SM. Cancer-associated IDH1 mutations produce 2-hydroxyglutarate. Nature 2009;462(7274):739–44. Available from: https://doi.org/10.1038/nature08617.

[58] Xu T, Stewart KM, Wang X, Liu K, Xie M, Ryu JK, Li K, Ma T, Wang H, Ni L, Zhu S, Cao N, Zhu D, Zhang Y, Akassoglou K, Dong C, Driggers EM, Ding S. Metabolic control of TH17 and induced Treg cell balance by an epigenetic mechanism. Nature 2017;548(7666):228–33. Available from: https://doi.org/10.1038/nature23475.

[59] Xu W, Patel CH, Alt J, Zhao L, Sun I-H, Oh M-H, Sun I-M, Wen J, Blosser RL, Tam AJ, Powell JD. GOT1 constrains TH17 cell differentiation, while promoting iTreg cell differentiation. Nature 2023;614 (7946):E1–11. Available from: https://doi.org/10.1038/s41586-022-05602-3.

[60] Yan H, Parsons DWilliams, Jin Genglin, McLendon Roger, Rasheed BAhmed, Yuan Weishi, Kos Ivan, Batinic-Haberle Ines, Jones Siân, Riggins Gregory J, Friedman Henry, Friedman Allan, Reardon David, Herndon James, Kinzler Kenneth W, Velculescu Victor E, Vogelstein Bert, Bigner Darell D. IDH1 and IDH2 Mutations in Gliomas. New England Journal of Medicine 2009;360(8):765−73. Available from: https://doi.org/10.1056/NEJMoa0808710.

[61] Figueroa ME, Abdel-Wahab O, Lu C, Ward PS, Patel J, Shih A, Li Y, Bhagwat N, Vasanthakumar A, Fernandez HF, Tallman MS, Sun Z, Wolniak K, Peeters JK, Liu W, Choe SE, Fantin VR, Paietta E, Löwenberg B, et al. Leukemic IDH1 and IDH2 Mutations Result in a Hypermethylation Phenotype, Disrupt TET2 Function, and Impair Hematopoietic Differentiation. Cancer Cell 2010;18(6):553−67. Available from: https://doi.org/10.1016/j.ccr.2010.11.015.

[62] Turcan S, Rohle D, Goenka A, Walsh LA, Fang F, Yilmaz E, Campos C, Fabius AWM, Lu C, Ward PS, Thompson CB, Kaufman A, Guryanova O, Levine R, Heguy A, Viale A, Morris LGT, Huse JT, Mellinghoff IK, Chan TA. IDH1 mutation is sufficient to establish the glioma hypermethylator phenotype. Nature 2012;483(7390):479−83. Available from: https://doi.org/10.1038/nature10866.

[63] Notarangelo G, Spinelli JB, Perez EM, Baker GJ, Kurmi K, Elia I, Stopka SA, Baquer G, Lin J-R, Golby AJ, Joshi S, Baron HF, Drijvers JM, Georgiev P, Ringel AE, Zaganjor E, McBrayer SK, Sorger PK, Sharpe AH, et al. Oncometabolite d-2HG alters T cell metabolism to impair CD8+ T cell function. Science 2022;377(6614):1519−29. Available from: https://doi.org/10.1126/science.abj5104.

[64] Hanahan D, Weinberg RA. Hallmarks of Cancer: The Next Generation. Cell 2011;144(5):646−74. Available from: https://doi.org/10.1016/j.cell.2011.02.013.

[65] Colegio OR, Chu N-Q, Szabo AL, Chu T, Rhebergen AM, Jairam V, Cyrus N, Brokowski CE, Eisenbarth SC, Phillips GM, Cline GW, Phillips AJ, Medzhitov R. Functional polarization of tumour-associated macrophages by tumour-derived lactic acid. Nature 2014;513(7519):559−63. Available from: https://doi.org/10.1038/nature13490.

[66] Husain Z, Huang Y, Seth P, Sukhatme VP. Tumor-derived lactate modifies antitumor immune response: Effect on myeloid-derived suppressor cells and NK cells. J Immunol 2013;191(3):1486−95. Available from: https://doi.org/10.4049/jimmunol.1202702 PubMed.

[67] Brand A, Singer K, Koehl GE, Kolitzus M, Schoenhammer G, Thiel A, Matos C, Bruss C, Klobuch S, Peter K, Kastenberger M, Bogdan C, Schleicher U, Mackensen A, Ullrich E, Fichtner-Feigl S, Kesselring R, Mack M, Ritter U, et al. LDHA-Associated Lactic Acid Production Blunts Tumor Immunosurveillance by T and NK Cells. Cell Metabolism 2016;24(5):657−71. Available from: https://doi.org/10.1016/j.cmet.2016.08.011.

[68] Kumagai S, Koyama S, Itahashi K, Tanegashima T, Lin Y, Togashi Y, Kamada T, Irie T, Okumura G, Kono H, Ito D, Fujii R, Watanabe S, Sai A, Fukuoka S, Sugiyama E, Watanabe G, Owari T, Nishinakamura H, et al. Lactic acid promotes PD-1 expression in regulatory T cells in highly glycolytic tumor microenvironments. Cancer Cell 2022;40(2):201−218.e9. Available from: https://doi.org/10.1016/j.ccell.2022.01.001.

[69] Watson MJ, Vignali PDA, Mullett SJ, Overacre-Delgoffe AE, Peralta RM, Grebinoski S, Menk AV, Rittenhouse NL, DePeaux K, Whetstone RD, Vignali DAA, Hand TW, Poholek AC, Morrison BM, Rothstein JD, Wendell SG, Delgoffe GM. Metabolic support of tumour-infiltrating regulatory T cells by lactic acid. Nature 2021;591(7851):645−51. Available from: https://doi.org/10.1038/s41586-020-03045-2.

[70] Isaacs JS, Jung YJ, Mole DR, Lee S, Torres-Cabala C, Chung Y-L, Merino M, Trepel J, Zbar B, Toro J, Ratcliffe PJ, Linehan WM, Neckers L. HIF overexpression correlates with biallelic loss of fumarate hydratase in renal cancer: Novel role of fumarate in regulation of HIF stability. Cancer Cell 2005;8(2):143−53. Available from: https://doi.org/10.1016/j.ccr.2005.06.017.

[71] Cheng J, Yan J, Liu Y, Shi J, Wang H, Zhou H, Zhou Y, Zhang T, Zhao L, Meng X, Gong H, Zhang X, Zhu H, Jiang P. Cancer-cell-derived fumarate suppresses the anti-tumor capacity of CD8+ T cells in the tumor microenvironment. Cell Metabolism 2023;35(6):961−978.e10. Available from: https://doi.org/10.1016/j.cmet.2023.04.017.

[72] Zhao H, Teng D, Yang L, Xu X, Chen J, Jiang T, Feng AY, Zhang Y, Frederick DT, Gu L, Cai L, Asara JM, Pasca di Magliano M, Boland GM, Flaherty KT, Swanson KD, Liu D, Rabinowitz JD, Zheng B. Myeloid-derived itaconate suppresses cytotoxic CD8+ T cells and promotes tumour growth. Nature Metabolism 2022;4(12):1660−73. Available from: https://doi.org/10.1038/s42255-022-00676-9.
[73] Lin H, Tison K, Du Y, Kirchhoff P, Kim C, Wang W, Yang H, Pitter M, Yu J, Liao P, Zhou J, Vatan L, Grove S, Wei S, Vigil T, Shah YM, Mortensen R, Kryczek I, Garmire L, et al. Itaconate transporter SLC13A3 impairs tumor immunity via endowing ferroptosis resistance. Cancer Cell 2024;42(12):2032−2044.e6. Available from: https://doi.org/10.1016/j.ccell.2024.10.010.
[74] Fan Y, Dan W, Wang Y, Ma Z, Jian Y, Liu T, Li M, Wang Z, Wei Y, Liu B, Ding P, Lei Y, Guo C, Zeng J, Yan X, Wei W, Li L. Itaconate transporter SLC13A3 confers immunotherapy resistance via alkylation-mediated stabilization of PD-L1. Cell Metabolism 2025;. Available from: https://doi.org/10.1016/j.cmet.2024.11.012.
[75] Aso K, Kono M, Kanda M, Kudo Y, Sakiyama K, Hisada R, Karino K, Ueda Y, Nakazawa D, Fujieda Y, Kato M, Amengual O, Atsumi T. Itaconate ameliorates autoimmunity by modulating T cell imbalance via metabolic and epigenetic reprogramming. Nature Communications 2023;14(1):984. Available from: https://doi.org/10.1038/s41467-023-36594-x.
[76] Baumann T, Dunkel A, Schmid C, Schmitt S, Hiltensperger M, Lohr K, Laketa V, Donakonda S, Ahting U, Lorenz-Depiereux B, Heil JE, Schredelseker J, Simeoni L, Fecher C, Körber N, Bauer T, Hüser N, Hartmann D, Laschinger M, et al. Regulatory myeloid cells paralyze T cells through cell−cell transfer of the metabolite methylglyoxal. Nature Immunology 2020;21(5):555−66. Available from: https://doi.org/10.1038/s41590-020-0666-9.

CHAPTER 10

Omics metabolism tools in antiaging drug discovery

Rafael Tiburcio[1], Jay Rappaport[2,3] and Clovis Palmer[2,3]

[1]Division of Experimental Medicine, Department of Medicine, University of California, San Francisco, CA, United States, [2]Tulane National Primate Research Center, Covington, LA, United States, [3]Department of Microbiology and Immunology, Tulane University School of Medicine, New Orleans, LA, United States

Introduction

Recent technological advances in high-throughput methods, such as next-generation sequencing and mass spectrometry, have revolutionized biomedical research and significantly improved drug discovery efforts. These innovations, along with the development of sophisticated bioinformatic techniques for analyzing large multidimensional data, have provided comprehensive insights into complex disruptions in metabolic processes that underlie the development of comorbidities associated with infections as well as aging. These processes amenable to pharmacologic manipulation represent a new era of drug discovery. Artificial intelligence (AI)-driven target discovery platforms such as the genomic-based PandaOmics have been used to identify dual-purpose gerotherapeutic drug candidates that may also have anticancer benefits [1]. Conceptually, "omics" encompasses a collection of disciplines that uses high-throughput analysis of biomolecules, such as nucleic acids, proteins, and metabolites, to identify and interrogate biological processes associated with diseases [2,3]. The research fields associated with the study of these biomolecules mainly include genomics/transcriptomics, proteomics, and metabolomics (integrative omics), which have identified complex nuances in pathological processes, as well as identifying influential mechanistic pathway(s) that may be therapeutically targeted.

Immunometabolism has matured into an important interdisciplinary field that has transformed our understanding of how systemic and immune cell intrinsic metabolic processes regulate immunity and inflammatory-related diseases, including those driven by viral infections and aging [4]. Rapid advances in multiomic techniques such as spatial transcriptomics and metabolic-flow cytometry (MET-flow) have been used to identify targetable tissue-specific disease processes. Historically, "omics" has been broadly viewed from a technological vantage point (technology-based) that uses experimental tools such as genomics, transcriptomics, proteomics, and metabolomics to study biological systems. Now, knowledge-based omics describes the systematic integration of multiple omics data to understand how interacting processes regulate biological phenotypes. Hence, omics can provide a large-scale molecular perspective on human diseases and redundancies in druggable pathways. An important facet of omics is computational biology which supplies the tools and algorithms necessary for processing and gaining key mechanistic insights from omics data. In this chapter, we discuss how omics is being used to identify new drug targets primarily related to aging diseases and discuss empirical evidence that omics can inform a new era of gerotherapeutic unbiased drug discovery. Where applicable, we will also examine how viruses can disrupt metabolic processes relevant to long-term aging comorbidities.

Genomics in disease prognosis and personalized medicine

Genomic analysis is an important component of many drug discovery programs, including repurposing. Next-generation sequencing can integrate disease-associated genetic variants with clinical datasets to provide new insight into disease pathogenesis as well as guide drug discovery for complex immune and metabolic diseases associated with infections and aging. While selective pressure of the host immune system can affect viral evolution and resistance to antiviral therapy, such as in the case of HIV infection, genome-wide genotyping has identified variations in genes encoding chemokine receptors and human leukocyte antigen that are associated with HIV susceptibility and progression [5].

As well, systematic strategies have linked variations in genes that encode metabolic signaling proteins with complex age-related diseases such as rheumatoid arthritis (RA) [6]. Such genes are the target of many approved drugs, supporting a common strategy of repurposing drugs to treat many viral and age-related diseases. In fact, RA risk genes have been connected to several drug, including tofacitinib, a Janus kinase (JAK1,2,3) pathway inhibitor or "Jakinib," used for treating a plethora of inflammatory conditions, including moderate-to-severe rheumatoid arthritis. Interestingly, JAK1 is an important redox-sensitive target for the Krebs cycle-derived metabolite itaconate and its derivative 4-octyl-itaconate (4-OTC), which suppresses pro-inflammatory macrophage activation by inhibiting JAK1 activation and glycolytic remodeling [7]. 4-OTC also attenuates inflammatory processes in SARS-CoV-2 and influenza virus infections indicating how omics can be used to identify multipurpose drug targets [8,9].

Genome-wide association study (GWAS) metaanalysis studying millions of single nucleotide polymorphisms (SNPs) has also identified significant connections between RA risk SNPs and their associating pathways, including the peroxisome proliferator-activated receptor gamma (PPARγ) and FKBP1A which are targeted by sulfasalazine and tacrolimus, respectively [6]. PPARγ plays crucial roles in lipid and glucose metabolism and has been implicated in the pathology of numerous age-related diseases such as diabetes, obesity, and neurodegenerative conditions. FKBP1A is a mitochondrial-related gene that encodes the FK506-binding protein 1 A which can form a ternary complex with rapamycin to inhibit the mechanistic target of rapamycin (mTOR), an evolutionarily conserved serine/threonine-protein kinase that has spurred significant interest as a potential target for life extension [10–13].

These pharmacogenomics approaches foster the development of more targeted and safer therapies based on a person's genetic profiles to improve treatment outcomes. This was the case observed by leveraging GWAS metaanalysis of glucose measurements in individuals of diverse ancestries where analysis of glucagon-like peptide-1 receptor (GLP1R) coding variation confirms its role as a key blood glucose regulator and also shows that treatment responses to GLP1R-targeting type 2 diabetes drug such as semaglutide, tirzepatide, and exendin-4 may be influenced by genetic variations [14].

Transcriptomics and repurposing of drugs for antiaging effects

Transcriptomics is an important drug discovery tool transforming our understanding on the molecular mechanism associated with diseases. Knowledge can also be gained on how drugs regulate important biological networks to identify potential off-targets and predict side effects. Transcriptomics aids in drug target identification, identifying new diagnostic and prognostic markers, as well as uncovering novel mode of action for drugs.

Gene expression microarray and high-throughput bulk RNA sequencing have been widely adopted in the basic sciences, translational and clinical medicine, and the biopharmaceutical industry for drug discovery. The advent of single-cell RNA sequencing (scRNA-seq) makes it more feasible to study gene regulation in cellular heterogenous tissues to zoom in on the cell-specific regulation of genes within a complex cellular environment.

Cellular metabolism intrinsically regulates immune cell functions and inflammation. The TCA cycle enzyme cis-aconitate decarboxylase (ACOD1/IRG1) encoded by the Irg1 gene catalyzes the conversion of cis-aconitate into the antiinflammatory metabolite itaconate. Itaconate accumulates in activated macrophages exposed to inflammatory substances such as bacterial lipopolysaccharide (LPS), an immunoregulatory mechanism that limits prolonged and adverse inflammatory reactions [15]. Cholesterol-lowering drugs, including statins, have been the corner stone in the primary care of cardiovascular diseases (CVD) patients, or those at risk. At the cellular level, reprogramming of macrophage metabolism and elevated activation have been linked to increased CVD risk and disease [16,17]. Thus harnessing macrophage metabolism to subdue inflammation has gained significant traction as a genuine therapeutic promise to prevent and treat age-associated diseases such as atherosclerosis.

In fact, utilizing patient-matched scRNA-seq data and validatory immunostaining experiments showed Irg1 and ACOD1 to be enriched in monocytes and macrophages within atherosclerotic lesions and carotid plaque from human specimens. In diet-induced atherosclerosis in mice, Irg1 expression was high in early infiltrating monocytes and neutrophils in atherosclerosis lesions, but its levels decrease with advanced disease, suggesting deficiency of the inflammatory ACOD1-itaconate axis with disease advancement [18]. In validating a critical role of ACOD1 in CVD pathogenesis, supplementation with the itaconate-derivative 4-octyl itaconate (4-OI) had beneficial impact on atherosclerosis [18].

In a system-level drug repurposing approach, transcriptomics utilizing gene expression data from patients' brain was used to discover drugs that could combat neurological aging. The concept is to first identify a gene expression signature of aging brains and then identify drug targets using the Connectivity Map (CMap), a database of drug-regulated gene expression profiles. CMap has been used to identify drugs that regulate similar transcriptional profiles as those seen in caloric-restricted rats and rhesus macaques [19]. Caloric restriction entails reducing calorie intake without malnutrition, and CR mimetics are drugs that can provide the benefits of CR without dietary restrictions. One advantage of harnessing the transcriptome of specific tissue across the age span is to understand how organ-specific age-regulated genes may contribute to development of organ-specific age-related conditions such as Alzheimer's disease. Thus by identifying a robust human brain aging transcriptomic signature consisting of 100 upregulated (enriched in bone mineralization and cell proliferation processes) and 117 downregulated (enriched in synaptic and acyl-CoA biosynthetic processes) genes, and using CMap, it was possible to identify potential neuroprotective therapeutic candidates [20]. These include previously described potential pro-longevity drugs such as resveratrol, a sirtuin and PPARγ target, and an established mTOR inhibitor rapamycin, trichostatin A an antibiotic antifungal agent, levothyroxine sodium for hypothyroidism, and the heat shock protein 9 (HSP9) target geldanamycin. Newly proposed antiaging candidates included HSP9 inhibitors alvespimycin and tanespimycin, rifabutin, an antibiotic that also targets B-cell lymphoma 6 (BCL6), and quinostatin predicted to target the Phosphoinositide 3-kinase (PI3K) pathway [20]. On the other hand, the same transcriptomic analysis predicted the topoisomerase inhibitors camptothecin, irinotecan, and daunorubicin to have pro-aging effects.

Machine learning utilizing differentially expressed genes can also be used to identify drugs that can be repurposed or re-positioned to target aging diseases. The concept of CMap, for example, is where genes, drugs, and disease states are linked by virtue of common gene expression profiles. The rationale and advantage of this approach is that each drug regulates unique gene expressions, which can be matched against the gene expression profile of a specific disease. A limitation of this technique is the gene expression data that may not be available for the diseases or drug of interest. Moreover, the complexities of gene expression associated with a particular disease may not be replicated by a single drug. To help address this limitation, a two-step CMap strategy was used to identify multidrug combinations with potentially superior antiaging effects when drugs such as trichostatin A, vorinostat, or anisomycin typically used to treat fungal infection were paired with a secondary drug. These include the antidiabetic treatments metformin and glibenclamide, danazol used for treating endometriosis, the antiinflammatory metabolite ampyrone, and a muscle relaxant chlorzoxazone used to treat pain [21]. Intriguingly, danazol elongates telomere in human, and metformin improves mitochondrial functions and inhibits telomere attrition [22,23]. Although these drug combinations have not been validated for their antiaging effects, CMap-based machine learning holds promise for combinational drug repositioning for treating a cluster of age-related diseases.

Overlapping mechanisms between viral infection and aging

The realization that viral infections, including HIV and SARS-CoV-2, cause age-related complications, many relating to metabolic and neurocognitive dysfunctions [24–27] has prompted considerable interests in understanding the overlapping mechanisms associated with infections and aging. Indeed, the distortions of inflammatory, metabolic, and gut-related markers associated with these infections are shared with aging [28,29]. Differentially expressed genes between uninfected and SARS-CoV-2-infected lung cells and between young and old individuals were used to discover mechanisms that overlap SARS-CoV-2 host responses and aging [30] Gene ontology analysis showed that SARS-CoV-2-regulated genes are associated with type I interferon signaling, defense responses, and electron transport chain, while genes associated with tissue developmental processes and amino acid metabolic processes were highly regulated between young and old individuals [30]. Nevertheless, 219 were found to significantly intersect SARS-CoV-2 infection and aging. By utilizing a reverse disease gene signature and CMap analysis, FDA-approved drugs with potential anti-SARS-CoV-2 activities were uncovered, including the antihistamine clemastine, the antipsychotic drug, haloperidol, the anti-HCV medication ribavirin, the high blood pressure treatment quinapril, and niacin. By analyzing concordant regulating genes between SARS-CoV-2 infection and aging, serine/threonine and tyrosine kinase inhibitors such as dasatinib, imatinib, and sorafenib were identified as drugs that intersect SARS-CoV-2 and aging. Notably, the serine/threonine–protein kinase RIPK1 targeted by pazopanib and sunitinib, and implicated in tissue fibrosis, was highlighted as a master player in this SARS-CoV-2-aging interaction [30].

This computational approach also identified histone deacetylase (HDAC1) targets vorinostat and belinostat and the heat shock protein 90 (HSP90) targets formoterol and primaquine at the SARS-CoV-2-aging intersection. Collectively, this transcriptomic approach identified protein kinase inhibitors, as main targets that intersect SARS-CoV-2 infection and aging [30].

RIPK1 (serine kinase) has been highlighted as being upstream of the largest number of genes that were differentially expressed. Collectively, this combined analysis approach identifies protein kinase inhibitors such as RIPK1, a serine/threonine–protein kinase (sunitinib, pazopanib, axitinib), as one of the main targets against SARS-CoV-2 infections with a highly age-dependent role and the largest number of downstream differentially expressed genes in the combined SARS-CoV-2 and aging interactome [30].

Proteomics for senolytic biomarkers and drug discovery

Proteomics is important in both target identification and validation stages of drug discovery. During target identification, techniques like flow cytometry, CyTOF, and mass spectrometry are used to profile protein expression and interactions within biological systems, helping to identify potential therapeutic targets [31]. In the target validation stage, proteomics can provide confirmation that modifying the expression or activity of a specific protein can have potential favorable disease outcomes. Further downstream validation approaches include structural analysis and protein interactions and loss-of-function or gain-of-function through mutagenesis. This section shows how proteomic workflow is used to study signatures of senescence and aging and how they are exploited for translational senotherapeutics.

Senotherapeutics and aging

Advances in proteomic workflows involving mass spectrometry-based techniques have enabled comprehensive analysis of cellular proteins and their associations with diseases. It has been used to study the biology of aging, and in particular, the identification of senescence-associated proteins and their involvement in aging and robustly identify senescence-targeting therapies, or the catch-all term "senotherapeutics." Cellular senescence is a state of irreversible growth arrest often defined by the senescence-associated secretory phenotype (SASP), increased metabolic activity, resistance to apoptosis, and arrest of cell proliferation. Accumulation of senescent cell occurs in many age-related pathologies such as neurocognitive diseases and type 2 diabetes. Therefore the selective removal of senescent cells holds promise as a translatable antiaging strategy and improves health span. Interventions that disrupt upstream instigators of senescence, such as inflammation, oxidative stress, and metabolic imbalance, may confer senotherapeutic benefits. For example, the combination of dasatinib and quercetin has shown powerful senolytic effects in humans, nonhuman primates, and mice and significantly reduced SARS-CoV-2-related adverse symptoms and mortality in mice [32–37]. Another potent senolytic, fisetin, a flavonoid polyphenol, extended life in mice [38]. Other FDA-approved drugs, such as the metabolic-regulating drugs metformin and rapamycin, used to treat type 2 diabetes and cancer, also possess senolytic properties.

Characterization of senescence-associated secretory phenotype and senescence-associated proteins

SASP has gained considerable interest due to its causative links to aging, and its characterization has been leveraged to identify new biomarkers for senescence burden, targetable mechanisms, and tools to test the efficacy of senotherapeutic. The goal continues to be to understand the heterogenicity of SASP and other senescence-associated proteins which are governed by cell type, method of senescence induction, and duration of senescence. Proteomics has been vital in identifying SASP in circulating plasma and associating it with aging and age-related pathologies, as well as prognosing such diseases. Indeed, circulating plasma levels of the SASP factors differentiation factor 15 (GDF15) and ACTIVIN A were strongly associated with chronological age independent of BMI and sex and associated with frailty index [39]. Besides circulating SASP, senescence signatures in tissues and other biofluids overlap with known aging biomarkers and have been linked to age-related pathologies. Unbiased mass spectrometry has been used to broaden and refine our understanding of the heterogenicity of ASAP, which is dependent on the senescence-inducing signal and the cell type involved. In one experimental design, exposure of lung fibroblasts and renal cortical epithelial cells to X-irradiation (IR), or atazanavir (anti-HIV medication) significantly induced senescence which was verified by β-galactosidase (SA-β-Gal) activity, p16INK4a protein, and interleukin-6 (IL-6) transcript [40]. Core shared pathways associated with SASPs include those related to tissue structure and extracellular matrix organization, neurodegeneration, and growth and metabolism. The chemokine C-X-C motif ligand 1 (CXCL1), Matrix Metallopeptidase 1 (MMP1), and stanniocalcin 1 (STC1) were all induced by these stimuli, suggesting their potential as general SASP biomarkers to measure senescent cell burden to study the efficacy of senolytics, as well as potential peripheral blood biomarker for age-related conditions such as idiopathic pulmonary fibrosis [40–42]. On the other hand, assignment of SASP to a specific tissue, inducer, or disease conditions could identify biomarkers with a higher degree of selectivity for aging diseases and avenues for novel drug discovery and interventions.

High-throughput proteomic technologies for novel SASP and senescence-associated proteins

Senotherapeutic studies in humans using the combination of dasatinib and quercetin demonstrate compelling feasibility and tolerability. However, the reports of nonserious adverse events such as nausea and fatigue underscore the need for further refinement of antiaging approaches. Proteomics has been leveraged for development of new drugs, including senotherapeutics, and includes the identification of intracellular and cell surface proteins uniquely expressed by senescent cells, as well as proteomic profiling of proteins that interact with senolytic drug candidates [43]. One of the most prominent proteomic target discovery approaches has been the quantitative unbiased analysis by mass spectrometry. For example, limited proteolysis coupled to mass spectrometry (LiP-MS) compares peptide fragments between untreated and drug-treated complex samples such as cell lysates, where the peptide profile is governed by protein conformational changes that alter accessibility to a protein's cleavage sites based on drug–protein interactions [43]. Other approaches such as thermal denaturation-based target discovery, pulse proteolysis, and stability of proteins from rates of oxidation (SPROX) take advantage of increased stability of a cognate protein-drug interaction in complex supernatants, which is preserved from degrading conditions, and subsequent analysis of remaining proteins by untargeted mass spectrometry analysis [43].

Proteomics also comprises surfaceome analysis to study cell surface proteins, which classically involves immunophenotyping by flow cytometry. This can integrate intracellular protein analysis to study metabolic targets by metabolic-flow cytometry (MET-flow) [44,45].

Metabolomics and metabolite profiling

Metabolites are biochemical products of cell processes and comprise substrates, intermediates, and products of multifactorial biochemical reactions that are found intracellularly and in body fluids such as blood, cerebrospinal fluids, saliva, and urine. The composition of a metabolite profile is also influenced by the microbiome present in the gut, tissues, and saliva. Hence, metabolite concentrations and signatures provide invaluable insights into the physiological and pathological states of an organism, such as infections and aging [46]. Metabolites are highly variable molecules that include highly heterogeneous lipid (lipidomics) classes such as sphingolipids and glycerophospholipids implicated in aging diseases. Sphingolipids are a class of lipids known for their roles in cell membrane structure and signaling, while glycerophospholipids, including phosphatidylcholines (PCs) and lysophosphatidylcholines (LysoPCs), serve as essential components of cell membranes and play critical roles in lipid metabolism and cell signaling. Nonlipid metabolites, on the contrary, lack a lipid head and include amino acids and their metabolic intermediates of the urea cycle linked to neurocognitive decline [47].

Metabolites are essential for many physiological processes, including energy production, growth, and cellular maintenance. Consequently, comparative analysis of the metabolome has been harnessed for drug discovery and disease diagnosis and prognosis. By complementing genomics, transcriptomics, and proteomics, metabolomics may be used to validate disease mechanisms and drug discovery.

High-throughput metabolomic techniques such as Nuclear Magnetic Resonance (NMR), Liquid Chromatography-Mass Spectrometry (LC-MS), and Gas Chromatography-Mass Spectrometry (GC-MS) are used to profile the metabolome of body fluids to elucidate metabolic processes associated with diseases, to identify drug targets, and to monitor the efficacy of drugs [48]. Mass spectrometry-based metabolomics involves targeted or untargeted analysis. Targeted metabolomics provides higher sensitivity and selectivity than untargeted analysis, requires prior knowledge of the metabolites of interest, and is used to interrogate a specific hypothesis. In contrast, untargeted metabolomics requires no prior knowledge of the metabolites of interest and is a nonhypothesis-driven approach to gain knowledge on unknown phenomena [48].

A major challenge in metabolomics analysis is the handling of vast amount of complex data. To address this, statistical and bioinformatics software and AI are being used to assess data quality and generate logical biological information. An important analysis step in metabolomics involves data normalization, which reduces technical biases such as sample quantities, batch effects, and background noise to ensure accurate downstream statistical analysis such as principal component analysis (PCA) and hierarchical clustering, which are used to identify patterns and relationships between metabolites and the biological phenomenon in question [49].

Metabolites in aging diseases

Blood biomarkers seek to link signals in the blood to global pathological conditions such as frailty or certain pathologies affecting specific tissues such as the brain. In one example, scientists use brain autopsies and blood samples to investigate how the metabolite concentrations in brain tissue and blood of the elderly associates with specific endophenotypes of Alzheimer's disease (AD), and along the way discovered important metabolic pathways associated with the disease. Quantitative and targeted metabolomics on brain tissue identified a signature comprising 26 metabolites that discriminated between AD patients and controls. Analysis of these metabolites in patients' blood evaluated their associations with CSF biomarkers of AD, MRI measures, and found higher blood concentrations of sphingolipids subclass (sphingomyelin) associated with disease severity and progression. Indeed, clinically, a greater decline in cognition was associated with higher baseline blood levels of sphingolipids, and specifically higher baseline blood concentration of SM C18:1 and SM C26:1 prognosed greater declines in attention and language skills, respectively [50]. Likewise, higher blood concentrations of certain glycerophospholipids also predicted greater declines in attention and language, while greater declines in visuospatial ability were associated with lower blood concentration of the polyamine, spermidine. Intriguingly, blood concentrations of several sphingolipid species (e.g., SMC (OH) C14:1 and SM 16:0) have been shown to be significantly associated with the CSF AD endophenotypes t-tau (total tau), p-tau (tau phosphorylation), and amyloidβ1−42 (Aβ metabolism), as well as brain atrophy and cognitive decline [50,51].

In assessment of their prognostic values, higher blood levels of the sphingolipid, SM C18:1, were associated with a significantly greater risk of conversion to incident AD among individuals with mild cognitive impairment, as well as significantly associating with elevated risk of conversion to incident AD among cognitively normal individuals. On the contrary, plasma levels of certain sphingolipids, such as many containing long aliphatic chains, were significantly lower in AD compared to controls. Thus beyond expanding our insights into the mechanisms of AD, metabolomics opens new potential avenues for novel disease-modifying treatments for AD, as well as delaying the disease at the prodromal stage.

SMs are a subclass of sphingolipids highly enriched in the brain and regulate several pathological processes linked to AD endophenotype such as processing of the amyloid precursor protein.

In this regard, modulating networks associated with sphingolipid metabolism may be a plausible strategy for innovative drug discovery to delay or treat AD. It follows that sphingosine-1-phosphate (S1P)-metabolizing enzymes and S1P analogs may be pursued to target AD linked to Aβ-related pathology [50]. More broadly, an understanding of the interactions between metabolites through network analysis is critical to identify tangible drug targets. As such, the formation of ceramides from sphingomyelin via sphingomyelinase, and the interconnecting nodes that feed into the biosynthesis of phosphatidylcholines and LysoPCs through the Kennedy pathway and Land's cycle, respectively, also represent potential targets for drug discovery to treat AD [50].

Sphingomyelin is the most abundant membrane sphingolipids, which are structural components of cell membranes and important for membrane fluidity, homeostasis, and brain synaptic plasticity. Ceramide, which induce neuronal death, is a central product in the sphingolipid biosynthesis pathway and is also generated from the catabolism of sphingomyelin by sphingomyelinases. Therefore approaches to pharmacologically reduce ceramide represent a genuine therapeutic opportunity to combat neurological diseases. Subsequently, altered sphingolipid metabolism underpins AD pathogenesis, whereby increased sphingomyelinase and ceramide synthase activities in the brain of AD patients increase the production of the pro-apoptotic ceramide and reduce sphingomyelin and S1P levels in the brain [52]. Ceramides may have detrimental effects by promoting mitochondrial dysfunction by breaking down mitochondrial membrane potential and impairing oxidative phosphorylation [53]. The neurotoxic peptide Aβ can increase neutral sphingomyelinase activity and increase the conversion of sphingomyelin into ceramide. On the contrary, ceramide can itself provoke Aβ formation by affecting the cleavage of amyloid precursor protein or by affecting cytoskeletal integrity [53]. While it remains unclear whether increased ceramide is a triggering factor in AD pathophysiology or a consequence of Aβ accumulation, the consensus postulates a consequential link between sphingolipid metabolism, Aβ formation, and neurotoxicity. Moreover, as a prognostic tool, the specific species of sphingomyelin may be of greater value rather than generalization by class.

Targeting the sphingomyelin pathway in AD

Higher elevated ceramide concentrations in the brain have been postulated to drive Aβ formation, while increased levels of S1P provide neuroprotective signals and foster neurogenesis. Therefore therapeutic approaches to reduce ceramide levels through inhibition of de novo SL synthesis, as well as approaches to increase S1P signaling, are regarded as potential causative treatment and preventative treatments for AD. One known inhibitor of de novo SL synthesis is myriocin, a potent antibiotic derived from fungi. In rodents, myriocin inhibits serine palmitoyl transferase (SPT), the first enzyme for ceramide biosynthesis, reduces body weight, and improves insulin sensitivity and metabolic health [54,55].

While myriocin has not been approved for human use due to toxicity concerns, it is found abundantly in some fungal species such as Cordyceps consumed in traditional Chinese medicine to treat ailments such as diabetes. Moreover, in mice, commercially available Cordyceps extract approved for human consumption (4–6 nmol/g myriocin content) selectively inhibits synthesis of sphingolipids and its precursor ceramide, protects mice from diet-induced obesity, and attenuates metabolic impairments associated with obesity such as insulin resistance and hepatic steatosis [56].

Fingolimod is a S1P receptor modulator with potent immunosuppressive properties used to treat multiple sclerosis and repurposed for treating other neurodegenerative diseases in humans. Beyond regulating S1P receptor activity, in vitro studies show Fingolimod attenuates the production of Aβ peptide in cultured neuronal cells [57]. From a therapeutic standpoint, Fingolimod causes significant restored memory in AD rats suggesting new opportunities for AD management by modulating SL synthesis and signaling in the brain [58].

Bioinformatics: integrating omics data

High-throughput data integration is a crucial aspect of modern biomedical research, involving the amalgamation of data from various "Omics" sources to create a holistic view of a particular biological system under investigation [59]. Fig. 10.1 illustrates a comprehensive workflow for the utilization of omics data in drug discovery. This integration process can be achieved through knowledge-based methods or data-driven strategies. Knowledge-based approaches leverage existing biological knowledge and ontologies, such as gene ontology or KEGG pathways, to integrate and interpret data. These approaches rely on established biological frameworks and predefined relationships. Conversely, data-driven approaches can be categorized into step-wise and simultaneous integration. Step-wise integration involves merging different data types sequentially, such as first integrating genomic data and then incorporating transcriptomic data. Simultaneous

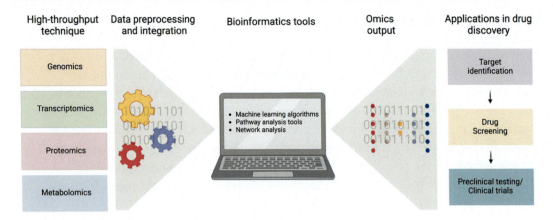

Figure 10.1: Comprehensive workflow integrating various omics techniques utilized in drug discovery.

Advancements in high-throughput techniques (e.g., genomics, transcriptomics, proteomics, and metabolomics) generate vast amounts of data that capture the biological complexity of organisms. By identifying differentially expressed genes, proteins, or metabolites, researchers can gain insights into the biological processes linked to specific conditions or treatments. To manage this data, various preprocessing and integration tools have been developed to standardize and clean it, ensuring statistical validity for analysis while minimizing noise and biases. Following preprocessing, bioinformatics approaches such as machine learning, pathway analysis, and network analysis reveal patterns and relationships within the data. Essentially, machine learning identifies predictive models, pathway analysis maps data onto known biological pathways, and network analysis clarifies interactions among biological components. Omics outputs, including gene sequences, expression levels, protein abundances, and metabolite profiles, provide a snapshot of a biological system molecular composition and activity. Collectively, these pieces of information contribute to target identification by revealing biomarkers and key regulatory proteins involved in disease pathways, allowing researchers to focus on the most promising therapeutic targets. In drug screening, omics data helps prioritize compounds based on their effects on specific targets, streamlining the identification of effective drug candidates. Integrating omics output into preclinical testing enhances the evaluation of drug candidates, leading to better predictions of their clinical performance and improving the efficiency of the drug development pipeline.

integration, on the other hand, involves the concurrent integration of multiple data layers, employing methods like canonical correlation analysis (CCA) or multiomics factor analysis (MOFA) to capture complex relationships between datasets [60].

Network analysis plays a significant role in understanding biological systems by examining relationships and interactions among various components, such as genes or proteins [61]. Techniques in network analysis include graph theory, which focuses on analyzing nodes (representing biological entities) and edges (representing interactions), and pathway analysis, which identifies and assesses key biological pathways and their alterations in disease states.

In the realm of machine learning and predictive modeling, several popular algorithms are used to analyze and interpret complex data. Supervised learning techniques, such as random forests and support vector machines (SVM), are employed for classification and regression tasks, allowing researchers to predict outcomes based on labeled data [62]. Neural networks, including deep learning models, are utilized for their ability to capture intricate patterns in large datasets [63]. Unsupervised learning methods, such as principal component analysis (PCA) and clustering algorithms like K-means, are used for dimensionality reduction and grouping similar data points without predefined labels. Ensemble methods, which combine multiple models to improve predictive performance, are also widely used, with gradient boosting being a prominent example [62].

Artificial intelligence (AI) is increasingly applied to predict drug efficacy, leveraging advanced algorithms and large datasets to forecast treatment responses [64]. Machine learning models analyze patient-specific data, such as genomic profiles, to predict how individuals will respond to different drugs. Deep learning techniques, including convolutional neural networks (CNNs), are utilized for their ability to process and interpret large-scale data, such as medical imaging [63]. Reinforcement learning, another AI approach, optimizes treatment strategies by learning from trial outcomes and adjusting recommendations accordingly. Additionally, AI-driven drug discovery platforms employ sophisticated algorithms to identify potential drug candidates and predict their efficacy, accelerating the drug development process and enhancing therapeutic outcomes [63].

Challenges and future directions

The field of omics and bioinformatics faces technical challenges such as managing data complexity and integration issues due to the vast and varied nature of datasets. Ethical considerations, particularly concerning data privacy and the responsible use of genetic information, are crucial for safeguarding individuals' rights. Looking ahead, the field is expected to focus on advancements in personalized medicine through multiomics integration, the enhancement of predictive modeling and drug discovery with AI, and innovations in real-time data analysis, all of which will drive future research and clinical applications.

Conclusion

The fusion of high-throughput technologies and advanced bioinformatics is transforming drug discovery and enabling innovative therapeutic strategies. The integration of various "omics" approaches helps researchers decode complex metabolic processes and their roles in infections and aging-related comorbidities. As immunometabolism advances, the use of multiomic technologies to identify more metabolic networks associated with diseases will be important to leverage such knowledge into drug development. By harnessing AI and multiomics analyzes, we are entering a promising era in drug development, with the potential to identify novel gerotherapeutic candidates. This chapter highlights these advancements and presents evidence supporting omics as a key driver of unbiased drug discovery, ultimately enhancing our capacity to identify safe and effective antiaging agents, combat age-related diseases and improve patient outcomes.

Acknowledgment

JR and CP were supported in part by P51OD011104-58 grant to the Tulane National Primate Research Center.

References

[1] Pun FW, Leung GHD, Leung HW, et al. A comprehensive AI-driven analysis of large-scale omic datasets reveals novel dual-purpose targets for the treatment of cancer and aging. Aging Cell 2023;22(12)e14017. Available from: https://doi.org/10.1111/acel.14017.

[2] Mogilenko DA, Sergushichev A, Artyomov MN. Systems immunology approaches to metabolism. Annu Rev Immunol 2023;41:317–42. Available from: https://doi.org/10.1146/annurev-immunol-101220-031513.

[3] Dai X, Shen L. Advances and trends in omics technology development. Front Med (Lausanne) 2022;9:911861. Available from: https://doi.org/10.3389/fmed.2022.911861. Published 2022 Jul 1.

[4] Palmer CS. Innate metabolic responses against viral infections. Nat Metab 2022;4(10):1245–59. Available from: https://doi.org/10.1038/s42255-022-00652-3.

[5] Tough RH, McLaren PJ. Interaction of the host and viral genome and their influence on HIV disease. Front Genet 2019;9:720. Available from: https://doi.org/10.3389/fgene.2018.00720. Published 2019 Jan 23.

[6] Okada Y, Wu D, Trynka G, et al. Genetics of rheumatoid arthritis contributes to biology and drug discovery. Nature 2014;506(7488):376–81. Available from: https://doi.org/10.1038/nature12873.

[7] Runtsch MC, Angiari S, Hooftman A, et al. Itaconate and itaconate derivatives target JAK1 to suppress alternative activation of macrophages. Cell Metab 2022;34(3):487–501.e8. Available from: https://doi.org/10.1016/j.cmet.2022.02.002.

[8] Ryan TAJ, Hooftman A, Rehill AM, et al. Dimethyl fumarate and 4-octyl itaconate are anticoagulants that suppress Tissue Factor in macrophages via inhibition of Type I Interferon. [published correction appears in Nat Commun. 2023 Jul 20;14(1):4374. doi: 10.1038/s41467-023-40034-1]. Nat Commun. 2023;14(1):3513. Available from: https://doi.org/10.1038/s41467-023-39174-1.

[9] Sohail A, Iqbal AA, Sahini N, et al. Itaconate and derivatives reduce interferon responses and inflammation in influenza A virus infection [published correction appears in PLoS Pathog. 2022 Nov 29;18(11):e1011002. doi: 10.1371/journal.ppat.1011002]. PLoS Pathog 2022;18(1)e1010219. Available from: https://doi.org/10.1371/journal.ppat.1010219.

[10] Dai J, Gao J, Dong H. Prognostic relevance and validation of ARPC1A in the progression of low-grade glioma. Aging (Albany NY) 2024;16(14):11162–84. Available from: https://doi.org/10.18632/aging.205952.

[11] Yang H, Rudge DG, Koos JD, Vaidialingam B, Yang HJ, Pavletich NP. mTOR kinase structure, mechanism and regulation. Nature 2013;497(7448):217–23. Available from: https://doi.org/10.1038/nature12122.

[12] Liu GY, Sabatini DM. mTOR at the nexus of nutrition, growth, ageing and disease [published correction appears in Nat Rev Mol Cell Biol. 2020 Apr;21(4):246. doi: 10.1038/s41580-020-0219-y]. Nat Rev Mol Cell Biol 2020;21(4):183–203. Available from: https://doi.org/10.1038/s41580-019-0199-y.

[13] Mannick JB, Lamming DW. Targeting the biology of aging with mTOR inhibitors Nat Aging 2023;3(6):642–60. Available from: https://doi.org/10.1038/s43587-023-00416-y.

[14] Lagou V, Jiang L, Ulrich A, et al. GWAS of random glucose in 476,326 individuals provide insights into diabetes pathophysiology, complications and treatment stratification. Nat Genet 2023;55(9):1448–61. Available from: https://doi.org/10.1038/s41588-023-01462-3.

[15] Mills EL, Ryan DG, Prag HA, et al. Itaconate is an anti-inflammatory metabolite that activates Nrf2 via alkylation of KEAP1. Nature 2018;556(7699):113–17. Available from: https://doi.org/10.1038/nature25986.

[16] Anzinger JJ, Butterfield TR, Angelovich TA, Crowe SM, Palmer CS. Monocytes as regulators of inflammation and HIV-related comorbidities during cART. J Immunol Res 2014;2014569819. Available from: https://doi.org/10.1155/2014/569819.

[17] Zhang X, Kapoor D, Jeong SJ, et al. Identification of a leucine-mediated threshold effect governing macrophage mTOR signalling and cardiovascular risk. Nat Metab 2024;6(2):359–77. Available from: https://doi.org/10.1038/s42255-024-00984-2.

[18] Cyr Y, Bozal FK, Barcia Durán JG, et al. The IRG1-itaconate axis protects from cholesterol-induced inflammation and atherosclerosis Proc Natl Acad Sci U S A 2024;121(15):e2400675121. Available from: https://doi.org/10.1073/pnas.2400675121 :e2400675121.

[19] Calvert S, Tacutu R, Sharifi S, Teixeira R, Ghosh P, de Magalhães JP. A network pharmacology approach reveals new candidate caloric restriction mimetics in C. elegans. Aging Cell 2016;15(2):256–66. Available from: https://doi.org/10.1111/acel.12432.

[20] Dönertaş HM, Fuentealba Valenzuela M, Partridge L, Thornton JM. Gene expression-based drug repurposing to target aging Aging Cell 2018;17(5):e12819. Available from: https://doi.org/10.1111/acel.12819.

[21] Kim SK, Goughnour PC, Lee EJ, et al. Identification of drug combinations on the basis of machine learning to maximize anti-aging effects. PLoS One 2021;16(1):e0246106. Available from: https://doi.org/10.1371/journal.pone.0246106. Published 2021 Jan 28.

[22] Townsley DM, Dumitriu B, Liu D, et al. Danazol treatment for telomere diseases. N Engl J Med 2016;374(20):1922–31. Available from: https://doi.org/10.1056/NEJMoa1515319.

[23] Kulkarni AS, Gubbi S, Barzilai N. Benefits of Metformin in Attenuating the Hallmarks of Aging. Cell Metab 2020;32(1):15–30. Available from: https://doi.org/10.1016/j.cmet.2020.04.001.

[24] Izadpanah A, Mudd JC, Garcia JGN, et al. SARS-CoV-2 infection dysregulates NAD metabolism. Front Immunol 2023;14:1158455. Available from: https://doi.org/10.3389/fimmu.2023.1158455.

[25] Palmer CS, Perdios C, Abdel-Mohsen M, et al. Non-human primate model of long-COVID identifies immune associates of hyperglycemia. Nat Commun 2024;15(1):6664. Available from: https://doi.org/10.1038/s41467-024-50339-4. Published 2024 Aug 20.

[26] Palmer CS, Henstridge DC, Yu D, et al. Emerging role and characterization of immunometabolism: relevance to HIV pathogenesis, serious non-AIDS events, and a cure. J Immunol 2016;196(11):4437–44. Available from: https://doi.org/10.4049/jimmunol.1600120.

[27] Yeoh HL, Cheng AC, Cherry CL, et al. Immunometabolic and lipidomic markers associated with the frailty index and quality of life in aging HIV + men on antiretroviral therapy. EBioMedicine 2017;22:112–21. Available from: https://doi.org/10.1016/j.ebiom.2017.07.015.

[28] Hearps AC, Maisa A, Cheng WJ, et al. HIV infection induces age-related changes to monocytes and innate immune activation in young men that persist despite combination antiretroviral therapy. AIDS 2012;26(7):843–53. Available from: https://doi.org/10.1097/QAD.0b013e328351f756.

[29] Giron LB, Dweep H, Yin X, et al. Plasma markers of disrupted gut permeability in severe COVID-19 patients [published correction appears in Front Immunol. 2021 Oct 04;12:779064. doi: 10.3389/fimmu.2021.779064]. Front Immunol 2021;12:686240. Available from: https://doi.org/10.3389/fimmu.2021.686240. Published 2021 Jun 9.

[30] Belyaeva A, Cammarata L, Radhakrishnan A, et al. Causal network models of SARS-CoV-2 expression and aging to identify candidates for drug repurposing. Nat Commun 2021;12(1):1024. Available from: https://doi.org/10.1038/s41467-021-21056-z. Published 2021 Feb 15.

[31] Yoshida M, Loo JA, Lepleya RA. Proteomics as a tool in the pharmaceutical drug design process. Curr Pharm Des 2001;7(4):291–310. Available from: https://doi.org/10.2174/1381612013398121.

[32] Hickson LJ, Langhi Prata LGP, Bobart SA, et al. Senolytics decrease senescent cells in humans: Preliminary report from a clinical trial of Dasatinib plus Quercetin in individuals with diabetic kidney disease [published correction appears in EBioMedicine. 2020 Feb;52:102595. doi: 10.1016/j.ebiom.2019.12.004]. EBioMedicine 2019;47:446–56. Available from: https://doi.org/10.1016/j.ebiom.2019.08.069.

[33] Ruggiero AD, Vemuri R, Blawas M, et al. Long-term dasatinib plus quercetin effects on aging outcomes and inflammation in nonhuman primates: implications for senolytic clinical trial design. Geroscience 2023;45(5):2785–803. Available from: https://doi.org/10.1007/s11357-023-00830-5.

[34] Islam MT, Tuday E, Allen S, et al. Senolytic drugs, dasatinib and quercetin, attenuate adipose tissue inflammation, and ameliorate metabolic function in old age. Aging Cell 2023;22(2):e13767. Available from: https://doi.org/10.1111/acel.13767.

[35] Xu M, Pirtskhalava T, Farr JN, et al. Senolytics improve physical function and increase lifespan in old age. Nat Med 2018;24(8):1246–56. Available from: https://doi.org/10.1038/s41591-018-0092-9.

[36] Novais EJ, Tran VA, Johnston SN, et al. Long-term treatment with senolytic drugs Dasatinib and Quercetin ameliorates age-dependent intervertebral disc degeneration in mice. Nat Commun. 2021;12(1):5213. Available from: https://doi.org/10.1038/s41467-021-25453-2. Published 2021 Sep 3.

[37] Pastor-Fernández A, Bertos AR, Sierra-Ramírez A, et al. Treatment with the senolytics dasatinib/quercetin reduces SARS-CoV-2-related mortality in mice. Aging Cell. 2023;22(3):e13771. Available from: https://doi.org/10.1111/acel.13771.

[38] Yousefzadeh MJ, Zhu Y, McGowan SJ, et al. Fisetin is a senotherapeutic that extends health and lifespan. EBioMedicine 2018;36:18–28. Available from: https://doi.org/10.1016/j.ebiom.2018.09.015.

[39] Schafer MJ, Zhang X, Kumar A, et al. The senescence-associated secretome as an indicator of age and medical risk. JCI Insight 2020;5(12):e133668. Available from: https://doi.org/10.1172/jci.insight.133668. Published 2020 Jun 18.

[40] Basisty N, Kale A, Jeon OH, et al. A proteomic atlas of senescence-associated secretomes for aging biomarker development. PLoS Biol 2020;18(1):e3000599. Available from: https://doi.org/10.1371/journal.pbio.3000599. Published 2020 Jan 16.

[41] Rosas IO, Richards TJ, Konishi K, et al. MMP1 and MMP7 as potential peripheral blood biomarkers in idiopathic pulmonary fibrosis. PLoS Med 2008;5(4):e93. Available from: https://doi.org/10.1371/journal.pmed.0050093.

[42] Ohkouchi S, Ono M, Kobayashi M, et al. Myriad functions of stanniocalcin-1 (STC1) cover multiple therapeutic targets in the complicated pathogenesis of idiopathic pulmonary fibrosis (IPF). Clin Med Insights Circ Respir Pulm Med 2015;9(Suppl 1):91–6. Available from: https://doi.org/10.4137/CCRPM.S23285. Published 2015 Dec 29.

[43] Dey AK, Banarjee R, Boroumand M, et al. Translating senotherapeutic interventions into the clinic with emerging proteomic technologies. Biol (Basel) 2023;12(10):1301. Available from: https://doi.org/10.3390/biology12101301. Published 2023 Oct 2.

[44] Palmer CS, Ostrowski M, Gouillou M, et al. Increased glucose metabolic activity is associated with CD4 + T-cell activation and depletion during chronic HIV infection. AIDS 2014;28(3):297–309. Available from: https://doi.org/10.1097/QAD.0000000000000128.

[45] Ahl PJ, Hopkins RA, Xiang WW, et al. Met-Flow, a strategy for single-cell metabolic analysis highlights dynamic changes in immune subpopulations. Commun Biol 2020;3(1):305. Available from: https://doi.org/10.1038/s42003-020-1027-9. Published 2020 Jun 12.

[46] Johnson CH, Ivanisevic J, Siuzdak G. Metabolomics: beyond biomarkers and towards mechanisms. Nat Rev Mol Cell Biol 2016;17(7):451–9. Available from: https://doi.org/10.1038/nrm.2016.25.

[47] Posset R, Gropman AL, Nagamani SCS, et al. Impact of Diagnosis and Therapy on Cognitive Function in Urea Cycle Disorders. Ann Neurol 2019;86(1):116–28. Available from: https://doi.org/10.1002/ana.25492.

[48] Gowda GA, Djukovic D. Overview of mass spectrometry-based metabolomics: opportunities and challenges. Methods Mol Biol 2014;1198:3–12. Available from: https://doi.org/10.1007/978-1-4939-1258-2_1.

[49] Chen Y, Li EM, Xu LY. Guide to Metabolomics Analysis: A Bioinformatics Workflow. Metabolites 2022;12(4):357. Available from: https://doi.org/10.3390/metabo12040357.

[50] Varma VR, Oommen AM, Varma S, et al. Brain and blood metabolite signatures of pathology and progression in Alzheimer disease: a targeted metabolomics study. PLoS Med 2018;15(1):e1002482. Available from: https://doi.org/10.1371/journal.pmed.1002482. Published 2018 Jan 25.

[51] Toledo JB, Arnold M, Kastenmüller G, et al. Metabolic network failures in Alzheimer's disease: A biochemical road map. Alzheimers Dement 2017;13(9):965–84. Available from: https://doi.org/10.1016/j.jalz.2017.01.020.

[52] He X, Huang Y, Li B, Gong CX, Schuchman EH. Deregulation of sphingolipid metabolism in Alzheimer's disease. Neurobiol Aging 2010;31(3):398–408. Available from: https://doi.org/10.1016/j.neurobiolaging.2008.05.010.

[53] Crivelli SM, Giovagnoni C, Visseren L, et al. Sphingolipids in Alzheimer's disease, how can we target them? Adv Drug Deliv Rev 2020;159:214–31. Available from: https://doi.org/10.1016/j.addr.2019.12.003.

[54] Glaros EN, Kim WS, Wu BJ, et al. Inhibition of atherosclerosis by the serine palmitoyl transferase inhibitor myriocin is associated with reduced plasma glycosphingolipid concentration. Biochem Pharmacol 2007;73(9):1340–6. Available from: https://doi.org/10.1016/j.bcp.2006.12.023.

[55] Ussher JR, Koves TR, Cadete VJ, et al. Inhibition of de novo ceramide synthesis reverses diet-induced insulin resistance and enhances whole-body oxygen consumption. Diabetes 2010;59(10):2453–64. Available from: https://doi.org/10.2337/db09-1293.

[56] Li Y, Talbot CL, Chandravanshi B, et al. Cordyceps inhibits ceramide biosynthesis and improves insulin resistance and hepatic steatosis. Sci Rep 2022;12(1):7273. Available from: https://doi.org/10.1038/s41598-022-11219-3. Published 2022 May 4.

[57] Takasugi N, Sasaki T, Ebinuma I, et al. FTY720/fingolimod, a sphingosine analogue, reduces amyloid-β production in neurons. PLoS One 2013;8(5):e64050. Available from: https://doi.org/10.1371/journal.pone.0064050. Published 2013 May 7.

[58] Hemmati F, Dargahi L, Nasoohi S, et al. Neurorestorative effect of FTY720 in a rat model of Alzheimer's disease: comparison with memantine. Behav Brain Res 2013;252:415–21. Available from: https://doi.org/10.1016/j.bbr.2013.06.016.

[59] Vitorino R. Transforming clinical research: the power of high-throughput omics integration. Proteomes 2024;12(3):25. Available from: https://doi.org/10.3390/proteomes12030025. Published 2024 Sep 6.

[60] Argelaguet R, Velten B, Arnol D, et al. Multi-omics factor analysis-a framework for unsupervised integration of multi-omics data sets. Mol Syst Biol 2018;14(6):e8124. Available from: https://doi.org/10.15252/msb.20178124. Published 2018 Jun 20.

[61] Agamah FE, Bayjanov JR, Niehues A, et al. Computational approaches for network-based integrative multi-omics analysis. Front Mol Biosci 2022;9:967205. Available from: https://doi.org/10.3389/fmolb.2022.967205. Published 2022 Nov 14.

[62] Greener JG, Kandathil SM, Moffat L, Jones DT. A guide to machine learning for biologists. Nat Rev Mol Cell Biol 2022;23(1):40–55. Available from: https://doi.org/10.1038/s41580-021-00407-0.

[63] Zou J, Huss M, Abid A, Mohammadi P, Torkamani A, Telenti A. A primer on deep learning in genomics. Nat Genet 2019;51(1):12–18. Available from: https://doi.org/10.1038/s41588-018-0295-5.

[64] Pun FW, Ozerov IV, Zhavoronkov A. AI-powered therapeutic target discovery. Trends Pharmacol Sci 2023;44(9):561–72. Available from: https://doi.org/10.1016/j.tips.2023.06.010.

CHAPTER 11

Neuroimmunometabolism as a regulator of obesity

Charles A.P. Sweeney and Ana I. Domingos
Department of Physiology, Anatomy and Genetics, University of Oxford, Oxford, United Kingdom

Introduction

Obesity is classified as a global pandemic that lacks adequate response. Metabolic adaptation hinders lifestyle strategies to tackle obesity, such as caloric restriction and exercise. Therefore a pharmacological strategy is needed. Obesity predisposes individuals to coronary heart disease, atherosclerotic cardiovascular disease, hypertension, type 2 diabetes, cancer, and autoimmune disorders [1,2]. The cumulative effect of these disorders is termed metabolic syndrome (MetS). MetS, as a condition with multifaceted comorbidities is characterized by chronic systemic low-grade, thought to contribute to neurodegenerative pathology. For example, metabolic disease and its comorbidities have been shown to contribute to mouse models of Alzheimer's disease [3,4] and autoimmune encephalomyelitis [5]. Obesity and its comorbidities encapsulate a vast economic burden [2]. The economic appetite for pharmacological treatment of obesity is vast, as evidenced by Novo Nordisk's success with the GLP-1 agonist Ozempic [6]. The study of the autonomic nervous system (ANS) may elucidate new pharmacological treatment paradigms for obesity. The ANS is subdivided into the sympathetic nervous system (SNS) and the parasympathetic nervous system (PSNS). The SNS is classically thought to activate in response to stress or harm [7], readying the body for strenuous activity. Conversely, the PSNS arm supports antagonistic, rest, and digest functions [8]. This binary and antagonistic view of the autonomic nervous system is useful as an entry point but limited in its resolution because adipose tissues, namely, brown adipose tissue (BAT) and white adipose tissue (WAT), receive innervation from solely the SNS. Furthermore, limitations in anatomical and histological approaches have led to the identification of large SNS nerve bundles but failed to appreciate smaller tracts and SNS tracts containing mixed nerves. Of interest to our group is capitalizing on recent advances in single-cell RNA-sequencing and tissue clearing, combined with traditional immunofluorescence approaches to broaden our understanding of the neuroanatomical map of the SNS.

Over the course of this chapter, we will describe the well-known processes governing body weight homeostasis centrally and peripherally. We will recapitulate our understanding of the role of sympathetic innervation in various adipose depots and how this can affect the energetic state of adipose in terms of browning. We will discuss the various immunological forces at play in adipose tissue, how they become disrupted in obesity, and how this informs cellular metabolism in the context of glucose homeostasis. We will describe how a seminal paper from our laboratory provides the missing link between adipose neuroendocrinology and immunometabolism. Finally, we will theorize how well-characterized bioenergetics of central catecholaminergic neurons could also apply to, and contextualize, recent advances in sympathetic neuronal biology from our group.

Body weight homeostasis and thermogenesis

Central modulation

The hypothalamus is composed of nuclei that receive autonomic and neuroendocrine feedback signals, integrating stimuli to respond via regulation of appetite and sympathetic drive thereby modulating organism energy balance [9]. Leptin is encoded by the ob gene [10]. Leptin is a blood-borne hormone that mediates energy balance and body weight homeostasis through its central regulation of appetite and food intake. The discovery of leptin by Jeffrey Friedman's group, therefore, serves as a paradigm shift, where adipose tissue can be regarded, not just simply as an energy storage depot. Instead, adipose tissue is an endocrine organ in its own right, wherein leptin signaling encodes the state of body adiposity centrally. Plasma leptin levels increase with body weight on high-fat diets and conversely decline with weight loss [11,12]. Mutation of leptin-expressing neurons reveals upregulation of leptin and hyperglycemia [13]. Leptin receptor (LepR) is expressed throughout the brain but concentrated in hypothalamic nuclei, namely, the arcuate nucleus (ARC) [14,15]. Anorexigenic pro-opiomelanocortin (POMC) neurons express leptin receptors (LepR). The activation of LepR by POMC neurons inhibits neuropeptide Y (NPY) and agouti-related protein (AGRP) neurons. NPY and AGRP neurons centrally have dense projections to the paraventricular nucleus (PVH) of the hypothalamus. Melanocortin 4 receptor (MC4R) is highly expressed in the PVH where POMC or AGRP ligands have antagonistic relationships with MC4R. In turn, recombinase mice show differences in feeding behaviors along this bivalent relationship [16] but not energy expenditure [17]. Instead, MC4R agonism can increase energy expenditure downstream of the PVH [18], including at adipose tissue depots in the periphery [19]. Furthermore, the PVH neurons that are negative for MC4R expression regulate thermogenesis or energy expenditure, including oxytocin or nitric oxide synthase-1 neurons [20]. NPY neurons that project from the ARC to PVH catecholaminergic (TH$^+$) neurons modulate energy expenditure by reducing noradrenergic signaling to BAT [21]. Sympathetic outflow therefore takes place where

POMC and AGRP converge but double knockout studies of both brain regions have not been conducted. Wang and colleagues report that ob/ob mice show a significant reduction in sympathetic innervation of subcutaneous WAT (scWAT) and BAT with sympathetic signaling rescued by chronic leptin treatment [22]. Furthermore, the deletion of the leptin receptor affected AGRP and POMC neurons in the hypothalamic ARC, driving the denervation of fat peripherally. AGRP and POMC neurons in the arc act via brain-derived neurotrophic factor (BDNF) in the hypothalamus. Leptin therefore mediates BDNF neurogenesis. Hypothalamic leptin receptor activation therefore drives sympathetic innervation via a BDNF-dependent pathway [23] and sympathetic tone more generally [24]. Dysregulation of central leptin signaling and dysregulation of the afferent arm are critical for obesity. Dysregulation of leptin signaling in the ARC [25] and chronic serum hyperleptinemia [26] cause central leptin resistance. Reduction of leptin serum levels by leptin-neutralizing antibodies or temporally controlled knockdown of leptin receptors rescues leptin sensitivity and weight loss returning to physiological body weight homeostasis [27]. Leptin-neutralizing antibodies alone are somewhat limited as an antiobesity therapy due to the fact that one would expect an increase in appetite. O'Brien and colleagues reviewed recent evidence suggesting that the endoplasmic reticulum in the hypothalamus may underpin central leptin resistance [28]. Leptin activation increases sympathetic nerve activity, with the SNS serving as the efferent arm of leptin signaling.

Neuroanatomy of the sympathetic nervous system

All sympathetic innervation in the periphery derives from the paravertebral sympathetic chain in the spinal cord. Seminal work by Bartness and colleagues on rats and hamsters through the use of retrograde transsynaptic traces (PRV) allowed for the first virtualization of the representation of adipose tissue in the brain [29–35]. These neuronal tracing studies revealed differential representation of sympathetic innervated organs and fat pads centrally, laying the groundwork for the study of the SNS, in a similar fashion to how somatotopic maps were generated for somatosensory and motor neurons of the somatic nervous system. The specificity of PRV transmission as exclusively transsynaptic was undermined by reported PRV nonsynaptic exocytosis in the dendrites of pyramidal hippocampal neurons [36]. Huesing and colleagues repeated Bartness and colleagues' seminal studies taking advantage of advancements in immunolabelling-enabled three-dimensional imaging of solvent-cleared organs (iDISCO) (whole-tissue clearing) and three-dimensional (3D) light-sheet microscopy allowing imaging of whole torsos demonstrating PVR transduction and visualization within the paravertebral sympathetic chain in situ [35]. This report reinforced Bartness and colleagues original findings that in mice, subcutaneous WAT innervation originates from T12-L1 of the spinal cord with preganglionic acetylcholinergic neurons arising from the T7–T10 levels. Further advances in retrograde tracing approaches using pseudorabies virus and GFP-labeled mice [37] have further subdivided WAT innervation.

The white fat pad that runs from the dorsolateral to the ventromedial inguinal region, inguinal WAT (iWAT) is divided into dorsolateral WAT (dlWAT) and inguinal WAT (iWAT). The former, dlWAT, is postganglionic and innervated by T11-T13 paravertebral ganglia. In contrast, the latter, iWAT, may receive input from the anterior cutaneous branch of the femoral nerve of L1−2 of the sympathetic chain merging onto the lumbar plexus [35]. Retrograde tracing of gonadal WAT (gWAT) reveals that it receives sympathetic innervation from aortic renal ganglia at T13, but the origin of these fibers is yet to be elucidated [38]. Similarly, combining iDISCO whole-tissue clearing and PRV retrograde tracing has revealed that interscapular brown adipose tissue (iBAT) receives sympathetic preganglionic innervation from T2−6 and postganglionic projections from caudal stellate ganglion (T1) and T2−5 sympathethic chain ganglia [39]. Further refining these imaging approaches, Huesing and colleagues used TH reporter mice to further enhance resolution, reporting that iBAT receives sympathetic innervation from dorsal rami. SNS innervation from the dorsal rami favors and prefers iBAT over WAT from various sympathetic varicosities [40]. A paucity of literature exists regarding sympathetic innervation of human BAT as the technical advances in murine iBAT and WAT do not translate to humans.

Classical osmium, silver, and gold stainings of the liver in the 19th century revealed its profuse innervation associated with the vasculature and ramifications of parenchymal cells [41]. Yamada and colleagues utilized electron microscopy on hepatic innervation, reporting that dense core vesicle-containing neurons terminated on hepatocytes adjacent to the connective tissue of the portal triads in mouse liver [42]. These findings suggest sympathetic innervation of the liver. The cellular identity of hepatic innervation was difficult to define for many years due to limitations in neuroanatomical imaging techniques. Forsmann and Ito conducted experiments on the Northern treeshrew (*T. Belangeri*). Sympathetic fibers were reported as opposed to hepatocytes. Auto-radiography identified these nerves as sympathetic, and chemical sympathectomy caused degeneration of intralobular nerve fibers suggesting hepato-sympathethic junctions [43]. The application of retroviral PRV tracing to the liver revealed the coeliac superior mesenteric ganglion and coeliac ganglion project sympathetic nerves to the liver. Greater and lesser branches of the splanchnic nerves provide preganglionic innervation [44,45]. Further studies may be necessary to validate these findings.

In contrast to the liver, the pancreas receives both sympathetic and parasympathetic efferent fibers. Organs which are innervated by both arms of the ANS are the progenitor of the bivalent dogma in ANS study. Historic histological analysis of fixed pancreatic tissue by Langerhans, Cajal, and colleagues on domestic canines and felines provided the anatomical foundation for the study of pancreas [46,47]. Technical developments in immunostaining, fluorescent microscopy, and retrograde tracing allowed for further characterization of the origins of dense sympathetic projections to the pancreas. Nonviral [48] and PRV [49−51] retrograde tracing studies Preganglionic sympathetic fibers from T5 to T12 provide inputs to the cocliac ganglia. Post-ganglia lie sympathetic fibers innervating the pancreatic islets of the same name, the Islets of Langerhans. In particular, postganglionic SNS projections were reported to the islets of Langerhans, acinar tissue, ducts, and vasculature [52–55], defining peri-insular, periacinar, periductal, and perivascular sympathetic nerve plexus. Lindsay and colleagues [55] conducted a 3D reconstruction of the pancreas using confocal microscopy of fluorescently tagged TH$^+$ neurons across the entire pancreas. Lindsay reported even distribution and density of sympathetic fibers in the pancreas. Sympathetic fibers favor contact with glucagon-secreting alpha cells over insulin-secreting beta cells [52]. Application of up-to-date tissue clearing and light-sheet microscopy has revealed that sympathetic fibers closely follow vasculature and form perivascular plexuses that innervate capillaries in the islet core and peri-insular plexus that contact alpha cells [56–59]. Martinez-Sanchez and colleagues provide a comprehensive review of the history and developments in SNS neural tracing, functional studies, and neuro immuno metabolomic interplay, including the liver and pancreas [60]. Fig. 11.1 is an adapted neuroanatomical of known SNS innervation.

Physiology of white, brown and beige adipocytes

Nonshivering thermogenesis is particularly important in infants and rodents due to their large surface area to mass ratio, which attenuates the thermogenic effect of shivering [61]. BAT primarily contributes to nonshivering thermogenesis. BAT has unique cellular physiology, containing mitochondria that express thermogenic uncoupling protein 1 (UCP-1). Mitochondria generate, through oxidative phosphorylation, a chemiosmotic electrochemical gradient through the displacement of protons across the mitochondrial inner membrane [62]. Canonically, ATP-synthase dissipates this gradient in the form of ATP and therefore cellular energy. In BAT, this gradient is noncanonically dissipated via UCP1 in the form of heat. Immunohistochemistry taken together with positron emission tomography and computer tomography (PET-CT) has demonstrated the presence of BAT in humans. BAT is dispersed but found primarily in the neck, supraclavicular, axillary, and paravertebral regions [63–65]. The uncoupling effect of UCPr1 rapidly dissipates any chemiosmotic gradients allowing the kinetics of the electron transport chain to reach maximum oxidative capacity and therefore provide a significant energy sink. This explains why maximally stimulated BAT could account for 20% of daily energy expenditure in adult humans [66]. For reference, the brain is thought to use 20% of daily energy expenditure in homeostatic conditions. Surgical sympathectomy or pharmacological blockade of sympathetic signaling has shown decreased glucose transport, lipase, and mitochondrial protein markers suggesting slowed metabolic activity combined with reported increases in weight independent of food intake. Furthermore, the obesogenic effect of ceased sympathetic signaling could be rescued by noradrenaline (NA) injection (Timothy J. [66–68]; Takahashi et al. [69]). These findings have been further reinforced by optogenetic stimulation of sympathetic nerves which induced thermogenesis [70].

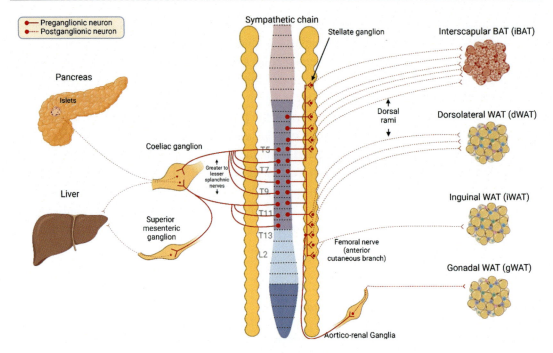

Figure 11.1

Neuroanatomical map of the known sympathetic nervous system
Preganglionic cholinergic neurons project from T5 to T13 of the sympathetic chain in the spinal cord to the coeliac and superior mesenteric ganglion. More superior projections make up the greater splanchnic nerves while more inferior projections constitute the lesser splanchnic nerves. Sympathetic postganglionic neurons project from the coeliac ganglion to the pancreas only. Sympathetic postganglionic neurons project from both the coeliac and superior mesenteric ganglion to the liver. Preganglionic cholinergic neurons project from T1 to T6 of the spinal cord, synapsing with postganglionic neurons forming the sympathetic chain. T6 preganglionic fibers project to the stellate ganglion. Postganglionic sympathetic dorsal rami project from the sympathetic chain to iBAT. Preganglionic cholinergic projections from T7 to T11 travel in an inferior fashion. These inferior cholinergic projections synapse with postganglionic sympathetic dorsal rami, projecting to dWAT. Furthermore, the sympathetic innervation of iWAT from the anterior cutaneous branch of the femoral nerve originates from this inferior portion of the sympathetic chain. At T13, a branch of the preganglionic cholinergic nerves travels further in an inferior fashion, synapsing at the aortico-renal ganglion. From the aortico-renal ganglion, sympathetic projections innervate gWAT. *dWAT*, Dorsolateral WAT; *gWAT*, gonadal WAT; *iBAT*, interscapular BAT; *iWAT*, inguinal WAT. Modified from Martinez-Sanchez, N., Sweeney, O., Sidarta-Oliveira, D., Caron, A., Stanley, S. A., & Domingos, A. I. (2022). The sympathetic nervous system in the 21st century: Neuroimmune interactions in metabolic homeostasis and obesity. Neuron, 110(21), 3597–3626. https://doi.org/10.1016/j.neuron.2022.10.017. Created with BioRender.com

As early as the 1960s Galton and colleagues [71] reported that WAT lipolysis is induced by adrenergic compounds. Gain-of-function experiments conducted via electrical stimulation of sympathetic nerves induced noradrenergic signaling and concomitant WAT lipolysis "zapping away fat." Loss of function experiments were conducted, the lipolytic effect of sympathethic nerve electrical stimulation being blocked by adrenergic antagonists [72] or upstream ganglionic blockade [73,74]. The aforementioned gain-of-function and loss-of-function approaches created a large body of early work implicating SNS signaling in WAT lipolysis. However, these reports were limited in their technical specificity as electrical stimulation will depolarize, nearby, non-TH$^+$ neurons. For example, we know that WAT is innervated by somatosensory nerves that travel together in the same nerve bundles [22]. In mice, Zeng and colleagues demonstrated that sympathetic nerves specifically drive lipolysis using intravital two-photon microscopy and optical projection tomography approaches to reconstruct 3D images of entire inguinal fat pads. They discovered that white adipocytes come into direct contact with sympathetic neurons, dubbed neuro-adipose junctions. Zeng and colleagues generated a transgenic mouse line that conditionally expressed channelrhodopsin in sympathethic neurons, TH^{CRE}Rosa26$^{LSL-Chr2}$ mice. Selective optogenetic stimulation of TH$^+$ neurons innervating subcutaneous WAT (scWAT) led to acute increases in levels of noradrenaline and lipolytic markers in scWAT and concomitant reduction in the mass of the fat pad after 4-week stimulation. Nerve crush injury of sympathethic nerves, acetylcholinergic ganlglion blockade, or diphtheria toxin—mediated TH$^+$ neuron ablation was used to undermine leptin-mediated noradrenergic signaling in WAT. Furthermore, Zeng and colleagues knocked-out dopamine β-hydroxylase, a key enzyme in the synthesis of noradrenaline, blocking leptin-induced lipolysis. Taken together, these studies highlight the critical importance of sympathetic innervation of WAT for adrenergic neuronal-induced lipolysis in response to leptin [75].

The neuro-adipose synapse and browning

As emphasized by the above loss-of-function studies, sympathetic innervation plays a critical role in the metabolism of surrounding adipose tissue. Cold challenge via exposure to 4°C for 12 hours is widely accepted as a conventional means of increasing sympathetic tone to study concomitant metabolic responses in adipose tissue. The notion that the density and localization of sympathetic axonal arborizations change within WAT in response to cold challenges is a question of some debate. Early reports indicated that increases in neuronal arborizations and increases in TH$^+$ neuron density have been reported post cold challenge [76,77]. Using contemporary tissue clearing techniques, Blaskiewicz and colleagues reported increased neural arborization in scWAT following cold challenge positing it could ameliorate obesity-induced neuropathy [78]. Jiang and colleagues similarly found increased arborization but did not engage in in-depth anatomical quantification. Taken together, both Blaskewicz and Jiang reported increased sympathetic neuronal arborization. In contrast, Chi and colleagues [79] reported no increase in nerve density in iWAT but instead reported significant increases in TH protein expression, suggesting an upregulation of synaptic function. The difference in these findings likely arises from methodological differences in the duration of cold challenge between both papers but Chi's western blotting results suggest increased arborization. Nguyen and colleagues [29] report that challenge sympathetic outflow is higher in iWAT compared to epididymal WAT (eWAT) after a 16-hour fasting challenge. In contrast, Brito and colleagues [80] reported that in response to cold exposure, sympathetic synaptic transmission increased in iWAT and eWAT but not in retroperitoneal WAT (rWAT). Collectively, these findings indicate differential activation of the SNS in a manner that's dependent on the challenge modality: cold or fasting. Brito and colleagues [80] further reported temporally dependent differential activation of branches of the SNS with the sympathetic tone of fibers innervating eWAT increasing early, but by day 12, evidence of sympathetic signaling to iWAT predominating. Although beyond the scope of this chapter, there's mounting evidence of parasympathetic, sensory innervation of thermogenic adipose depots. Leptin-sensitive sensory fibers innervate WAT [81]. Capsaicin-sensitive and calcitonin gene-related protein (CGRP)-expressing sensory nerves are present in WAT [82] and BAT [83], modulating BAT thermogenesis [84] and periovarian WAT browning [85]. Capsaicin-sensitive cells express TRPV1, a temperature-sensitive receptor, indicating that the PSNS is keeping taps on the local thermogenic activity of brown and beige adipose tissues. We speculate that there may be a complex feedback mechanism modulated by the hypothalamus or interneurons of the spinal cord that finely controls local thermogenesis within a given adipose depot. Wherein, TRPV1-expressing sensory fibers encode afferent temperature information, while leptin-sensitive fibers, for lack of a better phrase, encode afferent information on the amount of fuel available. This theoretical SNS and PSNS interplay could function similarly to a house's thermostat where feedback from the adipose sensory afferents fine-tunes noradrenergic signaling. Further work will be needed in this area, but collectively we can regard the SNS as a complex neuronal network, differentially and temporally modulating its output in response to challenge-specific stimuli.

Sympathetic nerves release noradrenaline into adipose tissues, phenocopying systemic effects of catecholaminergic release from the adrenal gland and therefore driving thermogenesis in BAT and browning in WAT and lipolysis in both cell types. Westfall and colleagues reported stimulation of sympathetic nerves pro-lipolytic effect by inhibition of NA uptake or agonism of adrenoreceptors [86]. These compounds are termed sympathomimetics; however, their potential antiobesity therapeutic effects have been hindered by cardiovascular toxicity and addictive effects [87]; R. [88]. Mahu and colleagues demonstrated that the use of PEGylated amphetamines (PEGyAMPH) increases the activity of thermogenic adipocytes by increasing SNS tone, while promoting vasodilation to dissipate heat and, critically, having no central or cardiovascular effects [89]. As alluded to by Mahu and colleagues, thermogenesis is also regulated by vasomotor modulation which can be challenging to untangle from noradrenergic signaling. Immune cells are classically studied in the context of injury and autoimmunity; however, uncovering the heterogeneity in the physiological role of macrophages in a tissue-dependent context concerning catecholaminergic metabolism has become an interest of our group. For example, a recent preprint from our group describes two distinct subsets of adrenal macrophages—dendritic-like and "foamy" lipid-laden macrophages that accumulate cholesterol, therefore regulating adrenal hormone output in the murine adrenal cortex in an age- and diet-dependent manner [90]. Concerning sympathetic neurons, in 2017, Pirzgalska and colleagues within our group discovered a distinct population of sympathetic neuron-associated macrophages (SAMs). SAMs, as per their name, are associated with sympathetic nerves in scWAT and other SNS compartments and characteristically, heavily express noradrenaline transporter SLC6A2 and degradation enzyme MAOa relative to other macrophages. SAMS imports and degrades noradrenaline; therefore SAM acts as a sink at the neuro-adipose synapse with SAM activity decreasing lipolysis. SAM recruitment is upregulated in obesity implying a local dysregulation of AT innervation caused by an immunogenic. Loss of function of SLC6A2 in obese mice attenuates obesity, promoting restoration of lipolysis and thermogenesis [91]. Taken together, SAMs modulate noradrenaline availability and therefore signaling at the neuro-adipose junction.

The binary divide between energy storage WAT versus thermogenic, energetically active BAT no longer holds. UCP-1 expression has been observed in WAT. UCP-1 expression can be induced in WAT by increasing sympathetic tone via an aforementioned cold challenge [92] or chronic β-adrenergic signaling [93] or finally via treatment with thiazolidinediones which activate PPARγ signaling [94], which will be discussed further in the section on immunometabolism. Wu and colleagues discovered beige adipocytes do not share a myf-5 lineage, unlike their BAT counterparts. Beige adipocytes have low basal expression of UCP-1 but can rapidly upregulate UCP-1 expression [95]. WAT can phenotypically remodel itself in response to chronic β-adrenergic signaling [93] and too-cold challenge, taking on a beige adipocyte phenotype, termed "browning" [96,97]. Sympathetic neurons innervate fat pads with a higher propensity for browning, namely iWAT, to a greater degree than other fat pads [79]. Taken together, we can regard leptin as the afferent arm in a negative feedback loop that regulates AT mass by reducing food intake [12,98–101]. The SNS serves as the effector arm in response to leptin's afferent signals, driving WAT lipolysis, BAT thermogenesis, and browning in adipose tissue [75]. Several other hypothalamic-acting, blood-borne hormones, including active thyroid hormone, estrogen, and glucagon-like peptide-1, have been reported to regulate obesity but this falls beyond this chapter's scope; see review [102]. We have only touched on the immunometabolomic interactions in adipose tissues concerning SAMs but other immunocytes play a key regulatory function at these sites. This will be the subject of the next section of this chapter.

Immunometabolism

With an overview of the neuroendocrine loop of leptin action and an understanding of the vast extent of sympathetic innervation throughout the body, we can begin to increase the resolution of understanding by describing the immunological players within adipose tissue and how they modulate the inflammatory state and metabolic function of adipose tissue.

Most components of the immune system receive input from the SNS. For example, primary lymphoid organs like the thymus and bone marrow, as well as secondary lymphoid tissues like the spleen, lymph nodes and arteries, tonsils, adenoids, skin, and liver, express adrenergic receptors, facilitating SNS input [103,104]. Furthermore, a broad range of leukocytes serve as components of innate and adaptive immune responses and express adrenergic receptors, including monocytes, neutrophiles, eosinophils, basophils, dendritic cells, and NK cells, which in turn allows the SNS to modulate the activation state, differentiation, survival, and chemotaxis of these leukocytes [102]. Leukocytes express leptin receptor and insulin receptors, allowing them to sense whole-body weight homeostasis, sense glycemic states, and modulate cell differentiation and polarization [105] accordingly and play a role in both these processes.

Macrophages role in insulin resistance in white adipose tissue and brown adipose tissue

Ontologically, there are two distinct macrophage populations. First, macrophages derived from the hematogenic wave of the yolk sac, which seeds tissue with tissue-resident macrophages, and second, monocytes differentiated through hematopoietic pluripotent stem cells [106]. Tissue macrophages develop in their independent microenvironment, surveying it for antigens to fulfilll their immunological role while facilitating the function of the tissue. Obesity has deleterious effects on systemic endocrine function but also local inflammatory processes within adipose tissue. This double shock leads to immunogenic cytokine signaling release, an increase in free fatty acid concentration, and concomitant deleterious effects on whole-body metabolism. Weisberg and colleagues [107] utilized profiled mRNA transcript expression in perigonadal adipose tissue from cohorts of mice that varied in sex and diet and compared WT versus obese mutant mice (Lep_{ob} and Agouti). This analysis revealed that 30% of the 100 most significantly correlated genes in various adipose depots are characteristic of macrophages. Immunohistochemical (IHC) analysis of pariogonadal, perineal, mesenteric, and subcutaneous adipose tissue revealed that the percentage of cells expressing murine macrophage marker F4/80 + and adipocyte size was significantly positively correlated with an increase in body mass. Weisberg reported similar findings in human subcutaneous tissue, stained for monocyte marker CD68. Furthermore, bone marrow transplant studies from macrophage-deficient mice (*Csf1op/op*) indicated that these F4/80 + cells in adipose tissue are CSF-1 dependent, bone marrow-derived macrophages and are responsible for almost all pro-inflammatory signaling in adipose tissue via TNF-α, iNOS, and IL-6 expression. After chronic exposure of adipocytes to low concentrations of TNF-α, a significant decrease is observed in the activation of the insulin receptor by insulin; therefore adipose tissue macrophages are also implicated in obesity. Xu and colleagues [108] further reinforced these findings using transcriptional profiling using multiple adipose tissues from depots from genetically modified (ob/ob, db/db, agouti, tubby) or diet-induced obese mice. Expression levels of macrophage-specific genes ADAM8, MIP-1α, MCP-1, MAC-1, F4/80, and CD68 were significantly upregulated in WAT of diet-induced obese mice after 16 weeks before the onset of hyperinsulinemia. IHC confirmed that macrophages, not other immune cells, were recruited to adipose tissue. After 26 weeks of diet-induced obesity, Xu reported further upregulation of chemotactic genes MIP-1α and MCP-1 before and after the onset of hyperinsulinemia. In vitro studies of MCP-1 showed impaired insulin-stimulated glucose uptake and adipogenic gene expression (LpL, adipsin, GLUT-4, aP2, beta3-adrenergic receptor, and PPARγ [109]). Xu's seminal report establishes a timeline, where infiltrating macrophage activity occurs before insulin resistance in adipose tissue. Further reinforcing this temporal sequence is that the administration of insulin-sensitizing drugs (PPARγ agonist rosiglitazone) downregulated the aforementioned genes to a significant degree except for chemotaxis. Collectively, this implicates the activation of macrophages in obese adipose as an initiating event that then drives macrophage recruitment, macrophage activation, and insulin resistance.

Pro-inflammatory cytokines released by adipose tissue macrophages like TNF-α stimulate lipolysis in human adipocytes via mitogen-activated protein kinase (MEK), and extracellular signal-related kinase (ERK)-dependent process leading to increases in intracellular cAMP and therefore PKA [110]. Furthermore, TNF-α production is implicated in insulin resistance [111]. In ob/ob or DIO obese mice, null mutation of the gene encoding TNF-α improved insulin sensitivity [112] and decreased levels of free fatty acid circulation. Similarly, functional knockout of the p55 TNF receptor (TNFR) improved insulin resistance over multiple models of obesity [113]. Preadipocytes and macrophages share functional and antigenic properties. Injection of labeled stroma-vascular cells from murine WAT or 3T3-L1 preadipocyte cell lines into nude mice took up phagocytic activity and expression of macrophage antigen (F4/80, Mac-1, CD80, CD86, and CD45) indicating that preadipocytes can differentiate into macrophages [114], and Xu and colleagues suggest that this differentiation is caused by TNF signaling. Within adipose tissue macrophages, a complex interplay occurs between immunogenic alpha-adrenergic receptors (α-ARs) counterbalanced by immunomodulatory beta-adrenergic signaling (β-ARs). Pongratz and colleagues [115] posit that adipocytes' distance from en-passant axonal signaling or sympathetic nerve terminals modulates this balance of cytokine output in adipocytes; see Fig. 11.2. α-ARs bind with higher affinity to noradrenaline (NA) than β-ARs. Near sympathetic neurons, there will be areas of high NE concentration which favor B-ARs binding affinity, driving immunomodulatory IL-10 excretion and inhibiting TNF-α cytokine excretion. If sympathetic fibers are denervated, zones of inflammation will occur with low NE concentration favoring α-ARs binding affinities leading to their activation and the production of TNF-α and the inhibition of IL-10 secretion. This becomes very relevant in the context of obesity and our later discussion on sympathetic perineurial cells.

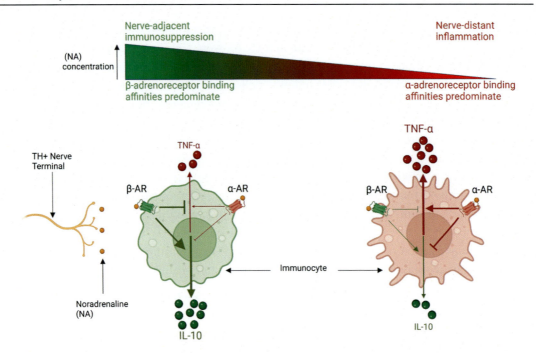

Figure 11.2

Local availability of catecholamines may determine immunocyte inflammatory profile in adipose tissue.

NA is the main neurotransmitter released from sympathetic nerves. Within the microenvironment of adipose tissue, NA concentration is higher near sympathetic nerves relative to further away. Immune cells within adipose tissue, including macrophages, simultaneously express α-ARs and β-AR. NA binds with higher affinity to α-ARs relative to β-ARs. Immunocytes close to sympathetic fibers will have a local NA availability sufficient to activate β-ARs. The differential spatial activation of α-ARs and β-ARs in immunocytes will affect the cytokines secretory profile. β-AR activation and signal transduction within macrophages close to the catecholaminergic source will cause increased IL-10 expression and an antiinflammatory profile. In contrast, α-ARs signal transduction will predominate in macrophages distant from the catecholamine source leading to the release of pro-inflammatory cytokine TNF-α. As previously discussed, TNF-α can promote preadipocytes to differentiate into macrophages and promote insulin resistance. α-ARs, α-Adrenoreceptors; β-AR, β-adrenoreceptors; NA, noradrenaline. Modified from Pongratz G, Straub RH. The sympathetic nervous response in inflammation. Arthritis Res Ther 2014;16(1). https://doi.org/10.1186/s13075-014-0504-2. Created using Biorender.

Adipose tissue macrophages also play a homeostatic role in thermogenic brown adipose tissue. Wolf and colleagues utilized two complementary conditional mutagenesis approaches to knockout Mecp2 in the Cx3Cr1 subpopulation of BAT-resident macrophages. This leads to significant decreases in the expression of UCP-1 and compromised sympathetic innervation. Mecp2 KO macrophages in iBAT overexpressed plexina4 which repulses axons accounting for the sympathethic denervation. There are indications that brown adipocyte can modulate their innervation by sympathetic nerves via the production of NGF [116]. A similar relationship has been observed between muscularis macrophages and enteric neurons [117], demonstrating the interplay between these two homeostatic regulatory systems across the plexin-semaphorin axis.

Aging effect on lipolysis

The lipolytic effect of NE in adipose depots declines with age, both in terms of the hydrolysis of triglycerides via beta-oxidation. Aged individuals have concomitant increases in visceral adipose tissue and loss of BAT thermoregulatory capacity which culminate in systemic effects such as decreased exercise and starvation tolerance. This is in part driven by the upregulation of monoamine oxidases and downstream dehydrogenases in ATM over lifecourse. Aging upregulates monoamine oxidases [118,119]. Camell and colleagues demonstrated that aged mice have significantly reduced serum-free fatty acid levels when compared to controls [120]. Visceral adipose tissue (VAT) from aged fasted mice failed to induce Hsl and Atgl, which account for 90% of triglyceride hydrolysis [121]. Similarly, Camell and colleagues cocultured adipocytes generated from progenitor cells of young mice and stimulated them with noradrenaline and cocultured macrophages sorted from the VAT of aged mice. Aged ATMS inhibited FFA release from noradrenaline-stimulated young adipocytes when cocultured. ATMS from young mice rescued lipolysis in VAT explants. BMDMs were stimulated with LPS and ATP and then cocultured with young VAT and stimulated by NA. Activation of the NLRP3 inflammasome by LPS in ATMS decreased the release of FFA, therefore reducing lipolysis. Whole-transcriptome analysis revealed that the growth factor controlling adiposity, Gdf3, was upregulated with age but this age-related upregulation could be ablated to youthful levels by knocking out the NLRP3 inflammasome [120]. MAO is known to upregulate with aging, where MAO ablation restored age-related attenuation of noradrenaline availability and concomitantly increased expression of lipolytic enzymes (ATGL, HSL) [122,123]. Taken together, these findings further indicate that therapeutic targeting of the intersection between the SNS and adipose tissue could attenuate age-related chronic inflammation in fat and the downstream effects on systemic low-grade inflammation and obesity.

Eosinophils

Eosinophils were first studied in the context of helminth immunity, and they are often associated with alternatively activated macrophages. As previously established, adipose tissue macrophages interact with adipocytes to maintain glucose homeostasis and are activated by IL-4. Eosinophils produce the majority of IL-4 in WAT. Functional knockout of IL-4-producing eosinophils leads to attenuation of ATM. ATM is reconstituted via an IL-4- and IL-33-dependent process. Diet-induced obese mice, with eosinophil knockout, show increased adiposity in fat depots and insulin insensitivity suggesting eosinophils maintain the aforementioned homeostasis mediated by ATMs. Eosinophils are present to a higher degree in individuals living in rural developing countries due to the helminth parasitism in the intestine correlating with countries where incidences of metabolic syndrome are rare [124]. Wu speculates that intestinal parasitism optimizes metabolic homeostasis. This sits in contrast to the insulin-resistant state in acute microbial infection of adipose tissue [125]. Further work will be needed to support this conclusion as it is perfectly feasible that, in developing nations, where parasitism is prominent, the critical threshold of adiposity needed to dysregulate body weight homeostasis is simply not met. Furthermore, nutritional dietary factors, such as the processing of food in developing nations, further complicate this conclusion. Regardless, modulation of eosinophil numbers could prove a therapeutic target for obesity if systemic eosinophil count was not affected, possibly by some small molecule intervention that only targeted adipose tissue.

Bridging the neuroendocrine-immunometabolomic gap

We have previously discussed the fields of neuroendocrinology and immunometabolism in a mutually exclusive fashion within the context of the cellular study of obesity. Haberman and colleagues from our group bridged the gap by mechanistically explaining how the neuroendocrine loop of leptin action interacts with immunometabolism. Haberman utilized mice wherein the expression of the leptin receptor (LepR) resulted in the expression of yellow fluorescent protein, termed LepR^{eYFP} reporter mice. Immuno-electron microscopy on cross sections of sympathetic ganglia and axon bundles derived from LepR^{eYFP} reporter mice revealed a LepR$^+$ cell barrier ensheathing sympathetic ganglia and axon bundles innervating both subcutaneous white adipose tissue (scWAT) and brown adipose tissue (BAT). A second round of immunofluorescent imaging showed that eYFP was not present in adipose tissue neurons costained with β-3 tubulin, ruling out nonsympathetic neuronal involvement [126].

Haberman and colleagues conducted cell sorting to isolate the LepR$^+$ cells from the superior cervical ganglia LepR^{eYFP} reporter mice and performed bulk RNA-sequencing on the isolated cells. Gene expression profiling revealed that the identity of this LepR$^+$ cell was largely perineurial (Cldn1, Cav1, Dcn, Igfbp6, Tjp1, Vcl) with some mesenchymal cell markers (Pdgfra, Vim, Pdpn, Cd34, and Ly6a). In addition, the gene expression profiling showed low expression of endothelial markers (Pecam1, Cdh5, Tek, and Kdr) and an absence of expression of the epithelial markers Epcam and Muc1. Haberman further validated these findings using flow cytometry, which showed that these barrier cells ensheathing sympathetic tissue stained positive for fibroblastic and perineurial markers, PDGFRα and ITGβ4, further reinforcing the perineurial identification of these specialized LepR-positive barrier cells. Single-nuclei sequencing on sympathetic ganglia acquired from humans indicated that only the perineurial cell clusters coexpressed LepR and IL-33 further validating these findings. Haberman termed this newly discovered cell type, sympathetic perineurial cells (SPCs) [126].

Sympathetic perineurial cells critical immunomodulatory signaling in adipose tissue

Where there is smoke, there is fire. Similarly, where there are immunogenic cytokines expressed in adipose tissue, there must be a relative underexpression of antiinflammatory signals. Haberman's RNA-sequencing of these SPCs reported high expression of antiinflammatory cytokines interleukin-33 (IL-33), transforming growth factor-beta 2 (TGF-β2), and interleukin-4 (IL-4) [126]. As previously described, the innate and adaptive immune systems exert powerful control over the pro-inflammatory or antiinflammatory state of adipose tissue. For example, in visceral adipose tissue (VAT), Foxp3$^+$CD4$^+$ regulatory T cells (T$_{regs}$) [124] and group 2 innate lymphoid cells (ILC2s) [127] immunomodulate local inflammation in VAT in an IL-33-dependent manner. The maintenance of this immunomodulatory population of T$_{regs}$ and ILC2s and therefore the antiinflammatory state is critically dependent on IL-33 signaling [127,128]. Using single-cell RNA-sequencing Spallanzani and colleagues identified distinct mesenchymal stromal cell subtypes that produce IL-33 to modulate VAT. They posit that these mesothelial stromal cells serve a rheostat function, where the physiological expansion of the fat pad during aging leads to a mechanosensitive-induced expression of IL-33 [129] to immunomodulate VAT inflammation. Subcutaneous white adipose tissue does not have this spatial limitation; thereby the absence of these IL-33-expressing stromal cells in that population means SPCs could have still been present but undiscovered at that time due to imaging limitations. Mahlakoiv and colleagues [130] provide additional insight into IL-33 expression in other depots. They reported that WAT-resident mesenchyme-derived stromal cells produced the majority of IL-33 with adipose stem and progenitor cells (ASPCs) producing IL-33 in all WAT depots with mesothelial stromal cells serving as an additional contributor of IL-33. Furthermore, they found that ASPC's found distributed between adipocytes produce IL-33, regulating ILC2s and eosinophils populations [130]. Collectively, Haberman's report of IL-33-producing SPCs adds another player to the pitch concerning IL-33 production in adipose tissue [126]. Fig. 11.3 recapitulates the neuroimmunometabolomic interactions within adipose tissue, including the SPC barrier. Hence, with IL-33 immunomodulatory role being well evidenced in the literature, one could conclude SPCs served a similar function in physiologic homeostasis. What about in obesity?

Haberman and colleagues became particularly interested in SPC's IL-33 and LepR coexpression with LepR being completely novel, not seen in the arcuate nucleus or any other organ tissue within the tabula muri's database. This data served as a proof-of-concept to encourage Haberman to generate a new transgenic mouse model that conditionally ablated IL-

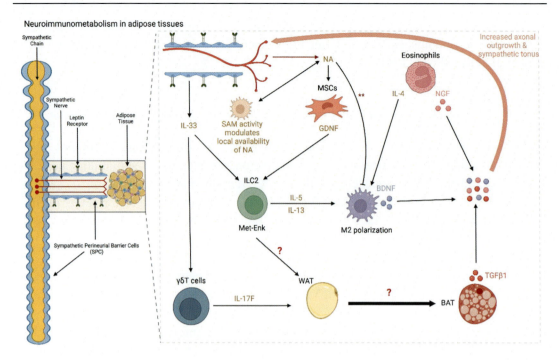

Figure 11.3
Neuroimmunometabolism in adipose tissue.
NA is exocytosed by sympathetic nerve terminals within adipose tissue or at sympathetic axonal varicosities in an en-passant fashion. Sympathetic neurons are enclosed by a specialized leptin receptor-positive perineurial cell barrier (SPC) that releases IL-33. IL-33 signaling drives an antiinflammatory phenotype by stimulating ILC2 and T-Cells. NA released by neighboring sympathetic nerves activates β-2 adrenergic receptor causing adipose MSCs to signal via GDNF, which modulates the activity of ILC2s in visceral fat. In turn, ILC2s produce type 2 innate cytokines and Met-enkephalin (Met-Enk), which may contribute to the browning of WAT to BAT but this is subject to debate. Type 2 innate cytokines and eosinophil-derived IL-4 induce M2 polarization in macrophages, but this can be inhibited by direct NA stimulation. **NA signaling can promote or inhibit an M2 state in adipose tissue macrophages depending on the degree of adjacency to the sympathetic nerve terminal (see Fig. 11.2). M2 polarization leads to BDNF secretion by macrophages, promoting neurogenesis via axonal outgrowth and increased sympathetic tone. The same neurogenic effect is elicited by nerve growth factor (NGF) produced by T cells stimulating beiging via IL-17F signaling to adipocytes, producing transforming growth factor-beta 1 (TGF). The activity of SAMs imports and metabolizes NA therefore regulating the local availability of NA. High SAM activity will attenuate NA-induced lipolysis, driving obesity. *GDNF*, Glial-derived neurotrophic factor; *MSCs*, mesenchymal stromal cells; *NA*, noradrenaline; *SAMs*, sympathetic neuron-associated macrophages; *SPCs*, sympathetic perineurial cells. *Modified from Martinez-Sanchez N, Sweeney O, Sidarta-Oliveira D, Caron A, Stanley SA, Domingos AI. The sympathetic nervous system in the 21st century: neuroimmune interactions in metabolic homeostasis and obesity. Neuron 2022;110(21):3597–3626. https://doi.org/10.1016/j.neuron.2022.10.017. Created using Biorender.com*

33 in SPC cells termed SPC$^{\Delta Il33}$. This was achieved by crossing Lep^{CRE} with IL33$^{fl/fl}$ mice. Habermann reported a significant decrease in T-regulatory cells, eosinophils, and CD45$^+$cells in BAT of SPC$^{\Delta Il33}$ mice on normal diet when compared to IL33$^{fl/fl}$ controls. qPCR of the same BAT showed increased expression of the pro-inflammatory cytokine IL-1b. Haberman also reported that SPC$^{\Delta Il33}$ mice on a high-fat diet (HFD) significantly increased in body weight without necessitating an increase in food intake. Similarly, increased expression in pro-inflammatory cytokines IL-1b and interleukin-6 (IL-6) was reported in HFD-fed SPC$^{\Delta Il33}$ mice. Hence, this suggests that the production of IL-33 by SPCs is protective against diet-induced obesity but begs the question of the role these SPCs play in BAT-induced thermogenesis. Haberman and colleagues found no significant differences between SPC$^{\Delta Il33}$ and IL33$^{fl/fl}$ controls in terms of BAT temperature, core temperature, energy expenditure, or expression of BAT thermogenic genes. A mouse housing regime of 10 days at thermoneutrality, followed by an additional 8-hour cold challenge, was found to cause a cold-challenged-induced upregulation of BAT thermogenic genes in WT mice, namely, Ucp1, Pgc1a, Elovl3, Dio2, Lpl, and Gpr3. When SPC$^{\Delta Il33}$ and IL33$^{fl/fl}$ control mice underwent the same housing regime to induce cold challenge-induced thermogenesis, expression of Elovl3 and Gpr3 was significantly ablated in SPC$^{\Delta Il33}$ mice when compared to I IL33$^{fl/fl}$ and WT controls. Elovl3 is an mRNA transcript involved in the biosynthesis of very long-chain fatty acids. Elovl3 expression is induced in BAT upon cold stimulation [131]. Westerberg and colleagues demonstrated that Elovl3-ablated mice were unable to generate heat or recruit fat to their brown adipose tissue, instead relying solely on shivering to thermoregulate under cold challenge. Gpr3 was reported by Sveidahl Johansen and colleagues to encode continuous Gs-coupled receptors without an exogenous ligand within BAT and beige adipose tissue. Cold stimulation stimulates Gpr3 transcription and upregulates lipolysis and thermogenesis independent of adrenergic ligand signaling to fat [132]. With the added context of Elovl3 and Gpr3 cellular function within BAT, we can conclude that Haberman's observation that SPC$^{\Delta Il33}$ mice ablation of Elovl3 and Gpr3 transcription after cold challenge indicates that the production of IL-33 by SPCs is required for cold-induced thermogenesis [126].

This begs the question, what is the physiological role of SPC-derived IL-33? Metabolic adaptation is a key characteristic of obesity, wherein energy expenditure decreases in response to fasting to conserve energy stores. Hence, the metabolic adaptation of obesity blunts the effect of diet restriction [133]. Haberman and colleagues developed a protocol to test metabolic adaptation in obesity, wherein 14-hour fasted mice were injected with leptin or sham injection, and after one hour had their BAT thermally imaged. qPCR showed expression of thermogenic genes (Elovl3, Ucp1, and Dio2) in SPC$^{\Delta Il33}$ mice had reduced compared to Il33$^{fl/fl}$ controls after a 14-hour fast, indicating curtailed thermogenic capacity with calorie restriction. Administration of leptin after the fast aimed to recover thermogenesis after the fasting-induced metabolic adaptation. Leptin injection rescued thermogenesis in Il33$^{fl/fl}$ mice after fasting as indicated by a significant relative temperature increase in BAT as captured by thermal camera when compared to PBS sham injection. In contrast, leptin was not able to rescue BAT thermogenesis after fasting in SPC$^{\Delta Il33}$ mice. In summary, SPC$^{\Delta Il33}$ takes on a pathological character during metabolic challenges with a high-fat diet and impaired BAT thermogenesis in response to cold, fasting, and leptin stimulation [126]. Taken together, these results unify the fields of neuroendocrinology and immunometabolism by characterizing SPCs, an upstream, immunomodulatory, sympathetic-associated stromal cell that bridges the gap between leptin and immunometabolism in the context of regulation of body weight in physiology and pathophysiology.

"Sailing under false colors": LepR$^+$ SPCs secrete IL-33 to mask the redox immunogenic niche they ensheathe

Chekov's gun is a narrative principle that states every element in a story must be necessary, and irrelevant elements should be removed. Evolutionary principals and mechanisms have a similar modus operandi. LepR$^+$ SPC's immunomodulatory function is clear in the context of the release of the cytokine IL-33, uniting two previously distinct fields. Adipose tissue homeostasis is dependent on IL-33-producing and IL-33-responsive immune cells [130,134,135]. SPCs are, therefore, not the sole producer of IL-33 in adipose tissue. IL-33 production as SPCs sole known functionality seems surplus to evolutionary requirements. Is there more to the picture? Furthermore, no explanation is given as to why SPCs have evolved to fully ensheath and insulate sympathetic ganglia and neurons, rather than just be associated with them like SAMs [91]. There is a lack of a high-resolution model, from molecule to organ system that explains SPC's full physiological function beyond being redundant IL-33-producing cells. Similarly, SPC$^{\Delta Il33}$ undoubtedly causes impaired BAT thermogenesis during cold, and the absence of SPCs causes BAT to have a more pro-inflammatory profile. However, there is a lack of a unified theory that describes how in obesity, a positive feedback loop occurs wherein concomitant signaling of the afferent arm of the neuroendocrine loop of leptin action leads to a constitutive increase in sympathetic tone, which in turn is deleterious to the efficacy of the afferent arm through leptin resistance and deleterious to the efferent arm, compromising noradrenergic signaling. Loss of function of the efferent arm will include loss of the SPC barrier, loss of noradrenergic lipolytic signaling, and concomitant compromise of thermogenesis in BAT and a pro-inflammatory phenotype in adipose tissue. Further examination into the well-studied biochemical features of catecholaminergic neurons with respect to oxidative stress could provide a window into SPC's barrier function paving the way for such a unified theory.

In the central nervous system (CNS), neurons are the stars of the show, celebrity-like in how their every need is catered by their entourage of glia. Like celebrities, some neuronal subtypes are more volatile than others, namely, dopaminergic neurons. Dopaminergic neurons are well studied in clinical neurology due to their role in motivation and addiction [136] and are well known for their "harsh" metabolic environment [137]. Dopaminergic neurons are "harsh" in the sense that they are heavily prone to oxidative stress due to their high rates of dopamine catabolism, low levels of antioxidants, and high iron content [138]. Dopamine catabolism is achieved through dopamine oxidation via monoamine oxidase (MAO) generating ROS and other injurious species [139]. Where dopamine production outstretches antioxidant capacity, conditions that increase the turnover of dopamine, such as an increase in TH^+ tone, will increase the formation of reactive metabolites like ROS [140]. A full appreciation of the importance of regulation of oxidative stress in neuronal cellular metabolism requires background knowledge of how the fields of oxidative stress, aging, and obesity synergize.

Oxidative stress is characterized by the generation of reactive oxygen species (ROS) by mitochondria as a byproduct of cell metabolism. ROS are highly transient and injurious oxygen or nitrogen (RNS) free radicals. ROS serve complex intracellular signaling functions at low concentrations ([141]) and are highly injurious at high concentrations, perturbing cell metabolism through oxidation of and damaging DNA. There are several sources for the generation of ROS [142] which is an excellent review. Most relevant to obesity research is the generation of ROS by the coupling of the electron transport chain (ETC) to oxidative phosphorylation (OX-PHOS). The ETC is arranged in order of increasing redox potential from complexes I to IV [143]. Electrons leak from the ETC to form ROS, primarily leaking from Complexes I and III of the chain [144,145] or intermediates of the ETC like the q-cycle. What causes electron leaking from the ETC and concomitant ROS generation? The intra-mitochondrial modulation of OX-PHOS is a field of its own, beyond our scope (review Vercellino et al. 2021 [146]). Quinlan and colleagues [147] report that the relative contribution of specific sites of the ETC to ROS production in isolated mitochondria much depends on the substrate type being oxidized, as is likely true in cells. Most relevant to obesity research is the suggestion that aberrant coupling that is nonoptimal "Mitchell-eonian" chemiosmotic pressure gradients can lead to a "traffic-jam" of intermediaries between complexes, like the q-cycle, leading to electron leak from these intermediaries and ROS generation. Similarly, the lack of local availability of the various substrates involved in the ETC could contribute to ROS generation. Furthermore, ROS generate more ROS in a positive feedback loop termed ROS-induced ROS release (RIRR). RIRR is caused by the collapse of the mitochondrial membrane potential leading to transient increases in ROS generated by the damaged mitochondria. RIRR can spread to neighboring mitochondria [148].

The entire family of uncoupling proteins is implicated in the regulation of local mitochondrial chemiosmotic gradients to modulate ROS generation. UCP-1 is expressed in brown and beige adipocytes, UCP-2 is expressed ubiquitously in all tissues [149],

UCP-3 in BAT, skeletal and cardiac muscle [150], and UCP-4 and UCP-5 [151] are expressed in the central nervous system. While UCP-1 function in thermogenesis is well known, the exact function of the other UCPs remains to be elucidated. Likely, they play a role in the modulation of intracellular ROS levels. ROS generation is also implicated in cellular senescence and aging. Rose and colleagues [152] reportthat genetic variability in UCP-2, UCP-3, and UCP-4 affects an individual's chances of surviving old age. Caloric restriction has long been known to slow aging [153]. Caloric restriction increases UCP-3 expression. Increased UCP-3 expression and concomitant uncoupling improve the very same metabolic processes that are impaired in obesity, including fatty acid oxidation [154], insulin sensitivity (UCP-2) [155], and whole-body energy balance [156]. On a cytosolic level, cells express scavenging enzymes like superoxide dismutase (SOD) and catalase to foil ROS. However, these endogenous antioxidant proteins are limited as ROS can rapidly combine with nitric oxide, at a diffusion-limited rate, to form equally injurious reactive nitrogen species (RNS). The formation of RNS from ROS is three to four times faster than the action of SOD [157], easily overtaking antioxidant enzymes. Possibly to counterbalance the increase in RNS over lifespan, senescence also upregulates monoamine oxidases and associated dehydrogenases in ATM. MAO upregulation and associated enzymes could further drive dysfunction in noradrenergic signaling to AT with concomitant implications for systemic inflammation driving aging [122,123]. ROS are immunogenic, damaging proteins, lipids, and nuclear DNA, generating a whole host of damage-associated molecular pathways (DAMPS). In response to extracellular DAMPS, macrophages increase intracellular ROS generation via NADPH oxidase or by oxidative phosphorylation. Increased intracellular ROS is sensed by Trx and thioredoxin interacting protein (TXNIP) which dissociate, enabling the binding of TXINP to NLRP3 leading to downstream activation of the NLRP3 inflammasome. Activated NLRP3 inflammasome propagates pro-inflammatory signaling by cleaving cytokines IL-18 and IL-1β into their active form via a caspase-mediated process [142,158–161]. NLRP3 inflammasome activation increases with age [162,163]. Taken together, this demonstrates that obesity and senescence are not mutually exclusive fields but symbiotic fields. Advances in one progress the other. Therefore study of obesity should not neglect mitochondria as synergies therein could lie a "fountain of youth."

How are ROS and intra-mitochondrial and cytosolic antioxidant mechanisms relevant to the degeneration of dopaminergic or sympathetic neurons more generally? Parkinson's disease is the second most common neurodegenerative disease and is characterized by neuroinflammation and degeneration of dopaminergic neurons of the substantia nigra pars compacta and concomitant neurological symptoms [164]. Oxidative stress is well characterized in the pathogenesis of Parkinson's disease [165]. Transgenic upregulation of UCP-2 in tyrosine hydroxylase neurons protects dopaminergic neurons from acute 1,2,3,4-methyl-phenyl-tetrahydropyridine toxicity (MPTP), a model of PD, and delays

PD symptomology [166]. Similarly, microinjection of DJ-1 protein into the medial forebrain of rats decreased dopaminergic loss in the substantia nigra in two other toxin-based models of PD (6-OHDA or MG-132). DJ-1 injection increased UCP-4, UCP-5, and SOD-2 mRNA transcripts and SOD-2 protein expression and therefore protected dopaminergic neurons by increasing antioxidative capacity [167]. DJ-1 is a protein encoded by the PARK7 gene that isoelectrically shifts in conditions of oxidative stress and translocates to the mitochondria where it is implicated in autophagy via chaperoning α-synuclein, apoptosis, cell survival, and clearance of ROS [168]. DJ-1 is expressed both in dopaminergic neurons [169] and to a greater extent in the associated reactive astrocytes [170]. This is natural as astrocytes engage in OX-PHOS, shuttling nutrients to their glycolytic dopaminergic counterparts. PARK7 mutation leads to early-onset familial PD and DJ-1s involvement in other models of PD and associated neuroinflammation detailed in the following review [171]. Dopamine is a critical part of the biosynthetic pathway of noradrenaline in sympathetic neurons (see Fig. 11.4). As sympathetic neurons must synthesize dopamine, the same "harsh" metabolic energetic demands placed on dopaminergic neurons apply to their less well-studied sympathetic cousins. Any budding hypothesis on neuronal cells must take into account the interplay with the parenchyma.

Although a paucity of literature exists, a bioenergetic relationship may exist between sympathetic neurons of the peripheral nervous system and satellite glia that is parallel to the relationships between astrocytes and dopaminergic neurons of the CNS. Mapps and colleagues [172] findings support this assumption, reporting that adult ablation of satellite glia impairs mTOR signaling, causes sympathetic soma atrophy, reduces expression of noradrenergic enzymes, and causes loss of sympathetic neurons. Furthermore, adult ablation of satellite glia in mice increased heart rate and pupil dilation indicating that the persisting "solo" sympathetic neurons have elevated activity. This is likely caused by an increase in sympathetic tone to compensate for the 25% loss of adult sympathetic neurons due to glial ablation. The biasing of any neuronal network toward excitability is considered a harbinger of neurodegeneration via energy deficiency, oxidative stress, mitochondrial dysfunction, and calcium overload leading to death by excitotoxicity [173]. Overexcitability in neuronal networks causes a rapid firing of action potentials and concomitant neuronal membrane depolarization and repolarization which places heavy energetic demands on neuronal-astrocyte energetics, making a harsh catecholaminergic environment even harsher. A key function of astrocytes is to serve as a sink for potassium cations in the extracellular space via astrocytic expression of inward-rectifying potassium channels, Kir4.1, which reduce energetic demands by maintaining ideal membrane potentials for action potential firing [174]. This potassium buffering capacity of astrocytes is further facilitated by connexin 43 gap junctions in the astrocytic syncytium allowing spatial regulation of extracellular potassium, returning excess to the cerebrovasculature

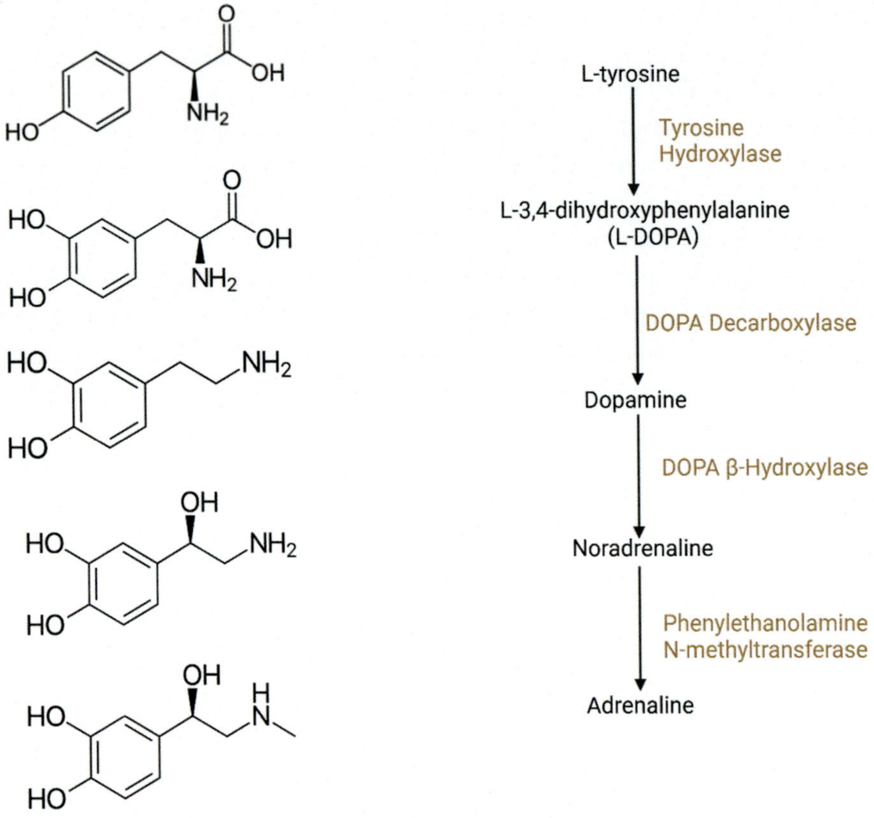

Figure 11.4
Bio-synthetic pathway of adrenaline.
As dopamine is a precursor to noradrenaline, synthesis of noradrenaline in sympathetic neuron's requires the same enzymes. Therefore the study of the harsh oxidative environment of central dopaminergic neurons is relevant to the study of sympathetic neurons. *Modified from Martinez-Sanchez N, Sweeney O, Sidarta-Oliveira D, Caron A, Stanley SA, Domingos AI. The sympathetic nervous system in the 21st century: neuroimmune interactions in metabolic homeostasis and obesity. Neuron 2022;110 (21):3597–3626. https://doi.org/10.1016/j.neuron.2022.10.017.*

[175]. Satellite glia also express Kir4.1 and Connexin 43. Mapps and colleagues [172] also found that satellite glia-specific deletion of Kir4.1 impaired catecholaminergic biosynthetic enzymes like TH and DBH in neuronal cell bodies. Furthermore, Connexin 43 is critical for propagating browning signals to WAT [96], possibly implicating satellite glia-to-adipocyte interactions in beiging. Collectively, these findings indicate that we can consider sympathetic neurons and associated satellite glia as a functional unit, with the latter supporting the energetics, metabolism, and function of the former, as is the case with astrocytes and dopaminergic neurons.

Is the sympathetic perineurial cell barrier a mediator of immune privilege?

How does comparison to central catecholaminergic neurons inform the functional of LepR$^+$, IL-33-producing SPC barrier cells? If the microenvironment adjacent to sympathetic nerves is increasingly immunogenic with increasing sympathetic tonus, containing a relatively high concentration of ROS and therefore DAMPs. SPCs could secrete IL-33 to quiesce surveying immune cells in adipose tissue, all the while masking and ensheathing the "harsh" oxidative and therefore immunogenic microenvironment of the sympathetic nerve. SPCs taken together with satellite glia could therefore buffer the harsh metabolic redox byproducts of an increase in sympathetic tone expected in overweight but not obese individuals. In overweight individuals with increasing body adipose from homeostasis, rising leptin concentrations, and concomitant increasing activation of the efferent arm of the neuroendocrine loop will continue to a point. We posit a point of obesity onset could be reached where SPC's/satellite glial buffering capacity of this redox environment is exhausted causing degeneration of the SPC barrier, ceasing IL-33 signaling, and exposing the immunogenic sympathetic neurons to immunocytes. Unsheathed DAMPS and ROS will activate the NLRP3 inflammasome in surveying immunocytes, and loss of IL-33 signaling will promote M1-like polarization (see Fig. 11.3). Loss of M2-like macrophages will attenuate sympathetic axonal outgrowth and may initiate sympathetic neuropathy in obesity. Sympathetic denervation lowers the concentration of NE which favors α-AT binding affinities driving TNF-α secretion and reducing IL-10 secretion from ATMs (Fig. 11.1) further polarizing adipose immunocytes. This will recruit macrophages to AT and may differentiate preadipocytes into macrophages increasing ATM populations. This could account for the metabolic adaptation seen in obesity as DAMP/ROS-initiated inflammation leads to runaway inflammation and sympathetic neuropathy. Adipose sympathetic neuropathy will dampen lipolytic signaling and, consequently, increase insulin resistance. Therefore we posit that one should consider everything within the SPC barrier a sympathetic immunogenic niche. Increased sympathetic output leads to a redox environment that degenerates the barrier, unsheathing DAMPS and ROS which initiate inflammatory sympathetic neuropathy. This theory is illustrated in Fig. 11.5.

Does the immunogenic niche the SPC barrier surrounds constitute an immune-privileged site? The brain, hair follicles, testes, the pregnant uterus, and the anterior chamber of the eye and cornea are classically considered immunological blindspots and therefore immune privileged to varying degrees. Although the application of this term can be controversial, compartmentalization alone does not constitute immune privilege; rather compartmentalization combined with the specialization of local immune responses [176]. As aptly put by Niderkorn [177], "immune privilege is the product of multiple anatomical, physiological, and immunoregulatory processes that conspire to restrict the immune systems recognition of foreign molecules (see no evil), to deviate the nature of the immune

(A) Overweight

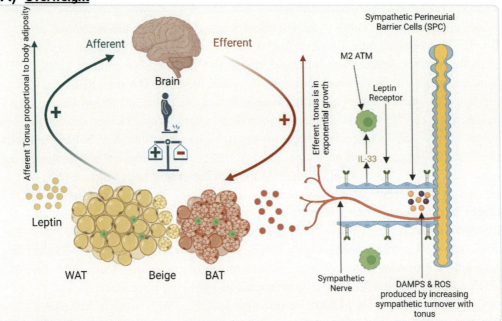

(B) Obese

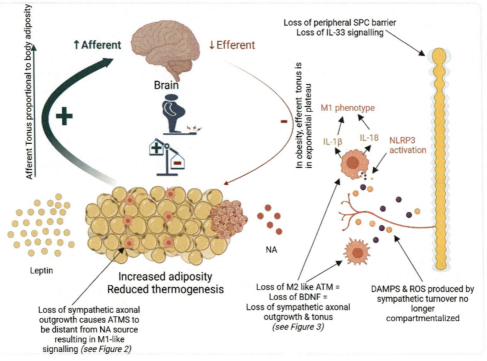

(Continued)

responses away from destructive inflammation (hear no evil), and to block the expression of immune-mediated inflammation that might occur in an immune-privileged site (do no evil)." Does the SPC barrier express cell membrane-bound (*CRP, FasL, MHC class Ib, TRAIL*) or secreted (*TGF-β, VIP, CGRP, α-MSH, SOM, MIF, SfasL, CRP, IDO*) immunomodulatory molecules classically associated with immune privilege? This area warrants further study as it could further our understanding of (neuro)immunometabolism function while further unveiling the etiology of obesity. How could SAMs respond to SPC degeneration at the onset of obesity? Further study is warranted to examine if SAMs crosstalk with adipose tissue immunocytes in a similar fashion to immunocyte crosstalk at other immune-privileged sites (e.g., microglia and peripheral immunocytes). For now, the SPC barrier enclosing an immunogenic niche is theoretical but highlights the exciting potential of (neuro)immunometabolism as a field of study.

Figure 11.5
Hypothesizing the function of the SPC barrier; ensheathing an immunogenic niche, shrouded by antiinflammatory IL-33 signaling.
(A) As adiposity increases, plasma leptin levels and leptin signaling will increase in a proportional manner. This will cause constitutive increases in efferent signaling via the sympathetic nervous system, leading to increases in sympathetic output and tonus. Sympathetic nerves are harsh metabolically and immunogenic, and DAMPS and ROS will be produced in the microenvironment of sympathetic nerves but can be possibly compartmentalized and buffered by the SPC barrier and satellite glia (not shown). Simultaneously, SPC's IL-33 signaling to ILC2 cells promotes M2-like phenotypes in surveying macrophages (see Fig. 11.3) promoting sympathetic axonal outgrowth and tonus. Sympathetic nerves innervate WAT, BAT, and beige adipocytes. (B) A point of critical onset of obesity is reached when sympathetic tone is lost. SPC knockout mice are obese. We hypothesize that sympathetic tone continues to increase in a positive feedback loop in overweight individuals until the SPC barrier cells are lost by apoptosis or metabolic failure. This point is the onset of obesity where the redox- and DAMP-prone microenvironment of sympathetic nerves is exposed to surveying immunocytes. Surveying adipose tissue macrophages or other immunocytes will take on an M1-like phenotype. M1 state could be achieve by activation of the NLRP3 inflammasome by ROS and DAMPS present near sympathetic nerves. Loss of the M2 state leads to loss of BDNF signaling depressing axonal outgrowth and tonus (see Fig. 11.3). With low sympathetic axonal outgrowth, α-adrenergic signaling and therefore pro-inflammatory M1-like macrophage states (see Fig. 11.2) will predominate as the distance between adipose tissue-resident or invading macrophages increases from the sympathetic catecholamine source. The following is not shown in the figure for the sake of brevity, and α-adrenergic signaling predominating in macrophages will cause the release of TNF-α which propagates the pro-inflammatory environment characteristic of adipose tissue in obesity. Central leptin resistance is also not shown in this figure as it's unknown if central leptin resistance happens before or after loss of efferent arm signaling in obesity. BAT, Brown adipose tissue; SPC, sympathetic perineurial cell; WAT, white adipose tissue. *Modified from Martinez-Sanchez N, Sweeney O, Sidarta-Oliveira D, Caron A, Stanley SA, Domingos AI. The sympathetic nervous system in the 21st century: neuroimmune interactions in metabolic homeostasis and obesity. Neuron, 2022;110(21):3597–3626. https://doi.org/10.1016/j.neuron.2022.10.017. Created using Biorender.com.*

References

[1] Versini M, Jeandel PY, Rosenthal E, Shoenfeld Y. Obesity in autoimmune diseases: Not a passive bystander. Autoimmunity Rev 2014;13(9):981−1000. Available from: https://doi.org/10.1016/j.autrev.2014.07.001, http://www.elsevier.com/locate/autrev.

[2] Chu DT, Minh Nguyet NT, Dinh TC, Thai Lien NV, Nguyen KH, Nhu Ngoc VT, et al. An update on physical health and economic consequences of overweight and obesity. Diabetes Metab Syndrome: Clin Res Rev 2018;12(6):1095−100. Available from: https://doi.org/10.1016/j.dsx.2018.05.004, http://www.journals.elsevier.com/diabetes-and-metabolic-syndrome-clinical-research-and-reviews/.

[3] Tyagi A, Mirita C, Taher N, Shah I, Moeller E, Tyagi A, et al. Metabolic syndrome exacerbates amyloid pathology in a comorbid Alzheimer's mouse model. Biochimica et Biophysica Acta (BBA) - Mol Basis Dis 2020;1866(10):165849. Available from: https://doi.org/10.1016/j.bbadis.2020.165849.

[4] Flores-Cordero JA, Pérez-Pérez A, Jiménez-Cortegana C, Alba G, Flores-Barragán A, Sánchez-Margalet V. Obesity as a risk factor for dementia and Alzheimer's disease: the role of leptin. Int J Mol Sci 2022;23(9):5202. Available from: https://doi.org/10.3390/ijms23095202.

[5] Sanna V, Di Giacomo A, La Cava A, Lechler RI, Fontana S, Zappacosta S, et al. Leptin surge precedes onset of autoimmune encephalomyelitis and correlates with development of pathogenic T cell responses. J Clin Investig 2003;111(2):241−50. Available from: https://doi.org/10.1172/JCI200316721.

[6] Wilding JPH, Batterham RL, Calanna S, Davies M, van Gaal LF, Lingvay I, et al. Once-weekly semaglutide in adults with overweight or obesity. N Engl J Med 2021;384(11):989−1002. Available from: https://doi.org/10.1056/NEJMoa2032183, http://www.nejm.org/medical-index.

[7] Winslow, Quaestio Medico-Chirurgica, (nd.)An Mortis Incertae Signa Minus Incerta a Chirurgicis, Quam Ab Aliis Experimentis? Quillau; 1740.

[8] Cannon WB. Bodily Changes in Pain, Hunger, Fear, and Rage. D. Appleton Co 1915;1915.

[9] Myers MG, Olson DP. Central nervous system control of metabolism. Nature 2012;491(7424):357−63. Available from: https://doi.org/10.1038/nature11705.

[10] Zhang Y, Proenca R, Maffei M, Barone M, Leopold L, Friedman JM. Positional cloning of the mouse obese gene and its human homologue. Nature 1994;372(6505):425−32. Available from: https://doi.org/10.1038/372425a0, http://www.nature.com/nature/index.html.

[11] AHRÉN. Plasma leptin and insulin in C57Bl/6J mice on a high-fat diet: relation to subsequent changes in body weight. Acta Physiol Scand 1999;165(2):233−40. Available from: https://doi.org/10.1046/j.1365-201x.1999.00518.x.

[12] Maffei M, Halaas J, Ravussin E, Pratley RE, Lee GH, Zhang Y, et al. Leptin levels in human and rodent: Measurement of plasma leptin and ob RNA in obese and weight-reduced subjects. Nat Med 1995;1(11):1155−61. Available from: https://doi.org/10.1038/nm1195-1155.

[13] Cohen P, Zhao C, Cai X, Montez JM, Rohani SC, Feinstein P, et al. Selective deletion of leptin receptor in neurons leads to obesity. J Clin Invest 2001;108(8):1113−21. Available from: https://doi.org/10.1172/jci13914.

[14] Münzberg H, Flier JS, Bjørbæk C. Region-specific leptin resistance within the hypothalamus of diet-induced obese mice. Endocrinology 2004;145(11):4880−9. Available from: https://doi.org/10.1210/en.2004-0726.

[15] Scott MM, Lachey JL, Sternson SM, Lee CE, Elias CF, Friedman JM, et al. Leptin targets in the mouse brain. J Comp Neurol 2009;514(5):518−32. Available from: https://doi.org/10.1002/cne.22025, http://www3.interscience.wiley.com/cgi-bin/fulltext/122211182/PDFSTART United States.

[16] Garfield AS, Li C, Madara JC, Shah BP, Webber E, Steger JS, et al. A neural basis for melanocortin-4 receptor-regulated appetite. Nat Neurosci 2015;18(6):863−71. Available from: https://doi.org/10.1038/nn.4011, http://www.nature.com/neuro/index.html.

[17] Balthasar N, Dalgaard LT, Lee CE, Yu J, Funahashi H, Williams T, et al. Divergence of melanocortin pathways in the control of food intake and energy expenditure. Cell 2005;123(3):493−505. Available from: https://doi.org/10.1016/j.cell.2005.08.035, https://www.sciencedirect.com/journal/cell.

[18] Vaughan CH, Shrestha YB, Bartness TJ. Characterization of a novel melanocortin receptor-containing node in the SNS outflow circuitry to brown adipose tissue involved in thermogenesis. Brain Res 2011;1411:17−27. Available from: https://doi.org/10.1016/j.brainres.2011.07.003.

[19] Voss-Andreae A, Murphy JG, Ellacott KLJ, Stuart RC, Nillni EA, Cone RD, et al. Role of the central melanocortin circuitry in adaptive thermogenesis of brown adipose tissue. Endocrinology 2007;148(4):1550−60. Available from: https://doi.org/10.1210/en.2006-1389, http://endo.endojournals.org/cgi/reprint/148/4/1550.

[20] Sutton AK, Pei H, Burnett KH, Myers MG, Myers MG, Rhodes CJ, et al. Control of food intake and energy expenditure by Nos1 neurons of the paraventricular hypothalamus. J Neurosci 2014;34(46):15306−18. Available from: https://doi.org/10.1523/JNEUROSCI.0226-14.2014, http://www.jneurosci.org/content/34/46/15306.full.pdf.

[21] Shi YC, Lau J, Lin Z, Zhang H, Zhai L, Sperk G, et al. Arcuate NPY controls sympathetic output and BAT function via a relay of tyrosine hydroxylase neurons in the PVN. Cell Metab 2013;17(2):236−48. Available from: https://doi.org/10.1016/j.cmet.2013.01.006.

[22] Wang Y, Leung VH, Zhang Y, Nudell VS, Loud M, Servin-Vences MR, et al. The role of somatosensory innervation of adipose tissues. Nature 2022;609(7927):569−74. Available from: https://doi.org/10.1038/s41586-022-05137-7.

[23] Wang P, Loh KH, Wu M, Morgan DA, Schneeberger M, Yu X, et al. A leptin−BDNF pathway regulating sympathetic innervation of adipose tissue. Nat Res, U S Nat 2020;583(7818):839−44. Available from: https://doi.org/10.1038/s41586-020-2527-y, http://www.nature.com/nature/index.html.

[24] Ozata M, Ozdemir IC, Licinio J. Human leptin deficiency caused by a missense mutation: Multiple endocrine defects, decreased sympathetic tone, and immune system dysfunction indicate new targets for leptin action, greater central than peripheral resistance to the effects of leptin, and spontaneous correction of leptin-mediated defects. J Clin Endocrinol Metab 1999;84(10):3686−95. Available from: https://doi.org/10.1210/jcem.84.10.5999, http://jcem.endojournals.org.

[25] Münzberg H, Huo L, Nillni EA, Hollenberg AN, Bjørbæk C. Role of signal transducer and activator of transcription 3 in regulation of hypothalamic Proopiomelanocortin gene expression by leptin. Endocrinology 2003;144(5):2121−31. Available from: https://doi.org/10.1210/en.2002-221037.

[26] Knight ZA, Hannan KS, Greenberg ML, Friedman JM. Hyperleptinemia is required for the development of leptin resistance. PLoS ONE 2010;5(6). Available from: https://doi.org/10.1371/journal.pone.0011376, http://www.plosone.org/article/fetchObjectAttachment.action?uri = info%3Adoi%2F10.1371%2Fjournal.pone.0011376&representation = PDF.

[27] Zhao S, Zhu Y, Schultz RD, Li N, He Z, Zhang Z, et al. Partial leptin reduction as an insulin sensitization and weight loss strategy. Cell Metab 2019;30(4):706. Available from: https://doi.org/10.1016/j.cmet.2019.08.005, http://www.cellmetabolism.org.

[28] O'Brien CJO, Haberman ER, Domingos AI. A tale of three systems: toward a neuroimmunoendocrine model of obesity. Annu Rev Cell Developmental Biol 2021;37:549−73. Available from: https://doi.org/10.1146/annurev-cellbio-120319-114106, http://www.annualreviews.org/journal/cellbio.

[29] Nguyen NLT, Randall J, Banfield BW, Bartness TJ. Central sympathetic innervations to visceral and subcutaneous white adipose tissue. Am J Physiol - Regulatory Integr Comp Physiol 2014;306(6):R375. Available from: https://doi.org/10.1152/ajpregu.00552.2013, http://ajpregu.physiology.org/content/ajpregu/306/6/R375.full.pdf.

[30] Pereira MMA, Mahú I, Seixas E, Martinéz-Sánchez N, Kubasova N, Pirzgalska RM, et al. A brain-sparing diphtheria toxin for chemical genetic ablation of peripheral cell lineages. Nat Commun 2017;8(1). Available from: https://doi.org/10.1038/ncomms14967.

[31] Bowers RR, Festuccia WTL, Song CK, Shi H, Migliorini RH, Bartness TJ. Sympathetic innervation of white adipose tissue and its regulation of fat cell number. Am J Physiol - Regulatory Integr Comp Physiol 2004;286(6):R1167. Available from: https://doi.org/10.1152/ajpregu.00558.2003.

[32] Youngstrom TG, Bartness TJ. Catecholaminergic innervation of white adipose tissue in Siberian hamsters. Am J Physiol-Regulatory, Integr Comp Physiology 1995;268(3):R744. Available from: https://doi.org/10.1152/ajpregu.1995.268.3.r744.

[33] Bamshad M, Aoki VT, Adkison MG, Warren WS, Bartness TJ. Central nervous system origins of the sympathetic nervous system outflow to white adipose tissue. Am J Physiol - Regulatory Integr Comp

[34] Bamshad M, Song CK, Bartness TJ. CNS origins of the sympathetic nervous system outflow to brown adipose tissue. Am J Physiol - Regulatory Integr Comp Physiol 1999;276(6):R1569. Available from: https://doi.org/10.1152/ajpregu.1999.276.6.r1569. Available from: ajpregu.physiology.org.

[Previous entry continues] Physiol 1998;275(1):R291. Available from: https://doi.org/10.1152/ajpregu.1998.275.1.r291. Available from: ajpregu.physiology.org.

[35] Huesing C, Qualls-Creekmore E, Lee N, François M, Torres H, Zhang R, et al. Sympathetic innervation of inguinal white adipose tissue in the mouse. J Comp Neurol 2021;529(7):1465–85. Available from: https://doi.org/10.1002/cne.25031.

[36] Patterson MA, Szatmari EM, Yasuda R. AMPA receptors are exocytosed in stimulated spines and adjacent dendrites in a Ras-ERK–dependent manner during long-term potentiation. Proc Natl Acad Sci 2010;107(36):15951–6. Available from: https://doi.org/10.1073/pnas.0913875107.

[37] Callaway EM, Luo L. Monosynaptic circuit tracing with glycoprotein-deleted rabies viruses. J Neurosci 2015;35(24):8979–85. Available from: https://doi.org/10.1523/JNEUROSCI.0409-15.2015, http://www.jneurosci.org/content/35/24/8979.full.pdf.

[38] Cardoso F, Wolterink RGJK, Godinho-Silva C, Domingues RG, Ribeiro H, Alves da Silva J, et al. Neuro-mesenchymal units control ILC2 and obesity via a brain–adipose circuit. Nature 2021;597 (7876):410–14. Available from: https://doi.org/10.1038/s41586-021-03830-7.

[39] François M, Torres H, Huesing C, Zhang R, Saurage C, Lee N, et al. Sympathetic innervation of the interscapular brown adipose tissue in mouse. Ann N Y Acad Sci 2019;1454(1):3–13. Available from: https://doi.org/10.1111/nyas.14119.

[40] Huesing C, Zhang R, Gummadi S, Lee N, Qualls-Creekmore E, Yu S, et al. Organization of sympathetic innervation of interscapular brown adipose tissue in the mouse. J Comp Neurol 2022;530(9):1363–78. Available from: https://doi.org/10.1002/cne.25281.

[41] Harting K. Über die feinere Innervation der Tube. Z für Zellforsch und Mikroskopische Anatomie 1929;9 (3):544–60. Available from: https://doi.org/10.1007/BF01266613.

[42] Eichi Y. Some observations on the nerve terminal on the liver parenchymal cell of the mouse as revealed by electron microscopy. Okajimas Folia Anatomica Japonica 1965;40(4-6):663–77. Available from: https://doi.org/10.2535/ofaj1936.40.4-6_663.

[43] Forssmann WG, Ito S. Hepatocyte innervation in primates. J Cell Biol 1977;74(1):299–313. Available from: https://doi.org/10.1083/jcb.74.1.299.

[44] Torres H, Huesing C, Burk DH, Molinas AJR, Neuhuber WL, Berthoud HR, et al. Sympathetic innervation of the mouse kidney and liver arising from prevertebral ganglia. Am J Physiol - Regulatory Integr Comp Physiol 2021;321(3):R328. Available from: https://doi.org/10.1152/ajpregu.00079.2021, https://journals.physiology.org/doi/full/10.1152/ajpregu.00079.2021.

[45] Yi CX, la Fleur SE, Fliers E, Kalsbeek A. The role of the autonomic nervous liver innervation in the control of energy metabolism. Biochimica et Biophysica Acta - Mol Basis Dis 2010;1802(4):416–31. Available from: https://doi.org/10.1016/j.bbadis.2010.01.006.

[46] Cajal S. Terminacion de los nervios y tubos glandulares del pancreas de los vertebrados. Trab Lab Histol Faculd Med Barc 1981;1981.

[47] Langerhans P, Morrison H. Contributions to the microscopic anatomy of the pancreas. Bull Inst Hist Med 1937;5(3):259–97 1937.

[48] Quinson N, Robbins HL, Clark MJ, Furness JB. Locations and innervation of cell bodies of sympathetic neurons projecting to the gastrointestinal tract in the rat. Arch Histology Cytology 2001;64(3):281–94. Available from: https://doi.org/10.1679/aohc.64.281, https://www.jstage.jst.go.jp/browse/aohc/.

[49] Rosario W, Singh I, Wautlet A, Patterson C, Flak J, Becker TC, et al. The brain–to–pancreatic islet neuronal map reveals differential glucose regulation from distinct hypothalamic regions. Diabetes 2016;65 (9):2711–23. Available from: https://doi.org/10.2337/db15-0629.

[50] Buijs RM, Chun SJ, Niijima A, Romijn HJ, Nagai K. Parasympathetic and sympathetic control of the pancreas: a role for the suprachiasmatic nucleus and other hypothalamic centers that are involved in the regulation of food intake. J Comp Neurol 2001;431(4):405–23. Available from: https://doi.org/10.1002/1096-9861(20010319)431:4<405::AID-CNE1079>3.0.CO;2-D.

[51] Jansen ASP, Hoffman JL, Loewy AD. CNS sites involved in sympathetic and parasympathetic control of the pancreas: a viral tracing study. Brain Res 1997;766(1-2):29–38. Available from: https://doi.org/10.1016/s0006-8993(97)00532-5.

[52] Rodriguez-Diaz R, Abdulreda MH, Formoso AL, Gans I, Ricordi C, Berggren PO, et al. Innervation patterns of autonomic axons in the human endocrine pancreas. Cell Metab 2011;14(1):45–54. Available from: https://doi.org/10.1016/j.cmet.2011.05.008.

[53] Ulas M, Penkowski A, Łakomy M. Adrenergic and cholinergic innervation of the chicken pancreas. Folia Morphologica 2003;62(3):243–6.

[54] Hisatomi A, Maruyama H, Orci L, Vasko M, Unger RH. Adrenergically mediated intrapancreatic control of the glucagon response to glucopenia in the isolated rat pancreas. J Clin Investigation 1985;75(2):420–6. Available from: https://doi.org/10.1172/JCI111716.

[55] Lindsay TH, Halvorson KG, Peters CM, Ghilardi JR, Kuskowski MA, Wong GY, et al. A quantitative analysis of the sensory and sympathetic innervation of the mouse pancreas. Neuroscience 2006;137(4):1417–26. Available from: https://doi.org/10.1016/j.neuroscience.2005.10.055.

[56] Tang SC, Peng SJ, Chien HJ. Imaging of the islet neural network. Diabetes, Obes Metab 2014;16:77–86. Available from: https://doi.org/10.1111/dom.12342, http://onlinelibrary.wiley.com/journal/10.1111/(ISSN)1463-1326.

[57] Tang SC, Shen CN, Lin PY, Peng SJ, Chien HJ, Chou YH, et al. Pancreatic neuro-insular network in young mice revealed by 3D panoramic histology. Diabetologia 2018;61(1):158–67. Available from: https://doi.org/10.1007/s00125-017-4408-y, link.springer.de/link/service/journals/00125/index.htm.

[58] Chien HJ, Chiang TC, Peng SJ, Chung MH, Chou YH, Lee CY, et al. Human pancreatic afferent and efferent nerves: mapping and 3-D illustration of exocrine, endocrine, and adipose innervation. Am J Physiol - Gastrointest Liver Physiol 2019;317(5):G694. Available from: https://doi.org/10.1152/AJPGI.00116.2019, https://www.physiology.org/doi/10.1152/ajpgi.00116.2019.

[59] Chiu YC, Hua TE, Fu YY, Pasricha PJ, Tang SC. 3-D imaging and illustration of the perfusive mouse islet sympathetic innervation and its remodelling in injury. Diabetologia 2012;55(12):3252–61. Available from: https://doi.org/10.1007/s00125-012-2699-6.

[60] Martinez-Sanchez N, Sweeney O, Sidarta-Oliveira D, Caron A, Stanley SA, Domingos AI. The sympathetic nervous system in the 21st century: neuroimmune interactions in metabolic homeostasis and obesity. Neuron 2022;110(21):3597–626. Available from: https://doi.org/10.1016/j.neuron.2022.10.017, http://www.cell.com/neuron/home.

[61] Cannon B, Nedergaard J. Brown adipose tissue: function and physiological significance. Physiological Rev 2004;84(1):277–359. Available from: https://doi.org/10.1152/physrev.00015.2003.

[62] Mitchell P. Vectorial chemiosmotic processes. Annu Rev Biochem 1977;46(1):996–1005. Available from: https://doi.org/10.1146/annurev.bi.46.070177.005024.

[63] Cypess AM, Lehman S, Williams G, Tal I, Rodman D, Goldfine AB, et al. Identification and importance of brown adipose tissue in adult humans. N Engl J Med 2009;360(15):1509–17. Available from: https://doi.org/10.1056/NEJMoa0810780, http://content.nejm.org/cgi/reprint/360/15/1509.pdf.

[64] Ikeda K, Maretich P, Kajimura S. The common and distinct features of brown and beige adipocytes. Trends Endocrinol & Metab 2018;29(3):191–200. Available from: https://doi.org/10.1016/j.tem.2018.01.001.

[65] Lidell ME, Betz MJ, Leinhard OD, Heglind M, Elander L, Slawik M, et al. Evidence for two types of brown adipose tissue in humans. Nat Med 2013;19(5):631–4. Available from: https://doi.org/10.1038/nm.3017.

[66] Rothwell NJ, Stock MJ. Effects of age on diet-induced thermogenesis and brown adipose tissue metabolism in the rat. Int J Obes 1983;7(6):583–9.

[67] Bartness TJ, Wade GN. Effects of interscapular Brown adipose tissue denervation on body weight and energy metabolism in ovariectomized and estradiol-treated rats. Behav Neurosci 1984;98(4):674–85. Available from: https://doi.org/10.1037//0735-7044.98.4.674.

[68] Benzi RH, Shibata M, Seydoux J, Girardier L. Prepontine knife cut-induced hyperthermia in the rat - Effect of chemical sympathectomy and surgical denervation of brown adipose tissue. Pflügers Arch Eur J Physiol 1988;411(6):593–9. Available from: https://doi.org/10.1007/BF00580853.

[69] Takahashi A, Shimazu T, Maruyama Y. Importance of sympathetic nerves for the stimulatory effect of cold exposure on glucose utilization in brown adipose tissue. Japanese J Physiol 1992;42(4):653–64. Available from: https://doi.org/10.2170/jjphysiol.42.653.

[70] Lyons CE, Razzoli M, Larson E, Svedberg D, Frontini A, Cinti S, et al. Optogenetic-induced sympathetic neuromodulation of brown adipose tissue thermogenesis. FASEB J 2020;34(2):2765–73. Available from: https://doi.org/10.1096/fj.201901361rr.

[71] Galton DJ, Bray GA. Studies on lipolysis in human adipose cells. J Clin investigation 1967;46(4):621–9. Available from: https://doi.org/10.1172/JCI105564.

[72] Fredholm B, Rosell S. Effects of adrenergic blocking agents on lipid mobilization from canine subcutaneous adipose tissue after sympathetic nerve stimulation. J Pharmacology Exp Therapeutics 1968;159(1):1–7.

[73] Bogdonoff MD, Weissler AM, Merritt FL. The effect of autonomic ganglionic blockade upon serum free fatty acid levels in man. J Clin invest 1960;39:959–65. Available from: https://doi.org/10.1172/JCI104117.

[74] Goodner CJ, Tustison WA, Davidson MB, Chu PC, Conway MJ. Studies of substrate regulation in fasting. I. Evidence for central regulation of lipolysis by plasma glucose mediated by the sympathetic nervous system. Diabetes 1967;16(8):576–89. Available from: https://doi.org/10.2337/diab.16.8.576.

[75] Zeng W, Pirzgalska RM, Pereira MMA, Kubasova N, Barateiro A, Seixas E, et al. Sympathetic neuro-adipose connections mediate leptin-driven lipolysis. Cell Press, Port Cell 2015;163(1):84–94. Available from: https://doi.org/10.1016/j.cell.2015.08.055, https://www.sciencedirect.com/journal/cell.

[76] Murano I, Barbatelli G, Giordano A, Cinti S. Noradrenergic parenchymal nerve fiber branching after cold acclimatisation correlates with brown adipocyte density in mouse adipose organ. J Anat 2009;214 (1):171–8. Available from: https://doi.org/10.1111/j.1469-7580.2008.01001.x.

[77] Vitali A, Murano I, Zingaretti MC, Frontini A, Ricquier D, Cinti S. The adipose organ of obesity-prone C57BL/6J mice is composed of mixed white and brown adipocytes. J Lipid Res 2012;53(4):619–29. Available from: https://doi.org/10.1194/jlr.m018846.

[78] Blaszkiewicz M, Willows JW, Dubois AL, Waible S, DiBello K, Lyons LL, et al. Neuropathy and neural plasticity in the subcutaneous white adipose depot. PLOS ONE 2019;14(9):e0221766. Available from: https://doi.org/10.1371/journal.pone.0221766.

[79] Chi J, Wu Z, Choi CHJ, Nguyen L, Tegegne S, Ackerman SE, et al. Three-dimensional adipose tissue imaging reveals regional variation in beige fat biogenesis and PRDM16-dependent sympathetic neurite density. Cell Metab 2018;27(1):226. Available from: https://doi.org/10.1016/j.cmet.2017.12.011, http://www.cellmetabolism.org/.

[80] Brito NA, Brito MN, Bartness TJ. Differential sympathetic drive to adipose tissues after food deprivation, cold exposure or glucoprivation. Am J Physiol - Regulatory Integr Comp Physiol 2008;294(5):R1445. Available from: https://doi.org/10.1152/ajpregu.00068.2008Brazil, http://ajpregu.physiology.org/cgi/reprint/294/5/R1445.

[81] Murphy KT, Schwartz GJ, Nguyen NLT, Mendez JM, Ryu V, Bartness TJ. Leptin-sensitive sensory nerves innervate white fat. Am J Physiol Endocrinol Metab 2013;304(12). Available from: https://doi.org/10.1152/ajpendo.00021.2013.

[82] Bartness TJ, Shrestha YB, Vaughan CH, Schwartz GJ, Song CK. Sensory and sympathetic nervous system control of white adipose tissue lipolysis. Mol Cell Endocrinol 2010;318(1-2):34–43. Available from: https://doi.org/10.1016/j.mce.2009.08.031.

[83] Bartness TJ, Vaughan CH, Song CK. Sympathetic and sensory innervation of brown adipose tissue. Int J Obes 2010;34(S1):S36. Available from: https://doi.org/10.1038/ijo.2010.182.

[84] Garretson JT, Szymanski LA, Schwartz GJ, Xue B, Ryu V, Bartness TJ. Lipolysis sensation by white fat afferent nerves triggers brown fat thermogenesis. States Molecular Metabolism 2016;5(8):626–34. Available from: https://doi.org/10.1016/j.molmet.2016.06.013, http://www.elsevier.com/wps/find/journaldescription.cws_home/728618/description.

[85] Garofalo MAR, Kettelhut IC, Roselino JES, Migliorini RH. Effect of acute cold exposure on norpinephrine turnover rates in rat white adipose tissue. J Autonomic Nerv Syst 1996;60(3):206–8. Available from: https://doi.org/10.1016/0165-1838(96)00037-9, www.elsevier.com/locate/jans.

[86] Westfall TC. Sympathomimetic drugs and adrenergic receptor antagonists. Elsevier BV; 2009. p. 685–95. Available from: 10.1016/b978-008045046-9.01156-6.

[87] Finer N. Sibutramine: its mode of action and efficacy. Int J Obes 2002;26(S4):S29. Available from: https://doi.org/10.1038/sj.ijo.0802216.

[88] Araujo JR, Martel F. Sibutramine effects on central mechanisms regulating energy homeostasis. Curr Neuropharmacol 2012;10(1):49–52. Available from: https://doi.org/10.2174/157015912799362788.

[89] Mahú I, Barateiro A, Rial-Pensado E, Martinéz-Sánchez N, Vaz SH, Cal PMSD, et al. Brain-sparing sympathofacilitators mitigate obesity without adverse cardiovascular effects. Cell Metab 2020;31(6):1120. Available from: https://doi.org/10.1016/j.cmet.2020.04.013.

[90] O'Brien CJO, Sidarta-Oliveira D, Stawiarski A, Ratti G, Loyher PL, Makhlouf M, et al. Distinct adrenal gland macrophages regulate corticosteroid production. bioRxiv, U Kingd bioRxiv 2023;. Available from: https://doi.org/10.1101/2023.09.05.556330, https://www.biorxiv.org.

[91] Pirzgalska RM, Seixas E, Seidman JS, Link VM, Sánchez NM, Mahú I, et al. Sympathetic neuron-associated macrophages contribute to obesity by importing and metabolizing norepinephrine. Nat Med 2017;23(11):1309–18. Available from: https://doi.org/10.1038/nm.4422, http://www.nature.com/nm/index.html.

[92] Young P, Arch JRS, Ashwell M. Brown adipose tissue in the parametrial fat pad of the mouse. FEBS Lett 1984;167(1):10–14. Available from: https://doi.org/10.1016/0014-5793(84)80822-4.

[93] Cousin B, Cinti S, Morroni M, Raimbault S, Ricquier D, Pénicaud L, et al. Occurrence of brown adipocytes in rat white adipose tissue: molecular and morphological characterization. J Cell Sci 1992;103(4):931–42. Available from: https://doi.org/10.1242/jcs.103.4.931.

[94] Fukui Y, Masui SI, Osada S, Umesono K, Motojima K. A new thiazolidinedione, NC-2100, which is a weak PPAR-γ activator, exhibits potent antidiabetic effects and induces uncoupling protein 1 in white adipose tissue of KKAy obese mice. Am Diabetes Assoc Inc, Jpn Diabetes 2000;49(5):759–67. Available from: https://doi.org/10.2337/diabetes.49.5.759, http://diabetes.diabetesjournals.org/.

[95] Wu J, Boström P, Sparks LM, Ye L, Choi JH, Giang AH, et al. Beige adipocytes are a distinct type of thermogenic fat cell in mouse and human. Cell 2012;150(2):366–76. Available from: https://doi.org/10.1016/j.cell.2012.05.016, https://www.sciencedirect.com/journal/cell.

[96] Zhu Y, Gao Y, Tao C, Shao M, Zhao S, Huang W, et al. Connexin 43 mediates white adipose tissue beiging by facilitating the propagation of sympathetic neuronal signals. Cell Metab 2016;24(3):420–33. Available from: https://doi.org/10.1016/j.cmet.2016.08.005.

[97] Harms M, Seale P. Brown and beige fat: development, function and therapeutic potential. Nat Med 2013;19(10):1252–63. Available from: https://doi.org/10.1038/nm.3361.

[98] Pelleymounter MA, Cullen MJ, Baker MB, Hecht R, Winters D, Boone T, et al. Effects of the obese gene product on body weight regulation in ob/ob mice. Science 1995;269(5223):540–3. Available from: https://doi.org/10.1126/science.7624776.

[99] Campfield LA, Smith FJ, Guisez Y, Devos R, Burn P. Recombinant mouse OB protein: Evidence for a peripheral signal linking adiposity and central neural networks. Science 1995;269(5223):546–9. Available from: https://doi.org/10.1126/science.7624778.

[100] Friedman JM. Leptin and the endocrine control of energy balance. Nat Metab 2019;1(8):754–64. Available from: https://doi.org/10.1038/s42255-019-0095-y, https://www.nature.com/natmetab/.

[101] Halaas JL, Gajiwala KS, Maffei M, Cohen SL, Chait BT, Rabinowitz D, et al. Weight-reducing effects of the plasma protein encoded by the obese gene. Science 1995;269(5223):543–6. Available from: https://doi.org/10.1126/science.7624777.

[102] Larabee CM, Neely OC, Domingos AI. Obesity: a neuroimmunometabolic perspective. Nat Rev Endocrinol 2020;16(1):30–43. Available from: https://doi.org/10.1038/s41574-019-0283-6, http://www.nature.com/nrendo/index.html.

[103] Bulloch K, Pomerantz W. Autonomic nervous system innervation of thymic-related lymphoid tissue in wildtype and nude mice. J Comp Neurol 1984;228(1):57–68. Available from: https://doi.org/10.1002/cne.902280107.

[104] Felten DL, Felten SY, Carlson SL, Olschowka JA, Livnat S. Noradrenergic and peptidergic innervation of lymphoid tissue. J Immunology 1985;135(2):755−65. Available from: https://doi.org/10.4049/jimmunol.135.2.755.

[105] van Niekerk G, Christowitz C, Conradie D, Engelbrecht AM. Insulin as an immunomodulatory hormone. Cytokine Growth Factor Rev 2020;52:34−44. Available from: https://doi.org/10.1016/j.cytogfr.2019.11.006, www.elsevier.com/inca/publications/store/8/6/8/index.htt.

[106] Ginhoux F, Jung S. Monocytes and macrophages: developmental pathways and tissue homeostasis. Nat Rev Immunology 2014;14(6):392−404. Available from: https://doi.org/10.1038/nri3671.

[107] Weisberg SP, McCann D, Desai M, Rosenbaum M, Leibel RL, Ferrante AW. Obesity is associated with macrophage accumulation in adipose tissue. J Clin Investigation 2003;112(12):1796−808. Available from: https://doi.org/10.1172/JCI200319246.

[108] Xu H, Barnes GT, Yang Q, Tan G, Yang D, Chou CJ, et al. Chronic inflammation in fat plays a crucial role in the development of obesity-related insulin resistance. J Clin Invest 2003;112(12):1821−30. Available from: https://doi.org/10.1172/jci19451.

[109] Sartipy P, Loskutoff DJ. Monocyte chemoattractant protein 1 in obesity and insulin resistance. Proc Natl Acad Sci U S Am 2003;100(12):7265−70. Available from: https://doi.org/10.1073/pnas.1133870100.

[110] Zhang HH, Halbleib M, Ahmad F, Manganiello VC, Greenberg AS. Tumor necrosis factor-α stimulates lipolysis in differentiated human adipocytes through activation of extracellular signal-related kinase and elevation of intracellular cAMP. Diabetes 2002;51(10):2929−35. Available from: https://doi.org/10.2337/diabetes.51.10.2929.

[111] Moller DE. Potential role of TNF-α in the pathogenesis of insulin resistance and type 2 diabetes. Trends Endocrinol Metab 2000;11(6):212−17. Available from: https://doi.org/10.1016/S1043-2760(00)00272-1.

[112] Uysal KT, Wiesbrock SM, Marino MW, Hotamisligil GS. Protection from obesity-induced insulin resistance in mice lacking TNF- α function. Nature 1997;389(6651):610−14. Available from: https://doi.org/10.1038/39335.

[113] Uysal KT, Wiesbrock SM, Hotamisligil GS. Functional analysis of tumor necrosis factor (TNF) receptors in TNF-α- mediated insulin resistance in genetic obesity. Endocrinology 1998;139(12):4832−8. Available from: https://doi.org/10.1210/endo.139.12.6337, https://academic.oup.com/endo/issue.

[114] Charrière G, Cousin B, Arnaud E, André M, Bacou F, Pénicaud L, et al. Preadipocyte conversion to macrophage: evidence of plasticity. J Biol Chem 2003;278(11):9850−9855,. Available from: https://doi.org/10.1074/jbc.M210811200.

[115] Pongratz G, Straub RH. The sympathetic nervous response in inflammation. Arthritis Res Ther 2014;16(1). Available from: https://doi.org/10.1186/s13075-014-0504-2, http://arthritis-research.com/.

[116] Nisoli E, Tonello C, Benarese M, Liberini P, Carruba MO. Expression of nerve growth factor in brown adipose tissue: implications for thermogenesis and obesity. Endocrinology 1996;137(2):495−503. Available from: https://doi.org/10.1210/endo.137.2.8593794.

[117] Muller PA, Koscsó B, Rajani GM, Stevanovic K, Berres ML, Hashimoto D, et al. Crosstalk between muscularis macrophages and enteric neurons regulates gastrointestinal motility. Cell 2014;158(2):300−13. Available from: https://doi.org/10.1016/j.cell.2014.04.050, https://www.sciencedirect.com/journal/cell.

[118] Balter NJ, Schwartz SL. Accumulation of norepinephrine by macrophages and relationships to known uptake processes. J Pharmacology Exp Therapeutics 1977;201(3):636−43.

[119] Czimmerer Z, Varga T, Poliska S, Nemet I, Szanto A, Nagy L. Identification of novel markers of alternative activation and potential endogenous PPARγ ligand production mechanisms in human IL-4 stimulated differentiating macrophages. Immunobiology 2012;217(12):1301−14. Available from: https://doi.org/10.1016/j.imbio.2012.08.270.

[120] Camell CD, Sander J, Spadaro O, Lee A, Nguyen KY, Wing A, et al. Inflammasome-driven catecholamine catabolism in macrophages blunts lipolysis during ageing. Nature 2017;550(7674):119−23. Available from: https://doi.org/10.1038/nature24022.

[121] Bertrand HA, Anderson WR, Masoro EJ, Yu BP. Action of food restriction on age-related changes in adipocyte lipolysis. J Gerontol 1987;42(6):666—73. Available from: https://doi.org/10.1093/geronj/42.6.666.

[122] Rogers NH, Landa A, Park S, Smith RG. Aging leads to a programmed loss of brown adipocytes in murine subcutaneous white adipose tissue. Aging Cell 2012;11(6):1074—83. Available from: https://doi.org/10.1111/acel.12010.

[123] Vega A, Chacón P, Monteseirín J, El Bekay R, Álvarez M, Alba G, et al. A new role for monoamine oxidases in the modulation of macrophage-inducible nitric oxide synthase gene expression. J Leukoc Biol 2004;75(6):1093—101. Available from: https://doi.org/10.1189/jlb.1003459.

[124] Feuerer M, Herrero L, Cipolletta D, Naaz A, Wong J, Nayer A, et al. Lean, but not obese, fat is enriched for a unique population of regulatory T cells that affect metabolic parameters. Nat Med 2009;15(8):930—9. Available from: https://doi.org/10.1038/nm.2002.

[125] Emilsson V, Thorleifsson G, Zhang B, Leonardson AS, Zink F, Zhu J, et al. Genetics of gene expression and its effect on disease. Nature 2008;452(7186):423—8. Available from: https://doi.org/10.1038/nature06758.

[126] Haberman ER, Sarker G, Arús BA, Ziegler KA, Meunier S, Martínez-Sánchez N, et al. Immunomodulatory leptin receptor + sympathetic perineurial barrier cells protect against obesity by facilitating brown adipose tissue thermogenesis. Immunity 2024;57(1):141. Available from: https://doi.org/10.1016/j.immuni.2023.11.006.

[127] Molofsky AB, Nussbaum JC, Liang HE, Dyken SJV, Cheng LE, Mohapatra A, et al. Innate lymphoid type 2 cells sustain visceral adipose tissue eosinophils and alternatively activated macrophages. J Exp Med 2013;210(3):535—49. Available from: https://doi.org/10.1084/jem.20121964, http://jem.rupress.org/content/210/3/535.full.pdf United States.

[128] Vasanthakumar A, Moro K, Xin A, Liao Y, Gloury R, Kawamoto S, et al. The transcriptional regulators IRF4, BATF and IL-33 orchestrate development and maintenance of adipose tissue—resident regulatory T cells. Nat Immunology 2015;16(3):276—85. Available from: https://doi.org/10.1038/ni.3085.

[129] Kakkar R, Hei H, Dobner S, Lee RT. Interleukin 33 as a mechanically responsive cytokine secreted by living cells. J Biol Chem 2012;287(9):6941—8. Available from: https://doi.org/10.1074/jbc.M111.298703, http://www.jbc.org/content/287/9/6941.full.pdf + html.

[130] Mahlakõiv T, Flamar A-L, Johnston LK, Moriyama S, Putzel GG, Bryce PJ, et al. Stromal cells maintain immune cell homeostasis in adipose tissue via production of interleukin-33. Sci Immunol 2019;4(35). Available from: https://doi.org/10.1126/sciimmunol.aax0416.

[131] Westerberg R, Månsson JE, Golozoubova V, Shabalina IG, Backlund EC, Tvrdik P, et al. ELOVL3 is an important component for early onset of lipid recruitment in brown adipose tissue. J Biol Chem 2006;281(8):4958—68. Available from: https://doi.org/10.1074/jbc.M511588200Sweden, http://www.jbc.org/cgi/reprint/281/8/4958.pdf.

[132] Sveidahl Johansen O, Ma T, Hansen JB, Markussen LK, Schreiber R, Reverte-Salisa L, et al. Lipolysis drives expression of the constitutively active receptor GPR3 to induce adipose thermogenesis. Cell 2021;184(13):3502. Available from: https://doi.org/10.1016/j.cell.2021.04.037, https://www.sciencedirect.com/journal/cell.

[133] Chouchani ET, Kajimura S. Metabolic adaptation and maladaptation in adipose tissue. Nat Metab 2019;1(2):189—200. Available from: https://doi.org/10.1038/s42255-018-0021-8.

[134] Spallanzani RG, Zemmour D, Xiao T, Jayewickreme T, Li C, Bryce PJ, et al. Distinct immunocyte-promoting and adipocyte-generating stromal components coordinate adipose tissue immune and metabolic tenors. Sci Immunol 2019;4(35). Available from: https://doi.org/10.1126/sciimmunol.aaw3658, https://immunology.sciencemag.org/content/4/35/eaaw3658/tab-pdf.

[135] Goldberg EL, Shchukina I, Youm YH, Ryu S, Tsusaka T, Young KC, et al. IL-33 causes thermogenic failure in aging by expanding dysfunctional adipose ILC2. Cell Metab 2021;33(11):2277. Available from: https://doi.org/10.1016/j.cmet.2021.08.004, http://www.cellmetabolism.org/.

[136] Volkow ND, Wise RA, Baler R. The dopamine motive system: Implications for drug and food addiction. Nat Rev Neurosci 2017;18(12):741−52. Available from: https://doi.org/10.1038/nrn.2017.130, http://www.nature.com/nrn/.

[137] Chinta SJ, Andersen JK. Dopaminergic neurons. Int J Biochem Cell Biol 2005;37(5):942−946,. Available from: https://doi.org/10.1016/j.biocel.2004.09.009, http://www.elsevier.com/locate/biocel.

[138] Halliwell B. Reactive oxygen species and the central nervous system. J Neurochem 1992;59(5):1609−23. Available from: https://doi.org/10.1111/j.1471-4159.1992.tb10990.x.

[139] Graham DG, Tiffany SM, Bell WR, Gutknecht WF. Autoxidation versus covalent binding of quinones as the mechanism of toxicity of dopamine, 6-hydroxydopamine, and related compounds toward C1300 neuroblastoma cells in vitro. Mol Pharmacology 1978;14(4):644−53.

[140] Hastings TG, Zigmond MJ. Identification of Catechol-Protein Conjugates in Neostriatal Slices Incubated with [3 H]Dopamine: impact of Ascorbic Acid and Glutathione. J Neurochemistry 1994;63(3):1126−32. Available from: https://doi.org/10.1046/j.1471-4159.1994.63031126.x.

[141] Reactive oxygen species in cell signaling. American Journal of Physiology-Lung Cellular and Molecular Physiology. Accessed. (2024), doi: 10.1152/ajplung.2000.279.6.L10052024.

[142] Mittal M, Siddiqui MR, Tran K, Reddy SP, Malik AB. Reactive oxygen species in inflammation and tissue injury. Antioxid Redox Signal 2014;20(7):1126−67. Available from: https://doi.org/10.1089/ars.2012.5149.

[143] Handy DE, Loscalzo J. Redox regulation of mitochondrial function. Antioxid Redox Signal 2012;16(11):1323−67. Available from: https://doi.org/10.1089/ars.2011.4123.

[144] Tretter L, Sipos I, Adam-Vizi V. Initiation of Neuronal Damage by Complex I Deficiency and Oxidative Stress in Parkinson's Disease. Neurochem Res 2004;29(3):569−77. Available from: https://doi.org/10.1023/B:NERE.0000014827.94562.4b.

[145] O'Malley Y, Fink BD, Ross NC, Prisinzano TE, Sivitz WI. Reactive oxygen and targeted antioxidant administration in endothelial cell mitochondria. J Biol Chem 2006;281(52):39766−75. Available from: https://doi.org/10.1074/jbc.M608268200, http://www.jbc.org/cgi/reprint/281/52/39766 United States.

[146] Vercellino I, Sazanov LA. The assembly, regulation and function of the mitochondrial respiratory chain. Nat Rev Mol Cell Biol 2022;23(2):141−61. Available from: https://doi.org/10.1038/s41580-021-00415-0, http://www.nature.com/molcellbio.

[147] Quinlan CL, Perevoshchikova IV, Hey-Mogensen M, Orr AL, Brand MD. Sites of reactive oxygen species generation by mitochondria oxidizing different substrates. Redox Biology 2013;1(1):304−12. Available from: https://doi.org/10.1016/j.redox.2013.04.005, http://www.journals.elsevier.com/redox-biology.

[148] R.-I.R. Mitochondrial, Release, An update and review - Google Search. (2024), 2024.

[149] Pecqueur C, Couplan E, Bouillaud F, Ricquier D. Genetic and physiological analysis of the role of uncoupling proteins in human energy homeostasis. J Mol Med 2001;79(1):48−56. Available from: https://doi.org/10.1007/s001090000150.

[150] Vidal-Puig A, Solanes G, Grujic D, Flier JS, Lowell BB. UCP3: An uncoupling protein homologue expressed preferentially and abundantly in skeletal muscle and brown adipose tissue. Biochem Biophys Res Commun 1997;235(1):79−82. Available from: https://doi.org/10.1006/bbrc.1997.6740, http://www.sciencedirect.com/science/journal/0006291X.

[151] Smorodchenko A, Rupprecht A, Sarilova I, Ninnemann O, Bräuer AU, Franke K, et al. Comparative analysis of uncoupling protein 4 distribution in various tissues under physiological conditions and during development. Biochimica et Biophysica Acta (BBA) - Biomembranes 2009;1788(10):2309−19. Available from: https://doi.org/10.1016/j.bbamem.2009.07.018.

[152] Rose G, Crocco P, De Rango F, Montesanto A, Passarino G, Vina J. Further Support to the uncoupling-to-survive theory: the genetic variation of human UCP Genes is associated with longevity. PLoS ONE 2011;6(12):e29650. Available from: https://doi.org/10.1371/journal.pone.0029650.

[153] Sohal RS, Weindruch R. Oxidative Stress, Caloric Restriction, and Aging. Science 1996;273(5271):59−63. Available from: https://doi.org/10.1126/science.273.5271.59.

[154] Darcy MacLellan J, Gerrits MF, Gowing A, Smith PJS, Wheeler MB, Harper M-E. Physiological increases in uncoupling protein 3 augment fatty acid oxidation and decrease reactive oxygen species production without uncoupling respiration in muscle cells. Diabetes 2005;54(8):2343−50. Available from: https://doi.org/10.2337/diabetes.54.8.2343.

[155] Chan CB, Kashemsant N. Regulation of insulin secretion by uncoupling protein. Biochemical Soc Trans 2006;34(5):802−5. Available from: https://doi.org/10.1042/bst0340802.

[156] Bézaire V, Seifert EL, Harper ME. Uncoupling protein-3: clues in an ongoing mitochondrial mystery. FASEB J 2007;21(2):312−24. Available from: https://doi.org/10.1096/fj.06-6966revCanada, http://www.fasebj.org/cgi/reprint/21/2/312.

[157] Beckman JS. Oxidative damage and tyrosine nitration from peroxynitrite. Chem Res Toxicol 1996;9 (5):836−44. Available from: https://doi.org/10.1021/tx9501445, http://pubs.acs.org/journal/crtoec.

[158] Schroder K, Tschopp J. The Inflammasomes. Cell 2010;140(6):821−32. Available from: https://doi.org/10.1016/j.cell.2010.01.040.

[159] Zhou R, Tardivel A, Thorens B, Choi I, Tschopp J. Thioredoxin-interacting protein links oxidative stress to inflammasome activation. Nat Immunology 2010;11(2):136−40. Available from: https://doi.org/10.1038/ni.1831.

[160] Dostert C, Pétrilli V, Van Bruggen R, Steele C, Mossman BT, Tschopp J. Innate immune activation through Nalp3 inflammasome sensing of asbestos and silica. Science 2008;320(5876):674−7. Available from: https://doi.org/10.1126/science.1156995.

[161] Martinon F, Mayor A, Tschopp J. The inflammasomes: guardians of the body. Annu Rev Immunology 2009;27(1):229−65. Available from: https://doi.org/10.1146/annurev.immunol.021908.132715.

[162] Spadaro O, Goldberg EL, Camell CD, Youm YH, Kopchick JJ, Nguyen KY, et al. Growth hormone receptor deficiency protects against age-related NLRP3 inflammasome activation and immune senescence. Cell Reports 2016;14(7):1571−80. Available from: https://doi.org/10.1016/j.celrep.2016.01.044, http://www.sciencedirect.com/science/journal/22111247.

[163] Youm YH, Grant RW, McCabe LR, Albarado DC, Nguyen KY, Ravussin A, et al. Canonical Nlrp3 inflammasome links systemic low-grade inflammation to functional decline in aging. Cell Metab 2013;18(4):519−32. Available from: https://doi.org/10.1016/j.cmet.2013.09.010, http://www.cellmetabolism.org/.

[164] Parkinson J. An essay on the shaking palsy. J Neuropsychiatry Clin Neurosci 2002;14(2):223−36. Available from: https://doi.org/10.1176/jnp.14.2.223.

[165] Jenner P, Olanow CW. Oxidative stress and the pathogenesis of Parkinson's disease. Neurology 1996;47 (6):S161. Available from: https://doi.org/10.1212/wnl.47.6_suppl_3.161s, http://www.neurology.org.

[166] Conti B, Sugama S, Lucero J, Winsky-Sommerer R, Wirz SA, Maher P, et al. Uncoupling protein 2 protects dopaminergic neurons from acute 1,2,3,6-methyl-phenyl-tetrahydropyridine toxicity. J Neurochem 2005;93(2):493−501. Available from: https://doi.org/10.1111/j.1471-4159.2005.03052.x.

[167] Sun SY, An CN, Pu XP. DJ-1 protein protects dopaminergic neurons against 6-OHDA/MG-132-induced neurotoxicity in rats. Brain Res Bull 2012;88(6):609−16. Available from: https://doi.org/10.1016/j.brainresbull.2012.05.013.

[168] Mencke P, Boussaad I, Romano CD, Kitami T, Linster CL, Krüger R. The role of dj-1 in cellular metabolism and pathophysiological implications for parkinson's disease. Cells 2021;10(2):1−17. Available from: https://doi.org/10.3390/cells10020347, https://www.mdpi.com/2073-4409/10/2/347/pdf.

[169] Bandopadhyay R, Kingsbury AE, Cookson MR, Reid AR, Evans IM, Hope AD, et al. The expression of DJ-1 (PARK7) in normal human CNS and idiopathic Parkinson's disease. Brain 2004;127(2):420−430,. Available from: https://doi.org/10.1093/brain/awh054.

[170] Rizzu P, Hinkle DA, Zhukareva V, Bonifati V, Severijnen LA, Martinez D, et al. DJ-1 colocalizes with tau inclusions: a link between Parkinsonism and Dementia. Ann Neurol 2004;55(1):113−18. Available from: https://doi.org/10.1002/ana.10782.

[171] MacMahon Copas AN, McComish SF, Fletcher JM, Caldwell MA. The Pathogenesis of Parkinson's Disease: A Complex Interplay Between Astrocytes, Microglia, and T Lymphocytes? Front Neurol

2021;12. Available from: https://doi.org/10.3389/fneur.2021.666737, http://www.frontiersin.org/ Neurology.

[172] Mapps AA, Boehm E, Beier C, Keenan WT, Langel J, Liu M, et al. Satellite glia modulate sympathetic neuron survival, activity, and autonomic function. elife Sci Publ Ltd, U S elife 2022;11. Available from: https://doi.org/10.7554/eLife.74295, https://elifesciences.org/articles/74295.

[173] Mehta A, Prabhakar M, Kumar P, Deshmukh R, Sharma PL. Excitotoxicity: Bridge to various triggers in neurodegenerative disorders. Eur J Pharmacol 2013;698(1-3):6—18. Available from: https://doi.org/10.1016/j.ejphar.2012.10.032.

[174] Higashi K, Fujita A, Inanobe A, Tanemoto M, Doi K, Kubo T, et al. An inwardly rectifying K+ channel, Kir4.1, expressed in astrocytes surrounds synapses and blood vessels in brain. Am J Physiol-Cell Physiol 2001;281(3):C922. Available from: https://doi.org/10.1152/ajpcell.2001.281.3.c922.

[175] Bellot-Saez A, Kékesi O, Morley JW, Buskila Y. Astrocytic modulation of neuronal excitability through K+ spatial buffering. Neurosci Biobehav Rev 2017;77:87—97. Available from: https://doi.org/10.1016/j.neubiorev.2017.03.002, www.elsevier.com/locate/neubiorev.

[176] Galea I, Bechmann I, Perry VH. What is immune privilege (not). Trends Immunol 2007;28(1):12—18. Available from: https://doi.org/10.1016/j.it.2006.11.004.

[177] Niederkorn JY. See no evil, hear no evil, do no evil: The lessons of immune privilege. Nat Immunol 2006;7(4):354—9. Available from: https://doi.org/10.1038/ni1328.

CHAPTER 12

Clinical stage drugs utilizing cellular metabolism pathways

Tristram A.J. Ryan[1], Luke A.J. O'Neill[2] and Zbigniew Zasłona[3]

[1]Harvard Medical School, and Division of Immunology, Division of Gastroenterology, Boston Children's Hospital, Boston, MA, United States, [2]Trinity College Dublin, School of Biochemistry and Immunology, Dublin, Ireland, [3]Molecure SA, Warsaw, Poland

Introduction

We have gathered sufficient evidence to claim that inhibition of glycolysis impairs proinflammatory responses whilst favoring antiinflammatory outcomes. Specifically, modulation of glycolytic reprogramming can predominantly affect inflammatory immune or cancer cells, offering low on-target toxicity. Not surprisingly, this has been exploited by researchers focused on the development of novel therapeutic interventions. Therapies targeting glycolysis include both pharmacologic inhibitors of key enzymes and receptors antagonists, while approaches focused on the citric acid—or tricarboxylic acid cycle (TCA)—cycle additionally explore analogs of metabolites that possess cytokine-like properties [1]. There are numerous preclinical programs and patents generated at university start-ups in addition to many biotech and big pharma-led projects aimed at targeting glycolysis and citric acid pathways clinically. Contrary to expectations, programs based on modulation of glycolysis and the citric acid cycle seem to hold the most promise in cancers, genetic, and autoimmune diseases, rather than the classical definition of physiological metabolic diseases.

Metabolites as clinical biomarkers

Diagnostic techniques, which are used to identify the primary endpoint in clinical trials as well as determine the efficacy of clinical interventions, may also be manipulated and utilized to set the context for drug development. A prime example, which highlights how exploiting immunometabolism can filter into clinical use, is an increase in the use of positron emission tomography/computed tomography (PET/CT) with the use of 18F-fluoro-2-deoxy-D-glucose (18F-FDG) in the diagnosis of inflammatory diseases, a technique that traditionally was used in oncology [2–4]. In this technique, 18F-FDG glucose analog is taken up by cells using membrane glucose transporter (GLUT) proteins, and the glucose analog is subsequently phosphorylated by hexokinase. Accumulation of 18F-FDG is observed at sites of inflammation where activation of proinflammatory cells depends on glycolysis and is accompanied by overexpression of GLUT1 and GLUT3 as well as the activity of hexokinase [2]. Thus the accumulation of 18F-FDG enables the imaging of inflammation and can allow for the future assessment of the efficacy of antiinflammatory drugs. Hence, the popularity of 18F-FDG PET/CT for the diagnosis of various inflammatory diseases such as sarcoidosis, inflammatory bowel disease, or vasculitis is increasing among clinicians [5]. CT provides additional information on the tissue remodeling, such as during fibrosis which can occur during chronic inflammation.

This approach has been used in clinical trials. 18F-FDG PET/CT was used as an endpoint readout for monitoring patients with sarcoidosis who had been treated with antibodies against macrophage-specific cytokines, such as Canakinumab (anti-IL-1b antibody) or CMK389 (anti-IL-18 antibody), from Novartis Pharmaceuticals [6]. These are examples of metabolic monitoring used for disease diagnosis but more importantly for the assessment of disease progression and the efficacy of tested drugs. Specifically, 18F-FDG PET/CT allowed for the examination of the activity of macrophages which were target cells in these studies, present at the center of granulomas and defined as an underlying factor determining the process of inflammation. In addition, an ongoing, first-in-human proof-of-concept Phase II clinical study assessing the chitinase-1 (CHIT1) inhibitor, OATD-01, which effectively mitigates inflammation driven by macrophages, is utilizing 18F-FDG PET/CT to assess the efficacy of the drug. OATD-01 is currently being tested in patients with pulmonary sarcoidosis (NCT06205121) [7] in a study with a readout utilizing an analog of glucose. Results from Phase II will provide valuable functional information on the glycolysis of granulomas, after treatment with a drug with a potential to reverse a proinflammatory phenotype of macrophages in the lungs of sarcoidosis patients. These studies demonstrate how modern approaches that target dysregulated immunometabolism as an underlying driver of disease are "flipping the script" by also using metabolites themselves as biomarkers to track both disease progression and treatment efficacy.

Targeting—and manipulating—immunometabolism for clinical therapies

Although observations that activated immune cells rely on glycolysis were made over 60 years ago, only recently we have seen an explosion in publications focused on the mechanistic insights on this process and cellular metabolism in general. It has resulted in the heightened interest of biotechs and big pharma, which has further elevated the whole immunometabolism field, offering new ideas to tackle human diseases. Below we will list and discuss some examples of newly approved drugs whose mechanism of action involves inhibition of enzymes involved in glycolysis or the citric acid/TCA cycle pathways (Fig. 12.1). Moreover, new studies are assessing marketed drugs that are used as a standard of care treatment and are revealing new and often unexpected mechanism of actions of approved drugs proving their ability to directly modulate cellular metabolism pathways, providing a hitherto unknown mechanism by which they exert their efficacy. Such historical clinical proof-of-concept experiments for medicines, developed at times when no mechanism of action was needed for their approval, provide strong encouragement for

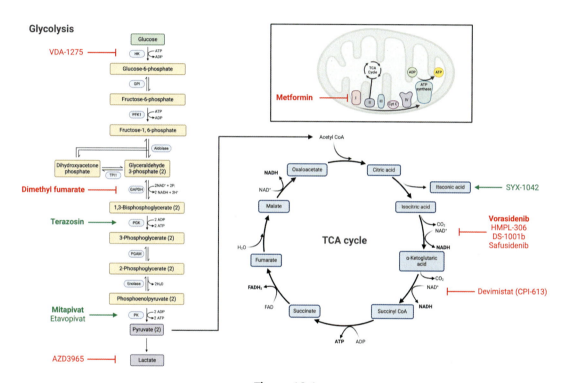

Figure 12.1

Clinical stage drugs utilizing cellular metabolism pathways. A selection of clinically approved drugs and compounds currently in clinical trials that either activate or inhibit metabolic processes to exert their effects. Existing, approved antiinflammatory drugs such as DMF and metformin suppress glycolysis and complex I of the electron transport chain, respectively—both critical metabolic processes—to suppress inflammation. Promisingly for the immunometabolism field, the IDH1/2 inhibitor vorasidenib was recently approved for IDH mutation-induced gliomas, with further IDH1/2 inhibitors also being currently evaluated in clinical trials. This demonstrates the exciting, translational potential that targeting metabolic processes holds for developing new, specific, and effective drugs for the clinic. Key: Compounds in red block, and compounds listed in green activate specific metabolic enzymes. Compounds in bold are clinically approved. AZD3965 and SYX-1042 are in Phase I clinical trials. VDA-1275, HMPL-306, DS-1001b, Safusidenib, and Devimistat (CPI-613) are in Phase II clinical trials. Etavopivat is currently being assessed in Phase III clinical trials. *DMF*, Dimethyl fumarate.

further development of drugs exploring the possibilities of modulation of glycolysis and cellular metabolism in general.

Drugs modulating glycolysis

The boosting or inhibition of glycolysis is context-dependent in the clinic, as enzymes involved in the process of glycolysis have also been extensively studied as direct therapeutic targets, and several drug development programs—reflected by hundreds of patents—are currently ongoing. In particular, metabolic checkpoint modulators are now being assessed for clinical utility.

One such example is the targeting of the very beginning of glycolysis, including glucose receptors and the very first enzyme in the glycolytic pathway. Preclinical studies have focused on the beneficial effects of therapeutically targeting immunometabolism via the glucose transporters (GLUT1 and, to a lesser extent, GLUT3). Its inhibition, in various labs, has been proven to demonstrate antiinflammatory effects by blockage of glycolysis induction. Full inhibition of glucose uptake is deadly, which can explain why none of the compounds have made it to the clinic so far; however, the number of emerging patents and small molecules targeting GLUT1 or dual GLUT1/GLUT3 indicates elevated current interest in modulation of glycolysis by targeting glucose uptake.

Hexokinase (HK) is an enzyme and the first step in glycolysis that catalyzes the phosphorylation of six-carbon sugars. Vidac Pharma is developing **VDA-1275**, a drug targeting HK2 preventing it from interacting with the voltage-dependent anion channel (VDAC) [8], which controls the passage of ions and metabolites between the mitochondria and the cytosol of cells. HK has different isoforms. HK1 is expressed widely to support glycolysis, for example, during anaerobic exercise, while the expression of HK2 is limited mostly to malignant tissues that overexpress HK2. Pharmacological inhibition of HK2 results in its translocation back into the cytosol, restoring cellular metabolism. In principle, this interaction is supposed to occur in cancer cells, but not others, as detachment of HK2 reduces glycolysis and triggers apoptosis in cancer cells, without affecting HK1-expressing normal cells. Currently, the drug is undergoing assessment in patients with early carcinoma and a lymphomatic form of skin cancer as part of a Phase II clinical study.

A prime example where we have harnessed the innate properties of endogenous metabolites to generate therapeutics is **dimethyl fumarate** (DMF), a methyl ester of the endogenous TCA cycle immunometabolite fumarate. Its mechanism of action involves the inhibition of glycolysis. DMF inhibits the glycolytic enzyme glyceraldehyde 3-phosphate dehydrogenase (GAPDH), suppressing aerobic glycolysis in myeloid and lymphoid cells, thereby limiting immune cell activation [9]. Originally identified as a treatment for psoriasis in 1959, DMF, marketed as Tecfidera, has been developed as an oral treatment by Biogen and was approved in 2013 by the US Food and Drug Administration (FDA) for multiple sclerosis (MS) and in 2017 by the EU for psoriasis. In line with its foundations spawning from an immunomodulatory metabolite, DMF therefore possesses immunomodulatory properties without causing immunosuppression. DMF also induces a disequilibrium in global T-cell numbers in MS, reducing memory T-cells and decreasing proinflammatory Th1/Th17 cells while increasing antiinflammatory Th2 cell numbers [10]. This results in shifting the profile of peripheral lymphocyte subsets toward an antiinflammatory genotype in MS patients which reduces the rate of MS relapse [11]. This is supported by DMF improving clinical scores in a mouse model of experimental autoimmune encephalomyelitis (which mimics MS) compared with wild-type control mice [9]. Furthermore, it was recently identified that DMF inhibits excessive type I interferon (IFN) production and signaling, resulting in the suppression of IFN- and tissue factor-mediated coagulation and thrombosis induced by bacterial or viral infections [12]. This has important potential clinical translation, as growing evidence indicates IFNs are important regulators of blood coagulation [13].

Therefore DMF acts broadly with multiple antiinflammatory effects. This may be in part due to DMF's innate electrophilicity, making it a potent cysteine-modifying agent. Thus DMF can covalently modify cysteine residues on proteins in a process termed succination. DMF blocks pyroptosis—a proinflammatory, lytic form of cell death—via succination of five cysteines on human gasdermin D (GSDMD) and ten cysteines on mouse GSDMD, forming S-(2-succinyl)-cysteine [14,15]. These include the cysteine residues, human Cys191 and mouse Cys192, which are critical for oligomerization of the N-terminal of GSDMD, with DMF subsequently protecting against LPS-induced lethality in vivo in mice [14]. DMF also succinates Cys151 on kelch-like ECH-associated protein 1 (KEAP1) in macrophages [16]. This activates the master regulator of the antioxidant response, nuclear factor erythroid-derived 2-related factor 2 (NRF2) [17], which is antiinflammatory and has been shown to suppress type I IFN signaling [18]. DMF also succinates JAK1 [19] and further blocks type I IFN in humans by targeting IRAK4-MyD88 interactions and IRAK4-mediated cytokine production in a Cys13-dependent manner [20]. In addition, DMF blocks activation of the NLRP3 inflammasome in a mouse model of experimental colitis via activation of NRF2 [21].

Collectively, this in turn brought interest into NRF2 as a therapeutic target and a transcription factor that is activated to inhibit inflammation. Since then, other antiinflammatory drugs have shown a potential to activate NRF2 which can transcriptionally regulate multiple genes that regulate production of mitochondrial ATP. A recent first-in-class drug which is an NRF2 activator and NF-kB inhibitor is Omaveloxolone (brand name Skyclarys®), developed by Reata Pharmaceuticals and then sold to Biogen. It was approved for medical use for the neurological indication Friedreich ataxia in the United States in 2023 and in the EU a year later, with potential to treat other diseases [22]. Omaveloxolone, in addition to the effects observed by commonly used antioxidants, can directly increase mitochondrial biogenesis and bioenergetics through NRF2 [22]. While evidence for the use of NRF2 activators for the treatment of inflammatory disorders and initiation of resolution of inflammation accumulates, preclinical work suggests that treatment of certain cancers can also benefit from the work on the development of NRF2 inhibitors.

While the aforementioned compounds inhibit various glycolytic enzymes to suppress glycolysis, enhancing glycolysis has also been proven to be beneficial in specific contexts. **Terazosin** (Hytrin) is an a1-adrenergic receptor antagonist that has been used since 1985 to treat high blood pressure and enlarged prostates in men. It has recently demonstrated efficacy in neurodegenerative diseases, by enhancing glycolysis and activation of phosphoglycerate kinase to produce ATP [23]. The working hypothesis is based on observations that the increase in energy availability in the brain may slow neurodegeneration processes, specifically via reductions in the accumulation of alpha-synuclein, a protein that causes neuronal death in neurodegenerative conditions such as Parkinson's disease. The neuroprotective effect of terazosin has been demonstrated in Parkinson's and potentially in dementia in preclinical and human studies [24]. This breakthrough data has caused enthusiasm and a positive shift toward drugs that enhance glycolysis among neurologists working on Parkinson's disease.

Pyruvate kinase is the enzyme involved in the last step of glycolysis which catalyzes the transfer of a phosphate group from phosphoenolpyruvate (PEP) to adenosine diphosphate (ADP), yielding pyruvate and ATP. **Mitapivat** (trade name Pyrukynd®), developed by Agios Pharmaceuticals, is a pyruvate kinase activator for the treatment of hemolytic anaemia in adults with pyruvate kinase deficiency (PKD) approved in 2022 by the FDA and the European Medicines Agency (EMA) in the EU as a first-in-class drug [25]. Unlike other cells, red blood cells (RBCs)—also called erythrocytes—rely mainly on anaerobic glycolysis for ATP production. In PKD, the shortage of ATP causes destruction of RBCs, leading to hemolytic anemia and ineffective erythropoiesis. Mitapivat has shown promising results in upregulating the pyruvate kinase enzyme, leading to increased ATP production.

Pyruvate kinase M2 (PKM2) is an isoenzyme of the glycolytic enzyme pyruvate kinase. An example of a clinical-stage PKM2 drug in development is **Etavopivat**, which has been developed by Forma Therapeutics (acquired by NovoNordisk in 2022) for sickle cell anemia and other blood disorders and is currently being tested in Phase III clinical trials [26]. In anemia, the body increases the production of 2,3-diphosphoglycerate (2,3-DPG), a glycolytic intermediate that helps transport oxygen into tissues, causing more defective hemoglobin to cluster. Reducing 2,3-DPG allows oxygen to better bind hemoglobin. Etavopivat activates metabolic energy causing 2,3-DPG levels to drop allowing stronger binding of oxygen to the faulty hemoglobin [27]. This prevents RBCs from taking on a sickle-like shape, thereby prolonging RBC survival and easing anemia symptoms.

Finally, a terminal product of glycolysis is lactate, an emerging immunomodulatory metabolite which is secreted by glycolytic cells. Lactate is the best known byproduct of glucose metabolism and specifically glycolysis. Monocarboxylate transporters (MCTs) are membrane proteins responsible for the transport of lactate, but also pyruvate and ketone bodies. The expression of MCTs is increased when glycolysis is induced, for example, in cancers and inflammation. Specifically, MCT1 has been on the radar of researchers since it is responsible for influx and efflux of lactate, while its expression is induced in cancer in inflammatory conditions. The dependence of cancer cells on glycolysis compared with normal cells provides a therapeutic niche to target MCT1.

AZD3965, developed by Astra Zeneca and currently being tested in Phase I clinical trials, is a selective and potent MCT1 inhibitor with activity against MCT2 but not MCT3/MCT4 and has demonstrated growth inhibition of various tumor cell lines, particularly lymphoma [28]. MCT1 is also expressed in normal tissues, but the aerobic glycolysis pathway is not a major component of energy production in most normal cells and therefore should be unaffected by selective MCT1 inhibition, reducing the likelihood of off-target toxicity [28]. The hypothesis behind the use of AZD3965 stems from the fact that inhibiting lactate transport out of cells via MCT1 would result in a feedback inhibition of glycolysis and a pH imbalance that may lead to cytotoxicity. Phase I results demonstrated target engagement concentrations at tolerable doses of AZD3965 in patients with advanced solid tumors, supporting further continuation of studies in cancer types expressing high MCT1 and low MCT4.

Targeting mitochondrial biology

Metformin is a clinically approved drug and a first-line treatment for type 2 diabetes. Metformin was first introduced to the market in Europe in the 1950s, and it took over 40 years for its approval in the USA by the FDA. Metformin is known to decrease glucose production in the liver and increase insulin levels, resulting in lower blood sugar levels. Similarly to DMF, metformin has broadly antiinflammatory properties that involve immunometabolic regulation. In 2000 it was identified that metformin suppresses oxidative phosphorylation by inhibiting mitochondrial complex I of the electron transport chain [29,30]. The net effect of this is that metformin limits NADH oxidation and TCA cycle flux, which results in decreased ATP synthesis within mitochondria. This elevates the AMP:ATP ratio, which in turn activates the master metabolic regulator AMP-activated protein kinase (AMPK) [31]. AMPK activation by metformin suppresses expression of the transcription factor sterol regulatory element-binding protein 1 (SREBP-1) [31], an insulin-dependent transcription factor that is elevated in type 2 diabetes and is associated with lipogenesis and insulin resistance. Additionally, metformin modulates metabolism via appetite suppression. It does this by elevating serum and hepatic levels of the appetite suppressor growth differentiation factor 15 (GDF15) [32,33], as well as increasing circulating levels of the recently characterized appetite-suppressing metabolite *N*-lactoyl phenylalanine [34,35]. These recent mechanistic studies identify metformin's immunometabolic regulation as a key component of its beneficial effects on body weight and energy balance.

Targeting the tricarboxylic acid cycle

The rapid expansion of the field of immunometabolism has brought with it manifold immunomodulatory roles for metabolites themselves, including those in the TCA cycle, which has focused interest on manipulating specific TCA cycle metabolites and intermediates for potential therapeutic benefit.

Isocitrate dehydrogenases 1 and 2 (IDH1/2) are metabolic enzymes that catalyze oxidative decarboxylation of isocitrate to a-ketoglutarate (a-KG) in the TCA cycle. IDH1/2 mutations have been reported to promote oncogenesis in various human cancers, including gliomas via increased glucose uptake and lactate production and generally induced glucose metabolism [36]. Mutations in IDH1 and IDH2 result in the aberrant conversion of a-KG to 2-hydroxyglutarate (2-HG), which subsequently leads to a cascade of detrimental cellular events, including impaired cellular differentiation and increased proliferation of malignant cells [37]. The ongoing development of drugs specifically targeting the mutant enzymes provides a precise treatment option with potentially fewer off-target effects compared with conventional therapies.

Vorasidenib, developed by Servier, was approved by the FDA for medical use in the United States in August 2024 for astrocytoma or oligodendroglioma with a susceptible IDH1/2 mutation [38]. The primary endpoint in the clinical study focused on efficacy of the compound and was the concentration of 2-HG measured from tumors. This was very important information for the whole immunometabolism field since it increases the significance of metabolites in biomedical research. 2-HG, as the main product of tumors with mutated IDH genes, induces global DNA hypermethylation and attenuates antitumor immunity resulting in induced tumor growth. Vorasidenib, a brain-penetrant pan-mutant IDH inhibitor, significantly reduced 2-HG levels resulting in tumor growth reduction [38]. Cytoplasmic mutant IDH1 and mitochondrial mutant IDH2 can switch to the other form when targeted by selective IDH1 or IDH2 drugs, justifying utilization of dual IDH1 and IDH2 inhibitors. **HMPL-306** is another novel dual inhibitor of IDH1 and IDH2 mutations, developed by Hutchison MediPharma for patients afflicted with various forms of cancer, most notably hematologic malignancies like acute myeloid leukemia (AML) and certain solid tumors, such as gliomas [39]. It is currently in Phase II of clinical trials. Similarly to Vorasidenib, HMPL-306 reduces the production of 2-HG, thereby alleviating its oncogenic effects and allowing the immune system to restore normal cellular processes [39]. Emphasizing IDH1/2 as a major current target of clinical interest, Daiichi Sankyo is developing **DS-1001b,** and AnHeart Therapeutics is developing **Safusidenib**, which are both brain-penetrant IDH1-mutant inhibitors for glioma patients. Both drugs are currently being assessed in Phase II clinical trials [40,41].

Devimistat (CPI-613) from Cornerstone Pharmaceuticals is a lipoic acid derivative which is broadly described as a TCA cycle inhibitor. It has been shown to inhibit pyruvate dehydrogenase resulting in a decrease in glycolysis [42]. Devimistat impairs ATP synthesis and induces mitochondrial reactive oxygen species and turnover consistent with mitophagy [43]. Mechanistically, it disrupts mitochondrial membrane potential and severely impairs mitochondrial respiration, resulting in cancer cell death independent of p53. Devimistat is undergoing four clinical Phase II trials and has been granted orphan drug designation by the FDA for the following indications: Burkitt's lymphoma, biliary tract cancer, soft tissue sarcoma, myelodysplastic syndrome (MDS), and peripheral T-cell lymphoma.

Metabolism as a portal to new therapeutics

We are now in an era where new examples of immunometabolic drugs entering clinical development are continuously unveiled (Fig. 12.1). This stems from the fact that in the last 20 years, cellular metabolism has become an integral part of basic immunology which explains underlying pathological processes in our bodies. We have experienced a rapid progression and acceptance that metabolic changes are the basis for many inflammatory diseases and cancer, and metabolism now sits at the forefront of immunology and cancer biomedical research. In the early 2000s, sequencing of the human genome promised us that it would help to find cures for all diseases but it has not. Targeting specific genes and proteins can fully treat only a handful of monogenic genetic disorders. We now know that most diseases appear to be regulated on the metabolic level; therefore most diseases require therapies that involve modulation of multiple pathways. By intervening in cellular metabolism, we have the capacity to shift the phenotype of multiple cell types and therefore target a broader spectrum of diseases and subsequently reach more patients. Nowadays, genetic screening seems to be important for personalized medicine in a sense of inclusion or exclusion criteria for clinical trials that benefit patients with specific mutations. A good example mentioned here is Vorasidenib which specifically targets a mutated form of an IDH1/2 enzyme.

Our description of most diseases has shifted toward their multifaceted character rather than simply trying to identify monogenic diseases. Experimental data continues to grow for the role of metabolites as instrumental immune players. While we are yet to witness the first approved drug developed in this way, studying metabolites can already enrich ideas in the search for novel biomarkers. This is the reason why improved tools and reagents developed by basic research on immunometabolism are crucial. Biomarkers used in hospitals require simplicity and accessibility. For metabolites to reach the clinical settings as biomarkers, interdisciplinary teams should be set up comprising clinicians, mathematicians, and bioinformaticians, as well as radiologists studying bioimaging to monitor metabolic changes driving diseases. Nowadays, a lot of discussion circles around the use of AI in biomedical research—in our opinion, one of the most needed tasks for AI would be to facilitate the understanding of metabolic networks. Such projects would be fundamental in expanding the knowledge of metabolites in health and disease. We are confident that research on metabolites will find applications in the faster diagnosis of the onset of certain diseases and help with patient stratification.

We have new therapies targeting glycolysis and the TCA cycle which have emerged using enzymes involved in these pathways as biologic targets. Some companies use metabolites that possess cytokine-like properties to form drug analogs—for example, Sitryx, in collaboration with Eli Lilly, currently has a Phase I program exploring itaconate mimetics for the treatment of autoimmune disorders. The most advanced drug candidate is **SYX-1042**, which is about to start Phase I [44]. Simultaneously, repurposing existing drugs with novel mechanism of actions involving cellular metabolism is taken as an approach by others. Establishing drugs discovery programs based on assays focused on cellular metabolic states can expand the list of new drugs even further. Each of these approaches builds immunometabolism as a new and emerging field in drug development. We have thus now entered into a new era, similar to when we realized that ATP mimetics can have profound cellular effects, which ultimately revolutionized the inhibition of kinases. Exciting.

Acknowledgments

The figure was created with BioRender.

References

[1] Zasłona Z, O'Neill LAJ. Cytokine-like roles for metabolites in immunity. Mol Cell 2020;78(5):814–23.
[2] Ward PS, Thompson CB. Metabolic reprogramming: a cancer hallmark even warburg did not anticipate. Cancer Cell 2012;21(3):297–308.
[3] Groheux D, Cochet A, Humbert O, Alberini JL, Hindié E, Mankoff D. ^{18}F-FDG PET/CT for staging and restaging of breast cancer. J Nucl Med 2016;57(Suppl 1):17S–26S.
[4] Sałyga A, Guzikowska-Ruszkowska I, Czepczyński R, Ruchała M. PET/MR-a rapidly growing technique of imaging in oncology and neurology. Nucl Med Rev Cent East Eur 2016;19(1):37–41.
[5] Jamar F, Buscombe J, Chiti A, Christian PE, Delbeke D, Donohoe KJ, et al. EANM/SNMMI guideline for 18F-FDG use in inflammation and infection. J Nucl Med 2013;54(4):647–58.
[6] Obi ON, Saketkoo LA, Russell AM, Baughman RP. Sarcoidosis: Updates on therapeutic drug trials and novel treatment approaches. Front Med (Lausanne) 2022;9:991783.
[7] Molecure S.A. Efficacy and Safety Study of OATD-01 in Patients With Active Pulmonary Sarcoidosis [Internet]. 2024. Report No.: NCT06205121. Available from: https://clinicaltrials.gov/study/NCT06205121?term = NCT06205121&rank = 1.
[8] Herzberg M., Becker O.M., Behar V., Yosef R., Dor-On E., Pahima H., et al. A novel chemical entity, that reverses Warburg metabolism by disrupting VDAC1/HK2 interaction through "Toposteric Effect" in Cancer. Research Square [Internet]. 2024; Available from: https://www.researchsquare.com/article/rs-4382720/v1.

[9] Kornberg MD, Bhargava P, Kim PM, Putluri V, Snowman AM, Putluri N, et al. Dimethyl fumarate targets GAPDH and aerobic glycolysis to modulate immunity. Science 2018;360(6387):449–53.

[10] Gross CC, Schulte-Mecklenbeck A, Klinsing S, Posevitz-Fejfár A, Wiendl H, Klotz L. Dimethyl fumarate treatment alters circulating T helper cell subsets in multiple sclerosis. Neurol Neuroimmunol Neuroinflamm 2016;3(1) e183.

[11] Mills EA, Ogrodnik MA, Plave A, Mao-Draayer Y. Emerging understanding of the mechanism of action for dimethyl fumarate in the treatment of multiple sclerosis. Front Neurol 2018;9:5.

[12] Ryan TAJ, Hooftman A, Rehill AM, Johansen MD, Brien ECO, Toller-Kawahisa JE, et al. Dimethyl fumarate and 4-octyl itaconate are anticoagulants that suppress Tissue Factor in macrophages via inhibition of Type I Interferon. Nat Commun 2023;14(1):3513.

[13] Ryan TAJ, O'Neill LAJ. An emerging role for type i interferons as critical regulators of blood coagulation. Cells 2023;12(5):778.

[14] Humphries F, Shmuel-Galia L, Ketelut-Carneiro N, Li S, Wang B, Nemmara VV, et al. Succination inactivates gasdermin D and blocks pyroptosis. Science 2020;369(6511):1633–7.

[15] Miglio G, Veglia E, Fantozzi R. Fumaric acid esters prevent the NLRP3 inflammasome-mediated and ATP-triggered pyroptosis of differentiated THP-1 cells. Int Immunopharmacol 2015;28(1):215–19.

[16] Brennan MS, Matos MF, Li B, Hronowski X, Gao B, Juhasz P, et al. Dimethyl fumarate and monoethyl fumarate exhibit differential effects on KEAP1, NRF2 activation, and glutathione depletion in vitro. PLoS One 2015;10(3) e0120254.

[17] Linker RA, Lee DH, Ryan S, van Dam AM, Conrad R, Bista P, et al. Fumaric acid esters exert neuroprotective effects in neuroinflammation via activation of the Nrf2 antioxidant pathway. Brain 2011;134(Pt 3):678–92.

[18] Ryan DG, Knatko EV, Casey AM, Hukelmann JL, Dayalan Naidu S, Brenes AJ, et al. Nrf2 activation reprograms macrophage intermediary metabolism and suppresses the type I interferon response. IScience 2022;25(2):103827.

[19] Schmitt A, Xu W, Bucher P, Grimm M, Konantz M, Horn H, et al. Dimethyl fumarate induces ferroptosis and impairs NF-κB/STAT3 signaling in DLBCL. Blood 2021;138(10):871–84.

[20] Zaro BW, Vinogradova EV, Lazar DC, Blewett MM, Suciu RM, Takaya J, et al. Dimethyl fumarate disrupts human innate immune signaling by targeting the IRAK4-MyD88 complex. J Immunol 2019;202(9):2737–46.

[21] Liu X, Zhou W, Zhang X, Lu P, Du Q, Tao L, et al. Dimethyl fumarate ameliorates dextran sulfate sodium-induced murine experimental colitis by activating Nrf2 and suppressing NLRP3 inflammasome activation. Biochem Pharmacol 2016;112:37–49.

[22] Pilotto F, Chellapandi DM, Puccio H. Omaveloxolone: a groundbreaking milestone as the first FDA-approved drug for Friedreich ataxia. Trends Mol Med 2024;30(2):117–25.

[23] Chen X, Zhao C, Li X, Wang T, Li Y, Cao C, et al. Terazosin activates Pgk1 and Hsp90 to promote stress resistance. Nat Chem Biol 2015;11(1):19–25.

[24] Simmering JE, Welsh MJ, Liu L, Narayanan NS, Pottegård A. Association of glycolysis-enhancing α-1 blockers with risk of developing Parkinson disease. JAMA Neurol 2021;78(4):407–13.

[25] Al-Samkari H, Galactéros F, Glenthøj A, Rothman JA, Andres O, Grace RF, et al. Mitapivat versus placebo for pyruvate kinase deficiency. N Engl J Med 2022;386(15):1432–42.

[26] Saraf SL, Hagar R, Idowu M, Osunkwo I, Cruz K, Kuypers FA, et al. Multicenter, phase 1 study of etavopivat (FT-4202) treatment for up to 12 weeks in patients with sickle cell disease. Blood Adv 2024;8(16):4459–75.

[27] Schroeder P, Fulzele K, Forsyth S, Ribadeneira MD, Guichard S, Wilker E, et al. Etavopivat, a pyruvate kinase activator in red blood cells, for the treatment of sickle cell disease. J Pharmacol Exp Ther 2022;380(3):210–19.

[28] Halford S, Veal GJ, Wedge SR, Payne GS, Bacon CM, Sloan P, et al. A phase I dose-escalation study of AZD3965, an oral monocarboxylate transporter 1 inhibitor, in patients with advanced cancer. Clin Cancer Res 2023;29(8):1429–39.

[29] El-Mir MY, Nogueira V, Fontaine E, Avéret N, Rigoulet M, Leverve X. Dimethylbiguanide inhibits cell respiration via an indirect effect targeted on the respiratory chain complex I. J Biol Chem 2000;275(1):223–8.

[30] Owen MR, Doran E, Halestrap AP. Evidence that metformin exerts its anti-diabetic effects through inhibition of complex 1 of the mitochondrial respiratory chain. Biochem J 2000;348(Pt 3):607–14.

[31] Zhou G, Myers R, Li Y, Chen Y, Shen X, Fenyk-Melody J, et al. Role of AMP-activated protein kinase in mechanism of metformin action. J Clin Invest 2001;108(8):1167–74.

[32] Day EA, Ford RJ, Smith BK, Mohammadi-Shemirani P, Morrow MR, Gutgesell RM, et al. Metformin-induced increases in GDF15 are important for suppressing appetite and promoting weight loss. Nat Metab 2019;1(12):1202–8.

[33] Coll AP, Chen M, Taskar P, Rimmington D, Patel S, Tadross JA, et al. GDF15 mediates the effects of metformin on body weight and energy balance. Nature 2020;578(7795):444–8.

[34] Scott B, Day EA, O'Brien KL, Scanlan J, Cromwell G, Scannail AN, et al. Metformin and feeding increase levels of the appetite-suppressing metabolite Lac-Phe in humans. Nat Metab 2024;6(4):651–8.

[35] Xiao S, Li VL, Lyu X, Chen X, Wei W, Abbasi F, et al. Lac-Phe mediates the effects of metformin on food intake and body weight. Nat Metab 2024;6(4):659–69.

[36] Parsons DW, Jones S, Zhang X, Lin JCH, Leary RJ, Angenendt P, et al. An integrated genomic analysis of human glioblastoma multiforme. Science 2008;321(5897):1807–12.

[37] Han S, Liu Y, Cai SJ, Qian M, Ding J, Larion M, et al. IDH mutation in glioma: molecular mechanisms and potential therapeutic targets. Br J Cancer 2020;122(11):1580–9.

[38] Mellinghoff IK, van den Bent MJ, Blumenthal DT, Touat M, Peters KB, Clarke J, et al. Vorasidenib in IDH1- or IDH2-mutant low-grade glioma. N Engl J Med 2023;389(7):589–601.

[39] Hutchison M.P. A Study of HMPL-306 in Advanced Solid Tumors With IDH Mutations [Internet]. 2024. Report No: NCT04762602. Available from: https://clinicaltrials.gov/study/NCT04762602.

[40] Natsume A, Arakawa Y, Narita Y, Sugiyama K, Hata N, Muragaki Y, et al. The first-in-human phase I study of a brain-penetrant mutant IDH1 inhibitor DS-1001 in patients with recurrent or progressive IDH1-mutant gliomas. Neuro Oncol 2023;25(2):326–36.

[41] Cain SA, Topp M, Rosenthal M, Tobler R, Freytag S, Best SA, et al. A perioperative study of Safusidenib in patients with IDH1-mutated glioma. Future Oncol 2024;1–12.

[42] Zachar Z, Marecek J, Maturo C, Gupta S, Stuart SD, Howell K, et al. Non-redox-active lipoate derivates disrupt cancer cell mitochondrial metabolism and are potent anticancer agents in vivo. J Mol Med (Berl) 2011;89(11):1137–48.

[43] Anderson R, Miller LD, Isom S, Chou JW, Pladna KM, Schramm NJ, et al. Phase II trial of cytarabine and mitoxantrone with devimistat in acute myeloid leukemia. Nat Commun 2022;13(1):1673.

[44] Sitryx. Pipeline [Internet]. [cited 2024 3]. Available from: https://www.sitryx.com/pipeline.

Index

Note: Page numbers followed by "*f*," "*t*," and "*b*" refer to figures, tables, and boxes, respectively.

A

Adaptive immune response, 157
  adenosine triphosphate (ATP), 157–158
  antigen-presenting cells, 158
  CD4$^+$ T cells
    metabolism of Tfh cells, 172–173
    metabolism of Th1 cells, 167
    metabolism of Th2 cells, 168–169
    metabolism of Th9 T cells, 169–170
    metabolism of Th17 T cells, 170–171
    metabolism of Treg cells, 164–166
    OXPHOS capacity, 165
    targeting Tfh cells, 173
    targeting Th1 cells, 168
    targeting Th2 cells, 169
    targeting Th17 cells, 171–172
    targeting Treg metabolism, 166–167
  CD8$^+$ T cells
    amino acid metabolism, 161
    effector and memory, 162–163
    fatty-acid metabolism, 161
    mitochondrial metabolism, 160
    Naive T cell metabolism, 158–159
    phosphoenolpyruvate (PEP), 160
    scavenge nucleotides, 160
    T cell activation, 159
  T cell exhaustion, 163–164
  humoral immunity
    B cell activation, 175–176
    B cell development, 174–175
    germinal center reaction, 176–178
Adenosine triphosphate (ATP), 157–158
Adipose tissue macrophages (ATMs), 42–43, 238–239
Amino acid L-arginine, 199
Amino acid metabolites
  arginase, 116
  arginine metabolism in immune cells, 115–116
  glutamine, 117
  homocysteine, 118
  inducible NOS (iNOS), 115
  tryptophan (Trp), 116–117
AMP-activated protein kinase (AMPK), 27–28
Antiaging drug discovery
  cellular metabolism, 211
  challenges and future directions, 221
  genomic analysis, 210
  immunometabolism, 209–210
  machine learning, 212–213
  metabolomics and metabolite profiling
    in aging diseases, 217–218
    sphingomyelin pathway, AD, 219
  overlapping mechanisms, 213–214
  overview, 209–210
  scRNA-seq data, 212
  senolytic biomarkers and drug discovery
    proteomic technologies, 215–216
    senescence associated proteins, 215
    senescence-associated secretory phenotype, 215
    senotherapeutics and aging, 214
  system-level drug repurposing approach, 212
  transcriptomics, 211–214
Antiinflammatory metabolites, 19–20
Antiinflammatory responses, blocking, 142–144
Apoptotic peptidase activating factor-1 (APAF-1), 64–65
Arachidonate 12-lipoxygenase (ALOX12), 68
Arginase, 116
Arginine metabolism in immune cells, 115–116
Atherosclerotic cardiovascular disease (ASCVD), 109–110
Atherosclerotic plaques, 110–111
ATP-binding cassette transporter G2 (ABCG2), 138–139
AZD3965, 269

B

B cell activation, 175–176
B cell development, 174–175
Bacterial infection, 9
Bioinformatics, 219–221

Body weight homeostasis and thermogenesis
  central modulation, 228–229
  sympathetic nervous system, 229–231, 232f
  white, brown and beige adipocytes, 231–233
Branched-chain amino acid (BCAA)-derived metabolites, 33
Bronchoalveolar lavage (BAL) fluid, 8
Butyrate and propionate, 120

C

CARD domain of caspase-11, 146
Cardiovascular diseases (CVDs)
  amino acid metabolites
    arginase, 116
    arginine metabolism in immune cells, 115–116
    glutamine, 117
    homocysteine, 118
    inducible NOS (iNOS), 115
    tryptophan (Trp), 116–117
  atherosclerotic plaques, 110–111
  cholesterol and lipid metabolites, 111–113
  eicosanoids, 112–113
  glucose metabolism and metabolites, 113–115
  glycation end products, 113
  HIF1α expression, 114
  lactate, 114
  low-density lipoproteins, 111–112
  pentose phosphate pathway (PPP), 115
  PKM2, 113–114
  immune cell metabolism, 111
  immune cells in, 109–110
  short-chain fatty acids (SCFAs), 120
  tricarboxylic acid cycle
    itaconate, 119
    succinate, 118–119
CD4$^+$ T cells
  metabolism of Tfh cells, 172–173
  metabolism of Th1 cells, 167
  metabolism of Th2 cells, 168–169
  metabolism of Th9 T cells, 169–170
  metabolism of Th17 T cells, 170–171
  metabolism of Treg cells, 164–166
  OXPHOS capacity, 165
  targeting Tfh cells, 173
  targeting Th1 cells, 168
  targeting Th2 cells, 169
  targeting Th17 cells, 171–172
  targeting Treg metabolism, 166–167
CD8$^+$ T cells
  amino acid metabolism, 161
  effector and memory, 162–163
  fatty-acid metabolism, 161
  mitochondrial metabolism, 160
  Naive T cell metabolism, 158–159
  phosphoenolpyruvate (PEP), 160
  scavenge nucleotides, 160
  T cell activation, 159
  T cell exhaustion, 163–164
Cellular metabolism, 211
Cellular metabolism pathways
  clinical biomarkers, 263–264, 265f
  drugs modulating glycolysis, 266–269
  mitochondrial biology, 269–270
  overview, 263
  portal to new therapeutics, 271–272
  targeting and manipulating immunometabolism, 264–266
  tricarboxylic acid cycle, 270–271
Ceramide, 218
CF transmembrane conductance regulator (CFTR), 11–12
CFTR-PTEN interaction, 11–12
Cholesterol metabolites
  eicosanoids, 112–113
  glucose metabolism and metabolites, 113–115
  glycation end products, 113
  HIF1α expression, 114
  lactate, 114
  low-density lipoproteins, 111–112
  pentose phosphate pathway (PPP), 115
  PKM2, 113–114
Citric acid cycle, 2–3
Class-switch recombination (CSR), 173–174
Constraint-based modeling
  single-cell RNA sequencing (scRNA-seq) data, 94–95
  tumor cells in preclinical settings, 92–93
COVID-19 pandemic, 4
Cytokine expression, 195
Cytokine secretion, 4
Cytokine secretion, immunometabolites
  IL-1β secretion, 191
  T cell cytokines, 199–201
  myeloid cell–derived metabolites, 201
  T cell-derived metabolites, 199–200
  Tumor cell-derived metabolites, 200–201
  TNF-α and IL-6, 195–196
  type I interferons, 196–199

D

Damage-associated molecular patterns (DAMPs)
  activated phagocytes, 130
  extracellular metabolites function
    block antiinflammatory responses, 142–144
    early metabolic reprogramming, 142–144
    high mobility group box 1 (HMGB1), 141
    lipids, 142
    oxPAPC modulates phagocytic responses, 142, 143f

oxPLs and hyperinflammation, 145–146
oxPLs and modulation of long-term metabolic process, 144–145
intracellular homeostasis, 129–130
intracellular metabolites function, 130–141
  depression of ETC activity, 131
  fumarate, 135–136
  immunomodulatory metabolites, 140–141
  itaconate, 136–139
  metabolites and derivatives, 139–140
  mitochondrial metabolites, 131
  succinate, 132–135
  tricarboxylic acid (TCA) cycle, 131
mitochondria, 132
pattern-recognition receptors (PRRs), 129
succinate's systemic signaling, 134
Devimistat (CPI-613), 271
Dihydroorotate dehydrogenase (DHODH), 168
Dimethyl fumarate (DMF), 266–267
DON treatment, 92

E

Early metabolic reprogramming, 142–144
Eicosanoids, 112–113
18F-FDG glucose analog, 263–264
Electron transport chain (ETC), 73–74
Endosomal sorting complex required for transport (ESCRT), 146
endothelial NOS (eNOS), 115
Eosinophils, 239–240
ESKAPE pathogens, 7–8, 20

Extracellular metabolites function, DAMPs
  blocking antiinflammatory responses, 142–144
  early metabolic reprogramming, 142–144
  high mobility group box 1 (HMGB1), 141
  lipids, 142
  oxPAPC modulates phagocytic responses, 142, 143f
  oxPLs and hyperinflammation, 145–146
  oxPLs and modulation of long-term metabolic process, 144–145

F

Fast tINIT (ftINIT), 91
Fatty acid oxidation (FAO), 40–41
Ferroptosis, 67–68
Fumarate
  accumulation, 71
  as damage-associated molecular pattern, 135–136
  pyroptosis by, 70–71, 72f

G

Gasdermin D, 194
GEM-based modeling approach, 95
General control nonderepressible 2 (GCN2), 38
Genome-scale metabolic models, 90, 90f
  constraint-based modeling, 90–92
  DON treatment, 92
Genome-wide association study (GWAS), 210–211
Germinal center reaction, 176–178
Glucose utilization, 15
Glutamine, 117
Glutaminolysis, 171
Glycolysis, 15
Glycolytic metabolism, 40–41
Granulocyte-macrophage colony-stimulating factor (GM-CSF), 40

H

Hemophilus influenzae, 8
Hereditary leiomyomatosis and renal cell carcinoma (HLRCC), 197
Heterozygous germline mutations, 200–201
Hexokinase (HK), 266
HIF1α deletion, 114
High mobility group box 1 (HMGB1), 141
Histone deacetylase (HDAC1) targets, 213
Homeostasis, 39–44
Homocysteine, 118
Host-microbe interactions
  bacterial infection, 9
  immunometabolites in infected airway, 8
  itaconate, 12, 17f
  Klebsiella pneumonia, 8
    antiinflammatory metabolites, 19–20
    clinical strains, 20
    in lungs, 18–19
    type 6 secretion system, 20–21
  overview, 7–8
  Pseudomonas aeruginosa
    biofilms in response to itaconate, 12–13
    succinate in lung, 10–12
    transcription factor RpoN, 13–14
  pulmonary immunometabolites, 9
  Staphylococcus aureus, 14–15
    airway immunometabolites, 14–15
    biofilm production, 16–18
    glucose utilization, 15
    glycolysis, 15
    neutrophils, 16
    proline, 15
    succinate, 9–10
Human plasma-like media (HPLM), 82–83
Humoral immunity
  B cell activation, 175–176
  B cell development, 174–175
  germinal center reaction, 176–178

Hypercholesterolemia, 44
Hyperglycemia, 114
Hypoxia-inducible factors (HIFs), 110

I

Immune cells, 83–89
Immunometabolic pathways, 4
Immunometabolism, 2–4, 209–210, 235–240
  adipose tissue macrophages, 238–239, 242f
  aging effect on lipolysis, 239
  eosinophils, 239–240
  LepR$^+$ SPCs and IL-33, 244–248
  sympathetic perineurial cell barrier, 249–251
Immunometabolites, cytokine secretion
  IL-1β secretion, 191
  T cell cytokines, 199–201
    myeloid cell–derived metabolites, 201
    T cell–derived metabolites, 199–200
    Tumor cell-derived metabolites, 200–201
  TNF-α and IL-6, 195–196
  type I interferons, 196–199
Inducible NOS (iNOS), 115
Inflammation drivers, 42–44
Influenza A virus (IAV) infection, 140
Intracellular metabolites function, DAMPs
  depression of ETC activity, 131
  fumarate, 135–136
  immunomodulatory metabolites, 140–141
  itaconate, 136–139
  metabolites and derivatives, 139–140
  mitochondrial metabolites, 131
  succinate, 132–135
  tricarboxylic acid (TCA) cycle, 131
Ischemia-reperfusion injury (IRI), 134

Itaconate, 119
  as damage-associated molecular pattern, 136–139
  in immunoregulation, 12
  itaconation, 71–73, 73f
  P. aeruginosa biofilms formation in response to, 12–13

J

JAK/STAT signaling, 97–98

K

Klebsiella pneumonia, 8
  antiinflammatory metabolites, 19–20
  clinical strains, 20
  in lungs, 18–19
  type 6 secretion system, 20–21

L

Lactate, 114
  functions, 200
Large language models (LLM), 101
Legionella pneumophila, 32–33
LepR$^+$ SPCs and IL-33, 244–248
Leucyl-tRNA synthetase (LARS), 30–32
Limited proteolysis coupled to mass spectrometry (LiP-MS), 215–216
Lipid metabolites
  eicosanoids, 112–113
  glucose metabolism and metabolites, 113–115
  glycation end products, 113
  HIF1α expression, 114
  lactate, 114
  low-density lipoproteins, 111–112
  pentose phosphate pathway (PPP), 115
  PKM2, 113–114
Lipids, 142
Low-density lipoproteins, 111–112
Lysophosphatidylcholine (LPC), 111–112

M

Machine learning, 212–213
Macrophages
  ferroptosis, 67–68
  itaconation, 71–73, 73f
  metabolic regulation of cell death, 70
  metabolic state, 63
  mitochondrial reactive oxygen, 73–74
  phenotype plasticity, 2
  programmed cell death, 63–67, 64f
  pyroptosis by fumarate, 70–71, 72f
  tricarboxylic acid (TCA) cycle, 69
  tumor necrosis factor (TNF), 65
  Warburg effect, 69–70
Membrane trafficking, 35–36
Metabolic and innate immune signaling
  mTORC1, 30–33
  sterol regulatory element-binding proteins, 35–37
Metabolic and innate sensing pathways, 28–29, 28f
Metabolism
  of CD4$^+$ T cells
    Tfh cells, 172–173
    Th1 cells, 167
    Th2 cells, 168–169
    Th9 T cells, 169–170
    Th17 T cells, 170–171
    Treg cells, 164–166
  of CD8$^+$ T cells
    amino acid, 161
    fatty-acid, 161
    mitochondrial, 160
    Naive T cell, 158–159
  Naive T cell, 158–159
  in oncology
    applying metabolic models, 98–99
    CD4 T cells, 85–86
    CD8 T cells, 84–85
    computational models, 89–90
    CRISPR screens, 82–83

immune cells and stromal cells, 83–89
lymphocyte metabolism, 97
muon framework, 98
myeloid-derived suppressor cells, 87–89
natural killer (NK) cells, 87
single-cell metabolic modeling, 95–98
T regulatory cells, 86–87
target discovery and clinical development, 99–101
therapeutic avenue, 81
tumor-associated macrophages (TAMs), 87–89
uncovering potential targets, 82–83
revolution, 1
Metabolite profiling, 216–219
Metabolites, 27–30
in aging diseases, 217–218
Metabolome profiling strategies, 82b
METAflux, 94–95
Metformin, 269–270
Microbiota-derived metabolites, 41
Microenvironmental nutrient sensing, 42–43, 43f
Mitochondrial outer membrane permeabilization (MOMP), 64–65
Mitogen-activated protein kinase (MAPK) pathway, 28–29
Mitokines, 131
Mixed lineage kinase-like (MLKL), 65
mROS-induced palmitoylation, 74, 75f
mTORC1, 30–33
Myeloid cell–derived metabolites, 201
Myeloid cells, 29
functional programs in, 31f
in stress response, 37–39
Myeloid derived suppressor cells (MDSCs), 19, 35, 87–89

N

Na^+/dicarboxylate cotransporter (NaDC3), 138–139
Naive T cell metabolism, 158–159
National Center for Biotechnology Information's (NCBI), 3–4
Natural killer (NK) cells, 87
Necroptosis, 65–66
Neuroimmunometabolism, obesity
body weight homeostasis and thermogenesis
central modulation, 228–229
sympathetic nervous system, 229–231, 232f
white, brown and beige adipocytes, 231–233
immunometabolism, 235–240
adipose tissue macrophages, 238–239, 242f
aging effect on lipolysis, 239
eosinophils, 239–240
LepR$^+$ SPCs and IL-33, 244–248
sympathetic perineurial cell barrier, 249–251
macrophages role in insulin resistance, 236–239
neuroendocrine-immunometabolomic gap, 240–251
sympathetic perineurial cells, 241–244
overview, 227–228
Neutrophils, 16
NF-kB proinflammatory signaling, 10–11
NIMA-related kinase 7 (NEK-7), 71–72
Ninjurin-1 (NINJ1), 66–67

O

Obesity, (neuro) immunometabolism
body weight homeostasis and thermogenesis
central modulation, 228–229
sympathetic nervous system, 229–231, 232f
white, brown and beige adipocytes, 231–233
immunometabolism, 235–240
adipose tissue macrophages, 238–239, 242f
aging effect on lipolysis, 239
eosinophils, 239–240
LepR$^+$ SPCs and IL-33, 244–248
sympathetic perineurial cell barrier, 249–251
macrophages role in insulin resistance, 236–239
neuroendocrine-immunometabolomic gap, 240–251
sympathetic perineurial cells, 241–244
overview, 227–228
Oncogenic cancer cells, 68
Oncology, metabolism in
applying metabolic models to clinical data, 98–99
CD4 T cells, 85–86
CD8 T cells, 84–85
computational models, 89–90
CRISPR screens, 82–83
immune cells and stromal cells, 83–89
lymphocyte metabolism, 97
muon framework, 98
myeloid-derived suppressor cells, 87–89
natural killer (NK) cells, 87
single-cell metabolic modeling, 95–98
T regulatory cells, 86–87
target discovery and clinical development, 99–101
therapeutic avenue, 81
tumor-associated macrophages (TAMs), 87–89
uncovering potential targets, 82–83
Outer mitochondrial membranes (OMMs), 74
Oxidative phosphorylation (OXPHOS), 3, 11–12, 20, 40

oxPAPC modulates phagocytic responses, 142, 143f
oxPLs and hyperinflammation, 145–146
oxPLs and modulation of long-term metabolic process, 144–145

P

Pathogen- or damage-associated patterns (PAMPS/DAMPS), 27
Pattern recognition receptors (PRRs), 27
Pentose phosphate pathway (PPP), 115
Peripheral blood mononuclear cell (PBMC), 98–99
Phagocytosis, 35–36
Phosphoenolpyruvate (PEP), 160
Programmed cell death, 63–67, 64f
Pro-inflammatory cytokines, 237
Pro-inflammatory functions, 44
Proline, 15
Protein kinase R-activated (PKR), 38
Protein kinase R-like ER kinase (PERK), 38
Proton motive force, 3
Pseudomonas aeruginosa
　biofilms in response to itaconate, 12–13
　infection fueled by succinate in lung, 10–12
　transcription factor RpoN, 13–14
PTPN2/N1 inhibitor, 99
Pyroptosis, 66
　regulation, by fumarate, 70–71, 72f
Pyruvate kinase, 268

R

RAVEN Toolkit, 92–93
Reactive oxygen species (ROS), 69
Receptor-interacting protein kinase 1 (RIPK1), 65
Reverse electron transport (RET), 134
RIG-I-like receptors (RLRs), 199
RNA GEM customization, 93f

S

scRNA-seq data, 212
Seahorse technology, 3–4
Senolytic biomarkers and drug discovery
　proteomic technologies, 215–216
　senescence associated proteins, 215
　senescence-associated secretory phenotype, 215
　senotherapeutics and aging, 214
Short-chain fatty acids (SCFAs), 120
Single cell spatially resolved metabolic (scSpaMet) framework, 100–101
Single nucleotide polymorphisms (SNPs), 210–211
Single-cell RNA sequencing (scRNA-seq) data, 94–95, 94t
Sphingomyelin pathway, AD, 219
SREBP signaling, 37
SREBP-dependent lipid metabolism, 40
Stability of proteins from rates of oxidation (SPROX), 215–216
Staphylococcus aureus, 2
　airway immunometabolites, 14–15
　biofilm production, 16–18
　glucose utilization, 15
　glycolysis, 15
　neutrophils, 16
　proline, 15
Sterol regulatory element-binding proteins (SREBPs), 29–30, 35–37
Stress response in myeloid cells, 37–39
Stromal cells, 83–89

Succinate
　as damage-associated molecular pattern, 132–135
　P. aeruginosa infection fueled by, 10–12
　and pathogenesis of bacterial infection, 9–10
　in pathogenesis of cardiovascular disease, 118–119
　systemic signaling, 134
Sympathetic nervous system, 229–231, 232f
Sympathetic perineurial cells (SPCs), 241–244
　barrier, 249–251
System-level drug repurposing approach, 212

T

T cell cytokines
　myeloid cell–derived metabolites, 201
　T cell-derived metabolites, 199–200
　tumor cell-derived metabolites, 200–201
T cell-derived metabolites, 199–200
T regulatory cells, 86–87
Targeting $CD4^+$ T cells
　Tfh cells, 173
　Th1 cells, 168
　Th2 cells, 169
　Th17 cells, 171–172
　Treg metabolism, 166–167
TCA cycle-derived metabolites, 133f
Ten-eleven translocation (TET) family, 165
Terazosin (Hytrin), 268
Thermogenesis and body weight homeostasis
　central modulation, 228–229
　sympathetic nervous system, 229–231, 232f
　white, brown and beige adipocytes, 231–233
Tissue microenvironment, 39

Tissue-resident macrophages (TRMs), 39
Tissue-resident myeloid cells, 29
TNF-induced cell death, 82–83
Toll-like receptor 4 (TLR4), 130–131
Trafficking myeloid cells, 29
Transcription factor E (TFE), 32
Transcription factor EB (TFEB), 139
Transcriptomics, 211–214
Transferrin receptor 1 (TfR1), 68
Transmembrane protein 30A (TMEM30A), 145–146
Tricarboxylic acid (TCA) cycle, 2–3, 69, 131
   intermediates, 118–119
   itaconate, 119
   succinate, 118–119
   targeting, 270–271
Tryptophan (Trp), 116–117
Tumor cell-derived metabolites, 200–201
Tumor interstitial fluid (TIF), 88
Tumor necrosis factor (TNF), 65
Tumor-associated macrophages (TAMs), 87–89
Type I interferons, 196–199
Type 6 secretion system, 20–21

V

Vascular cell adhesion molecule-1 (VCAM-1), 120
Ventilator-associated pneumonias (VAP), 7–8
Viral exposure, 40–41
Vorasidenib, 270

W

Warburg effect, 2, 69–70
White adipose tissue (WAT), 42–43

Printed in the United States
by Baker & Taylor Publisher Services

BREEDING DISEASE-RESISTANT HORTICULTURAL CROPS

BREEDING DISEASE-RESISTANT HORTICULTURAL CROPS

PAUL W. BOSLAND
Plant & Environmental Sciences Department, New Mexico State University (NMSU), Las Cruces, NM, United States

DEREK W. BARCHENGER
Scientist-Pepper Breeding, World Vegetable Center, Tainan, Taiwan

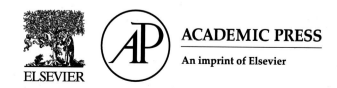

Academic Press is an imprint of Elsevier
125 London Wall, London EC2Y 5AS, United Kingdom
525 B Street, Suite 1650, San Diego, CA 92101, United States
50 Hampshire Street, 5th Floor, Cambridge, MA 02139, United States
The Boulevard, Langford Lane, Kidlington, Oxford OX5 1GB, United Kingdom

Copyright © 2024 Elsevier Inc. All rights reserved.

No part of this publication may be reproduced or transmitted in any form or by any means, electronic or mechanical, including photocopying, recording, or any information storage and retrieval system, without permission in writing from the publisher. Details on how to seek permission, further information about the Publisher's permissions policies and our arrangements with organizations such as the Copyright Clearance Center and the Copyright Licensing Agency, can be found at our website: www.elsevier.com/permissions.

This book and the individual contributions contained in it are protected under copyright by the Publisher (other than as may be noted herein).

Notices

Knowledge and best practice in this field are constantly changing. As new research and experience broaden our understanding, changes in research methods, professional practices, or medical treatment may become necessary.

Practitioners and researchers must always rely on their own experience and knowledge in evaluating and using any information, methods, compounds, or experiments described herein. In using such information or methods they should be mindful of their own safety and the safety of others, including parties for whom they have a professional responsibility.

To the fullest extent of the law, neither the Publisher nor the authors, contributors, or editors, assume any liability for any injury and/or damage to persons or property as a matter of products liability, negligence or otherwise, or from any use or operation of any methods, products, instructions, or ideas contained in the material herein.

ISBN: 978-0-443-15278-8

For Information on all Academic Press publications
visit our website at https://www.elsevier.com/books-and-journals

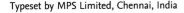

Publisher: Nikki P. Levy
Acquisitions Editor: Nancy J. Maragioglio
Editorial Project Manager: Dan Egan
Production Project Manager: Rashmi Manoharan
Cover Designer: Miles Hitchen

Typeset by MPS Limited, Chennai, India

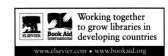

Contents

Preface xi

1 Introduction to breeding disease-resistant horticultural plants 1
Overview 1
Historical perspective 7
Koch's postulates 8
Terminology 13
A list of principal terms 13
References 17
Further reading 17

2 Resistance: the phenotype 21
Nonhost (innate) resistance 22
Plant defense to *Botrytis cinerea* 25
Effectors 30
Hypersensitive response 37
Systemic acquired resistance (SAR) 40
Induced systemic resistance 42
Cross-protection 44
Manipulation of plant architecture 46
Age-related resistance 51
Bibliography 57

3 Resistance: the genotype 67
Gene-for-gene theory 67
Lock and key concept 68
Nucleotide-binding and leucine-rich repeat receptors 69
Helper nucleotide-binding leucine-rich repeats 70
Classes of disease resistance (R) proteins 71
Quantitative disease resistance 73
Six characteristics of quantitative disease resistance 77
Marker-assisted selection 78
Loss-of-susceptibility concept 80
Inhibitor genes 84

Cytoplasmic inheritance 85
Resistance models 86
Molecular analysis 88
Bibliography 89

4 Resistance: the pathogen 97
Introduction 97
Pathogen acquisition and maintenance 98
Host differential 99
Culture collections 100
Specialized and working collections 101
Pathogenicity/virulence 102
Genetic variation of pathogens 103
Genetic variation of viroids and viruses 104
Genetic variation of bacteria 107
Genetic variation of oomycetes 113
Genetic variation of fungus 114
Bibliography 119

5 Resistance: the environmental interaction 127
Introduction 127
Protected cultivation 129
Growth chamber 130
Phytotron 131
Vertical farms 132
Environmental variables 135
Monitoring equipment 137
Relative humidity 138
Soil moisture 139
Light 140
Bibliography 141

6 Resistance: evaluating the interaction phenotype 145
Introduction 145
Disease screen/index 148
Evaluation of disease resistance 149
Quantifying host resistance 153

Scoring fatigue 156
Automated data collection 157
Area under the disease progress curve 161
Detached leaf screening 162
Rating scales 164
Statistics used for assessing disease resistance 167
Bibliography 169

7 Resistance sources 175
Natural sources of resistance 175
Species bridge 179
Embryo rescue 180
Germplasm repositories 181
Core collections 184
Mutation 186
Somaclonal variation 188
Genetic transformation 190
Bibliography 190

8 Resistance: Classical Breeding Methods 195
Introduction 195
Pure line selection 195
Single plant selection 196
Mass selection 196
Hybridization 196
Backcross method 197
Pedigree method 199
Recurrent selection 199
Somatic hybridization 199
Doubled haploids 201
Breeding symbols 201
Bibliography 203

9 Breeding for multiple disease resistance 205
Introduction 205
Interactions 206
Marker-assisted selection 210

Genome-wide association study 211
Marker serendipity 214
Disease-resistant rootstock 214
Bibliography 223

10 Resistance: biotechnology and molecular applications 227
Introduction 227
Tissue culture 228
Pyramiding resistance genes 229
Resistance gene analogs/comparative genetics/synteny 230
Pan-genomics 231
Direct gene transfer/transformation 232
Cisgenesis 234
CRISPR-Cas 9 system 235
Fungus-resistant GMO plants 236
Viral cross-protection 236
Metabolic engineering 237
Future of GMO and disease resistance 238
Bibliography 239

11 Resistance: gene deployment—durable resistance 245
Introduction 245
Emerging disease 251
Systems approach 252
Wise resistance management 254
Principles of disease control 255
Multilines 255
Anticipatory breeding/preemptive breeding 257
Evolutionary forces 257
Bibliography 259

12 Resistance: plant-parasitic nematodes 263
Introduction 263
Genetic variation for resistance 266
Evaluating the interaction phenotype 268
Sources of resistance 270
Biotechnology approaches to plant-parasitic nematode control 271

RNAi-based nematode resistance 272
Breeding for multiple pest resistance 275
Nematode-resistant rootstocks 276
Conclusion 278
Bibliography 280

Index 283

Preface

This book evolved from a course taught for more than three decades by P.W. Bosland at the New Mexico State University. On the first day of class the students hear that nothing will be harder for them in their careers as plant breeders than breeding disease-resistant plants. This is one area of plant breeding where understanding the genotype by environment interaction is crucial and essential; then add another layer of complexity, the genetic diversity of the pathogen causing the disease, and here is a relationship between a plant and a pathogen that is extraordinarily complex.

Breeding disease-resistant plants is not an end-all, but a beginning because of the ability of pathogens to overcome a plant's resistance. Plants and pathogens interact on a physical, chemical, and molecular level and changes in the genetics of either affect their interaction. With resistance, this results in a constant battle in which the pathogen evolves to overcome the resistance, instigating what has been called an evolutionary arms race between the pathogen and the plant. Depending on the complexity of the interaction between the pathogen and the host, the resistance may lose its efficacy rapidly or be durable through time.

In addition, climate change will affect durable resistance in crops and will require both a greater knowledge of pathogen population dynamics and plant host responses to temperature by the plant breeder. The alarming spread of devastating diseases, such as the bacterium *Xylella fastidiosa* that attacks olives (*Olea europaea*) and woody crops in southern Europe and the United States, or the *ug99* strain of stem rust fungus *Puccinia graminis* f. sp. *tritici* that affects wheat (*Triticum aestivum*) across parts of Africa, Asia, and the Middle East is attributed in part to warmer climates and presents a complex biogeographical and epidemiological problem. Because the environment plays a significant role in the development of disease and conversely the manifestation of resistance, changes in temperature can cause shifts from the resistant phenotype to a susceptible phenotype.

Another recent example is *Fusarium oxysporum* f. sp. *apii* race 4, a pathogen of celery (*Apium graveolens* var. *dulce*) that causes an emerging disease in California, United States. In approximately 2013 *F. oxysporum* f. sp. *apii* race 4 was noticed. This is highly aggressive at temperatures above 22°C. It has been spreading its geographic distribution within California and currently cannot be controlled via either host resistance or economical methods that reduce the pathogen abundance in infested soil. Although the organism *F. oxysporum* f. sp. *apii* has long been recognized, it is not as well-known as other forma speciales, such as f. sp. *lycopersici* on tomato (*Solanum lycopersicum*), f. sp. *cubense* on banana (*Musa acuminata*), and f. sp. *conglutinans* on cabbage (*Brassica oleracea* var. *capitata*). Lynn Epstein at the University of California-Davis believes that climate change will likely exacerbate Fusarium wilt disease severity and incidence in coastal California. At temperatures between 22°C and 26°C, *F. oxysporum* f. sp. *apii* race 4 is more aggressive than *F. oxysporum* f. sp. *apii* race 2, leading to the conclusion that the predicted climate change in California will increase the *F. oxysporum* f. sp. *apii* race 4 disease threat. Furthermore, climate change in California will also have a significant impact on the growth of multiple pathogens and consequently the need for disease-resistant crops in California.

Successful breeding for disease resistance is paramount for sustainable food production. Furthermore, a disease-resistant plant makes it possible to avoid or lessen the use of pesticides. Breeding disease-resistant plants can be considered a form of biological control, and their use is the first step in an integrated disease management program. Disease-resistant horticultural plants are a cornerstone of best management practices for organic growers. The development of disease-resistant plants is approached through both conventional breeding, where resistant traits are selected and incorporated into breeding lines over multiple generations, and through genetic engineering where genes for resistance are introduced into the plant genome. It is important to place breeding disease-resistant plants into the perspective of the whole cropping system. Resistance alone is not the sole means to achieve a disease-free crop and may lead to a rapid loss of the function of the resistance genes. One must use a resistant cultivar as part of an integrated system of production management.

Succinctly, one can say resistance is the absence of susceptibility, but it turns out not to be so simple or rational. There are a multitude of avenues to reach the phenotype called "resistant." However, growers see the concept of resistance and susceptibility as two sides of the same coin. Nevertheless, the importance of breeding disease-resistance plants cannot be overstated. The ever-growing world population plus rapidly evolving pathogen populations have increased the urgency of this task.

Introduction to breeding disease-resistant horticultural plants

Overview

US President Thomas Jefferson famously said, "the greatest service which can be rendered any country is to add a useful plant to its culture." Today, one can further elaborate adding "a disease-resistant plant is a godsend to a farmer." The Food and Agriculture Organization of the United Nations (FAO) estimates that between 20 and 40% of global crop yields are lost each year due to the damage wrought by plant pests and diseases. Whether it is a highly virulent strain of bacterial wilt of tomato (*Ralstonia solanacearum*), late blight of potato (*Phytophthora infestans*), or Panama disease (*Fusarium oxysporum* f.sp. *cubensis*) threatening banana (*Musa acuminata*) fields, disease is historically a multifarious menace to crop production.

Great strides have been made in developing disease-resistant horticultural cultivars that combine resistances to multiple diseases and pests. For example, a packet of tomato (*Solanum lycopersicum*) seeds may have the designation AVFFNT on it, indicating the cultivar has resistance to (A) anthracnose (*Colletotrichum phomoides*), (V) verticillium wilt (*Verticillium albo-atrum*), (FF) fusarium wilt (two races) (*F. oxysporum* f. sp. *lycopersici*), (N) nematodes (*Meloidogyne incognita*), and (T) tomato mosaic virus (ToMV; *Tobamovirus*). Other examples include garden pea (*Pisum sativum*), which may possess resistance to powdery mildew (*Erysiphe pisi*), fusarium wilt (*F. oxysporum* f. sp. *pisi*), pea enation mosaic virus (PEMV; *Enamovirus*), pea seedborne mosaic virus (PSbMV; *Potyvirus*), and bean leafroll virus (BLRV; *Luteovirus*), and cucumbers (*Cucumis sativus*) with resistance to angular leaf spot (*Pseudomonas syringae* pv. *lachrymans*), Alternaria leaf spot (*Alternaria alternata* f.sp. *cucurbitae*), anthracnose (*Colletotrichum orbiculare*), downy mildew (*Pseudoperonospora cubensis*), powdery mildew

(*Erysiphe cichoracearum*), Ulocladium leaf spot (*Ulocladium cucurbitae*), target spot (*Corynespora cassiicola*), scab (*Cladosporium cucumerinum*), cucumber mosaic virus (CMV, *Bromoviridae*), papaya ringspot virus (PRSV; *Potyvirus*), watermelon mosaic virus (WMV; *Potyvirus*), and zucchini yellow mosaic virus (ZYMV; *Potyvirus*).

There are still many disease challenges waiting for the plant breeder to conquer. As disease-resistant horticultural plants are deployed, evolution that is always occurring changes the pathogen population. Resistance makes it harder for the pathogen to survive and multiply, creating selection pressure for individuals in the pathogen population to develop novel ways to overcome the plant's resistance. It is said that a never-ending arms race drives coevolution between pathogen and host.

A second issue arises when crop production systems change. When cropping systems intensify and become more uniform, the microenvironment changes and pathogens may find a more optimal environment. For example, green bean (*Phaseolus vulgaris*) producers are using higher populations in the field to achieve higher yields, but greater plant densities create an environment favorable for white (*Sclerotinia sclerotiorum*) and gray mold (*Botrytis cinerea*).

Lastly, diseases can move to new locations by climatic events, such as typhoons, hurricanes, or transglobal winds; or with the assistance of animals, such as birds and most perilously humans moving seeds and plant parts. Viruses can be introduced by insect vectors spreading through a region. The oomycetes *P. infestans* that causes late blight on potatoes (*Solanum tuberosum*) can reproduce and spread both asexually (clonally) and sexually. Sexual reproduction occurs when induvial strains from different mating types (A1 and A2) are in proximity. While late blight has been present in the United States since at least the 1830s, there has historically been only one mating type (A1), so no sexual genetic recombination occurred. This made the pathogen remain uniform genetically, and resistance in the host remained effective and durable. In the 1990s, a new mating type (A2) arrived from Mexico, allowing for sexual recombination and the development of more virulent races.

An emerging viral threat to global tomato (*S. lycopersicum*) production is the tomato brown rugose fruit virus (ToBRFV, *Tobamovirus*). This is a new highly infectious virus that is currently causing great concern as it spreads to new tomato production areas. As stated earlier, monoculture conditions, intensive selection, international trade of infected propagating material and climate changes favor the rapid spread of new diseases. Among the different pathogens, viruses are the most threating, because of their rapid diffusion and production losses.

In 2015 ToBRFV was isolated for the first time in Jordan from greenhouse-grown tomato plants. The plants showed mild foliar symptoms and strong brown rugose symptoms on fruits, with a disease incidence close to 100%, suggesting a viral etiology based on symptoms. The tomato cultivars carrying the *Tm-2²* resistance gene that confers resistance to tobacco mosaic virus (TMV, *Tobamovirus*) and ToMV (*Tobamovirus*) showed mosaic patterns on leaves and occasionally narrowing of leaves and yellow-spotted fruits.

After the initial findings on tomato plants in Israel and Jordan, several reports were recorded in Europe, North America, Middle East, and Asia. Further concern about the tomato brown rugose fruit was raised when it was reported in pepper (*Capsicum* sp.) plants grown in Jordan, Italy, Turkey, Syria, and Lebanon. Since the first identification in 2015, laboratory inoculation experiments show that under certain circumstances, ToBRFV, can infect common grasses and weeds. Illustrating that weeds can act as a reservoir for the ToBRFV, which then could infect commercially cultivated crops. Weeds are often present in the production areas and, therefore, can act as potential sources of virus inoculum, representing a greater danger, especially if they are asymptomatic.

Dispersal of ToBRFV is mainly mechanical, but it can be carried for long distances, say from one country to another via contaminated seeds and fruits. During production, short-distance transmission occurs through infected propagation material, for example, cuttings and grafts. Direct plant-to-plant contact between an infected and a neighboring uninfected plant and in the process of ordinary cultivation practices, through wounds made to leaves or to the root system of seedlings. Infection can also happen through the transfer of infected sap from different surfaces, such as human body, clothes, work tools, gloves, shoes, and poles, as well as through irrigation or drainage water and/or nutrient solutions. Likewise, after harvesting, ToBRFV inoculum can remain infectious on surfaces and materials in a greenhouse, such as wires, glass, concrete, and soil. After transplanting in a greenhouse, only two infected plants are sufficient to reach a 100% infection rate because of the high plant-to-plant transmission rate.

The *Tm-2²* gene that for 50 years effectively controlled ToMV and TMV infections is ineffective against ToBRFV. Because the ToBRFV is capable of overcoming all known tobamovirus-resistance genes. Before ToBRFV, another tobamovirus that raised concern because of its rapid spread on resistant tomato genotypes was the tomato mottle mosaic virus (ToMMV, *Tobamovirus*), first described in 2013, infecting tomato crops in Mexico. It was subsequently found in the Americas, Asia, and Europe, causing infections on tomato and pepper crops. As ToMMV is an emerging virus with similarities to the ToBRFV, the European and Mediterranean Plant Protection Organization Panel on Phytosanitary Measures recommended that both be added to the European and Mediterranean Plant Protection Organization Alert List.

ToMMV raises less concern than tomato brown rugose fruit because some tomato genotypes were found to be totally resistant to ToMMV. In fact, an undefined genotype "E" of tomato, with resistance to ToMV and TMV, was also extremely resistant to ToMMV, although it is not specified in the work which tobamovirus-resistance gene is involved in the control of the virus.

Recently, Dr. Avner Zinger and colleagues (2021) at the Institute of Plant Sciences, Volcani Center, Israel, evaluated 160 genotypes for tolerance and resistance to ToBRFV, resulting in the identification of an unexpectedly high number of tolerant genotypes and a single genotype resistant to the virus. An analysis of the genetic inheritance revealed that a single recessive gene controls tolerance, whereas at least two genes control resistance.

The discovery of this resistance, determined by additive effects of a recessive gene and a dominant gene, represents a novelty in tomato genetics, because effective resistance to viruses described so far is controlled by single dominant genes, except for the resistance to Potato virus Y (PVY, *Potyviridae*) and tobacco etch virus (TEV, *Potyviridae*), both controlled by the same single recessive gene *pot-1*.

In the last few decades, ToMV, having spread rapidly throughout the world, has induced plant breeders to select tomato cultivars with genes of resistance to ToMV. This has led to the gradual abandonment of local cultivars. Similarly, the ToBRFV will motivate plant breeders to breed plants resistant to this pathogen.

Plant viruses spread by seed, such as ToBRFV, are particularly dangerous because of the possibility of long-distance movement of infected material in an extremely short time. Therefore suitable integrated management of ToBRFV requires monitoring of potential secondary hosts, hygiene, and prophylactic measures by agricultural personnel when handling plant material and other farm activities, followed by the removal of infected plants, and continuous monitoring of cultural practices. Unfortunately, even with the adoption of phytosanitary measures, ToBRFV was able to establish itself in production systems. Therefore the hope for the future is to introduce resistance of ToBRFV in tomato lines and hybrids, especially for those intended for cultivation in protected environments where the problem is particularly evident.

Resistance must not be observed as an "either—or" effect, rather it is a continuum of a resistance phenotype. The key take-home message for breeding disease-resistant horticultural plants is that components of resistance are like components of yield. Genes for yield do not exist per se; there are only genes for components of yield, and components of yield differ among crops. For example, the components of yield for sweet corn (*Zea mays*) depend on the number of plants per hectare, ears per plant, kernel rows per ear, kernels per row, and the kernel weight, while for peaches (*Prunus persica*), it depends on the weight of each fruit, number of flowers per fruiting shoot, number of fruiting shoots per branch, number of branches per tree, and the number of trees per hectare.

Similarly, genes for resistance differ among horticultural crops. While there are certain gene families that are often associated with host resistance, such as nucleotide-binding leucine-rich repeats (NB-LRR), there is no universal gene for resistance. There are genes that keep a pathogen from establishing itself on a plant, and these genes can be bred into a plant to make it a disease-resistant plant.

Breeding for disease-resistant horticultural crops is a broad concept. The first step is to learn everything about your crop. This includes production practices and quality components, the primary pathogens, and new and secondary pathogens that cause disease to the crop. There are many ways to learn this information. First is to attend everything from small meetings to large conferences dealing with the horticultural crop. With the advent of the internet, it has become easier to talk to people internationally. In fact, the best "reference library" is your computer and emailing colleagues, as they will know of new and evolving disease issues long before one reads about them in a scholarly journal.

A key step in setting up the disease-resistance breeding program is to set priorities; not every disease is an issue that must be addressed. For example, in New Mexico, USA, "chile wilt" caused by *Phytophthora capsici* is a prevalent disease, with every production field having the causal agent established in the soil. Breeding for disease-resistant chile peppers (*Capsicum annuum*) (Fig. 1.1) to phytophthora wilt is a major objective at

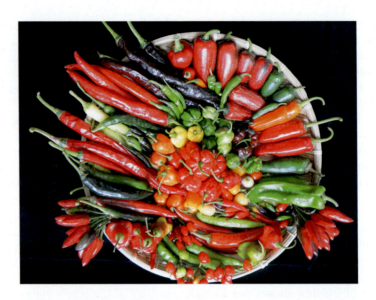

Figure 1.1 Bountiful plates and plants of healthy peppers (*Capsicum* sp.) at the World Vegetable Center. Courtesy of World Vegetable Center.

New Mexico State University, while bacterial leaf spot caused by four species of *Xanthomonas* is not a breeding objective in the New Mexico State University program because even though it is a major disease in the southeastern United States, it is less common in the semiarid region of New Mexico. This is because the pathogen favors 24°C–30°C and high humidity. In New Mexico, the temperature is warm, but the humidity is low; thus the disease is rare. When a chile pepper field does have infected plants, it is because either the grower planted contaminated seeds or the grower did not practice crop rotation. Thus breeding for bacterial leaf spot resistance in chile peppers is not a high priority in New Mexico.

The plant breeder must also be aware of "cryptic" diseases. These are diseases that are always present, and the crop must have resistance to be productive and profitable. For example, ToMV (*Tobamovirus*) has occurred in tomato (*S. lycopersicum*) for more than 75 years in the United States and the Netherlands and now occurs wherever tomato crops are grown, becoming a serious constraint on tomato production in most parts of the world. To the plant breeder's displeasure, ToMV has many host species and is readily spread mechanically. In addition, ToMV persists in seeds, plant debris, greenhouse benches, and clothing worn by people coming in contact with the infected plants. A study in the Netherlands disclosed that ToMV persisted for more than 3 years on clothing stored in a dark enclosed space. A survey of clothes worn by workers in tomato-growing nurseries showed that workers' outer clothing is seldom cleaned and is often worn from one season to the next. Fortunately, infection by ToMV is controlled by the durable resistance *Tm-22* gene, and growers plant only resistant cultivars, so one does not see symptoms and could wrongly assume that ToMV is not an issue.

Breeding disease-resistant horticultural crops is part of a strategy to assist the grower to achieve a sustainable and profitable production system. As the following chapters will illustrate, the plant breeder has an arduous task. Nevertheless, breeding for disease-resistance horticultural plants has been successful in the past and will be successful in the future using all the tools available to the plant breeder. An educated plant breeder is the first step to accomplishing this worthwhile goal, and it is our goal for this book to serve as a resource for plant breeders in developing disease-resistant cultivars of horticultural crops.

Historical perspective

A review of the history of breeding disease-resistance plants is important because it allows us to understand our past, which in turn, allows us to understand our present situation and plan for the future. If one studies the successes and failures of the past, it is possible to learn from the errors and avoid repeating them in the future, and the future looks promising for plant breeders using both classical and recent technologies to improve disease-resistance horticultural plants.

There are myths and historical accounts of disastrous disease epidemics. The ancient Romans had a festival called Robigalia, which was named for their God Robigus, where sacrifices were made to protect the wheat (*Triticum aestivum*) fields from a serious disease, rust (*Puccinia tritcina*) (Fig. 1.2). The concept of "disease resistance" may have started around 300 BCE when Theophrastus, the Greek philosopher, discussed that plants differed in resistance to disease. He observed that plants in low-lying areas of the field had higher levels of disease than those on higher ground. At the time, however, it was not realized that a pathogen caused the disease. The common concept was that disease arose from decaying plant material, an association with the idea of spontaneous generation. It was a common belief at the time that the causes of plant disease included divine power, religious belief, superstitions, and the effects of stars and wrath of God. Slowly, these ideas were replaced with the concept that other organisms caused plant diseases.

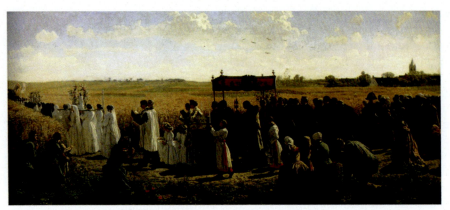

Figure 1.2 Blessing of the Wheat at Artois by Jules Breton (1857). Christian feast of Rogation replaces the Roman Robigalia on April 25 of the Christian calendar. Courtesy Wikiart, public domain.

In 1807 Isaac Benedict Prevost in Switzerland proved conclusively that the wheat bunt disease was caused by a fungus (*Tilletia tritici*) and could be controlled by dipping seed in copper sulfate. Unfortunately, the notion was not widely accepted until the German botanist and mycologist Heinrich Anton de Bary established that rusts and smut diseases are caused by pathogens. It would take a few more decades before the concept that bacteria can cause the disease would be accepted in 1877, when Thomas Burrill at the University of Illinois established that bacteria caused fire blight (*Erwinia amylovora*) of pear (*Pyrus communis*).

Robert Hermann Koch, a German physician, developed Koch's rules (today Koch's postulates) in 1882, stating that for an organism to cause disease, it needed to satisfy a set of three rules later changed to four rules by Erwin Frink Smith at the US Department of Agriculture.

Koch's postulates

1. An organism believed to cause disease must always be present in the host when the disease occurs.
2. The organism must be isolated and grown in pure culture.
3. The organism obtained from pure culture when inoculated must produce the symptoms of the disease.
4. (E. F. Smith added) An organism believed to cause the disease must be reisolated from the diseased plant and compared with the organism first isolated.

However, for some diseases, there are exceptions to Koch's postulates: obligate parasites, viruses, nematodes, and noninfectious causal agents (low temperatures, mineral excess, air pollution, etc.).

In 1894 Jakob Eriksson, a prominent Swedish mycologist and plant pathologist, using wheat rust (*Puccinia triticina*) showed that pathogens, although morphologically similar, differed from each other in their ability to attack different related host species. Eriksson's discovery of *formae speciales* (f.sp.) provided an enhancement to understanding the inheritance of resistance.

In 1900 the laws of inheritance developed by Gregor Mendel, an Augustinian friar and abbot, and biologist, were rediscovered, and the birth of genetics began aiding plant breeders to better understand the inheritance of resistance. Unfortunately, the new era of explaining disease-resistance traits by genetics had its distractors. The British botanist, mycologist, and plant pathologist, Harry Marshall Ward in 1902 promoted the "bridging-host" hypothesis. His theory encompassed the idea that bromegrass (*Bromus* sp.), grown for several generations with moderate resistance, allows the pathogen to become highly virulent. Thus the pathogen is plastic or malleable, and no matter what type of resistance the plant host has, the pathogen will overcome resistance in time. His observations had some legitimacy because resistance does fail, illustrating that not all resistance is durable.

Fortuitously, in 1905 Sir Rowland Biffen at the University of Cambridge, UK, demonstrated that resistance to yellow rust (*Puccinia striiformis* f. sp. *tritici*) in wheat (*T. aestivum*) was governed by a recessive gene segregating in a Mendelian ratio one resistant to three susceptible (1:3) in the F_2 generation. However, the "bridging" theory was so strong it hampered Biffen's important work. At the time, traditional breeding programs were identifying resistance sources and introgressing resistance genes into crops by hybridizing and selecting for traits well before understanding the mechanism of action of resistance genes. Also, in 1905 mycologists found that fungi have mating systems—allowing for genetic recombination. Later, in 1911 Mortier F. Barrus of Cornell University, USA, working with beans (*P. vulgaris*) and anthracnose (*Colletotrichum lindemuthianum*) demonstrated that different isolates of a microorganism differed in their ability to attack different cultivars of the same host species, this finding is the basis for the concept of physiological races and/or pathotypes. Barrus distinguished two races, alpha and beta, of anthracnose. It was subsequently established that the ability of a pathogen to infect a host strain, that is, virulence, is genetically determined. Thus both the ability of the host to resist invasion by a pathogen as well as the ability of a pathogen to invade its host are genetically controlled.

The concept of physiological differentiation was extensively applied to wheat stem rust (*Puccinia graminis* f. sp. *tritici*) by Elvin C. Stakman in 1910 at the University of Minnesota, USA, who coined the phrase, "physiological races," later to be shortened to race. Later in 1915 he coined the term "hypersensitive response" for the necrotic tissue reaction some plants show as resistance to a pathogen. Between 1918 and 1921, Paul R. Burkholder and Gordon P. McRostie, of Cornell University, USA, demonstrated the independent inheritance of resistance to different races of the pathogen. The understanding of disease resistance was heavily influenced in 1952, when Harold Henry Flor at North Dakota State University, USA, postulated the hypothesis of a gene-for-gene relationship between host and pathogen, which holds true in most cases and is widely accepted. His concept requires an avirulence (*Avr*) gene in the pathogen and a resistance (*R*) gene in the host plant for the resistant phenotype to manifest itself. At this point, the science of genetics could be applied to breeding for disease-resistant plants allowing breeders to consciously select for individual plants that had a resistant phenotype and know that at least some of that phenotype was genetically based. Usually, such resistance was developed as a second phase—a rescue operation—after new cultivars, selected primarily for high yield, was discovered to be susceptible to a particular disease. Plant breeders found early on that they could identify single genes (usually dominant) that conferred essentially complete resistance to the disease in question. Cultivars containing such excellent resistance were developed and released for large-scale use. But plant breeders then discovered, all too often, that the "perfect" resistance lost its effectiveness after a few seasons. They soon learned, with the aid of plant pathologists, that disease-causing pathogens are highly diverse genetically and that almost without fail a rare genotype will turn up that is not affected by the newly deployed resistance gene. The new pathogen genotype multiplies, and the horticultural crop's resistance loses its effectiveness or in the vernacular "breaks down."

Plant breeders change the genetic composition of horticultural crops as they select for disease resistance. One cannot say, categorically, that single gene resistance will always be undependable, or that multiple-factor resistance will always be durable. It is important to remember that the phrase "stability of resistance" refers to whether a previously resistant variety is overcome by a specific disease. A critical concept is that individual resistance genes do not lose their power to hold individual pathotypes in check. The resistance genes are stable and functioning, but previously undetected pathotypes appear, with types of virulence that are not curbed by the current resistance genes. The cultivar succumbs to the disease once again, albeit to a new race/pathotype/strain of the pathogen, and growers will say that the cultivar has broken down.

Toward the end of the 20th century, Brian J. Staskawicz and colleagues at University of California, Berkeley, USA, cloned the first avirulence gene in *P. syringae* pv. *glycinea*. Then in 1986 Roger N. Beachy and colleagues at Washington University, Missouri, USA created a transgenic plant expressing the coat protein of the TMV (*Tobamovirus*) that delayed the development of disease. Gurmukh S. Johal and Steven P. Briggs at Pioneer Hi-Bred International, Inc. reported the cloning of the first resistant gene, *Hm1* (NADPH-dependent reductase) in maize (*Z. mays*) by transposon tagging in 1992. The next year a second resistant gene, *Pto* (kinase type) in tomato (*S. lycopersicum*) was cloned by positional mapping at Cornell University, USA. More resistant genes were cloned in the following years belonging to a different class of genes; the leucine-rich repeat (LRR) motifs with a nucleotide-binding site (NBS) were the most common class. The LRR motifs implicate protein-to-protein interactions, while NBS implies a role in signal transduction pathways.

In 1996 "genetically modified organisms" (GMO crops) began to be planted in agriculture. Plant genomes can be engineered by physical methods or by use of *Agrobacterium tumefaciens* for the delivery of sequences hosted in T-DNA binary vectors. This breakthrough opened a new chapter in plant breeding, allowing the introduction of a new trait that does not occur naturally in the species. Two years later, Dennis Gonsalves at Cornell University, USA released a GMO papaya cultivar, Rainbow (*Carica papaya*) that is resistant to the devastating Papaya ringspot virus (PRSV, *Potyvirus*).

The 21st century began with *Arabidopsis thaliana* as the first plant genome to be sequenced. Many more crops and pathogens were then subsequently sequenced, bringing in a new era of scientific discovery. The first major crop to be sequenced was rice (*Oryza sativa*) in 2002. Currently, more than 350 reference genomes of plants have been sequenced, nearly 200 of which are horticultural plants, used as fruit, medicinal, ornamental, and vegetables. The advent of so many publicly available reference genomes has enabled more accurate identification of genes that confer resistance to pathogens and allowed researchers to have a better understanding of the genetic mechanism of resistance and host–pathogen interactions.

In the 1980s, a family of DNA sequences were discovered in the genomes of prokaryotic organisms known as clustered regularly interspaced short palindromic repeats (CRISPR) that are fragments of bacteriophages that previously infected the prokaryotes. These sequences play a role in detection of similar bacteriophages during subsequent infection and act as a defense system of acquired immunity for the prokaryote. Due to their highly accurate sequence recognition capacity, along with the CRISPR-associated protein 9 (Cas9), they were found useful in editing the genes within organisms to confer a missing phenotype. The gene editing tool of CRISPR-Cas9 has broad applications, from human medicine to biofuels and to modify the genomes of horticultural crop plants. The CRISPR-Cas9 technology has revolutionized plant breeding since its first application in 2013. The major breakthroughs were the generation of disease-resistant and environment-adaptive crops. For example, through the use of CRISPR-Cas9 resistance to Banana streak virus (BSV, *Badnavirus*) in banana (*M. acuminata*), Cucumber vein yellowing virus (CVYV, *Potyvirus*), ZYMV (*Potyvirus*), and PRSV (*Potyvirus*) in cucumber (*C. sativus*), powdery mildew (*Erysiphe necator*) and bunch rot (*B. cinerea*) in grape (*Vitis vinifera*), black pod rot (*Phytophthora tropicalis*) in cacao (*Theobroma cacao*), and fruit rot and root rot (*Phytophthora palmivora*) in papaya have been developed, just to list a few.

Unlike genetic modification via *Agrobacterium*, plants originating from the use of CRISPR-Cas9 are not considered GMO crops in the United States. In April 2016, the Food and Drug Administration (FDA) indicated that the CRISPR-edited mushroom (*Agaricus bisporus*) could enter the market without oversight, making it the first CRISPR-edited organism to receive such authorization from the United States government. In 2017 the FDA allowed the marketing of false flax (*Camelina sativa*), with enhanced omega-3 oil and drought-tolerant soybean (*Glycine max*), clearly indicating that CRISPR-edited plants can be cultivated and sold free from regulation. However, in other countries and regions, notably the large markets of the European Union, China, and Japan, there are still sociopolitical challenges, including consumer acceptable and governmental regulations associated with the technology. The CRISPR-Cas9 genome editing technique resulted in awarding the Nobel Prize in Chemistry in 2020 to Emmanuelle Charpentier at the Max

Planck Institute in Germany and Jennifer Doudna at Berkeley University in California, USA; however, the applications of CRISPR-Cas9 have yet to be fully realized in breeding for disease-resistant horticultural crops.

With the information gained over the last 2000 years or so, plant breeders have taken that cumulative knowledge and applied it to breeding for disease resistance. Using both classical and molecular approaches, tremendous gains have and will continue to be made. Classical plant breeding methods based on Mendel's laws of heredity, augmented with modern technologies have gained a prominent position in our discipline. A combination of new techniques with classical methods will lead to more efficient and successful breeding for disease-resistance procedures.

Terminology

The terminology in breeding disease-resistant horticultural plants can be confusing. Resistance is a broad term that has several definitions. Considered in a broad sense resistance to plant disease may be brought about by various mechanisms and be present in differing degrees. A general definition is that resistance is the ability of a plant variety to restrict the growth and development of a specified pathogen or the damage they cause when compared to susceptible plants under similar environmental conditions and pathogen pressure. Some people use immunity and resistance interchangeably, but resistant varieties may exhibit some disease symptoms or damage under heavy pathogen pressure, yet a grower would be satisfied and say the crop had resistance. Immunity is often associated with nonhost resistance.

A list of principal terms

Avirulence/virulence: Terms that consider the host. Avirulence genes are originally defined by their negative impact on the ability of a pathogen to infect their host plant. Characterization of avirulence genes has revealed that they encode an amazing assortment of proteins and belong to several gene families. Elucidation of the function of avirulence genes promises to provide insight into plant defense mechanisms, and new and improved strategies for the control of plant disease.

Antibiosis: Plant traits that adversely affect insect mortality, size, and life history. Sometimes used in disease resistance as a plant's chemical that may have an effect on the pathogen.

Biotypes: A variant group within a species that has a distinctive physiological characteristic, for example, forming a physiologically distinct race or variant.

Broad Spectrum Resistance: Resistance to most races, strains, or isolates of a pathogen species.

Constitutive Resistance: Plant defenses representing anatomical or biochemical features that are performed without any prior exposure to a pathogen.

Cross-protection: The phenomenon whereby a plant preinoculated with a mild virus strain becomes resistant to subsequent inoculation by a related severe strain.

Disease Triangle: Three factors, susceptible host, virulent pathogen, and conducive environment, that must be present and interact for disease to develop. Time is sometimes added as a four-essential factor.

Durability: Used to qualified resistance through time and across environments.

Effectors: Secreted molecules that enable microbes to interact with their hosts and to influence the outcome of the interaction. They are not distinguished by sharing similar chemical properties but are instead defined by their function within the biological context of an interaction.

Escapes (Pseudo-resistance): Phenotypically resistance resulting from transitory characters in susceptible host plants due to environmental conditions or host evasion.

Formae speciales (f. sp.): Meaning special form, an informal taxonomic grouping applied most frequently to a fungus that is adapted to a specific host. An example is *F. oxysporum* f. sp. *pisi*, which infects peas.

Founder Effect: Random change in genetic composition of a population due to an extreme reduction in its size during a colonization or infection episode.

Hypersensitive Response: Form of programmed cell death at the site of pathogen infection.

Immunity: Not subject to attack or infection by a specified pathogen.

Incubation Period: The time between inoculation and first visible symptoms, this often parallels the latent period, but not always.

Infection Efficiency: The proportion of spores successfully completing the infection process. Especially important in horticulture crops where one blemish could reduce the yield.

Infection Frequency: The proportion of spores that result in sporulation. Lowering infection frequency an important type of resistance, where only the reduction of spores is needed, for example, leaf blight of tomatoes.

Infectious Period: The time that the disease tissue sporulates.

Interaction Phenotype: The phenotype that is the result of host's genetic factors, environmental influences, and genotype of the pathogen. It is worth noting that the interaction phenotype is not stable in all environments.

Infection Type: Qualitative or quantitative description of the host reaction and/or pathogen growth in the infection court; principally measured on individual lesions, normally does not account for infection frequency, latent period, or infectious period; spore production per pustule is assessed in a qualitative sense because pustule size and spore production tend to be correlated.

Heterokaryon: A multinucleate cell that contains genetically different nuclei.

Latent Period: Measured as the time from infection to spore production.

Microbe-Associated Molecular Pattern (*MAMP*): Conserved microbe-specific molecules are recognized by the plant innate immune systems pattern recognition receptors (PRRs).

Necrotroph: Organism that actively kills the cells of its host to derive energy for its survival and multiplication.

Nucleotide-Binding and Leucine-Rich Repeat (*NB-LRR*) proteins: Proteins that function as intracellular receptors for the detection of pathogens in plants.

Nonhost (Innate) Resistance: Resistance exhibited by an entire plant species to all genetic variants of a nonadapted pathogen species and represents the most robust and durable form of plant resistance in nature. The presence of this defense system explains why plants are immune to most potential pathogens and are normally healthy.

Pathogen-Associated Molecular Pattern (PAMP): This term has been criticized on the premise that most microbes, not only pathogens, express the molecules detected; the term MAMP is preferred.

Pathogen-triggered Immunity (PTI): Basal resistance response induced upon perception of PAMPs by PRRs.

Pathogenicity: A term for the pathogen; the ability to cause disease. It does not consider the host.

Pathotypes: A disease-causing variant of a microorganism. It is distinguishable from other members of its species by its virulence and by unique molecular markers.

Pathovar (pv.): A pathological variant (pathovar) is a bacterial strain with similar characteristics that is differentiated at the subspecific level based on distinctive pathogenicity to one or more plant hosts. An example is *Xanthomonas campestris* pv. *vesicatoria* that causes bacterial spot disease in tomato (*S. lycopersicum*) and pepper (*C. annuum*).

Pattern Recognition Receptors (*PRR*): Specialized receptors that recognize the specific molecular structures on the surface of pathogens. These receptors are a key element of the innate immune system.

Phytoalexins: Low molecular weight, antimicrobial metabolites synthesized by the plant upon pathogen attack. Associated with antibiosis resistance.

Quantitative Trait Loci (*QTL*): Genomic region containing one or more genes that exhibits a statistically significant association between marker polymorphisms and quantitative trait variation.

Quantitative Disease Resistance (*QDR*): Resistance that confers a reduction in disease, not the absence of disease.

Quantitative Resistance Loci (*QRL*): Genetic loci associated with quantitative resistance characters.

Quantitative Trait Nucleotide (*QTN*): Causal molecular variant that affects variation in a quantitative trait.

Races: The concept of physiological differentiation among pathogens originally applied to wheat stem rust (*P. graminis* f. sp. *tritici*) by Stakman in 1910, who coined the phrase, physiological races, later to be shortened to race. Necessary to have a host differential to identify.

Reproduction Rate: A measure of a pathogen reproduction; major factors affecting reproduction rate are (1) infection frequency, (2) latent period, and (3) spore production.

Resistance: A term for the host that is a continuum from low to high resistance. The level of resistance needed by a grower will depend on the crop and the pathogen. Includes incomplete resistance where the resistance allows some spore production and partial resistance where spore production is reduced even though the host plants are susceptible to infection.

Spore Production: Measurement expressed as spore production per unit area of affected tissue, per lesion and/or per unit of time.

Sporulation Capacity: Number of spores produced during the lifetime of a colony, measured as the rate of cumulative sporulation over time.

Strain: A genetic variant based on host differential or genetic sequence.

Susceptibility: A term for the host and its inability to restrict the growth and development of a specified pathogen.

Tolerance: Can be designated either endurance or an intermediate level of observable resistance somewhere between immunity and full susceptibility. Maintaining both uses is confusing. Simons (1979) defines tolerance as a greater yield when disease present, but no yield difference if disease is absent. It is best to use tolerance to mean that the plant can endure severe disease without severe losses in yield or quality. It should not be used to describe partial or horizontal resistance.

Vertifolia Effect: Erosion of a crop's general (horizontal, minor gene, multigenic, polygenic) resistance in a cultivar after several generations of selection during which a major gene confers resistance to the dominant race or biotype of the pathogen. First described by Van der Plank (1963), who observed it in the potato cultivar Vertifolia with late blight resistance.

Virulence Profile: The number of virulence alleles within a specific population of the pathogen.

Virulence Source Population: Pathogen population, that is, heterogenous for virulence genes and represents a population in a particular locale or area; must be monitored for virulence in that population.

Wide hybridization: The crossing between two different species or genera, which has been used successfully to move resistance genes to pests and diseases into horticulturally adapted lines.

References

Simons, M.D., 1979. Modification of host–parasite interactions through artificial mutagenesis. Annual Review of Phytopathology 17, 75–96. Available from: https://doi.org/10.1146/annurev.py.17.090179.000451.

Van der Plank, J.E., 1963. Plant Diseases; Epidemics and Control. Academic Press, New York & London, p. 349.

Zinger, A., Lapidot, M., Harel, A., Doron-Faigenboim, A., Gelbart, D., Levin, I., 2021. Identification and mapping of tomato genome loci con-trolling tolerance and resistance to Tomato brown rugose fruit virus. Plants 10 (1), 179. Available from: https://doi.org/10.3390/plants10010179.

Further reading

Barnett, H.L., 1959. Plant disease resistance. Annual Review of Microbiology 13, 191–210. Available from: https://doi.org/10.1146/annurev.mi.13.100159.001203.

Barrus, M.F., 1911. Variation of varieties of beans in their susceptibility to anthracnose. Phytopathology 1, 190–195.

Bayer, P.E., Golicz, A.A., Scheben, A., Batley, J., Edwards, D., 2020. Plant pangenomes are the new reference. Nature Plants 6, 914–920. Available from: https://doi.org/10.1038/s41477-020-0733-0.

Bos, L., Parlevliet, J.E., 1995. Concepts and terminology on plant/pest relationships: Toward consensus in plant pathology and crop protections. Annual Review of Phytopathology 33, 69–102. Available from: https://doi.org/10.1146/annurev.py.33.090195.000441.

Boyd, L.A., Ridout, C., O'Sullivan, D.M., Leach, J.E., Leung, H., 2013. Plant–pathogen interactions: disease resistance in modern agriculture. Trends in Genetics 29, 233–240. Available from: https://doi.org/10.1016/j.tig.2012.10.011.

Broadbent, L., Fletcher, J.T., 1963. The epidemiology of tomato mosaic. IV. Persistence of virus on clothing and glasshouse structures. Annals of Applied Biology . Available from: https://doi.org/10.1111/j.1744-7348.1963.tb03747.x.

Brown, J.K.M., 2003. A cost of disease resistance: paradigm or peculiarity. Trends in Genetics 19, 667–671. Available from: https://doi.org/10.1016/j.tig.2003.10.008.

Brunt, A.A., 1986. Tomato mosaic virus. In: Van Regenmortel, M.H.V., Fraenkel-Conrat, H. (Eds.), The Plant Viruses. The Viruses. Springer, Boston, MA. Available from: https://doi.org/10.1007/978-1-4684-7026-0_9.

Caruso, A.G., Bertacca, S., Parrella, G., Rizzo, R., Davino, S., Panno, S., 2022. Tomato brown rugose fruit virus: A pathogen that is changing the tomato production worldwide. Annals of Applied Biology 181, 258–274. Available from: https://doi.org/10.1111/aab.12788.

Chen, F., Song, Y., Li, X., Chen, J., Mo, L., Zhang, X., et al., 2019. Genome sequences of horticultural plants: past, present, and future. Horticultural Research 6, 112. Available from: https://doi.org/10.1038/s41438-019-0195-6.

Collinge, D.B., Jørgensen, H.J.L., Lund, O.S., Lyngkjær, M.F., 2010. Engineering pathogen resistance in crop plants: Current trends and future prospects. Annual Review of Phytopathology 48, 269–291. Available from: https://doi.org/10.1146/annurev-phyto-073009-114430.

Epstein, L., Kaur, S., Henry, P.M., 2022. The emergence of *Fusarium oxysporum f.* sp. apii race 4 and *Fusarium oxysporum f.* sp. coriandrii highlights major obstacles facing agricultural production in coastal California in a warming climate: A case study. Frontiers in Plant Science . Available from: https://doi.org/10.3389/fpls.2022.921516.

Fister, A.S., Landherr, L., Maximova, S.N., Guiltinan, M.J., 2018. Transient expression of CRISPR/Cas9 machinery targeting TcNPR3 enhances defense response in *Theobroma cacao*. Frontiers in Plant Science 9, 268. Available from: https://doi.org/10.3389/fpls.2018.00268.

Francl, L.J., 2001. The disease triangle: a plant pathological paradigm revisited. The Plant Health Instructor . Available from: https://doi.org/10.1094/phi-t-2001-0517-01.

Gumtow, R., Wu, D., Uchida, J., Tian, M.A., 2018. A Phytophthora palmivora extracellular cystatin-like protease inhibitor targets papain to contribute to virulence on papaya. Molecular Plant-Microbe Interactions 31, 363–373. Available from: https://doi.org/10.1094/MPMI-06-17-0131-FI.

Gururani, M.A., Venkatesh, J., Upadhyaya, C.P., Nookaraju, A., Pandey, S.K., Park, S.W., 2012. Plant disease resistance genes: Current status and future directions. Physiological and Molecular Plant Pathology 78, 51–65. Available from: https://doi.org/10.1016/j.pmpp.2012.01.002.

Hoch, H., Staples, R.C., Whitehead, B., Comeau, J., Wolf, E.D., 1987. Signaling for growth orientation and cell differentiation by surface topography in

Uromyces. Science (New York, N.Y.) 235, 1659–1662. Available from: https://doi.org/10.1126/science.235.4796.1659.

International Seed Federation, 2012. Definition of the terms describing the reaction of plants to pests and abiotic stresses for the vegetable seed industry. http://www.worldseed.org/isf/diseases_resistance.html.

Langner, T., Kamoun, S., Belhaj, K., 2018. CRISPR crops: Plant genome editing toward disease resistance. Annual Review of Phytopathology 56, 479–512. Available from: https://doi.org/10.1146/annurev-phyto-080417-050158.

Malnoy, M., Viola, R., Jung, M.H., Koo, O.J., Kim, S., Kim, J.S., et al., 2016. DNA-free genetically edited grapevine and apple protoplast using CRISPR/Cas9 ribonucleoproteins. Frontiers in Plant Science 7, 1904. Available from: https://doi.org/10.3389/fpls.2016.01904.

McDonald, M.R., Gossen, B.D., Kora, C., Parker, M., Boland, G., 2013. Using crop canopy modification to manage plant diseases. European Journal of Plant Pathology 135, 581–593. Available from: https://doi.org/10.1007/s10658-012-0133-z.

Mishra, R., Nath, J., Bijayalaxmi, M., Raj, M., Joshi, K., 2021. A single transcript CRISPR/Cas9 mediated mutagenesis of CaERF28 confers anthracnose resistance in chilli pepper (*Capsicum annuum* L.). Planta 254, 5–17. Available from: https://doi.org/10.1007/s00425-021-03660-x.

Niks, R.E., Parlevliet, J.E., Lindhout, P., Bai, Y., 2011. Breeding crops with resistance to diseases and pests. Wageningen Academic Publishers, pp. 11–22. Available from: https://doi.org/10.3920/978-90-8686-171-2.

Panter, S.N., Jones, D.A., 2002. Age-related resistance to plant pathogens. Advances in Botanical Research 38, 251–280. Available from: https://doi.org/10.1016/S0065-2296(02)38032-7.

Parlevliet, J.E., 1979. Components of resistance that reduce the rate of epidemic development. Annual Review of Phytopathology 17, 203–222. Available from: https://doi.org/10.1146/annurev.py.17.090179.001223.

Pavan, S., Jacobsen, E., Visser, R.G.F., Bai, Y., 2010. Loss of susceptibility as a novel breeding strategy for durable and broad-spectrum resistance. Molecular Breeding 25, 1–12. Available from: https://doi.org/10.1007/s11032-009-9323-6.

Robinson, R.A., 1969. Disease resistance terminology. Review of Applied Mycology 48, 593–606.

Rouse, D., Nelson, R.R., MacKenzie, D.R., Armitage, C.R., 1980. Components of rate-reducing resistance in seedlings of four wheat cultivars and parasitic fitness in six isolates of Erysiphe graminis f.sp. tritici. Phytopathology 70, 1097–1100. Available from: https://doi.org/10.1094/Phyto-70-1097.

Savary, S., Ficke, A., Aubertot, J.-N., Hollier, C., 2012. Crop losses due to diseases and their implications for global food production losses and food security. Food Security 4, 519–537. Available from: https://doi.org/10.1007/s12571-012-0200-5.

Savary, S., Willocquet, L., Pethybridge, S.J., Esker, P., McRoberts, N., Nelson, A., 2019. The global burden of pathogens and pests on major food crops. Nature Ecology and Evolution 3, 430–439. Available from: https://doi.org/10.1038/s41559-018-0793-y.

Schenke, D., Cai, D., 2020. Applications of CRISPR/Cas to improve crop disease resistance: Beyond inactivation of susceptibility factors. iScience 23. Available from: https://doi.org/10.1016/j.isci.2020.101478.

Schulz, B., Boyle, C., 2005. The endophytic continuum. Mycological Research 109, 661–686. Available from: https://doi.org/10.1017/S095375620500273X.

Singh, S.P., Schwartz, H.F., 2010. Breeding common bean for resistance to diseases. A Review of Crop Science 50, 2199–2223. Available from: https://doi.org/10.2135/cropsci2009.03.0163.

Strange, R.N., Scott, P.R., 2005. Plant disease: a threat to global good security. Annual Review of Phytopathology 43, 83–116. Available from: https://doi.org/10.1146/annurev.phyto.43.113004.133839.

Tripathi, J.N., Ntui, V.O., Ron, M., Muiruri, S.K., Britt, A., Tripathi, L., 2019. CRISPR-Cas9 editing of endogenous banana streak virus in the B genome of *Musa* spp. overcomes a major challenge in banana breeding. Communications Biology 2 (46). Available from: https://doi.org/10.1038/s42003-019-0288-7.

Uhse, S., Djamei, A., 2018. Effectors of plant-colonizing fungi and beyond. PLoS Pathogens 14 (6), e1006992. Available from: https://doi.org/10.1371/journal.ppat.1006992.

van Schie, C.C.N., Takken, F.L.W., 2014. Susceptibility genes 101: How to be a good host. Annual Review of Phytopathology 52, 551–581. Available from: https://doi.org/10.1146/annurev-phyto-102313-045854.

Walters, D.R., 2009. Are plants in the field already induced? Implications for practical disease control. Crop Protection 28, 459–465. Available from: https://doi.org/10.1016/j.cropro.2009.01.009.

Wang, X., Tu, M., Wang, D., Liu, J., Li, Y., Li, Z., et al., 2018. CRISPR/Cas9-mediated efficient targeted mutagenesis in grape in the first generation. Plant Biotechnology Journal 16, 844–855. Available from: https://doi.org/10.1111/pbi.12832.

Wang, T., Zhang, H., Zhu, H., 2019. CRISPR technology is revolutionizing the improvement of tomato and other fruit crops. Horticultural Research 6, 77. Available from: https://doi.org/10.1038/s41438-019-0159-x.

Wingard, S.A., 1953. The nature of resistance to disease growing healthier plants. In: U.S.D.A. Yearbook of Agriculture. Plant Diseases, pp. 165–173. Available from: https://naldc.nal.usda.gov/download/IND43894315/PDF.

Yoder, O.C., Valent, B., Chumley, F., 1986. Genetic nomenclature and practice for plant pathogenic fungi. Phytopathology 76, 383–385. Available from: https://doi.org/10.1094/Phyto-76-383.

Zaidi, S.S.-A., Mukhtar, M.S., Mansoor, S., 2018. Genome editing: Targeting susceptibility genes for plant disease resistance. Trends in Biotechnology 36, 898–906. Available from: https://doi.org/10.1016/j.tibtech.2018.04.005.

Zhang, Y., Lubberstedt, T., Xu, M., 2013. The genetic and molecular basis of plant resistance to pathogens. Journal of Genetics and Genomics 40, 23–35. Available from: https://doi.org/10.1016/j.jgg.2012.11.003.

Resistance: the phenotype

Some of the most specialized life forms on Earth are plant pathogens. Based on molecular clock estimations plants and pathogens have been closely associated for more than 407 million years. During this long-term coevolution, the association between plants and pathogens assumes a dynamic and context-dependent association. Plants can recognize pathogens through specific receptors: cell surface–localized pattern-recognition receptors (PRRs) that perceive extracellular microbe–associated molecular patterns (MAMPs) and intracellular nucleotide-binding leucine-rich repeat receptors (NLRs) recognize specific effector molecules. Plant recognition of pathogens triggers a series of plant immune responses, including calcium ion influx, reactive oxygen species (ROS) burst, defense gene expression, and production of phytohormones and defensive specialized metabolites that collectively constitute the plant immune network. Meanwhile, in a shorter time scale, the dynamic arms race between plants and pathogens drives evolution of versatile virulence strategies by pathogens to escape plant recognition and/or interfere with plant immune responses that conversely also accelerate rapid evolutionary adaptation of plant immune sensory system for counteracting pathogen invasion.

The challenge of colonizing a living host cell comes from the evolutionary specificity that must exist for a pathogen to outmaneuver the plant's recognition and defense system. This relationship between a plant and a pathogen is complex with pathogens developing new biotypes, pathotypes, races, and strains that cause disease to plants that were considered resistant to the previous form of the pathogen. Plant breeders are fortunate that most plants are resistant to most organisms. Through domestication many crops were selected with some level of resistance, that is, those individual plants that did not succumb to disease were saved and propagated for the next generation. In effect, disease resistance was selected, and the crop's genetics were changed in favor of resistance genes. It is fundamentally important to remember that the pathogen and the disease it causes are not the same. We repeat—the pathogen and the disease it causes are not the same. Disease arises from the combination of the pathogen, the host it infects, the environment the host is growing in, and exposure time. Because of this complexity, the disease pyramid concept is always evolving.

A plant's phenotype is defined as the characteristics of the plant resulting from the interaction among genotype, environment, time, and crop management. For the plant breeder, a key concept in breeding for disease-resistant plants is that RESISTANCE IS A PHENOTYPE. A resistant plant is always from the point of view of the plant breeder, and subsequently the grower. Plant pathologists can determine resistance from different points of view, but a plant breeder must select for a level of resistance that is acceptable in the production system where the crop will be grown. Thus one needs to be aware that there is a continuum of disease outcomes, from mild to severe. Thought-provoking is the phenomenon of plants with a susceptible phenotype can produce resistant offspring. When it comes to genetic resistance, plant breeders have several general classes of genes based on their phenotypic effects to choose from, and not all forms of resistance are equal. If resistance is based on a biochemical constitutive, it can jeopardize the quality, palatability, or could be toxic to the consumer. In nature this type of resistance, works fine, but one cannot kill the consumer! The same can be said for morphological forms of resistance, where crops that are too fibrous or pubescent, for example, which would not be delectable to the consumers.

Nonhost (innate) resistance

Despite the omnipresence of potential pathogens in the environment and the constant threat of infection, disease is the exception, not the rule, generally most plants are healthy. In nature, an innate immune system protects plants from most pathogens in the environment because plants can only be infected by an extremely limited number of potential pathogens present in the environment. This innate resistance is commonly called nonhost resistance. Currently, the genetic and molecular evidence underlying molecular mechanisms of nonhost resistance are like the plant immune responses that occur in host plants following infection by adapted pathogens. Therefore it becomes apparent that all plants are nonhosts to most pathogens, highlighting the effectiveness of nonhost resistance.

Plants possess a sophisticated innate immunity involving various layers of defense responses. Some defense mechanisms are preformed/constitutive, while others are activated only after the attack by pathogens (pathogen induced). Based upon this fact, antimicrobial compounds derived from plants are classified into two main groups of phytoanticipins (constitutive) and phytoalexins (induced). The word phytoanticipins translates to the "plant anticipates." Phytoanticipins, such as saponins, phenylpropanoids, alkaloids, cyanogenic glycosides, and glucosinolates, are antimicrobial compounds presynthesized by plants. Phytoalexins are formed in response to a pathogenic attack and include various phenylpropanoids, alkaloids, and terpenes. An overlap between these groups of antimicrobial agents occurs because the phytoalexins of some plants can act as phytoanticipins in others.

Constitutive barriers like leaf hairs can be effective barriers to fungal infection. At the BAZ, Institute for Grapevine Breeding Siebeldingen, Germany the influence of leaf hairs during the interaction of downy mildew (*Plasmopara viticola*) on four *Vitis* species both under natural conditions and upon treatment with the detergent Tween 20, has been explored. The adaxial leaf sides with hydrophobic hairs repel water from the leaf surface preventing a successful penetration of the host via fungal germ tubes. Treatment with a detergent solution led to an enhanced attachment of water droplets. As a consequence of the detergent treatment, infection structures of *P. viticola* were formed on the field-resistant hosts, *Vitis doaniana* and *Vitis davidii* as in the susceptible *Vitis vinifera* hosts. It can be concluded that covering the leaf surface with hydrophobic hairs represents a major defense strategy and that the infection process is dependent on wetness. Although in *Vitis cinerea* and *Vitis labrusca* primary infection structures can be monitored after detergent treatment, the growth of the fungus was found to be restricted in these species indicating the action of additional or different defense strategies such as phytoanticipins or phytoalexins within the plant tissue.

In contrast, when Wesley E. Kloos and colleagues at North Carolina State University examined powdery mildew (*Golovinomyces cichoracearum*; formerly *Erysiphe cichoracearum*) resistance on gerbera daisy (*Gerbera hybrida*), they found the density of bristle macrohairs on the adaxial leaf surface as compared to wild type did not affect powdery mildew resistance.

Gray mold caused by *Botrytis cinerea* leads to substantial economic losses in strawberries (*Fragaria × ananassa*) worldwide. *B. cinerea* can infect multiple parts of the strawberry plant including fruit, flowers, and leaves. Currently, fungicides are used to control gray mold (*B. cinerea*) on strawberries that has led to increased development of fungicide-resistant strains of *B. cinerea*. An alternative management strategy and a solution to fungicide-resistant strains is to breed strawberries for gray mold (*B. cinerea*) resistant genotypes. When constitutive or innate resistance was examined in wild woodland strawberries (*Fragaria vesca*) for resistance to gray mold (*B. cinerea*), researchers at KU Leuven Plant Institute in Heverlee, Belgium found significant differences in the amount of total phenolics, total flavonoids, glucose, galactose, citric acid, hydrogen peroxide, and ascorbic acid. In addition, when the researchers screened different *F. vesca* genotypes for susceptibility to *B. cinerea*, two genotypes with different resistance levels were identified with a susceptible genotype *F. vesca* ssp. *vesca* Tenno 3 and a moderately resistant genotype *F. vesca* ssp. *vesca* Kreuzkogel 1. When these two genotypes were compared for fungal growth during early stages of infection in the leaves, they confirmed that the increased resistance in Kreuzkogel 1 as compared to Tenno 3 was due to the constitutive resistance mechanisms of Kreuzkogel 1 instead of the induction of defense responses. This study revealed that the innate resistance of strawberry (*Fragaria* × *ananassa*) leaves plays a major role in the resistance of woodland strawberry (*F. vesca*) leaves against *B. cinerea*. They suggested that plant breeders use this innate resistance in breeding gray mold resistance strawberries.

Exclusionary mechanisms that are preformed/constituency expression are a rigid cytoskeleton, production of secondary metabolites, epicuticular wax, trichome type, or density, to name just a few. Phytoanticipins are low molecular weight defense-related compounds present in plants even before the attack by pathogens or produced from preexisting precursors. Some of them are located at the plant surface (epidermal portion) while others are preformed compounds in vacuoles or organelles and are released only by the action of hydrolyzing enzymes after the pathogen attack. Hydrolyzing enzymes involved in liberation of final molecule are not synthesized de novo; therefore, these compounds are different from phytoalexins. Phytoanticipins include saponins, avenacin, and tomatine, for example, α-tomatine produced in tomato (*Solanum lycopersicum*) showing antimicrobial activity against many pathogenic fungi. In tomato, saponin shows specific resistance against *Fusarium oxysporum* f. sp. *lycopersici* and *Verticillium albo-atrum*. Despite significant efforts by researchers, confusion still exists and many of these phytochemicals that could be considered as phytoanticipins are reported as phytoalexins or vice versa.

Inclusionary resistance is defined as being inducible. For example, plants synthesize and accumulate an arsenal of antimicrobial secondary metabolites to protect themselves from the invasion of pathogens. Phytoalexins are chemically diverse and have a wide range of functions including antimicrobial activity acting as toxins to a pathogen. The suffix "alexin" literally means to "ward off." They are synthesized de novo and accumulate around the pathogen infection. These low molecular weight antimicrobial compounds are both synthesized by and accumulated in plants as a response to pathogen attacks. The concept of phytoalexins was introduced more than 80 years ago by Karl Otto Müller and H. Börger after observing that infection of potato (*Solanum tuberosum*) tubers with a strain of *Phytophthora infestans* capable of initiating hypersensitive reactions, significantly inhibited the effect of a subsequent infection by another strain of *P. infestans*. This inhibition was linked to a "principle" produced by the plant cells reacting hypersensitive that they named phytoalexin. Phytoalexins of grapevines (*V. vinifera*) belong mainly to the stilbene family, the skeleton of which is based on *trans*-resveratrol. Resveratrol represents a parent compound of a family of molecules, such as resveratrol glucosides (piceid), methylated derivatives (pterostilbene), and oligomers (a-viniferin and e-viniferin), with some expressing higher fungicide toxicity compared with resveratrol. Resistant grapevine (*Vitis* sp.) cultivars have been shown to react rapidly to downy mildew (*Plasmopara viticola*) infections by producing high concentrations of stilbenes at the site of infection, confirming their crucial role and effectiveness in grapevine resistance to downy mildew (*P. viticola*).

Plant defense to *Botrytis cinerea*

An example of the complex interaction between pathogen and host is illustrated with *B. cinerea*. *B. cinerea* is one of the most extensively studied necrotrophic plant pathogens. *B. cinerea* infects more than 200 plant species, causing gray mold, evident on the leaf surface as gray fluffy mycelium. Worldwide, it causes annual losses of anywhere from $10 billion to $100 billion (US). The fungus can counteract a broad range of plant defense systems.

A thorough review of how this sophisticated interaction between *B. cinerea* and host plays out was written by Dr. Kai Bi, the College of Life Science and Technology, Wuhan Polytechnic University, China and with colleagues Dr. Tesfaye Mengiste,

Department of Botany and Plant Pathology, Purdue University, United States, and Drs. Yong Liang and Amir Sharon School of the Plant Sciences and Food Security, Tel Aviv University, Israel. In the past decade, new details about the events and genes that control pathogenic and virulence development in *B. cinerea* have been discovered. While the story is far from complete, these discoveries lead to a paradigm shift for *B. cinerea* pathogenesis and virulence that instead of an aggressive attack governed mainly by the massive secretion of enzymes and toxins, to a complex, multifactorial, and multilayered process, including subtle mechanisms that can follow different infection routes.

The process begins with the breaching of the external layers of the plant, including the cuticle and cell wall, then *B. cinerea* must cope with preformed as well as pathogen-induced (phytoalexins) plant antimicrobial compounds that significantly affect disease development. *B. cinerea* has evolved various mechanisms to tolerate mycotoxic plant metabolites, such as the degradation of α-tomatine and the export of toxic glucosinolate degradation products. *B. cinerea* strains that are defective in their ability to cope with such plant defense compounds are hypovirulent, demonstrating the importance of these compounds in attenuating disease severity.

Botrytis cinerea is nonpathogenic on cereals. However, the Nep1-like proteins (NLPs), a class of noncatalytic cell-death–inducing proteins (CDIPs) interact with the glycosylinositol phosphorylceramide (GIPC) sphingolipids in the plant cell membrane and induce cell death in dicotyledonous plants. The lengths of the glycosylinositol phosphorylceramide head groups prevent the interaction of Nep1-like proteins with the glycosylinositol phosphorylceramide in monocots, making them insensitive to Nep1-like proteins. This difference might account for pathogenicity versus nonpathogenicity.

Once inside the plant, *B. cinerea* must cope with plant-resistant responses. The *B. cinerea* genome does not include host-specific toxins or *Avr* effectors. Therefore no single gene confers plant resistance against *B. cinerea*, and effector-triggered immunity (ETI) that is mediated by the specific interaction of a pathogen effector with a plant receptor resistance gene, is largely irrelevant. Thus the plant breeder cannot use the dominant major gene approach for resistance.

In the absence of complete or qualitative resistance, the quantitative virulence of *B. cinerea* is paralleled by quantitative plant defense responses based on the recognition of conserved pathogen-associated molecular patterns (PAMPs) by plant PRRs. Common PAMPs include molecules that are recognized as a fungal signal, such as chitin oligomers, as well as molecules that are vital for virulence, such as cell-death–inducing proteins that are recognized by plant receptor-like kinases (RLKs) and receptor-like proteins (RLPs) that activate a resistance response.

One of the earliest genes to be induced in the host following *B. cinerea* infection is the *Arabidopsis* receptor-like cytoplasmic protein kinases (*RLCK*) gene *BOTRYTIS-INDUCED KINASE 1* (*BIK1*). The *BIK1* gene integrates pattern-triggered immunity signals downstream of several plant PRRs independently of mitogen-activated protein kinases, connecting plant growth to resistance responses through its function in ethylene signaling. The resistance responses downstream of these signal cascades include the production of ROS, callose deposition, cell wall reinforcement, and the synthesis of the defense compounds, phytoalexins. These processes limit local infection and systemically increase resistance in uninfected parts of the plant, a systemic acquired resistance (SAR).

Bona fide classes of virulence factors include toxins, degradative enzymes (cutinases, proteases, and lipases), and cell-death–inducing proteins. Other verified factors include the detoxification of mycotoxic plant metabolites, such as α-tomatine and camalexin, by enzymatic modification or via efflux transporters. *B. cinerea* produces two major phytotoxic metabolites that are required for full virulence: the sesquiterpene botrydial and the polyketide botcinin. There are 275 predicted secreted carbohydrate-active enzymes (CAZymes) in *B. cinerea*, with many capable of degrading different types of sugar polymers in the plant cell wall. These secreted plant-cell-wall–degrading (PCWD) enzymes aid the fungus to conquer the cell wall barrier and utilize cell wall materials for nutrition. There is high redundancy among PCWD enzymes; however, the deletion of a single gene has a clear effect on pathogenicity. For example, the deletion of either of two endo-polygalacturonase (PG) genes, *bcpg1* and *bcpg2* (but not the four other polygalacturonase genes) reduced fungal virulence. A general reduction in pathogenicity was also observed following the deletion of a cellobiohydrolase and an endoglucanase gene, while the deletion of the endo-arabinanase gene, *bcara1*, reduced infection in *Arabidopsis* but not in other plant species.

When a T-DNA mutant library was created for *B. cinerea*, a hallmark of many of the nonpathogenic strains of *B. cinerea* were defects in the secretion of degradative enzymes, including PCWD enzymes. The *Snf1* kinase and the vesicular trafficking protein clathrin, both affect *B. cinerea* virulence through the regulation of activation and secretion of degradative enzymes, respectively. The transcription factor *XyrR1* regulates the expression of genes encoding PCWD enzymes, particularly xylanolytic and cellulolytic enzymes.

Cell-death–inducing proteins are generally regarded as virulence factors. However, like PCWD enzymes, cell-death–inducing proteins share high functional redundancy, and therefore their contribution to fungal virulence has been demonstrated in only a few cases. To overcome high functional redundancy, CRISPR-Cas9–mediated gene editing generated *B. cinerea* mutant strains with deletions of up to 10 cell-death–inducing proteins and two toxin genes. The effect on virulence varied depending on plant species and tissue, from no effect in tomatoes (*S. lycopersicum*) to up to a 40% reduction in virulence in apples (*Malus domestica*), suggesting that the effect of cell-death–inducing proteins is host-specific.

Cell-death–inducing proteins are secreted phytotoxic proteins that are regarded as virulence factors in hemibiotrophic and necrotrophic (*B. cinerea*) fungal and Oomycete plant pathogens. Similar to PCWD enzymes, cell-death–inducing proteins have high functional redundancy, and a clear contribution to fungal virulence has been shown in only a small number of cases. Nevertheless, more than 15 cell-death–inducing proteins have been characterized in *B. cinerea*. Of these, six are noncatalytic cell-death–inducing proteins and the rest are PCWD hydrolases, except for the transglycosylase *BcCrh1* that catalyzes the crosslinking of chitin and glucan polymers in the fungal cell wall. The plant cell-death–inducing activity of a number of catalytic cell-death–inducing proteins was found to be independent of their enzymatic activity, and in several cases, 20–40 aminoacid epitopes were found to be sufficient for the induction of cell death. Supporting a role for these cell-death–inducing proteins in pathogenicity are the deletion mutants of two genes, *bcxyn11a*, and *bcspl1*, that showed reduced virulence. Most cell-death–inducing proteins are recognized by plant receptors and elicit defense responses. A few protein derivatives that induce defense without inducing cell death have been produced, while there are no examples of the induction of cell death without the induction of the plant defense system. The contradicting activities and functional redundancy of cell-death–inducing proteins complicate their analysis; nevertheless, accumulating data strongly support their contribution to *B. cinerea* pathogenicity.

Another group of potential virulence factors are proteins that contribute to ROS metabolism and affect the cellular oxidative state, such as oxidoreductases. *B. cinerea* produces hydrogen peroxide (H_2O_2) that accumulates in hyphal tips and infection cushions, possibly facilitating host penetration by promoting the oxidation of cuticle polymers. Deletion of the *bcsod1* (superoxide dismutase) and *bcnoxb* (NADPH oxidase) genes reduced fungal virulence, supporting a role for H_2O_2 and other types of oxidizing agents in pathogenicity. However, no change in ROS production is observed in *bcnoxa* or *bcnoxb* single or double mutants. These findings suggest that NADPH oxidase might not contribute significantly to the oxidative burst in *B. cinerea*, and that reduced pathogenicity might be associated with changes in fungal development rather than a direct effect of ROS on the plant. Recent research revealed that *B. cinerea* secretes a cytochrome c-peroxidase that facilitates plant invasion by detoxification of host-derived ROS.

Another pathogenicity mechanism of host tissue is the local modulation of pH. Modulation of pH, including both acidification and alkalinization of the host tissue, is necessary for virulence and is achieved by the temporally and spatially controlled secretion of organic acids, primarily citric acid that acidifies the tissue, followed by accumulation of ammonia that alkalinizes it. Oxalic acid is produced at the late colonization stage; however, unlike *Sclerotinia sclerotiorum* (causal agent for white mold and Sclerotinia stem rot) in which oxalic acid is essential for pathogenicity, the role of oxalic acid in *B. cinerea* pathogenicity is unclear. It is clear that *B. cinerea* acidifies the host tissue and that this acidification is required for the proper progression of infection.

The transition from local to spreading lesions in the host is associated with a developmental switch from the production of small amounts of unoriented hyphae to the massive production of radiating mycelia that can spread as quickly as 0.5 mm per hour. Remarkably, the hyphae always remain behind the lesion edge that precedes a halo of dead cells. This process entails the activity of rapid cell death–inducing diffusible molecules, but candidate molecules have not yet been identified, and while they are assumed to originate in the *B. cinerea*, a plant origin cannot be ruled out.

Despite intensive research, *B. cinerea*-specific effector proteins that target the plant's defense system have not been discovered. The lack of candidate effectors might be due to technical difficulties in isolating them, but it is also possible that, in the case of a broad host range necrotrophic pathogen, "classical" effectors are inefficient or that their contributions are masked by other factors. Another possibility is that *B. cinerea* produces other types of immune-suppressing molecules.

One such molecule is sRNAs. Both pathogens and plants exchange sRNAs during their interaction, some will alter disease progression. *B. cinerea* contains two dicer homologs, *bccdl1* and *bccdl2*, both are required for virulence, and certain *B. cinerea* sRNAs have been shown to suppress defense-related *Arabidopsis* gene expression and affect disease levels.

It is apparent that disease resistance is a battle between the pathogen and plant, and even subtle changes can significantly affect disease progression, for example, changes in the fungal inoculum, timing of defense activation, or external conditions. As with most pathogen–host interactions the answer for resistance is an integrative approach combining the utilization of the plant defense systems, altering the plant environment, and impairing fungal development and pathogenic processes.

Effectors

It has been nearly four decades since the first pathogen avirulence gene was cloned and Flor's gene-for-gene hypothesis was confirmed by Staskawicz and colleagues at University of California, Berkeley. From all pathogen types, a plethora of pathogen molecules that are "avirulent" has been discovered. Because the term "avirulence" can be confusing, it has been eliminated and replaced by the neutral term "effector." Effectors include the so-called pathogen-associated molecular patterns PAMPs, host-specific toxin molecules, and nonspecific toxins produced by many pathogens.

It is accepted that disease incidence and disease severity are a function of all the interactions between a pathogen's effectors and the host receptors and the response that is induced or not, what is called resistance or susceptibility. Now, it is possible to use expressed pathogen genes or synthesized pathogen effectors to select responsive or nonresponsive host germplasm. The use of such effectors allows the dissection of complex quantitative traits into a series of quantifiable molecular interactions.

The first effectors were found in bacteria. The first fungal effectors discovered are the host-specific toxins recovered from culture filtrates and the leaf mold fungus, *Cladosporium fulvum* of tomato (*S. lycopersicum*). Now the approach to identifying effectors is with genome sequencing. Until a pathogen's effector suite is cloned, expressed, and deployed, it will be necessary to use the living pathogen to assess host resistance.

The term, antibiosis, is defined as the biological interaction between two organisms that can result in an adverse effect.

Typically, antibiosis occurs between plants and invertebrate pests or with herbivory; however, phytoalexins can be thought of antibiosis against pathogens. Although the relative importance of phytoalexins for disease resistance is still debated, plants contain a wealth of chemicals with some toxicity to pathogens or at least cause them to grow more slowly. Some chemicals, like jasmonic acid, may be produced by plants when first attacked by pathogens. However, their levels are sometimes too low to provide adequate protection.

Another method for the plant to protect itself is plant defense signaling, that is, wound induced. Recent observations show that wounding induces transient protection in tomato (*S. lycopersicum*) to pathogens. Researchers at the University of Turin in Italy demonstrated that wounded-induced resistance was positive against *B. cinerea* and *Phytophthora capsici*, but negative against *F. oxysporum* f. sp. *lycopersicum* and *Pseudomonas syringae* pv. *tomato*. They theorized that several defense markers are influenced locally and/or systemically by wounding and might be part of the core of conserved responses whereby wounding imparts coresistance to pathogens. They speculated that some of the physiological responses to wounding might contribute to the modulation of resistance in a more pathogen-specific manner. For example, responses to stresses like wounding and pathogen attack share potential coping denominators such as transducers, effectors of resistance, and hormones, among which ethylene is a possibility for cross-protection. Their results show that wounding reduces disease severity transiently giving the greatest protection 3–7 days before inoculation. Ethylene contributes to basal resistance either positively *B. cinerea* and *P. capsici*, or negatively for *F. oxysporum* f. sp. *lycopersicum* and *P. syringae* pv. *tomato*. The general phenomenon of wound-induced resistance is important because it proves that metabolic costs related to wound repair do not generally decrease the plant fitness if pathogen attack follows. Again, the reasons behind this common behavior in response to wounding are likely to be in the overlapping molecular responses to the both the abiotic and biotic stresses. This however does not exclude those specific mechanisms, both physiological and morphological, that may contribute to the final protective effect against each tested pathogen.

Endophytic bacteria are another interesting aspect of breeding disease–resistant horticultural crops. Endophytes are microbial entities that live within living tissues of plants. They often promote plant growth and protect their host plant against pathogens. In most cases their relationship with the host plant is symbiotic and probably mutualistic. Endophytes are a source of a plethora of biologically active substances. Many of the endophytes are capable of synthesizing bioactive compounds that the plant can use for defense against pathogenic fungi and bacteria. In Japan, researchers isolated a plant growth–promoting bacterium, *Azospirillum* sp. from rice (*Oryza sativa*), and colonized tomato (*S. lycopersicum*) with it to induce disease resistance against bacterial leaf spot (*P. syringae* pv. *tomato*) and gray mold (*B. cinerea*). The endophytic colonization by this strain induced disease resistance in tomato plants against these pathogens demonstrating that it can activate the innate immune system in tomato, which does not seem to be systemic acquired resistance (SAR). Therefore the plant breeder can select plants that encourage the endophytes to grow and produce these bioactive compounds as a way to get disease-resistant plants.

As one can expect, different plant species have different defense mechanisms; however, the most common form of defense mechanisms is through nonhost resistance. Nonhost resistance is sometimes referred to as "plant immunity" and involves the recognition of PAMPs or MAMPs, which are small molecular motifs from a vast array of molecules. Because nearly all microorganisms contain these molecular patterns and only very few are pathogenic, the use of MAMP is now preferred instead of PAMPs. The MAMP are molecular structures that are highly conserved among organisms and therefore are widely recognized by many organisms, often by the toll-like receptors (TLRs) or other PRRs. The recognition of MAMP by plants is often referred to as microbe-associated molecular patterns–triggered immunity (MTI), which is the initial defense response from the plant upon first encountering the microbe. Nonhost plants also have mechanisms to detect nonhost–pathogen effectors and can trigger a defense response referred to as ETI, which will be discussed further in later chapters. An interplay of both constitutive barriers and inducible reactions comprises the basis for this most durable form of plant disease resistance. However, the genetics of nonhost resistance between closely related plant species and their corresponding pathogens indicates that in these interactions, nonhost resistance primarily involves major genes that operate on a gene-for-gene principle, like that seen in host resistance.

Despite extensive research activities devoted to host and nonhost resistance, there is no unifying concept that connects these phenomena. A considerable body of research exists at the genetic and molecular level on some of the mechanisms underlying nonhost resistance. Previous definitions have attempted to qualitatively distinguish between host and nonhost interactions; however, many plant–pathogen systems cannot be neatly classified into these two extremes. A continuum of resistance outcomes is possible ranging from immunity to partial resistance with varying degrees of efficacy. Nevertheless, there is some evidence that host and nonhost resistance mechanisms can be the same, but not necessarily. To this end, relatively large portions of plant genomes are dedicated to defense against pathogens. With a relatively small genome (135 Mb), *Arabidopsis thaliana* contains 150 members of the nucleotide-binding site (NBS), leucine-rich repeat (LRR) family of resistance genes having more than 200 LRR kinases, for example. In the major Solanaceae crops of potato (*S. tuberosum*), tomato (*S. lycopersicum*), and pepper (*Capsicum annuum*) with larger genomes (840 Mb, 950 Mb, and 3.5 Gb, respectively), there have been 267, 443, and 755 NLR-encoding genes with potato, tomato, and pepper, respectively, identified.

Resistance involves, as an initial step, the recognition of the potential pathogen by way of chemical cues, originally termed "elicitors" or "general elicitors," followed by a response mechanism. Michelle C. Heath in the Botany Department at the University of Toronto suggested that there are numerous hurdles for the pathogen to overcome to establish a compatible interaction. These "event points" are designated points that are discreet events occurring between the pathogen and host that can be perceived as gene-for-gene events. This suggests that corresponding genes for host–parasite incompatibility act to produce a general and basic disorder that can be expressed at many stages in the host–parasite interaction.

Heath observed: (1) spore germination, (2) stomata contact, (3) appressoria, (4) haustoria, and (5) callus deposition, while examining the cowpea rust (*Uromyces phaseoli* var. *vignae*) interaction with the hosts, cowpea (*Vigna unguiculata*) cultivars; Early Ramshorn (susceptible host); Purple Hull Pinkeye (necrotic fleck resistance); and Queen Anne (immune); as well as in the nonhosts green bean (*Phaseolus vulgarus*), lima bean (*Phaseolus lunatus*), pea (*Pisum sativum*), fava/broad bean (*Vicia faba*), cabbage (*Brassica oleracea* var. *capitata*), tobacco (*Nicotiana tabacum*), and tomato (*S. lycopersicum*). She found that (1) uredospore germination and fungal development on leaf surface was not a determinant of resistance; (2) few stomatal contacts occurred in nonhosts; (3) topographical features aid in susceptibility; (4) many stages were recognized where interactions can take place; and (5) varietal resistance does not use prehaustoria incompatibility but induced after the formation of haustorium, which could be an example of gene-for-gene.

In most interactions, the cowpea rust pathogen frequently germinated and identified a stoma and produced an appressorium, with most infections terminating following the formation of a haustorial mother cell within the apoplast. Generally, haustoria were not observed, but in those rare cases where they did occur, they were usually associated with plant cell death (apoptosis). A distribution of infection site outcomes was observed on single leaves that ranged from germinated spores that did not locate a stoma to those that produced haustoria.

The underlying mechanism of nonhost immunity and host immunity involves the same nonself-detection systems, the combined action of nucleotide-binding and leucine-rich repeat (NB-LRR) proteins and PRRs. It is hypothesized that the relative contribution of NB-LRR and PRRs-triggered immunity to nonhost resistance changes as a function of phylogenetic divergence time between host and nonhost. Similarly, changes in pathogen–host range, for example, host range expansions, appear to be driven by variations in pathogen effector repertoires, leading to reproductive isolation and subsequent pathogen speciation.

Pathogens can range from highly specialized and only infect a single plant species (narrow host range) to others that are able to either colonize a few or a considerable number of hosts that can sometimes belong to different plant families (broad host range). Often, viruses have relatively narrow host ranges and infect closely related species or only a single species, although exceptions are common, particularly for some genera of viruses such as *Begomovirus*, which infects more than 1000 hosts. Conversely, pathogenic fungi, bacteria, and oomycetes typically have a much greater host range, for example, the fungus *B. cinerea* has a host range of more than 200 species. Pathogens rarely alter their host species range over recorded history; instead, speciation events and the development of forma specialis are more common. Forma specialis literally means "special form," and normally is abbreviated "f. sp." It is an informal taxonomic grouping that is applied to a pathogen, most frequently a fungus that is adapted to a specific host. An example is *F. oxysporum* f. sp. *pisi*, which causes wilt of pea (*P. sativum*). More than 100 formae speciales have been identified within *F. oxysporum*.

Because of the durability of nonhost resistance, it is commonly speculated that nonhost resistance should be exploited by plant breeders to improve disease resistance within host species. Thus plant phenotyping of nonhost resistance can operate at various levels of resolution and dimensionality, from the molecular to the whole plant, and in different environments, from controlled environments to field conditions. Although each level focuses on traits, the goal is to integrate knowledge from the bottom up to produce cultivars with higher levels of resistance. In that regard, the use of plant phenotyping methods as part of breeding programs has become a powerful research tool to help breeders generate cultivars more adaptable to diverse pathosystems.

Ideally, a plant species is classified as a nonhost if all accessions of the species are resistant to all isolates of the pathogen and uniform levels of resistance are observed in all interactions between both organisms. In practice, however, delimiting the host range of a pathogen is complicated by the quantitative nature of the resistance interaction phenotypes in the transition from host to nonhost. Interactions in this transitional phase may involve only a few accessions of a species being infected by a pathogen or only some isolates of a pathogen being able to infect a plant species. In addition, a continuum of disease phenotypes exists in the interaction with different plant species that range from full susceptibility (host) to complete immunity (nonhost).

The often-cited advantage of nonhost resistance is that it is a durable, broad-spectrum resistance against multiple strains of a pathogen. The possibility of transferring nonhost resistance to a horticultural plant is therefore an attractive objective. There are a limited number of examples of successful transfer of resistance from a nonhost species to a host. Although examples in horticultural crops are rare, one example of moving nonhost resistance into a host crop involves the transfer of the sweet corn (*Zea mays*) nucleotide-binding site leucine-rich repeat (NBS-LRR) motifs encoding gene *Rxo1* into rice (*O. sativa*). The causal agent of bacterial leaf streak of rice is *Xanthomonas oryzae* pv. *oryzicola*, but it is not a pathogen of maize. The maize gene, *Rxo1*, conferring a strong hypersensitive response was isolated by positional cloning and the NBS-LRR protein encoded by this gene conferred resistance to bacterial leaf streak when transferred to rice. Interestingly, *Rxo1* also provides protection in maize against maize bacterial leaf stripe (*Burkholderia andropogonis*) a completely different organism.

In *A. thaliana*, a leucine-rich repeat receptor-kinase (LRR) recognizes a conserved, abundant bacterial translation initiation factor protein, the Elongation factor Tu (Ef-Tu) that activates the pattern-triggered immunity (PTI) pathway. No equivalent receptor is present in solanaceous plants and transfer of this gene to tomato (*S. lycopersicum*) and *Nicotiana benthamiana* provided increased resistance against the bacterial diseases; bacterial canker (*Agrobacterium tumefaciens*), black speck (*P. syringae*), and bacterial wilt (*Ralstonia solanacearum*). It is noteworthy that a fully functional signaling pathway enabling effector function resistance (EFR) to function in these solanaceous species was preexisting.

These examples of the transfer of resistance genes from one nonhost species conferring resistance in another species against pathogens that do not parasitize the gene donor parent are important and could provide a basis for future research in breeding for resistance. Potentially, these genes may play a role in protecting the donor plants against these nonadapted pathogen species. This conclusion, however, is entirely presumptive because the absence of functional *Rxo1* allele in maize does not increase its susceptibility to nonadapted pathogens. Redundancy in nonhost resistance is likely to mask any individual contributions of these genes and adds difficulty in confirming their roles in nonhost resistance. In chile pepper (*C. annuum*), for example, *P. capsici* is a highly destructive pathogen; however, chile pepper is a nonhost to the pathogen famously known to cause late blight (*P. infestans*) of tomato (*S. lycopersicum*) and potato (*S. tuberosum*). Two different genes for capsidiol biosynthesis, 5-*epi*-aristolochene synthase (*EAS*) and 5-*epi*-aristolochene 1,3-dihydroxylase (*EAH*) have been found to be effective in nonhost resistance in chile pepper to *P. infestans*. Similarly, the *RB* gene from *Solanum bulbocastanum* that confers broad-spectrum resistance to *P. infestans* in both tomato and potato has been found to result in an elevated level of resistance in chile pepper when introduced via the development of an *A. tumefaciens* mediated transformation system. However, the combination of these three genes has not been deployed and therefore one is unable to predict how durable or broad spectrum the resistance might be to multiple species of *Phytophthora*, if at all.

An important question to ask is whether identifying single genes potentially involved in nonhost resistance and deploying them individually into host plants will result in durable resistance. Given the well-documented transient efficacy of these types of genes it seems unlikely that a single NBS-LRR encoding gene will be able to provide durable resistance, unless those members involved in nonhost resistance recognize are indispensable subset of either pathogen effector proteins or effector modifications of plant proteins. Conversely, a pattern-recognition receptor would seem to offer a greater chance of durability given the conservation of microbe-associated molecular patterns molecules, suggesting biological constraints act upon these molecules that prevent mutation or deletion for resistance avoidance. However, at least on an evolutionary time scale, MAMP immunity pathways are ultimately suppressed by the deployment of novel effectors. Moreover, the durability of an adult plant resistance gene like *Lr34* in providing resistance to pathogens of a different species after heterologous transfer would be exceedingly difficult to predict, as important factors such as the substrate of this transporter and the resulting mechanism of resistance are currently unknown.

A possibility is that single gene deployment of nonhost resistance genes in new species may result in loss of their efficacy due to pathogen adaptation, which in turn may make the gene donor species susceptible to a previously nonadapted pathogen. Is this scenario likely? While in some instances very few genes confer apparent immunity to a pathogen species, in other instances it appears that nonhost resistance is polygenic. The loss of a single nonhost resistance gene in this latter case is unlikely to result in the susceptibility of the donor gene species. An obvious approach to alleviate some of these concerns would be to treat cloned nonhost resistance genes like any other resistance gene and avoid their single gene deployment.

Hypersensitive response

The resistance phenomenon known as the hypersensitive response (HR) was first described by pioneering plant pathologists more than 100 years ago. H. Marshall Ward saw variable responses by wheat (*Triticum aestivum*) cultivars to leaf rust (*Puccinia dispersa*, a synonym for *Puccinia triticina*), while E.C. Gibson noted that varieties of *Chrysanthemum* that were resistant to *Puccinia chrysanthemi* hyphae exhibited a localized plant cell death. Similar observations were made by Dorothea Marryat in the wheat–leaf yellow rust (*Puccinia glumarum*) pathosystem. However, the actual definition of the HR arose from the work of Elvin C. Stakman who investigated the responses of various cereal crops to differing formae speciales of the black stem rust fungus, *Puccinia graminis*. He noted cases where "host plants exhibit a considerable degree of resistance to the fungus. ... the host plant in such cases is ... hypersensitive to the fungus." He further defined "hypersensitiveness ... to indicate the abnormally rapid host plant death when attacked by rust fungi." A very general definition of the HR could therefore be an area of cell death that forms at the point of attempted pathogen ingress and correlates with the exhibition of resistance. This retains Stakman's 1915 focus on a phenotype-based description, rather than defenses that have come to be associated with this cell death phenomenon; for example, a myriad of defense genes and the production of antimicrobial secondary metabolites such as phytoalexins.

HR is a plant mechanism to prevent the spread of infection. Hypersensitive response/resistance is found in all higher plants and is characterized by a rapid cell death (apoptosis) at the point of pathogen ingress and is associated with pathogen resistance. By inducing apoptosis, the plant imposes a reduction or ideally elimination of the available energy source for the pathogen, inhibiting further colonization of other plant cells and tissues. The ubiquity of this response among higher plants, despite its costs, exemplifies that it is an extremely effective component of the plant immune system. Due to the potentially severe costs of inappropriate activation, plants employ multiple mechanisms to suppress inappropriate activation of hypersensitive resistance. However, the necrosis associated with hypersensitive resistance is not effective to contain necrotrophic pathogens, those that can survive on dead tissue. Thus this type of resistance is activated only against biotrophic pathogens. They colonize and obtain energy from living cells or tissues rather than killing their host. The resistance is somewhat effective against hemibiotrophic pathogens. They initially colonize living tissue by way of biotrophic invasion and obtain energy from living host tissue but later switch to necrotrophic growth, rampantly killing host cells and obtaining nutrients from dead tissues.

The first idea of how the HR occurs came from Flor's gene-for-gene model. In 1955 Harold Henry Flor at North Dakota State University, United States, postulated that for every resistance gene (R) encoded by the plant, there is a corresponding avirulence (*Avr*) gene encoded by the microbe. This hypothesis was based on his work with rust (*Melampsora lini*) of flax (*Linum usitatissimum*), where he showed that based on inheritance patterns (ratios) in segregating populations containing one, two, three, or four resistance genes, the phenotypic response followed mono-, bi-, tri- or tetra-factorial ratios, respectively, indicating the presence of counteracting genes between the host and the pathogen. In other words, the plant is resistant to the pathogen if both the avirulence (*Avr*) and resistant (R) genes are present during the plant–pathogen interaction. The genes that are involved in the plant–pathogen interactions tend to evolve at a very rapid rate (Fig. 2.1).

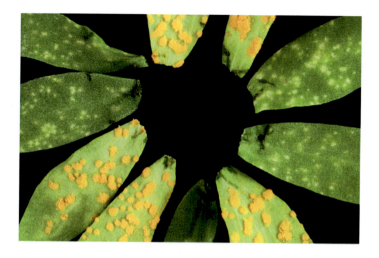

Figure 2.1 Flax (*Linum usitatissimum*) leaves displaying resistance and susceptibility to rust (*Melampsora lini*). Courtesy CSIRO, Photographer: Carl Davies.

A distinctive feature of the HR lesions is a sharp cellular delineation between the dead and surrounding living tissue. Despite these features, HR defies easy description. The HR forming during different plant–pathogen interactions can vary enormously in phenotype and timing. Such variation only partially relates to differing infection strategies adopted by the various types of pathogens that elicit a HR, for example, oomycetes, fungi, bacteria or viruses, and undoubtedly reflects differences in underlying HR cell death mechanisms. It is misleading to generalize among pathosystems and significant variation between differing HR mechanisms. Further, some models for the HR are based on the use of cell death elicitors from necrotizing pathogens; for example, cryptogein from *Phytophthora cryptogea* and victorin from *Cochiliobolus victoriae* are, in fact, elicitor factors. Although these can be thought to confuse HR studies there is clear evidence of overlap in necrotrophic pathogen–induced cell death and the HR.

It is self-evident that HR is an example of programmed cell death (PCD). Programmed cell death occurs as a regulated process, mediated by the dying cell and frequently with contributions from surrounding tissue. It is perhaps more easily understood by contrast with nonprogrammed death, which classically results from cell lysis, for example, following mechanical damage, and where the biochemical and genetic status of the cell is irrelevant.

Harold H. Flor with his gene-for-gene theory, first described the dependence of the HR and resistance on resistance gene interaction with pathogen-encoded avirulence (*avr*) gene production. Subsequently, a large number of resistance genes have been cloned. A near-ubiquitous feature of resistance gene products is the possession of variable numbers of leucine-rich repeats, and frequently nucleotide-binding sites. However, no interaction with obvious death effectors is known. A recent reinterpretation of resistance gene products function suggests that resistance gene products act to protect plant proteins against manipulation by pathogen-derived effectors. According to this hypothesis *Pto*, which is guarded by *Prf*, is the pathogenicity target of *AvrPto*, rather than a host resistance protein, and *Prf* is the host defense R protein that recognizes the *AvrPto:Pto* complex and initiates the HR.

An example of the gene-for-gene model and HR is for bacterial spot (*Xanthomonas* sp.) of pepper (*C. annuum*). There are at least six different bacterial spot resistance (*Bs*) genes in pepper and at least 10 different races of the bacterial spot pathogen. Extensive research has identified and characterized these *Bs* genes and establish host differentials to characterize the race structure of the pathogen. The *Bs1*, *Bs2*, *Bs3*, and *Bs4* genes are all dominant resistance genes and elicit a HR. Using genetic transformation, the *Bs2* gene from pepper was inserted into tomato (*S. lycopersicum*) and found to be highly effective, as the *AvrBs2* gene from bacterial spot is highly conserved across *Xanthomonas* species. However, mutations in the *avr* genes and shifting bacteria populations have overcome resistance conferred by many of the *Bs* genes, including *Bs2*. Recently, efforts have been made to identify and characterize more broad-spectrum resistance genes in pepper that do not elicit an HR and have recessive inheritance patterns, *bs5* and *bs6*, that when pyramided results in resistance to all known races of the pathogen (Fig. 2.2).

Hypersensitive resistance can induce SAR, a broad spectrum systemic enhanced resistance to pathogenic infection following a localized infection by a necrotizing pathogen or following treatment with various chemical agents. It is dependent on the phytohormone salicylate (salicylic acid) and associated with the accumulation of pathogenesis-related proteins.

Systemic acquired resistance (SAR)

Pathogens attacking plants activate specific resistance mechanisms collectively called induced resistance. Plant researchers have known for more than 100 years that plants can be preconditioned against diseases caused by a variety of pathogens. This induced resistance response is ubiquitous in plants, having been reported

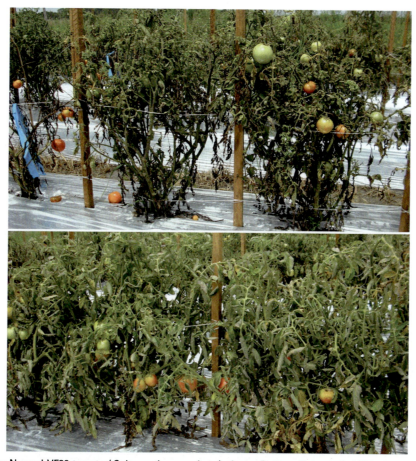

Figure 2.2 Top: Normal VF36 tomato (*Solanum lycopersicum*) plants. Bottom: Transgenic VF36 tomato plants with the pepper (*Capsicum annuum*) 35 S:Bs2 gene. Courtesy of PLoS ONE, https://doi.org/10.1371/journal.pone.0042036.g003.

in more than 100 plant species from 30 families. Induced resistance is a physiological "state of enhanced defensive capacity" and is effective against a broad range of organisms, including fungi, bacteria, viruses, nematodes, parasitic plants, and even arthropods.

The two most clearly defined forms of induced resistance are SAR and induced systemic resistance (ISR) that are differentiated based on the nature of the elicitor and the regulatory pathways involved. Australian researchers, Ian Alfred Murray Cruikshank and M. Mandryk, in 1960 demonstrated SAR in field-grown tobacco (*N. tabacum*) plants using stem injections of *Peronospora tabacina* (the causative agent of blue mold of tobacco), which triggered SAR against subsequent inoculations of the same pathogen. These landmark studies led to the development of the classic SAR models during the 1980s in other plants, such as cucumber (*Cucumis sativus*), green bean (*P. vulgaris*), rice (*O. sativa*), and *A. thaliana*, demonstrating that SAR is conserved across diverse plant families and is effective against a broad range of viral, bacterial, and fungal pathogens.

The recognition of the pathogen infection by the plant is the first step in the development of SAR. The classic form of SAR is triggered by exposing the plant to virulent, avirulent, and non-pathogenic microbes, or artificially with chemical inducers or elicitors. Any disruption in the plant's ability to accumulate salicylic acid results in the loss of pathogenesis-related gene expression and attenuation of the SAR response.

Once the plant reacts to the pathogen, signals are released that trigger resistance in adjacent as well as distant tissues. Currently, there is no common denominator that can be used to group inducing pathogens, and not all plant–pathogen interactions lead to SAR inducement. Conceivably, each taxonomic group of plants may have evolved its own set of SAR genes in response to evolutionary pressure from a specific spectrum of pathogens.

Induced systemic resistance

Unlike SAR, ISR does not involve the accumulation of pathogenesis-related proteins or salicylic acid, but instead, relies on pathways regulated by jasmonate and ethylene. However, these characterizations are based on a limited number of ISR systems.

The specificity of ISR to various organisms has been observed. There is evidence from in vivo studies that SAR and ISR pathways can interfere with one another. This negative cross-talk between responses of the SAR and ISR pathways was demonstrated by reducing phenylpropanoid biosynthesis that in turn reduced the expression of SAR. Additional evidence showed that jasmonate-induced responses, although benefiting plants under attack from a pathogen, are costly and result in reduced seed yield in plants not under pathogen pressure. Attempts to artificially stimulate, or genetically modify plants to express SAR and ISR pathways on demand may not result in the expected and desired outcome. The evidence points toward several possible negative scenarios such as, plants resistant to pathogens, but very susceptible to herbivore attack, and vice versa, while plants expend energy on protection from nonexistent threats. Additionally, the specificity in responses indicates that there are multiple systems of response in plant species and more studies are necessary to get a better understanding of the coordination by plants of multiple defense systems against multiple biotic threats.

Because induced resistance is a biological response, it should be amenable to breeding strategies to minimize its negative impact on horticultural traits, and perhaps even improve its overall effectiveness. Data exist supporting heritability in the induction of plant defenses and physiological costs incurred from maintaining plant defenses, opening the possibility of breeding plants with improved ISR responses with minimizing fitness costs. It is highly likely for plant breeders to select for variability that exists within plant populations for the induction, maintenance, and overall robustness (in terms of the number and effectiveness of individual biochemical components involved) of induced resistance responses. Interestingly, some limited studies evaluating SAR among cultivars that differed in their level of resistance toward a particular pathogen found improved efficacy in partially resistant cultivars over susceptible cultivars, whereas others reported just the opposite or few differences among cultivars. However, there is evidence from an ecological study using families of wild radish (*Raphanus raphanistrum*) derived from full-sibling or half-sibling mating that significant differences existed among families for fitness costs following induction, as measured by differences among various reproductive traits, suggesting that among the families there was either genetic variability for the induction of resistance or genetic variability for the physiological costs associated with the induced resistance response, which implies heritability.

A question that arises when ISR is discussed is why it is not used more in plant breeding programs. There are factors favorable and unfavorable for the development and use of ISR. Some of the favorable factors include problems with the resistance of pathogens to pesticides; the necessity to remove pesticides from the market because of the increased testing and cost of testing to meet requirements of regulatory agencies and the lack of substitutes for removed compounds; health and environmental problems with pesticides and the increased popularity of "organic crops" and "sustainable agriculture"; the inability of pesticides to effectively control some pathogens, for example, virus and soilborne pathogens; classical pesticides may not be economically feasible for farmers in developing countries. In these countries the level of awareness for the safe and effective application of classical pesticides is low, thus creating dangers to human health and the environment, resistance of the public to genetically modified plants. With ISR, foreign genes are not introduced.

The "traditional" genes for resistance in the plant are those that are expressed; ISR has a broad spectrum and is effective for a long time; many defenses are activated, when ISR is less likely to develop resistance in pathogens. Nevertheless, with all the favorable aspects there are few examples of cultivars released as having ISR as the mechanism for resistance.

Cross-protection

Cross-protection in plants is the phenomenon whereby a plant preinoculated with a mild virus strain becomes resistant to subsequent inoculation by a related severe virus strain. It has been used in cases where no resistant plants are available. Cross-protection has been developed at a commercial level to protect cucurbit crops against Zucchini yellow mosaic virus (ZYMV, *Potyvirus*). The mild or weak (WK) strain ZYMV-WK is a natural variant of a severe aphid nontransmissible isolate. Although efficient against most ZYMV isolates, ZYMV-WK does not protect against very divergent isolates such as those from Réunion Island indicating some specificity in the protection. A single amino acid change (R to I) in the severe strain (FRNK) conserved domain of the HC-Pro is responsible for symptom attenuation of ZYMV-WK. A complete technological package (mild strain production, quality control protocols, and inoculation machines) has been developed to implement commercial ZYMV cross-protection (Fig. 2.3).

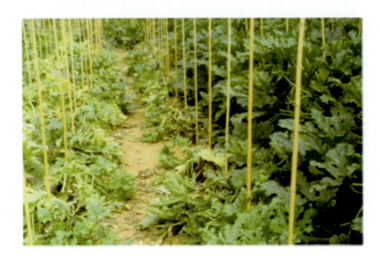

Figure 2.3 Cross-protected zucchini crop in greenhouse conditions. Left: unprotected plants infected with a severe strain of Zucchini yellow mosaic virus, ZYMV; right: plants preventively inoculated with the mild strain ZYMV-WK, protected against infection with severe strains. Courtesy: Desbiez, C., Lecoq, H., 2021. Viruses as infectious agents: plant viruses, in: Encyclopedia of Virology (Fourth Edition).

Although several hypotheses have been proposed to explain the molecular mechanism underlying cross-protection, no single hypothesis can account for all the data obtained. At Cornell University, United States, A. Frank Ross in 1961 using Tobacco mosaic virus (TMV; *Tobamovirus*) sensitized tobacco (*N. tabacum*) against subsequent "challenge" inoculations of TMV on infected leaves or on distal uninfected leaves. Clearly, one may remark that this method mirrors vaccination in animals.

System-acquired resistance and ISR pathways do not appear to apply selective pressure to pathogen populations based on any single genetic determinant or specific mode of action. Unlike race-specific resistance, induced resistance is quantitative because of the cumulative effects of numerous plant defense mechanisms. Because of its similarity to quantitative resistance, the effectiveness of induced resistance has the potential to "erode" over time as the pathogen population evolves.

The efficacy of SAR and ISR pathways also depend on the pathogen, and some pathogens do not respond to elicitors. For example, SAR induced by benzothiadiazole (BTH) was ineffective against fusarium wilt (*F. oxysporum* f. sp. *cucumerinum*) of cucumber (*C. sativus*). Preinoculation of green bean (*P. vulgaris*) plants with *Colletotrichum lindemuthianum* or foliar applications of 2,6 dichloroisonicotinic acid (INA) was ineffective against two root pathogens, *Fusarium solani* f. sp. *phaseoli* and pathogenic *Rhizoctonia* spp. Several elicitors of SAR and ISR also failed to reduce symptoms of late leaf spot (*Phaeoisariopsis personata*) of peanut (*Arachis hypogaea*) and in some cases exacerbated symptoms. It is conceivable that in the previous examples, the disease was unaffected because the pathogen was able to thwart host defenses or because the plant lacked effective defenses or lacked the capacity to initiate defenses against the pathogen.

Neither SAR nor ISR pathways are stand-alone methods for disease control, but merely add another tool for breeding disease—resistant horticultural crops. Each crop and disease will be unique in some regard. The effective use of either SAR or ISR will heavily depend on disease forecasting and the ability to activate plant defenses at critical developmental periods when the plant is most susceptible, because SAR and ISR are ineffective once the pathogen has established itself. There is also the risk of rendering the plant susceptible to other pathogens or insect herbivores, so it will be necessary to continuously monitor various pests during the growth of the crop.

The future use of SAR and ISR to control plant disease in conventional agriculture has potential. Synthetic elicitors do not exhibit any direct antimicrobial activity, unlike traditional pesticides, they provide a way to control disease without asserting direct selective pressure on pathogen populations. In addition, the use of synthetic elicitors seems to be environmentally benign relative to current pesticides. These characteristics make ISR, an attractive approach for managing plant diseases in a sustainable manner within the scope of a conventional agriculture system.

It is important to understand that SAR and ISR, as defined, are probably only two outcomes out of an array of possibilities. It is likely that other forms of induced resistance exist that vary in their reliance on salicylic acid, ethylene, brassinosteroids, and jasmonate and other yet discovered plant regulators.

Manipulation of plant architecture

Patterns of plant growth and characteristics of plant form may influence susceptibility to infection and subsequent disease expression. Dense foliage, resulting in insufficient aeration, may predispose fruit crops to diseases such as mildew rots (*B. cinerea*), rots of small fruits, brown rots (*Monilinia fructicola*) of stone fruits, and black rot (*Guignardia bidwelli*) of grapes that thrive in highly humid microenvironments. Of some consequence to the overall extent of infection is the number of infective site or the amount of susceptible tissue available at any one time. Flushes of stem growth of short duration, followed by a hardening-off of the tissue may, for example reduce the probability of fire blight (*Erwinia amylovora*) infection of some oriental pear species (*Pyrus calleryana*).

The number of growing points also may influence susceptibility to disease, because there is a direct relationship between the number of shoots and the number of possible sites for infection. A plant with many growing points may produce either more foliage, blossoms, or total surface area, leading to the possibility of more initial infection. There is also the possibility, however, that a greater number of growing points may prevent the complete destruction of extensive damage to a single plant, as a certain number of growing points may remain uninfected.

When genes for resistance are unknown, breeding for disease avoidance can be a solution. Plant breeders can select for altered plant architectural features to facilitate disease control by creating unfavorable environments for pathogen growth or limiting pathogen contact with the host. The morphology required to limit losses depends on the host plant and pathogen.

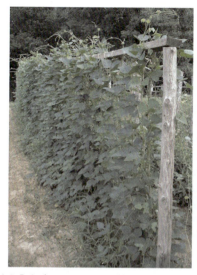
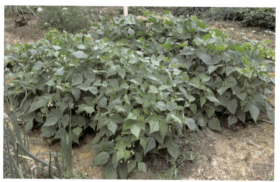

Figure 2.4 Pole (nondeterminacy) and bush (determinacy) beans (*Phaseolus vulgaris*) illustrating the two types of determinate plant growth.

Breeding for modified plant architecture depends on the underlying genetic basis for the trait. Diversity in architectural phenotypes can result from a single gene, a few genes, or quantitative factors. Determinacy, for example, can be conferred by a single major gene as in green bean (*Phaseolus vulgaris*). Other traits, such as internode length, vine length, and number of branches in cucumber (*C. sativus*), exhibit continuous variation among accessions, with an approximately 10-fold range in values (Fig. 2.4).

In general, any morphological feature that reduces humidity in the canopy has the potential to reduce infection by fungal and bacterial diseases. For example, in carrot (*Daucus carota*), lateral trimming of the canopy by 30%–40% after canopy closure reduced sclerotinia rot (*Sclerotinia sclerotiorum*) to zero under moderate disease pressure. Trimming reduced relative humidity within the carrot canopy and increased air and soil temperature. Trimming also severed infected petioles, which reduced the opportunity for infection to progress to the carrot crown. Similarly, breeding a plant so that its susceptible organs or tissues are not in direct contact with the pathogen can also reduce pathogen infection. Therefore if one bred a carrot with more upright and less spreading foliage, sclerotinia rot may be reduced.

Another example of resistance based on plant architecture is in asparagus (*Asparagus officinalis*) to *Stemphylium* leaf spots on fronds or purple spots on spears caused by *Stemphylium vesicarium*. Under field conditions for natural infection, various levels of resistance can be observed among cultivars with French cultivars more susceptible than North American cultivars because of distinct plant architectures. French cultivars are shorter, lower branched and more compact than North American cultivars, producing a microenvironment more favorable to the fungus.

Cucumbers (*C. sativus*) with shorter vines, reduced branching, and smaller leaves, reduced *P. capsici* fruit rot. Adjusting plant morphology to reduce viral disease incidence is more challenging, because the infection is less dependent on environmental factors like humidity; however, it is possible to select for morphological features that reduce the infection by the vectors of viral diseases. In onions (*Allium cepa*), thrips (*Thrips tabaci* or *Franklinella schultzei*) and the viruses they vector, most commonly members of *Tospovirus*, can be a major production limitation. However, it has been reported that onion plants with more blue-green colored foliage appear to be more attractive to thrips, while yellow-green leaves typically have less thrip infestation and lower levels of viral diseases. The nonpreference of arthropod pests toward certain plants based on morphological features is termed antixenosis and is an exceptionally durable form of resistance for host plants. It has been found that this blue color in some onions is associated with elevated levels of epicuticular waxes, while glossy or semiglossy onions have lower levels of wax and are more yellow in color (Fig. 2.5).

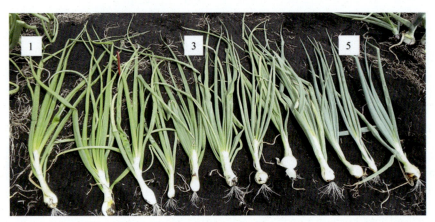

Figure 2.5 Onions (*Allium cepa*) with various levels of wax on the leaves. From left to right: 1 = glossy, 3 = semiglossy, and 5 = waxy. Courtesy: Munaiz, E.D., Groves, R.L., Havey, M.J. 2019. Amounts and Types of Epicuticular Leaf Waxes among Onion Accessions Selected for Reduced Damage by Onion Thrips. Journal of the American Society for Horticultural Science 145, 1; https://doi.org/10.21273/JASHS04773-19.

Some varieties of plums (*Prunus domestica*) resist brown rot (*Monilinia fructicola*) because the stomata soon become plugged with masses of small parenchymatous cells. The toughness of the skin, the firmness of the flesh, and high fiber content also are characteristics that make cultivars of plums resistant to brown rot. As ripening progresses, the texture of the resistant varieties remains firm, while that of the susceptible becomes softer.

With raspberry (*Rubus idaeus*), it has been reported that resistance to some fungal diseases is associated with distinctive morphological traits, most notable cane pubescence (fine hairs). Pubescence is determined by gene *H*; the recessive allele gives glabrous canes. Gene *H* is rarely homozygous (*HH*) because it is linked with a lethal recessive gene. Raspberry (*R. idaeus*) cultivars and selections with pubescent canes are more resistant to cane botrytis (*B. cinerea*) and spur blight (*Didymella applanata*) than nonpubescent ones, but more susceptible to cane spot (*Elsinoe veneta*), powdery mildew (*Sphaerotheca macularis*) and yellow rust (*Phragmidium rubi-idaei*). How gene *H* results in a large increase or decrease in disease resistance have not been determined. It has been suggested that it is due to linkage with major resistance genes or minor gene complexes that independently contribute to the resistance or susceptibilities of the six diseases affected. An alternative explanation is that the gene itself is responsible through pleiotropic effects on each of the resistances. The gene *H* is known to have other pleiotropic effects besides its main effect on cane pubescence: it is associated with a small increase in spine frequency and a decrease in spine size. Hairs and spines are both outgrowths of epidermal cells and their early development is interrelated. It would therefore seem likely that gene *H* acts early in development and affects several cell characteristics. Resistance to *B. cinerea* and *Didymella. applanata* is highest in immature tissues and it has postulated that the gene increases resistance by delaying cell maturity and this delay may reduce resistance to *E. veneta* and *P. rubi-idaei* as these fungi only invade immature tissues. Alternatively, cane hairiness itself could affect the ability of fungi to adhere and infect tissues.

Spur blight and cane botrytis occupy the same ecological niche on raspberry (*R. idaeus*) canes and often one or the other predominates. Spur blight infects mature or senescent leaves on young canes of raspberry (*R. idaeus*), then grows within the petioles to the nodes where the disease lesions develop. Buds at infected nodes are retarded in growth compared to those at noninfected nodes, and infection usually results in the failure of buds to develop into fertile lateral shoots the following spring. *B. cinerea* infects in a similar manner though with bud dwarfing more severe. Lateral shoot loss with these diseases is the most important factor for yield loss. It has been shown that a common resistance operates against these two pathogens. Whether resistance is caused by a major gene, a complex of dominant minor genes or a major gene in combination with minor genes has yet to be determined. Field screening either with natural infection or with a simple wound inoculation method remains the best method for analysis of resistance status, as glasshouse inoculations do not result in characteristic disease symptoms.

Cane spot can be expressed in leaves, fruits, and young canes but it is most easily recognized by the deeply penetrating sunken lesions it produces on second-year fruiting canes (floricanes) that lead to damaged vascular tissue and yield loss in susceptible cultivars. Natural infection of selections in field observation plots with a high disease incidence remains the most effective way of resistance breeding.

Gene *H* has been reported to be associated with high susceptibility to cane spots in European cultivars and originally it was thought that cultivars carrying the gene would inevitably be susceptible. However, several North American cultivars are good sources of resistance, despite carrying the gene.

Yellow rust (*P. rubi-idaei*) on raspberry (*R. idaeus*) has come to prominence with the expansion of raspberry (*R. idaeus*) production under plastic tunnels. The high humidity in plastic tunnels exacerbates the disease. Bait plants in commercial plantations in replicated field experiments have been used to assess genetic resistance. The American cultivar Latham is known to exhibit complete resistance transmissible through four generations and determined by gene *Yr*.

Dr. Julie Graham and colleagues at the Scottish Crop Research Institute, Dundee, United Kingdom used a population that segregates for gene *H* and for resistance to cane botrytis (*B. cinerea*), spur blight (*D. applanata*), powdery mildew (*S. macularis*), and yellow rust (*P. rubi-idaei*). They identified map regions associated with resistance to cane botrytis (*B. cinerea*), spur blight (*D. applanata*), cane spot (*E. veneta*), and yellow rust (*P. rubi-idaei*) and gene *H*. The map location for gene *H* was determined to be on linkage group 2 and associations with resistance to the cane botrytis (*B. cinerea*), and spur blight (*D. applanata*) complex. Gene *H* and a DNA marker associated with resistance to yellow rust (*P. rubi-idaei*) were also associated with spines. Hairs and spines are both outgrowths of epidermal cells and their early development is interrelated, hence such an association is not unexpected. A factor from the cultivar, Latham was identified on linkage group 3 that is associated with resistance to rust (*P. rubi-idaei*) as well as resistance to spur blight (*D. applanata*), botrytis (*B. cinerea*) and increased number of spines. In contrast to cane botrytis (*B. cinerea*) and spur blight (*D. applanata*), no significant associations between gene *H* and yellow rust (*P. rubi-idaei*) or cane spot (*E. veneta*) were determined. It may be that the presence of a resistance gene overcomes any effect of gene *H*. It does seem likely therefore that the gene *H* itself is having some effect on resistance to *Didymella. applanata* and *B. cinerea* and spine number by its action early in development affecting several cell characteristics. A reason for the resistance and pubescens may be that water run-off is more rapid on hairy canes than nonhairy ones and bud infection therefore occurred less often on canes with hairs. However, by direct inoculation of cane tissues, the effects on disease symptom expression could be demonstrated up to a year after infection. For cane spot (*E. veneta*), no association with gene *H* could be detected.

Age-related resistance

Age-related resistance traits are targets of breeding programs to enhance disease resistance. Juveniles are typically less resistant/more susceptible to infectious disease than adults, and this difference in susceptibility can help fuel the spread of pathogens.

One hypothesis is that natural selection has optimized resistance to peak at ages where disease exposure is greatest. A central assumption of this hypothesis is that hosts have the capacity to evolve resistance independently at different ages. This would mean that host populations have (1) standing genetic variation in resistance at both juvenile and adult stages, and (2) that this variation is not strongly correlated between age classes so that selection acting at one age does not produce a correlated response at the other age. Based on the heterogeneity of host species, host age, infected host organ, and causal pathogens, age-related resistance is also referred to as "ontogenic resistance," "developmental resistance," "mature seedling resistance," or "adult plant resistance." The complexity of nomenclature indicates that there are multiple mechanisms involved in developmentally acquired defense. For many horticultural plants, genetic tools that distinguish age-dependent innate immune response from secondary consequence caused by physiological and morphological changes, such as trichome density, cuticle thickness, and leaf curling, associated with developmental transitions are still limited.

Plant age is a crucial factor in determining the outcome of a host–pathogen interaction. The term "age-related resistance" describes the gain or reinforcement of disease resistance during the process of host maturation. Agricultural practices routinely adapt plant development knowledge in disease management strategy programs. For example, planting date can often be adjusted to minimize the cost of exposing plants at a susceptible age to a seasonally active pathogen. Therefore breeding for earliness is a way to provide disease resistance to a horticultural crop.

A team of international scientists examined age-related resistance in strawberry (*Fragaria* × *ananassa*) to powdery mildew (*Podosphaera aphanis*). They evaluated 10 strawberry (*Fragaria* × *ananassa*) cultivars using a diverse set of isolates of *P. aphanis*. They reported the rapid development of age-related resistance. Susceptibility of leaves and fruit declined exponentially with age. Receptacle tissue of berries inoculated at four phenological stages from bloom to ripe fruit became nearly immune to infection approximately 10–15 days after bloom, as fruit transitioned from the early green to the late green or early white stage of berry development, although the achenes remained susceptible for a longer period. Leaves also acquired ontogenic resistance early in their development, and they were highly resistant shortly after unfolding and before the upper surface was fully exposed. No significant difference was found in the susceptibility of the adaxial versus abaxial surfaces of the leaves. The rapid acquisition of age-related resistance by leaves and fruit revealed a narrow window of susceptibility to which breeding programs might be advantageously useful.

It is accepted that depending on the age of the plant tissue, differences in levels of resistance are observed. A positive correlation between host age and disease resistance is observed in many plants. For example, researchers in Portugal, found clear age-related resistance to downy mildew (*Hyaloperonospora parasitica*) a worldwide foliar disease of *Brassica* vegetables. Disease symptoms start from the lower leaves and progress upwards. The researchers studied the influence of leaf position, plant age, and leaf age on the expression of resistance to downy mildew (*H. parasitica*) in various *B. oleracea* genotypes. The upper leaves were more resistant than the lower leaves when 7–19-week-old broccoli and Tronchuda cabbage plants were assessed. Two broccoli lines, PCB21.32 and OL87123–2, were fully susceptible at the cotyledon stage, and showed a clear resistance increase from lower to upper leaves at 6 weeks and PCB21.32 was fully resistant 16 weeks after sowing. Immature leaves were more resistant than adjacent fully expanded mature leaves. Susceptibility increased with leaf age when the same leaf was evaluated at 2–4-week intervals. The progression of downy mildew (*H. parasitica*) from the base of the plant upwards on *B. oleracea* in the field could be due to differences in leaf resistance in addition to environmental variation.

In successive developmental stages throughout their life cycles, plants face dynamic changes in biotic and abiotic conditions that create distinct ecological niches for host–pathogen interactions. Many types of age-related resistance have similarities to known plant defense systems, including preformed defenses, race-specific gene-for-gene resistance, SAR, and ISR. Diana Cervantes at the University of Idaho in Moscow, Idaho, United States, and her colleagues provide an excellent example of age-related resistance with Honesty or Money Plant (*Lunaria annua*) and white rust (*Albugo candida*). In a multiyear study, they found juvenile plants had 20 times the sorus (blister) density of second-year, adult plants. They suggested that the phenology of adult plants with mature leaves is flowering and maturing seed, by the time white rust begins to build upon the leaves of juveniles. With white blister rusts, the interpretation of resistance can be complicated by the frequency of asymptomatic infections that adult plants would pass on to the next generation. However, they found no asymptomatic infection of seeds of *Lunaria annua* in their sampling of the plants in Idaho, United States (Fig. 2.6).

Researchers at the University of the West Indies in the Republic of Trinidad and Tobago investigated the effect of age of the plant, developmental stage of the leaf, and midrib versus lamina leaf tissue to resistance to bacterial leaf spot disease (*Acidovorax anthurii*) of anthurium (*Anthurium* sp.). They used a leaf-disk vacuum-infiltration inoculation toward developing a rapid nondestructive method of screening for resistance to bacterial leaf spot in segregating populations. The screening method consisted of a vacuum-infiltration of leaf lamina disks. Their technique quantitatively differentiates levels of resistance of anthurium cultivars, as early as 5 days postinoculation. Plant ages between 2 and 5 years did not influence resistance levels to bacterial leaf spot disease.

Richard C. Michelmore at University of California at Davis, United States, studying downy mildew (*Bremia lactucae*) of

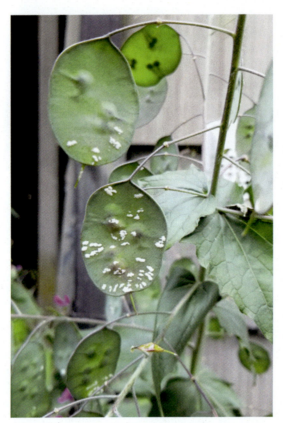

Figure 2.6 The seedpods or silicles of money plant (*Lunaria annua*) infected with white rust (*Albugo candida*) pathogen. Courtesy of Jay W. Pscheidt, Oregon State University.

lettuce (*Lactuca sativa*) observed that the deployment of resistant cultivars carrying dominant resistance genes (*Dm* genes) plays a crucial role in integrated downy mildew disease management; however, high variability in *B. lactucae* populations lead to the defeat of plant resistance conferred by *Dm* genes. Nevertheless, he observed some lettuce cultivars exhibiting field resistance that is only manifested in adult plants. The ability to use marker-assisted gene pyramiding of multiple *Dm* genes in combination with quantitative trait loci (QTLs) for adult field resistance provides the opportunity to develop cultivars with more durable resistance to *B. lactucae*.

Age-related resistance can be hard to quantify because plant age is not always straightforward. Plant age may refer to the developmental progression of individual organs (e.g., their size, color, and/or shape), known as ontogenesis. Plant organs undergo cell division, cell expansion, differentiation, ripening in the case of fruit, and finally, senescence. Leaves and fruits at early developmental stages are often protected by surrounding structures such as preexisting leaves, sepals, or petals that reduce the risk of pathogen attack.

Researchers at Michigan State University, United States, examined age-related resistance in winter squash fruit (*Cucurbita moschata*) to *P. capsici*. Winter squash (*C. moschata*) fruit as they mature acquire resistance to *P. capsici* and this age-related resistance could be exploited by plant breeders to limit crop loss due to fruit rot. The researchers wanted to determine whether preformed or pathogen-induced antifungal activity during fruit development is correlated with age-related resistance. They examined fruit peel methanol/ethanol extracts of three cultivars of *C. moschata* at different developmental stages with and without *P. capsici* inoculation. Results indicated the presence of compounds with antifungal activity in all fruit ages evaluated, but the antifungal activity decreased with age indicating a lack of association between preformed antifungal activity and age-related resistance in winter squash. In addition, no significant change was detected in the antifungal activity among fruit ages that were inoculated with *P. capsici* and examined at separate times post inoculation, suggesting no association between the induced antifungal activity and age-related resistance in winter squash. While the mechanism of age-related resistance can be structural or chemical, their study did not show an association between the production of either constitutive or induced antifungal activity and age-related resistance to *P. capsici*. These results may rule out a biochemical defense associated with age-related resistance of *C. moschata* fruits and suggest that other structural or genetic factors control age-related resistance. Nevertheless, age-related resistance may be an approach for plant breeders to use to manage fruit rot disease.

Chronological age of a plant can be defined by the exact amount of time postplanting or postorganogenesis, such as "weeks after planting" or "days after pollination." The timing of age-related resistance activation and the progression of plant maturation are heavily influenced by environmental conditions. Hence, in addition to chronological age, assessing the physiological age of a plant is also useful in determining the timing of age-related resistance onset.

Physiological age of a plant can be defined by the appearance of characteristic morphological and physiological features, such as "flowering stage" or "adult vegetative stage." Most flowering plants go through successive developmental transitions in a predictable temporal pattern. The first transition is from the embryonic stage to the juvenile vegetative stage that is characterized by seed germination. Next, plants grow from the juvenile vegetative stage to the adult vegetative stage that is associated with significant and abrupt change in form and function. Characteristics affected include internode length and stem structure as well as leaf form, size, and arrangement. It should not be confused with seasonal change, where early and late growth in a season is markedly different. A plant further enters reproductive stage that eventually results in production of an inflorescence and fruit. Age-related resistance is often associated with transitions among these developmental stages.

Breeding for age-related resistance is challenging due to complex interactions between environmental conditions, plant physiology, and pathogen life cycle. The plasticity of morphological traits under varying environmental conditions (temperature, humidity, ultraviolet light exposure, etc.) complicates the quantification of "plant age." Distinct environmental conditions associated with each developmental stage may influence the outcome of disease resistance in addition to the action of an age-dependent immune response. More typically, plant breeders will focus on breeding for earliness, instead of age-related resistance. Some have called this earliness, as "disease-escaping" or "avoidance." It involves avoiding disease by planting at a time when, or in areas where inoculum is absent or ineffective due to environmental conditions. The major aim is to enable the host to avoid contact with the pathogen or to ensure that the susceptible stage of the plant does not coincide with favorable conditions for the pathogen. The main practices under avoidance are choice of geographical area, selection of the field, choice of sowing/planting time, selection of seed and planting material, short duration/disease-escaping cultivars, and modification of production practices.

The basis for breeding for earliness as a mechanism of disease resistance is that the less time the plant is in the field the lower the exposure time to pathogens and the possibility of avoiding a window of time when the pathogen is active. For example, a noticeably short duration cultivar could be developed where the grower can harvest before a disease becomes a problem. Extra early maturing cowpeas (*V. unguiculata*) mature before the soil warms to allow wilt (*F. oxysporum* f. sp. *tracheiphilum*) and root knot nematodes (*Meloidogyne incognita* and *Meloidogyne javanica*) to infect the plants. Cultivars that depend on earliness can be susceptible when planted later in a season. With early maturing potatoes (*S. tuberosum*) that mature before the appearance of the late blight disease (*P. infestans*), are among the first to succumb to this disease if planted late as to be still immature when the moist weather of the late summer or early fall enables late blight to spread. Furthermore, when Dutch hyacinth (*Hyacinthus orientalis*) was investigated for earliness as a mechanism for resistance to yellow disease of hyacinth (*Xanthomonas hyacinthi*), it was not effective. Professor Van Tuyl at the Institute for Horticultural Plant Breeding, Wageningen University and Research, the Netherlands assessed 14 hyacinth cultivars and four wild accessions of *H. orientalis* he found that the degree of earliness itself was not associated with the degree of resistance.

Bibliography

Ahuja, I., Kissen, R., Bones, A.M., 2012. Phytoalexins in defense against pathogens. Trends in Plant Science 17, 73–90. Available from: https://doi.org/10.1016/j.tplants.2011.11.002.

Alonso-Villaverde, V., Voinesco, F., Viret, O., Spring, J.-L., Gindro, K., 2011. The effectiveness of stilbenes in resistant vitaceae: ultrastructural and biochemical events during *Plasmopara viticola* infection process. Plant Physiology and Biochemistry 49, 265–274. Available from: https://doi.org/10.1016/j.plaphy.2010.12.010.

Alzohairy, S.A., Hammerschmidt, R., Hausbeck, M.K., 2021. Antifungal activity in winter squash fruit peel in relation to age related resistance to *Phytophthora capsici*. Physiological and Molecular Plant Pathology 114, 101603. Available from: https://doi.org/10.1016/j.pmpp.2021.101603.

Ando, K., Grumet, R., Terpstra, K., Kelly, J.D., 2007. Manipulation of plant architecture to enhance crop disease control. CAB Reviews: Perspectives in Agriculture, Veterinary Science, Nutrition and Natural Resources 2 (26). Available from: https://doi.org/10.1079/PAVSNNR20072026.

Ando, K., Hammar, S., Grumet, R., 2009. Age-related resistance of diverse cucurbit fruit to infection by *Phytophthora capsici*. Journal of the American Society of Horticultural Science 134, 176–182. Available from: https://doi.org/10.21273/JASHS.134.2.176.

Andolfo, G., Ercolano, M.R., 2015. Plant innate immunity multicomponent model. Frontiers in Plant Science 6. Available from: https://doi.org/10.3389/fpls.2015.00987.

Asalf, B., Gadoury, D.M., Tronsmo, A.M., Seem, R.C., Dobson, A., Peres, N.A., et al., 2014. Ontogenic resistance of leaves and fruit, and how leaf folding influences the distribution of powdery mildew on strawberry plants colonized by *Podosphaera aphanis*. Phytopathology 104, 954–963. Available from: https://doi.org/10.1094/PHYTO-12-13-0345-R.

Bagga, S., Lucero, Y., Apodaca, K., Rajapakse, W., Lujan, P., Ortega, J.L., et al., 2019. Chile (*Capsicum annuum*) plants transformed with the RB gene from *Solanum bulbocastanum* are resistant to *Phytophthora capsici*. PLoS One 14 (10), e0223213. Available from: https://doi.org/10.1371/journal.pone.0223213.

Baldwin, I.T., 1998. Jasmonate-induced responses are costly but benefit plants under attack in native populations. Proceedings of the National Academy of Science USA 95, 8113–8118. Available from: https://doi.org/10.1073/pnas.95.14.8113.

Balint-Kurti, P., 2019. The plant hypersensitive response: concepts, control, and consequences. Molecular Plant Pathology 20, 1163–1178. Available from: https://doi.org/10.1111/mpp.12821.

Baruaha, A., Sivalingamb, P.N., Urooj, F., Senthil-Kuma, M., 2020. Nonhost resistance to plant viruses: what do we know? Physiological and Molecular Plant Pathology 111, 01506. Available from: https://doi.org/10.1016/j.pmpp.2020.101506.

Benhamou, N., Nicole, M., 1999. Cell biology of plant immunization against microbial infection: the potential of induced resistance in controlling plant diseases. Plant Physiology Biochemistry 37, 703–719. Available from: https://doi.org/10.1016/S0981-9428(00)86684-X.

Bennett, F.G.A., 1981a. The expression of resistance to powdery mildew infection in winter wheat cultivars I. Seedling resistance. Annals of Applied Biology 98, 295–303. Available from: https://doi.org/10.1111/j.1744-7348.1981.tb00762.x.

Bennett, F.G.A., 1981b. The expression of resistance to powdery mildew infection in winter wheat cultivars II. Adult plant resistance. Annals of Applied Biology 98, 305–317. Available from: https://doi.org/10.1111/j.1744-7348.1981.tb00763.x.

Bi, K., Liang, Y., Mengiste, T., Sharon, A., 2023. Killing softly: a roadmap of *Botrytis cinerea* pathogenicity. Trends in Plant Science 28, 211–222. Available from: https://doi.org/10.1016/j.tplants.2022.08.024.

Bostock, R.M., 1999. Signal conflicts and synergies in induced resistance to multiple attackers. Physiological and Molecular Plant Pathology 55, 99–109. Available from: https://doi.org/10.1006/pmpp.1999.0218.

Boutrot, F., Zipfel, C., 2017. Function, discovery, and exploitation of plant pattern recognition receptors for broad-spectrum disease resistance. Annual Review of Phytopathology 55, 257–286. Available from: https://doi.org/10.1146/annurev-phyto-080614-120106.

Broadhurst, P.G., 1996. Stemphylium disease tolerance in *Asparagus officinalis* L. Acta Horticulturae 415, 387–391. Available from: https://doi.org/10.17660/ActaHortic.1996.415.55.

Buonaurio, R., Scarponi, L., Ferrara, M., Sidoti, P., Bertona, A., 2002. Induction of systemic acquired resistance in pepper plants by acibenzolar-S-methyl against bacterial spot disease. European Journal of Plant Pathology 108, 41–49. Available from: https://doi.org/10.1023/A:1013984511233.

Cervantes, D., Ridout, M., Nischwitz, C., Newcombe, G., 2021. Adult plant resistance to white rust in *Lunaria annua*. Phytopathologia Mediterranea 60, 381–385. Available from: https://doi.org/10.36253/phyto-12805.

Chang, M., Chen, H., Liu, F., Qing Fu, Z., 2022. PTI and ETI: convergent pathways with diverse elicitors. Trends in Plant Science 27, 113–115. Available from: https://doi.org/10.1016/j.tplants.2021.11.013.

Cheng, X., Luan, Y., Wu, X., 2021. Chapter 2 – Plant non-host resistance against viruses: current status and future prospects. In: Kumar Gaur, R., Khurana, S.M.P., Sharma, P., Hohn, T. (Eds.), Plant Virus-Host Interaction (Second Edition) Molecular Approaches and Viral Evolution. Academic Press, pp. 45–57.

Coelho, P.S., Valério, L., Monteiro, A.A., 2009. Leaf position, leaf age and plant age affect the expression of downy mildew resistance in *Brassica oleracea*. European Journal of Plant Pathology 125, 179–188. Available from: https://doi.org/10.1007/s10658-009-9469-4.

Cohen, R., Pivonia, S., Burger, Y., Edelstein, M., Gamliel, A., Katan, J., 2000. Toward integrated management of *Monosporascus wilt* of melon in Israel. Plant Disease 84, 496–505. Available from: https://doi.org/10.1094/PDIS.2000.84.5.496.

Damon, S.J., Groves, R.L., Havey, M.J., 2014. Variation for epicuticular waxes on onion foliage and impacts on numbers of onion thrips. Journal of the American Society of Horticultural Science 139, 495–501. Available from: https://doi.org/10.21273/HORTSCI15414-20.

Dann, E.K., Deverall, B.J., 1996. 2,6-dichloro-isonicotinic acid (INA) induces resistance in green beans to the rust pathogen, *Uromyces appendiculatus*, under field conditions. Australasian Plant Pathology 25, 199–204. Available from: https://doi.org/10.1071/AP96034.

Dempsey, D.M.A., Shah, J., Klessig, D.F., 1999. Salicylic acid and disease resistance in plants. Critical Reviews in Plant Science 18, 547–575. Available from: https://doi.org/10.1080/07352689991309397.

Develey-Rivière, M.-P, Galiana, E., 2007. Resistance to pathogens and host developmental stage: a multifaceted relationship within the plant kingdom. New Phytologist 175, 405–416. Available from: https://doi.org/10.1111/j.1469-8137.2007.02130.x.

Dong, X., 2001. Genetic dissection of systemic acquired resistance. Current Opinion in Plant Biology 4, 309–314. Available from: https://doi.org/10.1016/S1369-5266(00)00178-3.

Durrant, W.E., Dong, X., 2004. Systemic acquired resistance. Annual Review of Phytopathology 42, 185–209. Available from: https://doi.org/10.1146/annurev.phyto.42.040803.140421.

Ellis, J., 2006. Insights into nonhost disease resistance: can they assist disease control in agriculture? The Plant Cell 18, 523–528. Available from: https://doi.org/10.1105/tpc.105.040584.

Fan, J., Doerner, P., 2012. Genetic and molecular basis of nonhost disease resistance: complex, yes; silver bullet, no. Current Opinion in Plant Biology 15, 400–406. Available from: https://doi.org/10.1016/j.pbi.2012.03.001.

Francia, D., Demaria, D., Calderini, O., Ferraris, L., Valentino, D., Arcioni, S., et al., 2008. Do pathogen-specific defense mechanisms contribute to wound-induced resistance in tomato? Plant Signaling and Behavior 3, 340–341. Available from: https://doi.org/10.4161/psb.3.5.5351.

Fravel, D.R., 1988. Role of antibiosis in the biocontrol of plant diseases. Annual Review of Phytopathology 26, 75–91. Available from: https://doi.org/10.1146/annurev.py.26.090188.000451.

Fu, Z.Q., Dong, X., 2013. Systemic acquired resistance: turning local infection into global defense. Annual Review of Plant Biology 64, 839–863. Available from: https://doi.org/10.1146/annurev-arplant-042811-105606.

Fujita, M., Kusajima, M., Okumura, Y., Nakajima, M., Minamisawa, K., Nakashita, H., 2017. Effects of colonization of a bacterial endophyte, Azospirillum sp. B510, on disease resistance in tomato. Bioscience, Biotechnology, and Biochemistry 81, 1657–1662. Available from: https://doi.org/10.1080/09168451.2017.1329621.

Ganoid, T., Métraux, J.P., 1999. Cross-talk in plant cell signaling structure and function of the genetic network. Trends in Plant Science 4, 503–507. Available from: https://doi.org/10.1016/S1360-1385(99)01498-3.

García, Y.H., Zamora, O.R., Troncoso-Rojas, R., Tiznado-Hernández, M.E., Báez-Flores, M.E., Carvajal-Millan, E., et al., 2021. Toward understanding the molecular recognition of fungal chitin and activation of the plant defense mechanism in horticultural crops. Molecules (Basel, Switzerland) 26, 6513. Available from: https://doi.org/10.3390/molecules26216513.

Glazebrook, J., 2005. Contrasting mechanisms of defense against biotrophic and necrotrophic pathogens. Annual Review of Phytopathology 43, 205–227. Available from: https://doi.org/10.1146/annurev.phyto.43.040204.135923.

Gozzo, F., 2003. Systemic acquired resistance in crop protection: from nature to a chemical approach. Journal of Agricultural and Food Chemistry 51, 4487–4503. Available from: https://doi.org/10.1021/jf030025s.

Graham, J., Smith, K., Tierney, I., MacKenzie, K., Hackett, C.A., 2006. Mapping gene H controlling cane pubescence in raspberry and its association with resistance to cane botrytis and spur blight, rust and cane spot. Theoretical and Applied Genetics 112, 818–831. Available from: https://doi.org/10.1007/s00122-005-0184-z.

Guo, W., Chen, L., Herrera-Estrella, L., Cao, D., Tran, L.-S.P., 2020. Altering plant architecture to improve performance and resistance. Trends in Plant Science 25, 1154–1170. Available from: https://doi.org/10.1016/j.tplants.2020.05.009.

Hammerschmidt, R., Kuc, J., 1995. Induced resistance to disease in plants. Kluwer, Dordrecht, the Netherlands.

Han, X., Tsuda, K., 2022. Evolutionary footprint of plant immunity. Current Opinion in Plant Biology 67, 102209. Available from: https://doi.org/10.1016/j.pbi.2022.102209.

Heath, M.C., 1974. Light and electron microscope studies of the interactions of host and non-host plants with cowpea rust – *Uromyces phaseolli* var. vignae. Physiological Plant Pathology 4, 403–414. Available from: https://doi.org/10.1016/0048-4059(74)90025-3.

Heath, M.C., 2000a. Non-host resistance and nonspecific plant defenses. Current Opinion in Plant Biology 3, 315–319. Available from: https://doi.org/10.1016/S1369-5266(00)00087-X.

Heath, M.C., 2000b. Hypersensitive response-related death. Plant Molecular Biology 44, 321–334. Available from: https://doi.org/10.1023/A:1026592509060.

Heath, M.C., 2000c. The First Touch. Physiological and Molecular Plant Pathology 56, 49–50. Available from: https://doi.org/10.1006/pmpp.2000.0257.

Heath, M.C., 2001. Non-host resistance to plant pathogens: Nonspecific defense or the result of specific recognition events. Physiological and Molecular Plant Pathology 58, 53–54. Available from: https://doi.org/10.1006/pmpp.2001.0319.

Heil, M., 2001. The ecological concept of costs of induced systemic resistance. European Journal of Plant Pathology 107, 137–146. Available from: https://doi.org/10.1023/A:1008793009517.

Heil, M., Hilpert, A., Kaiser, W., Linsenmair, K.E., 2000. Reduced growth and seed set following chemical induction of pathogen defence: does systemic acquired resistance (SAR) incur allocation costs? Journal of Ecology 88, 645–654. Available from: https://doi.org/10.1046/j.1365-2745.2000.00479.x.

Hijwegen, T., Verhaar, M.A., 1994. Effects of cucumber genotype on the induction of resistance to powdery mildew, *Sphaerotheca fuliginea*, by 2,6-dichloroisonicotinic acid. Plant Pathology 44, 756–762. Available from: https://doi.org/10.1111/j.1365-3059.1995.tb01700.x.

Hofius, D., Munch, D., Bressendorff, S., Mundy, J., Petersen, M., 2011. Role of autophagy in disease resistance and hypersensitive response-associated cell death. Cell Death and Differentiation 18, 1257–1262. Available from: https://doi.org/10.1038/cdd.2011.43.

Holub, E.B., Cooper, A., 2004. Matrix, reinvention in plants: how genetics is unveiling secrets of non-host disease resistance. Trends in Plant Science 9, 211–214. Available from: https://doi.org/10.1016/j.tplants.2004.03.002.

Horvath, D.M., Stall, R.E., Jones, J.B., Pauly, M.H., Vallad, G.E., Dahlbeck, D., et al., 2012. Transgenic resistance confers effective field level control of bacterial spot disease in tomato. PLoS One 7, e42036. Available from: https://doi.org/10.1371/journal.pone.0042036.

Hu, L., Yang, L., 2019. Time to fight: molecular mechanisms of age-related resistance. Phytopathology 109, 1500–1508. Available from: https://doi.org/10.1094/PHYTO-11-18-0443-RVW.

Ishii, H., Tomita, Y., Horio, T., Narusaka, Y., Nakazawa, Y., Nishimura, K., et al., 1999. Induced resistance of acibenzolar-S-methyl (CGA 245704) to cucumber and Japanese pear diseases. European Journal of Plant Pathology 105, 77–85. Available from: https://doi.org/10.1023/A:1008637828624.

Jeandet, P., Clément, C., Courot, E., Cordelier, S., 2013. Modulation of phytoalexin biosynthesis in engineered plants for disease resistance. International Journal of Molecular Sciences 14, 14136–14170. Available from: https://doi.org/10.3390/ijms140714136.

Johnson, L.E.B., Bushnell, W.R., Zeyen, R.J., 1979. Binary pathways for analysis of primary infection and host response in populations of powdery mildew fungi. Canadian Journal of Botany 57, 497–511. Available from: https://doi.org/10.1139/b79-065.

Jones, J., Minsavage, G., Roberts, P., Johnson, R., Kousik, C., Subramanian, S., et al., 2002. A non-hypersensitive resistance in pepper to the bacterial spot pathogen is associated with two recessive genes. Phytopathology 92, 273–277. Available from: https://doi.org/10.1094/PHYTO.2002.92.3.273.

Kloos, W.E., George, C.G., Sorge, L.K., 2005. Inheritance of powdery mildew resistance and leaf macrohair density in *Gerbera hybrida*. HortScience: a Publication of the American Society for Horticultural Science 40, 1246–1251. Available from: https://doi.org/10.21273/HORTSCI.40.5.1246.

Kortekamp, A., Zyprian, E., 1999. Leaf hairs as a basic protective barrier against downy mildew of grape. Journal of Phytopathology 147, 453–459. Available from: https://doi.org/10.1111/j.1439-0434.1999.tb03850.x.

Kroon, B.A.M., Scheffer, R.J., Elgersma, D.M., 1991. Induced resistance in tomato plants against *fusarium wilt* invoked by *Fusarium oxysporum* f. sp. *dianthi*. Netherlands Journal of Plant Pathology 97, 401–408.

Kuc, J., 2000. Development and future direction of induced systemic resistance in plants. Crop Protection 19, 8–10. Available from: https://doi.org/10.1016/S0261-2194(00)00122-8.

Lacombe, S., Rougon-Cardoso, A., Sherwood, E., Peeters, N., Dahlbeck, D., van Esse, H.P., et al., 2010. Interfamily transfer of a plant pattern-recognition receptor confers broad-spectrum bacterial resistance. Nature Biotechnology 28, 365–369. Available from: https://doi.org/10.1038/nbt.1613.

Lawton, K., Weymann, K., Friedrich, L., Vernooij, B., Uknes, S., Ryals, J., 1995. Systemic acquired resistance in Arabidopsis requires salicylic acid but no ethylene. Molecular Plant-Microbe Interactions 6, 863–870.

Lee, S., Kim, S.Y., Chung, E., Joung, Y.H., Pai, H.S., Hur, C.G., et al., 2004. EST and microarray analyses of pathogen-responsive genes in hot pepper (*Capsicum annuum* L.) non-host resistance against soybean pustule pathogen (*Xanthomonas axonopodis* pv. glycines). Functional and Integrative Genomics 4, 196–205. Available from: https://doi.org/10.1007/s10142-003-0099-1.

Lee, H.A., Kim, S., Kim, S., Choi, D., 2017. Expansion of sesquiterpene biosynthetic gene clusters in pepper confers nonhost resistance to the Irish potato famine pathogen. New Phytologist 215, 1132–1143. Available from: https://doi.org/10.1111/nph.14637.

Leeman, M., den Ouden, F.M., van Pelt, J.A., Dirkx, F.P.M., Steijl, H., Bakker, P.A.H.M., et al., 1996. Iron availability affects induction of systemic resistance to *Fusarium wilt* of radish by *Pseudomonas fluorescens*. Phytopathology 86, 149–155. Available from: https://doi.org/10.1094/Phyto-86-149.

Leskovar, D.I., Kolenda, K., 2002. Strobilurin + acibenzolar-S-methyl controls white rust without inducing leaf chlorosis in spinach. Annals of Applied Biology 140, 171–175. Available from: https://doi.org/10.1111/j.1744-7348.2002.tb00170.x.

Li, W., Xu, Y.P., Zhang, Z.X., Cao, W.Y., Li, F., Zhou, X., et al., 2012. Identification of genes required for nonhost resistance to *Xanthomonas oryzae* pv. oryzae reveals novel signaling components. PLoS One 7 (8), e42796. Available from: https://doi.org/10.1371/journal.pone.0042796.

Li, P., Lu, Y.-J., Chen, H., Day, B., 2020. The lifecycle of the plant immune system. Critical Reviews in Plant Sciences 39, 72–100. Available from: https://doi.org/10.1080/07352689.2020.1757829.

Louws, F.J., Wilson, M., Campbell, H.L., Cuppels, D.A., Jones, J.B., Shoemaker, P.B., et al., 2001. Field control of bacterial spot and bacterial speck of tomato using a plant activator. Plant Disease 85, 481–488. Available from: https://doi.org/10.1094/PDIS.2001.85.5.481.

Lyon, G.D., Reglinski, T., Newton, A.C., 1995. Novel disease control compounds: the potential to 'immunize' plants against infection. Plant Pathology 44, 407–427.

Maleck, K., Levine, A., Eulgem, T., Morgan, A., Schmid, J., Lawton, K.A., et al., 2000. The transcriptome of *Arabidopsis thaliana* during systemic acquired resistance. Nature Genetics 26, 403–410. Available from: https://doi.org/10.1038/82521.

McDowell, J.M., Dangl, J.L., 2000. Signal transduction in the plant immune response. Trends in Biochemical Sciences 25, 79–82. Available from: https://doi.org/10.1016/S0968-0004(99)01532-7.

Mellersh, D.G., Heath, M.C., 2004. Cellular expression of resistance to fungal plant pathogens. In: Punja, Z.K. (Ed.), Fungal Disease Resistance in Plants: Biochemistry, Molecular Biology, and Genetic Engineering. Food Products Press, NY, pp. 31–55. 266 pages.

Mengiste, T., 2012. Plant immunity to necrotrophs. Annual Review of Phytopathology 50, 267–294. Available from: https://doi.org/10.1146/annurev-phyto-081211-172955.

Miedes, E., Vanholme, R., Boerjan, W., Molina, A., 2014. The role of the secondary cell wall in plant resistance to pathogens. Frontiers in Plant Science 5, 358. Available from: https://doi.org/10.3389/fpls.2014.00358.

Müller, K.O., Börger, H., 1940. Experimentelle untersuchungen über die *Phytophthora resistenz* der Kartoffel (Experimental studies on the phytophthora resistance of the potato) Arbeit. Biol. Reichsant Land Forstwirtsch 23, 189–231.

Mur, L.A.J., Kenton, P., Lloyd, A.J., Ougham, H., Prats, E., 2008. The hypersensitive response; the centenary is upon us but how much do we know? Journal of Experimental Botany 59, 501–520. Available from: https://doi.org/10.1093/jxb/erm239.

Murphy, J.F., Zehnder, G.W., Schuster, D.J., Sikora, E.J., Polston, J.E., Kloepper, J.W., 2000. Plant growth-promoting rhizobacteria mediated protection in tomato against tomato mottle virus. Plant Disease 84, 779–784. Available from: https://doi.org/10.1094/PDIS.2000.84.7.779.

Mysore, K.S., Ryu, C.M., 2004. Non-host resistance: how much do we know? Trends in Plant Science 9, 97–104. Available from: https://doi.org/10.1016/j.tplants.2003.12.005.

Nazarov, A., Baleev, D.N., Ivanova, M.I., Sokolova, L.M., Karakozova, M.V., 2020. Infectious plant diseases: etiology, current status, problems and prospects in plant protection. Acta Naturae 12, 46–59. Available from: https://doi.org/10.32607/actanaturae.11026.

Ngou, B.P.M., Ding, P., Jones, J.D.G., 2022. Thirty years of resistance: zig-zag through the plant immune system. The Plant Cell 34, 1447–1478. Available from: https://doi.org/10.1093/plcell/koac041.

Nguyen, H.P., Chakravarthy, S., Velásquez, A.C., et al., 2010. Methods to study PAMP-triggered immunity using tomato and *Nicotiana benthamiana*. Molecular Plant-Microbe Interaction 23, 991–999. Available from: https://doi.org/10.1094/MPMI-23-8-0991.

Nurnberger, T., Lipka, V., 2005. Non-host resistance in plants: New insights into an old phenomenon. Molecular Plant Pathology 6, 335–345. Available from: https://doi.org/10.1111/j.1364-3703.2005.00279.x.

Oh, S., Choi, D., 2022. Receptor-mediated nonhost resistance in plants. Essays in Biochemistry EBC20210080, https://doi.org/10.1042/EBC20210080.

Oliver, R., 2009. Plant breeding for disease resistance in the age of effectors. Phytoparasitica 37, 1–5. Available from: https://doi.org/10.1007/s12600-008-0013-4.

Panter, S.N., Jones, D.A., 2002. Age-related resistance to plant pathogens. Advances in Botanical Research 38, 251–280. Available from: https://doi.org/10.1016/S0065-2296(02)38032-7.

Papik, J., Folkmanova, M., Polivkova-Majorova, M., Suman, J., Uhlik, O., 2020. The invisible life inside plants: deciphering the riddles of endophytic bacterial diversity. Biotechnology Advances 44. Available from: https://doi.org/10.1016/j.biotechadv.2020.107614.

Parra, L., Simko, I., Michelmore, R.W., 2021. Identification of major quantitative trait loci controlling field resistance to downy mildew in cultivated lettuce (*Lactuca sativa*. Phytopathology 111, 541–547. Available from: https://doi.org/10.1094/PHYTO-08-20-0367-R.

Pegg, G.F., Woodward, S., 1986. Synthesis and metabolism of α-tomatine in tomato isolines in relation to resistance to *Verticillium albo-atrum*. Physiological and Molecular Plant Pathology 28, 187–201. Available from: https://doi.org/10.1016/S0048-4059(86)80063-7.

Romero, A.M., Kousik, C.S., Ritchie, D.F., 2001. Resistance to bacterial spot in bell pepper induced by acibenzolar-S-methyl. Plant Disease 85, 189–194. Available from: https://doi.org/10.1094/PDIS.2001.85.2.189.

Ross, A.F., 1961a. Localized acquired resistance to plant virus infection in hypersensitive hosts. Virology 14, 329–339.

Ross, A.F., 1961b. Systemic acquired resistance induced by localized virus infections in plants. Virology 14, 340–358.

Schulze-Lefert, P., Panstruga, R., 2011. A molecular evolutionary concept connecting nonhost resistance, pathogen host range, and pathogen speciation. Trends Plant in Science 16, 117–125. Available from: https://doi.org/10.1016/j.tplants.2011.01.001.

Smith, C.A., MacHardy, W.E., 1982. The significance of tomatine in the host response of susceptible and resistant tomato isolines infected with two races of *Fusarium oxysporum* f. sp. *lycopersici*. Phytopathology 72, 415–419.

Stall, R.E., Jones, J.B., Minsavage, G.V., 2009. Durability of resistance in tomato and pepper to Xanthomonas causing bacterial spot. Annual Review of Phytopathology 47, 265–284. Available from: https://doi.org/10.1146/annurev-phyto-080508-081752.

Sticher, L., Mauch-Mani, B., Métraux, J.-P., 1997. Systemic acquired resistance. Annual Review of Phytopathology 35, 235–270. Available from: https://doi.org/10.1146/annurev.phyto.35.1.235.

Thordal-Christensen, H., 2003. Fresh insights into processes of non-host resistance. Current Opinion in Plant Biology 6, 351−357. Available from: https://doi.org/10.1016/S1369-5266(03)00063-3.

Tiku, A.R., 2020. Antimicrobial compounds (phytoanticipins and phytoalexins) and their role in plant defense. In: Mérillon, J.M., Ramawat, K. (Eds.), Co-evolution of secondary metabolites. Reference Series in Phytochemistry. Springer, Cham. Available from: https://doi.org/10.1007/978-3-319-96397-6_63.

Uma, B., Rani, T.S., Podile, A.R., 2011. Warriors at the gate that never sleep: non-host resistance in plants. Journal of Plant Physiology 168, 2141−2152. Available from: https://doi.org/10.1016/j.jplph.2011.09.005.

Vallad, G.E., Goodman, R.M., 2004. Systemic acquired resistance and induced systemic resistance in conventional agriculture. Crop Science 44, 1920−1934. Available from: https://doi.org/10.2135/cropsci2004.1920.

Vallejos, C.E., Jones, V., Stall, R.E., Jones, J.B., Minsavage, G.V., Schultz, D.C., et al., 2010. Characterization of two recessive genes controlling resistance to all races of bacterial spot in peppers. Theoretical and Applied Genetics 121, 37−46. Available from: https://doi.org/10.1007/s00122-010-1289-6.

Van de Weyer, A.-L., Monteiro, F., Furzer, O.J., Nishimura, M.T., Cevik, V., Witek, K., et al., 2019. A species-wide inventory of NLR genes and alleles in *Arabidopsis thaliana*. Cell 178, 1260−1272. Available from: https://doi.org/10.1016/j.cell.2019.07.038. e14.

Van Tuyl, J.M., 1982. Breeding for resistance to yellow disease of hyacinths. II. Influence of flowering time, leaf characters, stomata, and chromosome number on the degree of resistance. Euphytica 31, 621−628. Available from: https://doi.org/10.1007/BF00039200.

Vanden Langenberg, K.M., Wehner, T.C., 2016. Downy mildew disease progress in resistant and susceptible cucumbers tested in the field at different growth stages. HortScience: a Publication of the American Society for Horticultural Science 51, 984−988. Available from: https://doi.org/10.21273/HORTSCI.51.8.984.

VanEtten, H.D., Mansfield, J.W., Bailey, J.A., Farmer, E.E., 1994. Letter to the editor. Two classes of plant antibiotics:phytoalexins versus "phytoanticipins.". Plant Cell 6, 1191−1192. Available from: https://doi.org/10.1105/tpc.6.9.1191.

Vleeshouwers, V.G.A.A., Oliver, R.P., 2014. Effectors as tools in disease resistance breeding against biotrophic, hemibiotrophic, and necrotrophic plant pathogens. Molecular Plant-Microbe Interactions 27, 196−206. Available from: https://doi.org/10.1094/MPMI-10-13-0313-IA.

Walters, D.R., Ratsep, J., Havis, N.D., 2013. Controlling crop diseases using induced resistance: challenges for the future. Journal of Experimental Botany 64, 1263−1280. Available from: https://doi.org/10.1093/jxb/ert026.

Wei, G., Kloepper, J.W., Tuzun, S., 1996. Induced systemic resistance to cucumber diseases and increased plant growth by plant growth-promoting rhizobacteria under field conditions. Phytopathology 86, 221−224. Available from: https://doi.org/10.1094/Phyto-86-221.

Whalen, M.C., 2005. Host defence in a developmental context. Molecular Plant Pathology 6, 347−360. Available from: https://doi.org/10.1111/j.1364-3703.2005.00286.x.

Wulff, B.B.H., Horvath, D.M., Ward, E.R., 2011. Improving immunity in crops: new tactics in an old game. Current Opinion in Plant Biology 14, 468−476. Available from: https://doi.org/10.1016/j.pbi.2011.04.002.

Yan, Z., Reddy, M.S., Yyu, C.-M., McInroy, J.A., Wilson, M., Kloepper, J.W., 2002. Induced systemic protection against tomato late blight by plant growth-promoting rhizobacteria. Phytopathology 92, 1329–1333. Available from: https://doi.org/10.1094/PHYTO.2002.92.12.1329.

Zhao, Y., Vlasselaer, L., Ribeiro, B., Terzoudis, K., Van den Ende, W., Hertog, M., et al., 2022. Constitutive defense mechanisms have a major role in the resistance of woodland strawberry leaves against *Botrytis cinerea*. Frontiers in Plant Science . Available from: https://doi.org/10.3389/fpls.2022.912667.

Zehnder, G.W., Murphy, J.F., Sikora, E.J., Kloepper, J.W., 2001. Application of rhizobacteria for induced resistance. European Journal of Plant Pathology 107, 39–50. Available from: https://doi.org/10.1023/A:1008732400383.

Zhang, S., Reddy, M.S., Kokalis-Burelle, N., Wells, L.W., Nightengale, S.P., Kloepper, J.W., 2001. Lack of induced systemic resistance in peanut to late leaf spot disease by plant growth-promoting rhizobacteria and chemical elicitors. Plant Disease 85, 879–884. Available from: https://doi.org/10.1094/PDIS.2001.85.8.879.

Zhao, B., Lin, X., Poland, J., Trick, H., Leach, J., Hulbert, S., 2005. A maize resistance gene functions against bacterial streak disease in rice. Proceedings of the National Academy of Science USA 102, 15383–15388. Available from: https://doi.org/10.1073/pnas.0503023102.

3

Resistance: the genotype

Resistance as a "genotype" begins after the rediscovery of Mendel's Laws of Inheritance. At the University of Cambridge in 1905, Sir Rowland Harry Biffen stated that resistance to yellow rust (*Puccinia struformis* f. sp. *tritici*) in wheat (*Triticum aestivum*) was controlled by a single gene, and it has recessive inheritance patterns. Unfortunately, many plant breeders doubted his results because when they evaluated their resistance phenotype it would not behave as Sir Biffen reported. This is because the expression of resistance can occur with several genetic models. Resistance has been documented to be inherited as dominant, recessive, incomplete dominance, additive, epistasis, and influenced by suppressor genes with epistatic effects.

Investigations of plant genomes within and across species provide insight into the evolutionary forces that have shaped the architecture and function of genes related to resistance. The resistance genotypes in higher plants are normally classified into two classes: (1) preformed resistance mechanisms and (2) inducible resistance mechanisms. The first grouping is referred to as "major gene resistance," "gene-for-gene resistance," "race-specific resistance," and sometimes "seedling resistance." The genes in this group conform to Flor's gene-for-gene hypothesis. Plant breeders prefer to work with single genes with large effects because they are easy to screen and simple to transfer during the breeding process.

Plants, unlike animals, do not possess circulating immune cells to intercept microbial signals. Thus their innate immune system is cell autonomous meaning that each plant cell recognizes microbial signals and responds accordingly. To prevent infection by viruses, bacteria, oomycetes, or fungi plants possess two main types of immune receptors: pattern recognition receptors (PRRs) on the cell surface and intracellular nucleotide-binding and leucine-rich repeat receptors (NLR).

Gene-for-gene theory

As discussed in Chapter 2, Flor's central tenet in the classical gene-for-gene concept of plant disease resistance states that "for each gene that conditions resistance in the host gene (*R*-gene) there is a corresponding gene that conditions virulence in the pathogen (*Avr* gene)." The gene-for-gene theory states that two crucial genes are necessary for the expression of resistance: the resistant gene in the host and the corresponding avirulence (*Avr*) effector gene in the pathogen. Each resistance gene confers resistance to pathogen strains carrying the corresponding avirulence factor. In other words, the efficacy of resistance genes is pathogen strain dependent. The ability of the pathogen to overcome resistance is derived from mutation of the *Avr* gene leading to loss of recognition by the corresponding resistance gene. The resistance genes encode receptor proteins that either directly or indirectly recognize pathogen avirulence proteins. Therefore if "n" genes for resistance with two interaction phenotypes, then 2^n races can exist. Resistance genes have been isolated from many plant species. Numerous avirulence genes have been isolated from plant pathogens, and they typically encode proteins that are secreted into the host to promote infection.

Lock and key concept

The "Lock and Key Concept" explains the specificity of the resistance gene and the avirulence gene. Table 3.1 illustrates this lock and key concept.

The important aspect of the lock and key concept is its specificity. An interaction that results in infection is known as a compatible reaction, while a resistant reaction is referred to as incompatible. Plant pathogens that induce a resistance reaction have avirulence genes (*Avr*), dominant genes that produce a product that initiates a response from the plant. For there to be resistance, the plant must have a corresponding resistance gene (*R*) to recognize the product. Resistance genes are generally dominant; however, there are many exceptions to this rule. Infectious pathogens have a recessive avirulence gene (*Avr*) and do not produce any detectable product. They can evade the plant's resistance mechanisms undetected and cause disease. When such a plant pathogen has the avirulence gene (*Avr*), it does not matter if the plant has any resistance genes. In Table 3.1, the S* interactions show this possibility. The authenticity of gene-for-gene has profound consequences for breeding for resistance. Foremost among the arguments is whether all resistance operates on a gene-for-gene basis, and the simple answer is no. In fact, while gene-for-gene is common, in the real-world setting, plants are rarely infected by a single race or strain of a single pathogen, and therefore relying on the gene-for-gene model for breeding certainly has limitations.

Table 3.1 The interactions among genotypes of the host and pathogen and the outcome of the interaction.

	R1R2	R1r2	r1R2	r1r2
A1A2	R	R	R	S
A1a2	R	R	S*	S
a1A2	R	S*	R	S
a1a2	S	S	S	S

R, resistance phenotype; S, susceptible phenotype.

Nucleotide-binding and leucine-rich repeat receptors

Plant immunity is often triggered by the specific recognition of pathogen effectors by intracellular nucleotide-binding and leucine-rich repeat receptor (NLR) domains. Plant nucleotide-binding and leucine-rich repeat receptors contain an N-terminal signaling domain that is mostly represented by either a toll-interleukin-1 receptor (TIR) domain or a coiled-coil domain. In many cases, single nucleotide-binding and leucine-rich repeat receptor proteins are sufficient for both effector recognition and signaling activation. However, many paired nucleotide-binding and leucine-rich repeat receptors have now been identified where both proteins are required to confer resistance to pathogens. Recent detailed studies on *Arabidopsis thaliana* toll/interleukin-1 receptor intracellular nucleotide-binding leucine-rich repeat pair RRS1 and RPS4 and on the rice (*Oryza sativa*) coiled-coil intracellular nucleotide-binding leucine-rich repeat pair RGA4 and RGA5 have revealed for the first time how these protein pairs function together. In both cases, the paired partners interact physically to form a hetero-complex receptor in which each partner plays distinct roles in effector recognition or signaling activation, highlighting a conserved mode of action of nucleotide-binding and leucine-rich repeat receptor pairs across both monocotyledonous and dicotyledonous plants. An "integrated decoy" model for the function of these receptor complexes has been hypothesized. In this model, a plant protein targeted by an effector has been duplicated and fused to one member of the nucleotide-binding and leucine-rich repeat receptor pair, where it acts as a bait to trigger defense signaling by the second intracellular nucleotide-binding leucine-rich repeat upon effector binding. This mechanism may be common to many other plant intracellular nucleotide-binding leucine-rich repeat pairs.

Because plants are immobile, they have evolved numerous resistance genes, the majority of which encode the intracellular nucleotide-binding leucine-rich repeat. Genome sequences have revealed that higher plant species contain anywhere from 50 nucleotide-binding leucine-rich repeats in papaya (*Carica papaya*) to more than 1005 nucleotide-binding leucine-rich repeat genes hundred in wheat (*T. aestivum*). It is known that members of Solanaceae family typically have a larger number of the nucleotide-binding leucine-rich repeats than other species. Tomato (*Solanum lycopersicum*) has 267 nucleotide-binding leucine-rich repeat domains, potato (*Solanum tuberosum*) has 443 nucleotide-binding leucine-rich repeat-type genes, and chile pepper (*Capsicum annuum*) has 755 nucleotide-binding leucine-rich repeat encoding genes. The number, arrangement, and domain combinations of these genes can vary dramatically even among plant ecotypes, indicating that nucleotide-binding leucine-rich repeats can be rapidly gained or lost. Nucleotide-binding leucine-rich repeat proteins were discovered to be present in humans and other animals about 5 years after they were found in plants. Although both plant and animal nucleotide-binding leucine-rich repeats play roles in pathogen detection, they appear to have arisen independently through convergent evolution. In animals, nucleotide-binding leucine-rich repeats play a role much like plant membrane-localized PRRs, detecting pathogen-associated molecular patterns (PAMPs) or damage-associated molecular patterns (DAMPs). Plant nucleotide-binding leucine-rich repeats are also structurally distinct from animal nucleotide-binding leucine-rich repeats. Both plants and animals feature a nucleotide-binding domain believed to be involved in oligomerization, and a leucine-rich repeat domain that is thought to be involved in effector recognition and autoimmune. Most plant species have hundreds of genes that encode the intracellular nucleotide-binding leucine-rich repeat (Fig. 3.1).

Helper nucleotide-binding leucine-rich repeats

Recently "helper" nucleotide-binding leucine-rich repeat receptors have been discovered.

Jeffery L. Dangl at the University of North Carolina at Chapel Hill and colleagues suggest that helper nucleotide-binding leucine-rich repeat receptors (hNLRs) are downstream signaling element activating effector-triggered immune responses (ETI). The sensor nucleotide-binding leucine-rich repeat receptors (sNLRs)—hNLRshNLRs model differs from the paired model in that each

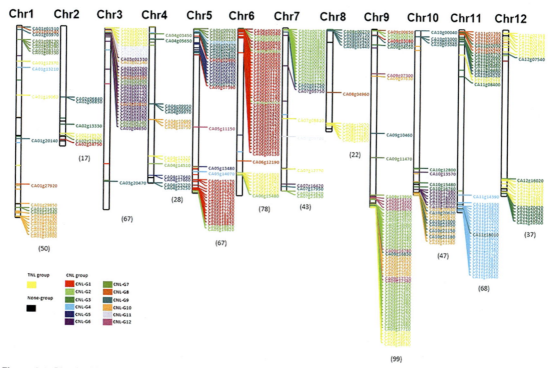

Figure 3.1 Physical localization of pepper (*Capsicum annuum*) nucleotide-binding leucine-rich repeat immune receptors (NLRs). White rectangular boxes symbolize the 12 pepper chromosomes. Line and letter colors indicate NLR subgroups. For ease of visualization, genes with intact NB domains are represented on the chromosomes. Numbers in parentheses represent the total numbers of mapped NB-encoding genes on each chromosome. Courtesy: Frontiers in Plant Science, https://doi.org/10.3389/fpls.2016.01205.

hNLR can transduce signals from multiple diverse sNLRs. To date three groups of hNLRs have been described, all of which are coiled-coil domain at their N-terminus. They include the activated disease resistance 1 (ADR1) family, the N required gene 1 (NRG1) family, and the nucleotide-binding leucine-rich repeat protein required for hypersensitive resistance-associated cell death.

Classes of disease resistance (R) proteins

Most disease resistance proteins that are activated upon effector recognition fall into five classes based primarily on their combination of a limited number of structural motifs.

Class 1 consists of just one member, *Pto* from tomato (*S. lycopersicum*), that has a serine/threonine kinase catalytic region and a myristylation motif at its N-terminus.

Class 2 comprises many proteins having a region of LRRs, a putative nucleotide-binding site (NBS), and an N-terminal putative leucine-zipper (LZ) or other coiled-coil (CC) sequence.

Class 3 is like Class 2 but instead of the CC sequence, these proteins have a region with similarity to the N-terminus of the homology with the cytoplasmic domains of the *Drosophila* toll protein and the mammalian interleukin-1 receptor proteins that are therefore referred to as the TIR region. The resistance proteins belonging to the first three classes lack transmembrane domains and all are thought to be localized intracellularly.

Class 4 are the *Cf* proteins from tomato (*S. lycopersicum*). They lack an NBS and instead have a transmembrane and an extracellular LRR receptor, and a small putatively cytoplasmic tail without obvious motifs.

Class 5 consists of just the *Xa21* protein from rice (*O. sativa*), that in addition to an extracellular LRR receptor and a transmembrane, has a cytoplasmic serine/threonine kinase region.

As with most things in biology, a few exceptions are noted with resistance proteins that do not fit into these five classes. A few examples include a toxin reductase, *Hm1*, in maize (*Zea mays*) that controls resistance to maize leaf spot (*Cochliobolus carbonum*), the *Mlo* gene in barley (*Hordeum vulgare*) is an apparent membrane protein where recessive mutant alleles confer resistance to powdery mildew (*Blumeria graminis* f. sp. *hordei*) and may be a negative regulator of defense responses, the *RPW8* protein conferring resistance in *Arabidopsis* to powdery mildew (*Golovinomyces orontii*) in a nonrace-specific way. Other resistance proteins may act in specific recognition but have novel structures. The *Ve* proteins for resistance to *Verticillium* in tomato (*S. lycopersicum*) are putative cell-surface glycoproteins with receptor-mediated endocytosis-like signals. The *RTM1* and *RTM2* restrict systemic movement of the Tobacco etch virus (TEV; *Potyvirus*) in resistant *A. thaliana* ecotypes and display jacalin-like sequences and similarity to a small heat shock-like protein, respectively. A toll-interleukin-1 receptor nucleotide-binding leucine-rich repeat protein, *RRS1-R*, is unusual in that it provides strain-nonspecific resistance to *Ralstonia solanacearum*, has recessive inheritance, and contains in its C terminus a putative nuclear localization signal and a 60-amino acid motif characteristic of the WRKY (pronounced "worky" family of plant transcriptional activator proteins that bind DNA). Recently, the *Rpg1* protein for resistance to barley stem rust (*Puccinia graminis*) was found to contain two tandem protein kinase domains and a predicted weak transmembrane domain.

Quantitative disease resistance

Quantitative disease resistance is widespread in horticultural plants. Literature for breeding disease-resistant plants is replete with terms referring to quantitative disease resistance in plants, examples include partial, complex, polygenic, oligogenic, horizontal, field, and durable. Quantitative traits exhibit a continuous distribution of phenotypic values in a genetically variable population that do not fit Mendelian segregation ratios. Furthermore, many economically important traits in horticultural crops are quantitatively inherited, such as yield and yield components, quality attributes, and pertinently resistance to diseases. Quantitative trait improvement employing phenotype-based selection has made significant selection gains. The development of molecular-based markers enables analysis of the relationship between marker genotypes and variation in phenotypes to dissect quantitative traits into quantitative trait loci (QTLs).

Definitions are essential to create a mutual understanding of a subject, but definitions tend to oversimplify complex biological phenomenon. Host–pathogen interactions are often complicated, and host resistance often cannot be described simply as either qualitative or quantitative, and in some cases may exist in a gray zone between the two. As Jesse A. Poland currently at King Abdullah University of Science and Technology, Saudi Arabia, and his colleagues state "qualitative and quantitative disease resistance might only be two ends of a continuum, with R-genes tending to lie toward one end of the spectrum and quantitative-resistant loci toward the other." Because of its more complex genetic basis, quantitative resistance is more difficult for breeders to manipulate because it requires population breeding strategies and statistical techniques to determine which progenies have improved resistance.

Classical quantitative genetics provide tools for studying complex disease resistance. Many disease resistance traits in plants have a polygenic background, and the disease phenotypes are modified by environmental factors. Therefore the phenotypic values usually show a quantitative variation. The phenotypes of such disease traits, however, are often measured in discrete but ordered categories. In terms of disease resistance, they are described as quantitative resistance traits (QRT) and are controlled by the quantitative-resistant loci (QRLs). Theoretically, QRL can be race-specific or not. For example, potato late blight (*Phytophthora infestans*) is a classic quantitative resistance and is the model James Edward Vanderplank of the Plant Protection Research Institute, Pretoria, South Africa, developed his ideas on "vertical" and "horizontal" resistance. Vanderplank proposed that a decline in horizontal resistance is due to the absence of selection pressure, especially during breeding for vertical resistance. Christiane Leonards-Schippers at the Max-Planck-Institute, Köln, Germany, and colleagues studying potato late blight found 11 genomic segments on nine chromosomes to be associated with resistance. They found three QRLs were race-specific, seven were specific to race 1; seven were specific to race 0; and four were nonspecific to these two races. Thus the classic nonrace-specific resistance was made up of a small number of race-nonspecific and other race-specific resistance loci. One QRL on chromosome 4 coincided in a location with a known qualitative resistance gene, *R1*.

Krishna Bhattarai and colleagues investigated the QTL for powdery mildew (*Golovinomyces cichoracearum*; formerly *Erysiphe cichoracearum*), resistance in gerbera daisy (*Gerbera hybrida*). Powdery mildew (*G. cichoracearum*) is one of the most devastating pathogens infecting gerbera and is one of the most challenging diseases in gerbera production. Reduction in visual appeal results in significant losses to both gerbera (*G. hybrida*) nurseries and the cut flower industry. In addition, reduced flower production and stunted plant growth are also caused by powdery mildew in greenhouse and field growing conditions. Again, host resistance is one of the most effective, environmentally friendly and cost-effective methods to control powdery mildew (*G. cichoracearum*) and minimize crop losses in gerbera (*G. hybrida*). Developing powdery mildew-resistant gerbera (*G. hybrida*) cultivars could offer a long-term solution to mitigate the disease, reduce the use of fungicides, and lower costs in gerbera production. A better understanding of the genetics underlying powdery mildew (*G. cichoracearum*) resistance in gerbera (*G. hybrida*) will facilitate the development of new powdery mildew-resistant cultivars.

The large genome size, large number of chromosomes ($2n = 50$), and limited availability of molecular markers have hindered the construction of linkage map in gerbera (*G. hybrida*). In this study, they showed that genotype-by-sequencing (GBS) can identify single nucleotide polymorphisms (SNPs) in gerbera (*G. hybrida*) to discover powdery mildew resistance loci by using a segregating F_1 population developed by hybridizing two gerbera (*G. hybrida*) breeding lines, one exhibiting powdery mildew (*G. cichoracearum*) resistance and one exhibiting susceptibility. The resistant parent is used in gerbera (*G. hybrida*) breeding programs as a source of powdery mildew (*G. cichoracearum*) resistance in developing new cultivars (*G. hybrida*). In total, 85 segregating individuals were genotyped by sequencing and the 3541 SNPs found in the progenies constructed a linkage map.

Individuals of the segregating population and its parents were evaluated for powdery mildew (*G. cichoracearum*) resistance in a greenhouse. Each progeny was asexually propagated to obtain four clonal plants that served as four biological replicates. All plants were arranged in four blocks on metal benches. Each block contained one replicate of all individuals and the parents randomly placed on the metal benches. The individuals were exposed to natural powdery mildew (*G. cichoracearum*) infection in the greenhouse. The greenhouse had been used to grow gerbera (*G. hybrida*) plants for more than 10 years, and severe powdery mildew (*G. cichoracearum*) was observed in the greenhouse during their testing period. To promote powdery mildew (*G. cichoracearum*) development in the greenhouse, two highly susceptible commercial cultivars were grown and placed among the gerbera (*G. hybrida*) individuals. Powdery mildew (*G. cichoracearum*) disease scoring began 30–45 days after moving gerbera (*G. hybrida*) plants into the greenhouse. Uniform distribution of the inoculum in the whole greenhouse was maintained by running circulation fans within the greenhouse. These actively growing foliar parts had equal chances for freely spreading powdery mildew (*G. cichoracearum*) spores to land and germinate on the foliar leaf surfaces. All individuals were phenotyped over 2 years to record the variation caused due to differences in growing conditions. Visual score rating was performed by evaluating the presence of powdery mildew (*G. cichoracearum*) spores and mycelial growth on the plant surfaces. Powdery mildew (*G. cichoracearum*) severity was rated using a scale of 1–10: 1 = no disease, 2 = trace to 10%, 3 = 10%–20%, 4 = 20%–30%, 5 = 30%–40%, 6 = 40%–50%, 7 = 50%–60%, 8 = 60%–70%, 9 = 70%–80%, and 10 = 80%–100%. The disease severity data were recorded for 4 weeks and following a weekly disease rating procedure. The means of the four replications were calculated and used for Area Under Disease Progress Curve (AUDPC) calculation. Each disease evaluation was performed every 7 days for four consecutive weeks. AUDPC scores for each year for every individual were calculated separately. No significant block (or replicate) effect was observed; therefore, the average of all evaluations within a year was calculated and used for QTL mapping.

Based on the phenotypic powdery mildew (*G. cichoracearum*) AUDPC values, QTLs were identified. One QTL explained approximately 17%–20% of the phenotypic variation for resistance. This locus and the two single nucleotide polymorphism-linked markers will be useful for breeding gerbera for powdery mildew (*G. cichoracearum*) resistance.

As the first GBS study in gerbera (*G. hybrida*), they observed interesting phenomena in this species. Out of the high-quality SNPs from GBS, only about 22% of them could be mapped to linkage groups. Many SNPs showed significant segregation distortion ratios, unexpectedly high recombination frequencies, or high nearest-neighbor stress values. These phenomena might have resulted from gerbera's highly heterozygous, complex genome and/or the lack of a high-quality reference genome for reliable variant calls. Although the cause(s) for this high portion (nearly 78%) of unmappable SNPs remains to be understood, it does suggest the need for the discovery of significantly more SNPs for genetic mapping in gerbera.

The powdery mildew development in resistant and susceptible gerbera (*G. hybrida*) has been studied and is determined that when the conidia land and establish on the leaf surfaces, they germinate in both resistant and susceptible gerbera (*G. hybrida*) lines. However, hyphal branching is observed in the susceptible lines, whereas it was significantly reduced in resistant lines 72 hours postinoculation. Similar reduction of haustoria and hyphal growths have been observed on the leaf surface of powdery mildew-resistant cucumbers (*Cucumis sativus*). Multiple powdery mildew resistance mechanisms in cucumber (*C. sativus*) are known to confer the resistance including recessive genes showing R-gene-like response including hypersensitivity reactions-like spots, accumulation of serine/threonine-protein kinase receptor (RPK2), or loss of function of CsMLO1 susceptibility gene. However, the molecular mechanisms underlying the resistance in both gerbera and cucumber (*C. sativus*) remain to be completely understood.

Plant nucleotide-binding and leucine-rich repeat receptors (NLR) play distinct roles within co-acting pairs to confer resistance. In the absence of pathogens, nucleotide-binding and leucine-rich repeat receptors proteins are in an inactive state, whereas, after avirulence recognition, they are activated and induce disease resistance signaling. The molecular mechanisms occurring during the transition from "inactive" to "active" state and the downstream signaling partners are still largely unknown. Current models of nucleotide-binding and leucine-rich repeat receptor function predict that, in the resting state, intramolecular interactions between different domains maintain resistance proteins in a closed auto-inhibited conformation. For several resistance proteins, this "off" state has been shown to be associated with "adenosine 5'-diphosphate" (ADP) binding. Simon J. Williams and his colleagues proposed that pathogen effector recognition favors a more open nucleotide-binding and leucine-rich repeat protein structure allowing nucleotide exchange and binding to adenosine triphosphate (ATP). These models based on nucleotide-binding and leucine-rich repeats functioning singly do not explain how two distinct nucleotide-binding and leucine-rich repeat proteins cooperate in pathogen recognition and signaling. However, the hNLR model explained above may assist in deciphering this phenomenon.

At the International Rice Research Institute in the Philippines, Zhi-Kang Li and his colleagues examined bacterial spot (*Xanthomonas oryzae* pv. *oryzae*) resistance in rice (*O. sativa*), and found four resistance genes (*Xa4, xa5, xa13,* and *Xa21*) and 12 races of *X. oryzae* pv. *oryzae*. The qualitative component of the resistance genes was reflected by their large effects against corresponding avirulent *X. oryzae* pv. *oryzae* races. The quantitative component of the resistance genes was their residual effects against corresponding virulent races and their epistatic effects that together could lead to high-level resistance in a race-specific manner. These results revealed important differences between the different types of resistance genes.

Two resistance genes, *Xa4* and *Xa21*, had complete dominance against the avirulent *X. oryzae* pv. *oryzae* races and had large residual effects against virulent ones. They acted independently and cumulatively, suggesting they are involved in different pathways of the rice defensive system. The third resistance gene, *xa5*, showed partial dominance or additivity to the avirulent *Xoo* races and had relatively small but significant residual effects against the virulent races. In contrast, *xa13* was completely recessive, had no residual effects against the virulent races, and showed more pronounced race specificity. There was a strong interaction leading to increased resistance between *xa13* and *xa5* and between either of them and *Xa4* or *Xa21*, suggesting their regulatory roles in the rice defensive pathway(s).

Six characteristics of quantitative disease resistance

Jesse A. Poland and colleagues hypothesize there are six characteristics that describe quantitative disease resistance. First, quantitative disease resistance is based on genes regulating morphology and developmental traits. Second, QRLs represent mutations or alleles at genes for basal defense. Third, QRLs affect the production of components of chemical antibiosis. Fourth, QRLs participate in defense signal transduction. Fifth, QRLs are weak or defeated resistance (R) genes, and last number six is that QRLs are unidentified genes. The authors noted that no single hypothesis accounts for all quantitative disease-resistant and QRLs, and multiple hypotheses for quantitative disease resistance are valid.

They continue that a quantitative disease resistance can be dissected with the genetic analysis methods of QTL mapping to localize QRLs that are regions of the host plant genome significantly associated with quantitative variation in disease resistance phenotypes. A QRL contains causal gene(s) and causal quantitative trait nucleotides (QTN) that are responsible for the phenotypic effect on quantitative disease resistant. The biological and molecular bases of QRLs are diverse, based on QRLs that have been cloned and functionally validated to date, as well as QRLs for which candidate genes have been identified and for which corroborative evidence for their role in QRLs has been obtained. Although none of the QRLs characterized to date has a gene structure similar to qualitative resistance R-genes or encodes R-gene type proteins with LRR motifs, it is certainly possible that future studies will reveal that some QRLs have similarities to R-gene structures and proteins. QRLs for which the phenotypic effects on QRLs have been verified and where tightly linked DNA-based markers have been determined are used in marker-assisted selection (MAS) breeding strategies for the development of cultivars.

Marker-assisted selection

MAS can augment or be used in lieu of phenotype-based selection for trait improvement. A DNA marker is a gene or other fragment of DNA whose location in the genome is known. It is a unique DNA sequence occurring near the gene or locus of interest, in this case, a resistance gene. For example, Partha Saha and colleagues at the Division of Vegetable Science, Indian Council of Agricultural Research-Indian Agricultural Research Institute, New Delhi, India, used a marker-assisted backcross breeding method to pyramid a black rot (*Xanthomonas campestris* pv. *campestris*) resistance gene (*Xca1bo*) and a downy mildew (*Hyaloperonospora parasitica*) resistance gene (*Ppa3*) into a cauliflower (*Brassica oleracea* var. *botrytis*) cultivar.

As a tool for breeding, MAS can be advantageous for traits with a complex inheritance that is difficult or expensive to phenotype, such as quantitative resistance to diseases. Isolate- or race specificity can also be a feature of quantitative disease resistance. For example, the polygenic resistance of chile pepper (*C. annuum*) to potyviruses consists of a combination of isolate-specific and broad-spectrum QTL. Despite many published QRL mapping studies, few studies have reported the cloning and functional validation of the causal gene(s) and causal QTNs underlying a QRL. Even though, both public and private breeding programs are using MAS for QRLs, the published literature underrepresents the efforts of the private sector due to intellectual property concerns. Examples of MAS for QRLs in horticultural crop plants from the literature include MAS for single QRL, multiple QRLs (pyramiding or stacking), and QRLs plus qualitative resistance genes.

Two bottlenecks for MAS breeding are genotyping costs and throughput rate of large sample numbers and phenotyping, evaluating large numbers of individuals or families in replicated field experiments across locations and seasons. Methods for genotyping are undergoing major changes due to innovative technologies that are increasing sample throughput and decreasing costs per sample. High-throughput genotyping platforms based on SNPs are being applied in the commercial sector and, as costs decrease, are likely to be feasible for use in breeding programs.

Regardless of how streamlined the genotyping pipeline becomes in breeding programs, the need for precise and reliable phenotype data on quantitative traits will remain and will require replicated field experiments to obtain the relevant information. The bottleneck will continue to be trait phenotyping. Novel approaches and methods to facilitate reliable and precise high-throughput phenotyping for quantitative traits, including quantitative disease resistance, are needed.

Whole genome sequencing has the potential to revolutionize genotype-based selection methods in breeding because of decreasing costs and increasing accessibility of high-throughput technologies. Whole genome sequencing can enable haplotype-based selection or selection based on the configuration of alleles present across many loci simultaneously. It may become feasible for breeding programs to adopt whole genome sequencing and haplotype-based selection on a large scale if costs and technological issues can be addressed.

Our understanding of quantitative disease resistance and QRLs will benefit greatly from the expansion of genomic resources and tools that enable the detailed study of various host–pathogen systems to unfold the biological bases for resistance. Genomic resources and new tools for higher-throughput functional testing of candidate genes will facilitate the identification and verification of the causal gene(s) and quantitative trait nucleotide(s) for QRLs and will determine whether QRLs do indeed have diverse biological and molecular bases.

Strategies for the deployment of quantitative disease resistance and QRLs in breeding need to be evaluated and managed to avoid the evolutionary arms race observed in several host–pathogen gene-for-gene systems in which widely deployed resistance R-genes experience loss of effectiveness. Questions that a plant breeder should ask are (1) should QRLs be deployed together with qualitative resistance genes in the same plant; (2) do QRLs serve as a backup system to resistant R-genes in providing some level of resistance to the crop in the event of resistant R-gene breakdown; (3) does resistant R-gene breakdown reduce the longevity of quantitative disease resistance conferred by deployed QRLs; and (4) what are best-practice strategies for QRLs deployment?

Loss-of-susceptibility concept

As mentioned earlier, growers view resistance and susceptibility as opposite sides of the same coin, and thus most studies have focused on the resistance side in search for plant resistance genes and other defense genes. However, a new paradigm at the beginning of the 21st century began to question whether plant genes are required for susceptibility. Therefore can the "loss of susceptibility" give a resistant phenotype? The simple answer is yes. These genes are referred to as susceptibility S-genes. Any plant gene that facilitates a compatible interaction with the pathogen can be considered an S-gene. More than 150 S-genes have been described in *Arabidopsis*, and there are S-gene orthologs present in diverse horticultural crop species.

It has been shown that to remove susceptibility genes can work to produce a resistant phenotype. The loss of susceptibility is sometimes referred to as loss of function. Some of the unique forms of resistance conferred by loss of function are genes like *Mlo*, *PMR6*, and *eIF4E*. The recessive barley mildew resistance locus o (*mlo*) mutant has been successfully employed for more than 80 years against powdery mildew (*B. graminis*) disease. Powdery mildew locus O (*Mlo*) gene family is one of the largest seven transmembrane protein-encoding gene families. The *Mlo* proteins act as negative regulators of powdery mildew (*B. graminis*) resistance and a loss-of-function mutation in *Mlo* confers broad-spectrum resistance to powdery mildew (*B. graminis*). For a long time, resistance conferred by loss of function of the barley (*H. vulgare*) mildew resistance locus (*Mlo*) gene was considered a unique type of plant immunity. Now there are many more examples, for example, the gene

PMR6 that encodes a pectate lyase–like protein with a novel C-terminal domain. Mutations in *PMR6* alter the composition of the plant cell wall. The recessive allele, *pmr6*, provides resistance to powdery mildew (*E. cichoracearum*) and requires neither salicylic acid nor the ability to perceive jasmonic acid or ethylene to function, indicating that the resistance mechanism does not require the activation of the well-known defense pathways. Thus *pmr6* resistance represents a novel form of disease resistance based on the loss of function of a gene required during a compatible interaction rather than the activation of known host defense pathways. The loss of function may be more commonplace in nature than previously known.

For example, powdery mildew is a common disease of cucumber (*C. sativus*) under field and greenhouse conditions globally and is a major threat to cucumber (*C. sativus*) yield and quality. Two pathogens, *Podosphaera xanthii* (previously known as *Sphaerotheca fuliginea*) and *G. cichoracearum* (formerly *E. cichoracearum*), have been reported as the most common fungi causing cucumber powdery mildew. So far, the application of protective fungicides has been the major way of controlling this disease. However, powdery mildew strains have become resistant to fungicides over the years. Thus breeding cultivars resistant to powdery mildew is the most effective and environment-friendly strategy for controlling the disease.

At least for obligate pathogens such as powdery mildew, the majority of resistance genes deliberately deployed by plant breeders are race-specific resistance (R) genes. However, because R-genes confer race-specific resistance that can easily be overcome by new pathogen races in a short period, R-gene resistance to powdery mildew is of limited horticultural value. In contrast, the loss-of-function *mlo* (mildew resistance locus o) confers almost complete, durable, and broad-spectrum resistance to powdery mildew in tomato (*S. lycopersicum*), muskmelon (*Cucumis melo*) and pea (*Pisum sativum*). Genetic analysis by Jingtao Nie at the School of Agriculture and Biology, Shanghai, China demonstrated that powdery mildew resistance in cucumber (*C. sativus*) is quantitatively inherited and controlled a gene that is MLO-like. This MLO-like gene, designated *CsMLO1*, mediates powdery mildew resistance in cucumber (*C. sativus*). Moreover, the mechanism of *CsMLO1* to mediate resistance in cucumber (*C. sativus*) was found not to involve the signaling molecules ethylene, jasmonic acid or salicylic acid. They confirmed using transgenic plants that *CsMLO1* is able to complement the susceptibility phenotype in *Arabidopsis*. They also discovered that when *CsMLO1* is defective in three independent natural mutations, it causes a loss of susceptibility. These three independent natural mutations causing loss of function of *CsMLO1* resulted in a durable and broad-spectrum powdery mildew resistance in cucumber (*C. sativus*).

Translation initiation factors 4E (commonly known as *eIF4E* gene) have long been known to be a susceptibility factor to potyviruses (*Potyviridae*), and the inactivation of the *eIF4E2* gene has provided resistance to Pepper veinal mottle virus (PVMV, *Potyvirus*) in tomato (*S lycopersicum*) plants.

Normally, with potato (*S. tuberosum*) a strategy to control late blight (*P. infestans*) is to introgress disease resistance (*R*) genes that are effective against diverse *P. infestans* isolates. More than 35 potato resistance genes conferring late blight resistance have been identified, most of which encode NLR proteins. These intracellular proteins mount successive defense responses when they recognize corresponding avirulence (*AVR*) proteins secreted by the pathogen. The avirulence proteins, known as RxLR (arginine–any amino acid–leucine–arginine) effectors, display high evolutionary rates, and as a result, *P. infestans* can rapidly escape nucleotide-binding domain, LRR-mediated resistance, thereby limiting the durability of genetic resistance in cultivars possessing a single resistance gene. *P. infestans* has more than 550 RxLR effector genes that evolve more rapidly in comparison to other genes in gene-dense regions. Hence, RxLR effectors are able to undergo rapid adaptation, thereby avoiding recognition by R-proteins. *P. infestans* overcomes R-gene-mediated resistance by adapting its matching effectors. Pyramiding or stacking resistance genes is a potential strategy to achieve broad-spectrum and durable late blight resistance. Potato being an autopolyploid (4x) can have several resistant genes; nevertheless, resistant potato cultivars can be overcome by the pathogen if no regional resistance gene strategy is developed.

Another approach to gain disease resistance in potato is the impairment of the susceptibility genes (S-genes). Researchers at Wageningen University and Research, the Netherlands, report that the genetic loss of host susceptibility in potato (*S. tuberosum*) is a new source of resistance to prevent or diminish pathogen infection. They showed that RNA interference (RNAi)-mediated silencing of the potato susceptibility (S) genes *StDND1*, *StDMR1*, and *StDMR6* led to increased late blight (*P. infestans*) resistance. Their research suggests that different defense mechanisms are involved in late blight (*P. infestans*) resistance and can be mediated by the functional impairment of different potato S-genes.

In addition, in the cultivar Gy14 cucumber (*C. sativus*) with the *STAYGREEN* (*CsSGR*) gene, where it was shown that the Gy14 cucumber (*C. sativus*) is resistant to oomyceteous downy mildew (*Pseudoperonospora cubensis*), bacterial angular leaf spot (*Pseudomonas syringae* pv. *lachrymans*), and fungal anthracnose pathogen (*Colletotrichum orbiculare*), by an SNP in the coding region resulted in a nonsynonymous amino acid substitution in the *CsSGR* protein, and thus disease resistance. Genes in the chlorophyll degradation pathway showed differential expression between resistant and susceptible lines in response to pathogen inoculation. The SNP was significantly associated with disease resistance in natural and breeding populations. Cucumber (*C. sativus*) breeders have made a selection for this resistance allele. This durable, broad-spectrum disease resistance is caused by a loss-of-susceptibility mutation of *CsSGR*.

The characterization and manipulation of host–pathogen infection processes for the establishment of disease can generate novel resistance mechanisms in horticultural crops that are not necessarily found in natural populations. As a cautionary note, some newly engineered crop lines have displayed unexpected phenotypes and vulnerabilities to disease, underscoring the need for rigorous performance testing of new breeding material in field settings over multiple seasons.

Ralph Panstruga at the Rheinisch-Westfälische Technische Hochschule Aachen University in Germany believes that *mlo*-based resistance and nonhost resistance are "two faces of the same coin," as both types of resistance share analogous features like prehaustoria resistance mechanisms to powdery mildew. This is because *mlo*-based resistance requires all three described *PEN* genes for nonhost resistance in *A. thaliana* and the *Ror2* genes (homolog of *PEN1*) in barley (*H. vulgare*). It has been demonstrated that mutations in these genes that affect nonhost resistance to powdery mildews compromise *mlo*-based resistance and vice versa. Thus the absence of the key host protein (*MLO*) converts a compatible interaction between an adapted powdery mildew pathogen and its respective host plant into an incompatible interaction having similar molecular mechanisms of nonhost resistance. There is also the possibility of using recessive gene resistance that can result from loss or modification of function of host genes that encode protein targets for pathogen effectors and therefore may be essential for virulence.

It must be remembered that the first reported plant disease resistance gene identified by Sir Biffen was yellow rust (*Puccinia striiformis* f. sp. *tritici*) in wheat (*T. aestivum*) that was governed by a recessive gene segregating in the ratio 3 resistant to 1 susceptible in F_2. The isolation and characterization of genes associated with disease susceptibility in the host have gained much interest. The initiative-taking deployment of modified susceptibility genes in crops will become possible as a geographical sampling of pathogen genomes increases.

Inhibitor genes

Another form of susceptibility is inhibitor genes. These genes inhibit the resistant R-gene from manifesting itself. An excellent example of this is the *Ipcr* (inhibitor of *Phytophthora capsici* resistance) gene in *Capsicum*. The gene inhibits resistance to *P. capsici* but not to other species of *Phytophthora*, or other bacteria and viruses. When a highly *P. capsici*-resistant plant is hybridized to a plant with the *Ipcr* gene, the resultant F_1 population, is completely susceptible to *P. capsici*, despite the dominance inheritance of *P. capsici* resistance in the *Capsicum* parent. The F_2 population segregates in a 3:13 resistant-to-susceptible (R:S) ratio. The testcross population segregates in a 1:1 R:S ratio, and a backcross population to *Ipcr* parent displays complete susceptibility. These results demonstrate the presence of a single dominant inhibitor gene affecting *P. capsici* resistance in *Capsicum*. Moreover, when accessions carrying the *Ipcr* gene were challenged against six *Phytophthora* species, the nonhost resistance was not overcome. Thus the *Ipcr* gene is interfering with host-specific resistance but not the pathogen- or microbe-associated molecular pattern nonhost responses. The obvious question then is, are there genes causing susceptibility in crop plants, and by replacing them with the recessive allele, a resistant phenotype is obtained?

To exploit susceptibility S-genes for resistance breeding, the S-gene orthologs need to be found across cultivated plant species, and knowledge of how to obtain and apply loss-of-function mutants of S-genes in resistance breeding. Sequence homology to characterize S-genes could be identified by mining available sequence databases in a plant species. Another potential approach is to use gene-silencing techniques such as virus-induced gene silencing, RNAi, or even possible clustered regularly interspaced short palindromic repeats-associated protein 9 (CRISPR-Cas9) system to observe altered phenotypes for susceptibility to a pathogen. Nowadays, virus-induced silencing is practiced in many plant species for large-scale functional analysis. A classic approach would be chemical or irradiation mutagenesis, which in the past has been disparaged as an approach for discovering resistance. As with the search for any trait, natural S-gene alleles can be obtained by screening the germplasm of the plant species.

The resistant phenotype can be achieved in many ways. There is the most common way: the presence of corresponding resistance R-genes to recognize pathogen effectors, and another one is by the absence of susceptibility S-genes. Loss of function of the S-genes leads to resistance that inherits recessively in normal plants and dominantly in plants where the S-gene is silenced by using the RNAi technique. In practice, most of the resistance breeding programs aim to introgress resistance (R)-genes from members of wild species into horticulturally adapted plants. Dominant resistance is highly effective and, unfortunately, often race-specific. In most cases, resistance conferred by dominant resistance genes can be overcome by pathogens resulting in outbreaks of large epidemics, which "bust" the once "booming" cultivars. Repeated boom-and-bust cycles in agriculture continuously force plant breeders to introduce cultivars with new resistance traits. In contrast, to dominate resistance genes, it has been shown that loss of function in S-genes often leads to durable and broad-spectrum resistance, such as *mlo*-based resistance. Thus exploitation of S-gene alleles that are insensitive to manipulation by pathogen effectors provides an alternative breeding strategy that is complementary to the R-gene conferred resistance.

Cytoplasmic inheritance

Occasionally, a plant trait conferring disease resistance or susceptibility is associated with a cytoplasmic characteristic, in which case the trait will be maternal, not paternally transmitted. Cytoplasmic inheritance is also known as non-Mendelian inheritance because the pattern of inheritance does not segregate in accordance with Mendel's laws. Cytoplasmic inheritance can be defined as the process that takes part in the process of inheritance that transfers the genetic characters by means of cytoplasmic elements in plants. The cytoplasm consists of autonomous organelles like mitochondria and plastids that have their own genomes, which are circular like bacterial genomes. These genomes encode their own proteins that can have functions within and outside the organelle. Normally, reciprocal hybridizations that are hybridizing in both directions, where the female parent is also used as the male parent and the male is used as the female, are the techniques plant breeders employ to learn if the trait of interest is inherited in a Mendelian fashion or not.

The most notorious resistance that is associated with cytoplasmic inheritance is the Texas, or T-cytoplasm (cms-T) of maize (*Z. mays*). This cytoplasmic male-sterility (CMS) system suppresses the production of viable pollen grains and is inherited in a non-Mendelian manner. The cms-T was first described in the cultivar, Golden June, in Texas. The discovery of the T-cms was important to maize breeders because the use of male-sterility traits in hybrid seed production made the process easier because hand emasculation was not necessary.

During the 1950s and 1960s, cms-T was used extensively to avoid the need for hand or mechanical emasculation in the production of hybrid corn. Unfortunately, in 1969 and 1970, the Southern corn leaf blight (*Bipolaris maydis* race T) struck the southern and midwestern regions of the United States, severely blighting maize (*Z. mays*) carrying the cms-T, which was more than 85% of the United States maize (*Z. mays*) acreage. Maize (*Z. mays*) plants carrying normal cytoplasm were generally only mildly affected by *B. maydis* race T. It was evident that the cms-T-cytoplasm was solely responsible for the susceptibility of the plants to the disease, and large-scale usage of cms-T for hybrid seed production was abandoned. Another fungal disease, Yellow leaf blight, (*Didymella zeae-maydis*) is also uniquely virulent to cms-T maize. Because this latter pathogen is restricted to the cooler northern regions of the United States, it was less serious than Southern corn leaf blight. The maize blight epidemic demonstrated the significance of the cytoplasm in providing resistance and/or susceptibility.

Resistance models

While extensive research has been carried out to understand plant–disease interactions, it is also useful for researchers to devise models to better understand the functionality of resistance genes that govern the resistant phenotype. Identifying a resistance gene, or more likely a locus on a chromosome that is statistically associated with disease resistance and developing molecular markers within the QTL for MAS is useful and where many plant breeders stop. However, understanding the genetics of resistance and characterizing the plant's response to attack by a pathogen can provide deeper insights into pathosystems and ultimately breed more durable resistant plants.

The "Elicitor-Receptor Model," proposed by Peter Albersheim and colleagues, states that disease resistance is associated with the perception by the plant of signal molecules, namely elicitors that are produced by the avirulent pathogen. This simplest mechanistic explanation of the genetic interaction between resistance genes with avirulence genes states that the latter encode or generate "specific ligands" that interact physically with a "receptor" that is encoded by the corresponding plant's resistance gene. This specific recognition event leads to the induction of effective defense responses, including a programmed cell death response termed the hypersensitive response. Even though the role of specific elicitors in race/cultivar-specific resistance has been well documented, the extent to which elicitor recognition contributes to other types of resistance, such as partial resistance and nonhost resistance, remains poorly defined, and experimental data to support this model are rare.

An alternative model, the "Guard Model (Hypothesis)" put forward by Erik Van der Biezen and Jonathan Jones in 1998 postulates that plant resistance proteins act by monitoring (guarding) the target of their corresponding pathogen effector. In only some cases is there direct interaction between the resistance gene product and the avirulence gene product. The lack of evidence for a direct interaction between the resistance gene and the avirulence gene product led to the formation of the guard hypothesis for the nucleotide-binding site leucine-rich repeat (NLR) motif class of resistance genes. This model proposes that the resistance gene proteins interact, or guard, a protein known as the guardee that is the target of the avirulence gene protein. When it detects interference with the guardee protein, it activates resistance.

Because neither the Elicitor-Receptor nor the Guard Model explained the resistance interaction completely, a third model was put forward the "Decoy Model." Renier A.L. van der Hoorn and Sophien Kamoun state that the key assumptions behind their Decoy Model are: (1) resistance genes are typically polymorphic in natural plant populations; (2) effector targets are under selection for decreased binding affinity to effectors and (3) in the presence of the resistance gene protein, there is selection on the guarded effector target to maintain or improve its interaction with the effector. This has not been shown directly, but this process should not be different from the adaptation of resistance gene proteins that physically interact with effectors (Fig. 3.2).

It is interesting to note that each of the four players in this antagonistic molecular interaction are under selection forces to adapt: (1) the operative target is under selection to evade manipulation by the effector; (2) the effector is under selection to target the adjusted operative targets while preventing interactions with the decoy, which would trigger defense responses in the presence of the resistance gene protein; (3) the decoy is under selection to adapt to adjusted effectors and is under additional selection to

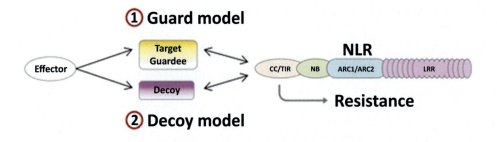

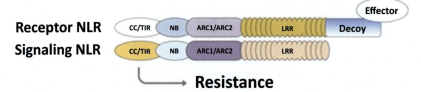

Figure 3.2 Model of integrated decoys in NLR Protein Pairs. Pathogen effectors target host proteins for manipulation to promote infection. Indirect recognition of these effectors occurs when these target proteins are guarded by host NLR proteins (1), or if duplicated target genes evolve into decoy proteins monitored by host NLRs (2). Alternatively, the decoy may be integrated into the structure of the receptor component of an NLR pair (3), allowing AVR recognition by direct binding. Courtesy Frontiers in Plant Science, https://doi.org/10.3389/fpls.2014.00606.

prevent autoimmune responses; and (4) the resistance gene protein is under selection to adapt to novel decoy-effector complexes while preventing autoimmune responses. As a result, each component is part of a molecular arms race in which each player is a target of the next. The Decoy Model remains to be experimentally demonstrated, but it is consistent with several recent observations and provides a challenging platform for future experiments. New data and more experiments will generate a better understanding of effector perception in plants, ultimately leading to novel approaches for plant breeders to manipulate innate immunity and improve pathogen resistance.

Molecular analysis

As has been discussed, the disease-resistant phenotype is often controlled by the gene-for-gene mechanism, where avirulence gene products encoded by pathogens are specifically recognized, either directly or indirectly by plant disease resistance gene products. Research arising from molecular cloning of resistance genes from several plant species conferring resistance to different pathogens and molecular cloning of corresponding avirulence genes from various pathogens has resulted in knowledge on the mode of action of gene-for-gene interaction. Disease resistance genes cloned from diverse plant species such as tomato (*S. lycopersicum*), rice (*O. sativa*), and *A. thaliana* encode proteins that share one or more similar structural motifs. These motifs include LRR regions, NBSs, and kinase domains. Especially, members of the NLR regions class of resistance genes encoding proteins containing a nucleotide-binding site and carboxyl-terminal LRRs confer resistance to quite different types of plant pathogens, such as bacteria, fungi, oomycetes, viruses, and nematodes.

Bibliography

Bai, Y., Pavan, S., Zheng, Z., Zappel, N.F., Reinstadler, A., Lotti, C., et al., 2008. Naturally occurring broad-spectrum powdery mildew resistance in a Central American tomato accession is caused by loss of Mlo function. Molecular Plant–Microbe Interactions 21, 30–39. Available from: https://doi.org/10.1094/MPMI-21-1-0030.

Beketova, M.P., Chalaya, N.A., Zoteyeva, N.M., Gurina, A.A., Kuznetsova, M.A., Armstrong, M., et al., 2021. Combination breeding and marker-assisted selection to develop late blight resistant potato cultivars. Agronomy 11, 2192. Available from: https://doi.org/10.3390/agronomy11112192.

Belcher, A.R., Zwonitzer, J.C., Santa Cruz, J., Krakowsky, M.D., Chung, C.L., Nelson, R., et al., 2012. Analysis of quantitative disease resistance to southern leaf blight and of multiple disease resistance in maize, using near-isogenic lines. Theoretical and Applied Genetics 124, 433–445. Available from: https://doi.org/10.1007/s00122-011-1718-1.

Bergelson, J., Kreitman, M., Stahl, E.A., Tian, D., 2001. Evolutionary dynamics of plant R-genes. Science (New York, N.Y.) 292, 2281–2284. Available from: https://doi.org/10.1126/science.1061337.

Bernoux, M., Ellis, J.G., Dodds, P.N., 2011. New insights in plant immunity signaling activation. Current Opinion in Plant Biology 14, 512–518. Available from: https://doi.org/10.1016/j.pbi.2011.05.005.

Bhattarai, K., Sharma, S., Verma, S., Peres, N.A., Xiao, S., Clark, D.G., et al., 2023. Construction of a genome-wide genetic linkage map and identification of quantitative trait loci for powdery mildew resistance in Gerbera daisy. Frontiers in Plant Science 13. Available from: https://doi.org/10.3389/fpls.2022.1072717.

Biffen, R.H., 1905. Mendel's laws of inheritance and wheat breeding. Journal of Agricultural Science 1, 4–48.

Brotman, Y., Normantovich, M., Goldenberg, Z., Zvirin, Z., Kovalski, I., Stovbun, N., et al., 2012. Dual resistance of melon to *Fusarium oxysporum* Races 0 and 2 and to Papaya ring-spot virus is controlled by a pair of head-to-head-oriented NB-LRR genes of unusual architecture. Molecular Plant 6, 235–238. Available from: https://doi.org/10.1093/mp/sss121.

Brouwer, D.J., Jones, E.S., St Clair, D.A., 2004. QTL analysis of quantitative resistance to Phytophthora infestans (late blight) in tomato and comparisons to potato. Genome/National Research Council Canada = Genome/Conseil National de Recherches Canada 47, 475–492. Available from: https://doi.org/10.1139/g04-001.

Brown, J.K.M., 2003. A cost of disease resistance: paradigm or peculiarity? Trends in Genetics 19, 667–671. Available from: https://doi.org/10.1016/j.tig.2003.10.008.

Buschges, R., Hollricher, K., Panstruga, R., Simons, G., Wolter, M., Frijters, A., et al., 1997. The barley Mlo gene: a novel control element of plant pathogen resistance. Cell 88, 695–705. Available from: https://doi.org/10.1016/S0092-8674(00)81912-1.

Cesari, S., Bernoux, M., Moncuquet, P., Kroj, T., Dodds, P., 2014a. A novel conserved mechanism for plant NLR protein pairs: the 'integrated decoy' hypothesis. Frontiers in Plant Science 5, 606. Available from: https://doi.org/10.3389/fpls.2014.00606.

Cesari, S., Kanzaki, H., Fujiwara, T., Bernoux, M., Chalvon, V., Kawano, Y., et al., 2014b. The NB-LRR proteins RGA4 and RGA5 interact functionally and physically to confer disease resistance. The EMBO Journal 33, 1941–1959. Available from: https://doi.org/10.15252/embj.201487923.

Christopoulou, M., McHale, L.K., Kozik, A., Reyes-Chin Wo, S., Wroblewski, T., Michelmore, R.W., 2015. Dissection of two complex clusters of resistance genes in lettuce (*Lactuca sativa*). Molecular Plant-Microbe Interactions 28, 751–765. Available from: https://doi.org/10.1094/MPMI-0614-0175-R.

Cook, D.E., Mesarich, C.H., Thomma, B.P.H.J., 2015. Understanding plant immunity as a surveillance system to detect invasion. Annual Review of Phytopathology 53, 541–563. Available from: https://doi.org/10.1146/annurev-phyto-080614-120114.

Corwina, J.A., Kliebensteina, D.J., 2017. Quantitative resistance: more than just perception of a pathogen. The Plant Cell 29, 655–665. Available from: https://doi.org/10.1105/tpc.16.00915.

Cui, H., Xiang, T., Zhou, J.M., 2009. Plant immunity: a lesson from pathogenic bacterial effector proteins. Cell. Microbiology 11, 1453–1461. Available from: https://doi.org/10.1111/j.1462-5822.2009.01359.x.

Dalio, R.J.D., Paschoal, D., Arena, G.D., Magalhães, D.M., Oliveira, T.S., Merfa, M. V., et al., 2020. Hypersensitive response: from NLR pathogen recognition to cell death response. Annals of Applied Biology 178, 268–280. Available from: https://doi.org/10.1111/aab.12657.

Darvill, A., Albersheim, P., 1984. Phytoalexins and their elicitors – a defense against microbial infection in plants. Annual Review of Plant Physiology and Plant Molecular Biology 35, 243–275. Available from: https://doi.org/10.1146/annurev.pp.35.060184.001331.

Day, P.R., 1974. Genetics of host-parasite interaction. Freeman, San Francisco, 238 pages.

Dodds, P.N., Lawrence, G.J., Catanzariti, A., The, T., Wang, C.A., Ayliffe, M.A., et al., 2006. Direct protein interaction underlies gene-for-gene specificity and co-evolution of the flax resistance genes and flax rust avirulence genes. Proceedings of the National Academy of Sciences of the USA 103, 8888–8893. Available from: https://doi.org/10.1073/pnas.0602577103.

Ellis, J., Dodds, P., Pryor, T., 2000a. The generation of plant disease resistance gene specificities. Trends in Plant Science 5, 373–379. Available from: https://doi.org/10.1016/S1360-1385(00)01694-0.

Ellis, J., Dodds, P., Pryor, T., 2000b. Structure, function, and evolution of plant disease resistance genes. Current Opinion in Plant Biology 3, 278–284. Available from: https://doi.org/10.1016/S1369-5266(00)00080-7.

Ender, M., Kelly, J.D., 2005. Identification of QTL associated with white mold resistance in common bean. Crop Science 45, 2482–2490. Available from: https://doi.org/10.2135/cropsci2005.0064.

Flor, H.H., 1955. Host-parasite interaction in flax rust-its genetics and other implications. Phytopathology 45, 680–685.

Flor, H.H., 1956. The complementary genic systems in flax and flax rust. Advanced in Genetics 8, 29–54. Available from: https://doi.org/10.1016/S0065-2660(08)60498-8.

Flor, H.H., 1965. Tests for allelism of rust resistance genes in flax. Crop Science 5, 415–417. Available from: https://doi.org/10.2135/cropsci1965.0011183X000500050013x.

Flor, H.H., 1971. Current status of the gene-for-gene concept. Annual Review of Phytopathology 9, 275–296. Available from: https://doi.org/10.1146/annurev.py.09.090171.001423.

Fraser, R.S.S., 1990. The genetics of resistance to plant viruses. Annual Review of Phytopathology 28, 179–200. Available from: https://doi.org/10.1146/annurev.py.28.090190.001143.

Fuchs, M., 2017. Pyramiding resistance-conferring gene sequences in crops. Current Opinion in Virology 26, 36–42. Available from: https://doi.org/10.1016/j.coviro.2017.07.004.

Gallois, J.-L., Moury, B., German-Retana, S., 2018. Role of the genetic background in resistance to plant viruses. International Journal of Molecular Sciences 19, 2856. Available from: https://doi.org/10.3390/ijms19102856.

Gao, Y., Wang, W., Zhang, T., Gong, Z., Zhao, H., Han, G.-Z., 2018. Out of water: the origin and early diversification of plant R-genes. Plant Physiology 177, 82–89. Available from: https://doi.org/10.1104/pp.18.00185.

Garcia-Ruiz, H., Szurek, B., Van den Ackerveken, G., 2021. Stop helping pathogens: engineering plant susceptibility genes for durable resistance. Current Opinion in Biotech 70, 187–195. Available from: https://doi.org/10.1016/j.copbio.2021.05.005.

Ghislain, M., Byarugaba, A.A., Magembe, E., Njoroge, A., Rivera, C., Román, M. L., et al., 2019. Stacking three late blight resistance genes from wild species directly into African highland potato varieties confers complete field resistance to local blight races. Plant Biotechnology Journal 17, 1119–1129. Available from: https://doi.org/10.1111/pbi.13042.

Gorshkov, V., Tsers, I., 2022. Plant susceptible responses: the underestimated side of plant–pathogen interactions. Biological Review 97, 45–66. Available from: https://doi.org/10.1111/brv.12789.

Gururani, M.A., Venkatesh, J., Upadhyaya, C.P., Nookaraju, A., Pandey, S.K., Park, S.W., 2012. Plant disease resistance genes: current status and future directions. Physiological and Molecular Plant Pathology 78, 51–65. Available from: https://doi.org/10.1016/j.pmpp.2012.01.002.

Hammond-Kosack, K., Parker, J.E., 2003. Deciphering plant-pathogen communication: fresh perspectives for molecular resistance breeding. Current Opinion in Biotechnology 14, 177–193. Available from: https://doi.org/10.1016/S0958-1669(03)00035-1.

Hashimoto, M., Neriya, Y., Yamaji, Y., Namba, S., 2016. Recessive resistance to plant viruses: potential resistance genes beyond translation initiation factors. Frontiers in Microbiology 7, 1–11. Available from: https://doi.org/10.3389/fmicb.2016.01695.

Hasley, J.A.R., Navet, N., Tian, M., 2021. CRISPR/Cas9-mediated mutagenesis of sweet basil candidate susceptibility gene ObDMR6 enhances downy mildew resistance. PLoS One 16, 1–17. Available from: https://doi.org/10.1371/journal.pone.0253245.

Hooker, A.L., 1974. Cytoplasmic susceptibility in plant disease. Annual Review of Phytopathology 12, 167–179. Available from: https://doi.org/10.1146/annurev.py.12.090174.001123.

Hückelhoven, R., Eichmann, R., Weis, C., Hoefle, C., Proels, R.K., 2013. Genetic loss of susceptibility: a costly route to disease resistance. Plant Pathology 62, 56–62. Available from: https://doi.org/10.1111/ppa.12103.

Hulbert, S.H., Webb, C.A., Smith, S.M., Sun, Q., 2001. Resistance gene complexes: evolution and utilization. Annual Review of Phytopathology 39, 285–312. Available from: https://doi.org/10.1146/annurev.phyto.39.1.285.

Jamann, T.M., Poland, J.A., Kolkman, J.M., Smith, L.G., Nelson, R.J., 2014. Unraveling genomic complexity at a quantitative disease resistance locus in maize. Genetics 198, 333–344. Available from: http://www.genetics.org/lookup/suppl/doi:10.1534/genetics.114.167486/-/DC1.

Jiang, H., Wang, C., Ping, L., Tian, D., 2007. Pattern of LRR nucleotide variation in plant resistance genes. Plant Science 173, 253–261. Available from: https://doi.org/10.1016/j.plantsci.2007.05.010.

Joshi, R.K., Nayak, S., 2013. Perspectives of genomic diversification and molecular recombination towards R-gene evolution in plants. Physiology and Molecular Biology of Plants 19, 1–9. Available from: https://doi.org/10.1007/s12298-012-0138-2.

Jubic, L.M., Saile, S., Furzer, O.J., El Kasmi, F., Dangl, J.L., 2019. Help wanted: helper NLRs and plant immune responses. Current Opinion in Plant Biology 50, 82–94. Available from: https://doi.org/10.1016/j.pbi.2019.03.013.

Keen, N.T., 1990. Gene-for-gene complementarity in plant-pathogen interactions. Annual Review of Genetics 24, 447–463. Available from: https://doi.org/10.1146/annurev.ge.24.120190.002311.

Kelly, J.D., Vallejo, V., 2006. QTL analysis of multigenic disease resistance in plant breeding. In: Tuzun, S., Bent, E. (Eds.), Multigenic and Induced Systemic Resistance in Plants. Springer, New York, pp. 21–48. 521 pages.

Kim, S.H., Qi, D., Helm, M., 2016. Using decoys to expand the recognition specificity of a plant disease resistance protein. Science (New York, N.Y.) 351, 684–687. Available from: https://doi.org/10.1126/science.aad3436.

Kim, S., Park, J., Yeom, S.-I., Kim, Y.-M., Seo, E., Kim, K.-T., et al., 2017. New reference genome sequences of hot pepper reveal the massive evolution of plant disease-resistance genes by retroduplication. Genome Biology 18, 210. Available from: https://doi.org/10.1186/s13059-017-1341-9.

Koseoglou, E., van der Wolf, J.M., Visser, R.G.F., Bai, Y., 2022. Susceptibility reversed: modified plant susceptibility genes for resistance to bacteria. Trends in Plant Science 27, 69–79. Available from: https://doi.org/10.1016/j.tplants.2021.07.018.

Kourelis, J., van der Hoorn, R.A.L., Sueldo, D.J., 2016. Decoy engineering: the next step in resistance breeding. Trends in Plant Science 21, 371–373. Available from: https://doi.org/10.1016/j.tplants.2016.04.001.

Kourelis, J., van der Hoorn, R.A.L., 2018. Defended to the nines: 25 years of resistance gene cloning identifies nine mechanisms for R protein function. The Plant Cell 30, 285–299. Available from: https://doi.org/10.1105/tpc.17.00579.

Kuroiwa, K., Thenault, C., Nogué, F., Perrot, L., Maziera, M., Gallois, J.-L., 2022. CRISPR-based knock-out of eIF4E2 in a cherry tomato background successfully recapitulates resistance to pepper veinal mottle virus. Plant Science 316, 111160. Available from: https://doi.org/10.1016/j.plantsci.2021.111160.

Lapin, D., Van den Ackerveken, G., 2013. Susceptibility to plant disease: more than a failure of host immunity. Trends in Plant Science 18, 546−554. Available from: https://doi.org/10.1016/j.tplants.2013.05.005.

Leonards-Schippers, C., Gieffers, W., Schaüfer-Pregl, R., Ritter, E., Knapp, S.J., 1994. Quantitative resistance to phytophthora infestans in potato: a case study for QTL mapping in an allogamous plant species. Genetics 137, 67−77. Available from: https://www.genetics.org/content/137/1/67.

Li, Z.-K., Sanchez, A., Angeles, E., Singh, S., Domingo, J., Huang, N., et al., 2001. Are the dominant and recessive plant disease resistance genes similar?: a case study of rice R genes and *Xanthomonas oryzae* pv. oryzae races. Genetics 159, 757−765. Available from: https://www.genetics.org/content/159/2/757.

Loegering, W.Q., 1978. Current concepts in interorganismal genetics. Annual Review of Phytopathology 16, 309−320. Available from: https://doi.org/10.1146/annurev.py.16.090178.001521.

Mäkinen, K., 2019. Plant susceptibility genes as a source for potyvirus resistance. Annals of Applied Biology 176, 122−129. Available from: https://doi.org/10.1111/aab.12562.

Martin, G.B., Brommonshenkel, S.H., Chunwongse, J., Frary, A., Ganal, M.W., Spivey, R., et al., 1993. Map-based cloning of a protein kinase gene conferring disease resistance in tomato. Science (New York, N.Y.) 262, 1432−1436. Available from: https://doi.org/10.1126/science.7902614.

Martin, G.B., Bogdanove, A.J., Sessa, G., 2003. Understanding the functions of plant disease resistance proteins. Annual Review of Plant Biology 54, 23−61. Available from: https://doi.org/10.1146/annurev.arplant.54.031902.135035.

McDowell, J.M., Woffenden, B.J., 2003. Plant disease resistance genes: recent insights and potential applications. Trends in Biotechnology 21, 178−183. Available from: https://doi.org/10.1016/S0167-7799(03)00053-2.

Merrick, L., Burke, A., Chen, X., Carter, A., 2021. Breeding with major and minor genes: genomic selection for quantitative disease resistance. Frontiers in Plant Science . Available from: https://doi.org/10.3389/fpls.2021.713667.

Meyers, B.C., Kaushik, S., Nandety, R.S., 2005. Evolving disease resistance genes. Current Opinion in Plant Biology 8, 129−134. Available from: https://doi.org/10.1016/j.pbi.2005.01.002.

Michelmore, R.W., Meyers, B.C., 1998. Clusters of resistance genes in plants evolve by divergent selection and a birth-and-death process. Genome Research 8, 1113−1130. Available from: https://doi.org/10.1101/gr.8.11.1113.

Monaghan, J., Zipfel, C., 2012. Plant pattern recognition receptor complexes at the plasma membrane. Current Opinion in Plant Biology 15, 349−357. Available from: https://doi.org/10.1016/j.pbi.2012.05.006.

Nass, H.A., Pedersen, W.L., MacKenzie, D.R., Nelson, R.R., 1981. The residual effects of some "defeated" powdery mildew resistance genes in isolines of winter wheat. Phytopathology 71, 315−318.

Nie, J., Wang, Y., He, H., Guo, C., Zhu, W., Pan, J., et al., 2015. Loss-of-function mutations in CsMLO1 confer durable powdery mildew resistance in cucumber (*Cucumis sativus* l.). Frontiers in Plant Science 6. Available from: https://doi.org/10.3389/fpls.2015.01155.

Nelson, R., Wiesner-Hanks, T., Wisser, R., Balint-Kurti, P., 2018. Navigating complexity to breed disease-resistant crops. Nature Reviews. Genetics 19, 21−33. Available from: https://doi.org/10.1038/nrg.2017.82.

Pavan, S., Jacobsen, E., Visser, R.G.F., Bai, Y., 2010. Loss of susceptibility as a novel breeding strategy for durable and broad-spectrum resistance. Molecular Breeding 25. Available from: https://doi.org/10.1007/s11032-009-9323-6.

Pedersen, W.L., Leath, S., 1988. Pyramiding major genes for resistance to maintain residual effects. Annual Review of Phytopathology 26, 369–378. Available from: https://doi.org/10.1146/annurev.py.26.090188.002101.

Petit-Houdenot, Y., Fudal, I., 2017. Complex interactions between fungal avirulence genes and their corresponding plant resistance genes and consequences for disease resistance management. Frontiers in Plant Science 8, 1072–1079. Available from: https://doi.org/10.3389/fpls.2017.01072.

Poland, J.A., Balint-Kurti, P.J., Wisser, R.J., Pratt, R.C., Nelson, R.J., 2009. Shades of gray: the world of quantitative disease resistance. Trends in Plant Science 14, 21–29. Available from: https://doi.org/10.1016/j.tplants.2008.10.006.

Price, J.S., Bever, J.D., Clay, K., 2004. Genotype, environment and genotype by environment interactions determine quantitative resistance to leaf rust (*Coleosporium asterum*) in Euthamia graminifolia (Asteraceae). New Phytologist 162, 729–743. Available from: https://doi.org/10.1111/j.1469-8137.2004.01082.x.

Pring, D.R., Lonsdale, D.M., 1989. Cytoplasmic male-sterility and maternal inheritance of disease susceptibility in maize. Annual Review of Phytophathology 27, 483–502. Available from: https://doi.org/10.1146/annurev.py.27.090189.002411.

Reeves, G., Monroy-Barbosa, A., Bosland, P.W., 2013. A novel capsicum gene inhibits host-specific disease resistance to *Phytophthora capsici*. Phytopathology 103, 472–478. Available from: https://doi.org/10.1094/PHYTO-09-12-0242-R.

Richter, T.E., Ronald, P.C., 2000. The evolution of disease resistance genes. Plant Molecular Biology 42, 195–204. Available from: https://doi.org/10.1023/A:1006388223475.

Saha, P., Ghoshal, C., Saha, N., Verma, A., Srivastava, M., Kalia, P., et al., 2021. Marker assisted pyramiding of downy mildew resistant gene Ppa3 and black rot resistant gene Xca1bo in popular early cauliflower variety *Pusa Meghna*. Frontiers in Plant Science. Available from: https://doi.org/10.3389/fpls.2021.603600.

Santillán Martínez, M.I., Bracuto, V., Koseoglou, E., Appiano, M., Jacobsen, E., Visser, R.G.F., et al., 2020. CRISPR/Cas9-targeted mutagenesis of the tomato susceptibility gene PMR4 for resistance against powdery mildew. BMC Plant Biology 20, 1–13. Available from: https://doi.org/10.1186/s12870-020-02497-y.

Seo, E., Kim, S., Yeom, S.I., Choi, D., 2016. Genome-wide comparative analysis reveal the dynamic evolution of nucleotide-binding leucine-rich repeat gene family among Solanaceae plants. Frontiers in Plant Science 7, 1205. Available from: https://doi.org/10.3389/fpls.2016.01205.

Slusarenko, A.J., Fraser, R.S.S., van Loon, L.C. (Eds.), 2000. Mechanisms of resistance to plant diseases. Kluwer Academic Pub., The Netherlands, p. 620.

Staskawicz, B.J., 2001. Genetics of plant-pathogen interactions specifying plant disease resistance. Plant Physiology 125, 73–76. Available from: https://doi.org/10.1104/pp.125.1.73.

St Clair, D.A., 2010. Quantitative disease resistance and quantitative resistance loci in breeding. Annual Review of Phytopathology 48, 247–268. Available from: https://doi.org/10.1146/annurev-phyto-080508-081904.

Sun, K., Schipper, D., Jacobsen, E., Visser, R.G.F., Govers, F., Bouwmeester, K., et al., 2022. Silencing susceptibility genes in potato hinders primary infection with *Phytophthora infestans* at different stages. Horticulture Research 9. Available from: https://doi.org/10.1093/hr/uhab058uhab058.

Sy, O., Steiner, R.L., Bosland, P.W., 2008. Recombinant inbred line differential identifies race-specific resistance to phytophthora root rot in *Capsicum annuum* L. Phytopathology 98, 867–870. Available from: https://doi.org/10.1094/PHYTO-98-8-0867.

Takabayashi, N., Tosa, Y., Oh, H.S., Mayama, S., 2002. A gene-for-gene relationship underlying the species-specific parasitism of avena/triticum isolates of *Magnaporthe grisea* on wheat cultivars. Phytopathology 92, 1182–1188. Available from: https://doi.org/10.1094/PHYTO.2002.92.11.1182.

Thomma, B.P.H.J., Nurnberger, T., Joostena, M.H.A.J., 2011. Of PAMPs and effectors: the blurred PTI-ETI dichotomy. The Plant Cell 23, 4–15. Available from: https://doi.org/10.1105/tpc.110.082602.

Thrall, P.H., Burdon, J.J., 2003. Evolution of virulence in a plant host-pathogen metapopulation. Science (New York, N.Y.) 299, 1735–1737. Available from: https://doi.org/10.1126/science.1080070.

Van der Hoorn, R.A.L., Kamoun, S., 2008. From guard to decoy: a new model for perception of plant pathogen effectors. The Plant Cell 20, 2009–2017. Available from: https://doi.org/10.1105/tpc.108.060194.

van Wersch, S., Tian, L., Hoy, R., Li, X., 2020. Plant NLRs: the whistleblowers of plant immunity. Plant Communications 1, 100016. Available from: https://doi.org/10.1016/j.xplc.2019.100016.

Wanderley-Nogueira, A.C., Bezerra-Neto, J.P., Kido, E.A., Tadeu de Araujo, F., Barbosa Amorim, L.L., Crovella, S., et al., 2017. Plant elite squad: first defense line and resistance genes – identification, diversity, and functional roles. Current Protein and Peptide Science 18. Available from: https://doi.org/10.2174/1389203717666160724193045.

Wang, Y., Tan, J., Wu, Z., VandenLangenberg, K., Wehner, T.C., Wen, C., et al., 2019. STAYGREEN, STAY HEALTHY: a loss-of-susceptibility mutation in the STAYGREEN gene provides durable, broad-spectrum disease resistances for over 50 years of U.S. cucumber production. New Phytologist 221, 415–430. Available from: https://doi.org/10.1111/nph.15353.

Williams, S.J., Sohn, K.H., Wan, L., Bernoux, M., Sarris, P.F., Segonzac, C., et al., 2014. Structural basis for assembly and function of a heterodimeric plant immune receptor. Science (New York, N.Y.) 344, 299–303. Available from: https://doi.org/10.1126/science.12473.

Zhang, Y., Lubberstedt, T., Xu, M., 2013. The genetic and molecular basis of plant resistance to pathogens. Genomics 40, 23–35. Available from: https://doi.org/10.1016/j.jgg.2012.11.003.

4

Resistance: the pathogen

Introduction

Pathogens are among the most specialized life forms on Earth. The challenge of colonizing a living host cell comes from the evolutionary specificity that must exist for a pathogen to outmaneuver the host immune system. In plants, most of the microbial attackers are inhibited by nonhost resistance and microbe-associated molecular pattern (MAMP) triggered immunity. Successful pathogens have evolved protein effectors to suppress pattern-triggered immunity (PTI) to infect, colonize, and cause disease. Plants have evolved resistance genes that encode resistance proteins that recognize specific pathogen protein effectors directly or indirectly and induce a rapid and robust immune response, known as effector-triggered immunity (ETI). In response, pathogens diversify the recognized effector gene or evolve new effector genes to diminish the ETI, whereas plants subsequently evolve new resistance proteins to recognize the new effectors and again induce ETI, continuing the endless evolutionary arms race between pathogen and host. One interesting example of this evolutionary arms race is for *Phytophthora parasitica* var. *nicotianae* in tobacco (*Nicotiana tabacum*). When Melinda J. Sullivan and her colleagues at the US Department of Agriculture in North Carolina, USA, planted cultivars that were completely resistant to race 0 in the field, a rapid shift in the population structure to race 1 was observed. Conversely, the use of partially resistant cultivars to both races resulted in a decrease in population levels of race 1 relative to race 0.

Pathogens are known to develop and form new biotypes, pathotypes, races, or strains that can cause disease in plants that remain unaffected by the original form of the pathogen. The host range of a pathogen (pathogenicity) is defined by the plant species it can infect and successfully complete its life cycle. Some pathogens rapidly evolve and new pathotypes or strains develop on a season-to-season basis, while others seem to mutate much more slowly with a single race or strain predominating a region for several years. For example, it has been found that in potatoes (*Solanum tuberosum*), one genotype of *Phytophthora infestans*, US-1, was likely the predominant strain causing late blight disease across the world and was persistent in North America for most of the 20th century.

As plant breeders, we typically consider our breeding strategy from the perspective of the host. However, it is becoming increasingly important to also consider the genome and genes of the pathogen in developing resistant cultivars. With this in mind, a novel approach to develop host resistance in plants has been established called effectoromics. This involves the identification of effectors that are highly expressed during infection, based on the genome sequence of the pathogen. This typically requires the identification of effectors from many isolates of the pathogen. The effectors are then cloned in expression vectors and subjected to iterative functional assays on host leaves, often through agroinfiltration. The leaves are then scored for the presence or absence of local hypersensitive response (HR), to determine resistance in the host. This approach is used to identify both isolate-specific and broad-spectrum resistance genes in the host through quantitative trait loci (QTLs) mapping or genome-wide association studies (GWAS). Juan Du and Vivianne G.a.a. Vleeshouwers at Wageningen University and Research, the Netherlands, state that effectoromics can assist in detecting resistance (R)-genes in plant germplasm. They list four advantages of effectoromics: (1) accelerating R-gene identification; (2) distinguishing functional redundancy; (3) detecting recognition specificity, and (4) assisting in R-gene deployment. To date, there have been limited reports using effectoromics in horticultural crops, with a few successful examples in the identification resistance genes to *P. infestans* in tobacco (*N. tabacum*) and *Phytophthora capsici* in potato (*S. tuberosum*).

In this chapter, the importance of understanding the pathogen and the benefits of having a strong understanding of the pathosystem when breeding for host resistance is discussed.

Pathogen acquisition and maintenance

For the plant breeder having isolates that are representative of the pathogen is most important to identify sources of resistance and for routine screening of segregating breeding populations. However, the selection of the most appropriate isolate for disease screening is complex. Often plant breeders will utilize the most virulent strain of a pathogen available to conduct their screening. Other plant breeders will select the most common strain of the pathogen in their target region. Both approaches have merit, but it is important to consider the implications of each option. Host resistance to a rare but highly virulent strain may not be useful if the race-specific resistance genes do not confer resistance to less virulent strains as well that are more common in each region.

The need to focus on the most appropriate strain or race becomes increasingly important when linkage drag is associated with host resistance. For example, the *FoI3* locus that confers resistance to fusarium wilt race 3 (*Fusarium oxysporum* f. sp. *lycopersici*) but is also associated with reduced fruit size and increased sensitivity to bacterial spot in tomato (*Solanum lycopersicum*). However, if race 3 is highly virulent but not that common in one's region, it may not be necessary to work with this resistance gene, reducing the need to break the linkages associated with the gene *FoI3*. Breeding for resistance to the most common race or isolate in a target region has additional challenges, as pathogen populations are constantly evolving, and new strains can also be introduced. The introduction of a new isolate or race to a region can result in devastating crop loss if the host resistance present in the population cannot recognize the new pathogen effectors, as described above.

Host differential

The plant breeder must be aware that the race of the pathogen is likely to change. Therefore, regular race surveys need to be accomplished on a known set of hosts, known as a host differential, which varies for resistance genes/alleles. This is important because the virulence analyses can detect new novel virulence. One of the most severe diseases of rose (*Rosa x hybrida*) in the outdoor landscape is black spot disease (*Diplocarpon rosae*). There are numerous races of the disease, and resistance is race-specific; however, race characterization was done in several countries each with different independent host differentials. Vance Whitaker at the University of Florida and colleagues developed a universal set of host differentials consisting of nine rose (*Rosa x hybrida*) cultivars that unified the nomenclature for the international collection of *D. rosae* races. This type of foundational research is critical for breeding host resistance because it effectively monitors pathogen populations and identifies new virulent races that can overcome host resistance.

Another important host differential is the New Mexico Recombinant Inbred Lines (NMRIL) that identifies races of

Phytophthora capsici. The NMRIL consists of 26 specific RILs that were generated from the hybridization of the highly resistant *Capsicum annuum* accession Criollo de Morelos-334 and a susceptible cultivar, Early Jalapeno. The establishment of the NMRIL has enabled researchers worldwide indentify the race of their *P. capsici* isolate.

When a new virulence is found, the plant breeder can begin to introduce resistance for it, such as "preemptive breeding or anticipatory breeding" approaches. As the name implies, anticipatory breeding is the method where the breeders develop host resistance for pathogen races that are anticipated to become widespread and cause major losses in the future. Anticipatory breeding is discussed in more detail in Chapter 11. Anticipatory breeding was established in wheat (*Triticum aestivum*) for rust (*Puccinia triticina*) disease by Robert McIntosh and Graham Brown in Australia; however, systems have been developed to apply anticipatory breeding in the horticultural crops of sunflower (*Helianthus annuus*) against rust (*Puccinia helianthin*), and in chile pepper (*Capsicum annuum*) against phytophthora blight (*P. capsici*).

In addition to the utilization of host differentials, pathogens are often characterized based on their genome sequences, allowing a better understanding of the diversity of the pathogen populations and phylogeny locally and globally. This type of study can also lead to the identification of effector genes that contribute to the increased virulence levels. The identification of effectors in the pathogen can also allow for the identification of the effector targets in the host, making breeding efforts more effective.

Culture collections

Currently, the most extensive living culture collection is the American Type Culture Collection (ATCC). In addition, it is a global bioresource center that holds plant pathology–related resources in a variety of categories including fungi, bacteria, and viruses. The bacterial collection contains 18,000 strains from 750 genera. The fungal collection contains 27,000 strains, while the virus collection has more than 1000 isolates. They also have antisera of plant viruses and a small collection of phytoplasma specimens. The ATCC has affiliates around the world and is supported by user fees as well as by grants from the National Science Foundation (NSF). CABI manages a collection of more than 30,000 living strains from 142 nations (90% unique to CABI). It is one of the world's largest Genetic Resource collections and holds the UK's National Collection of Fungus Cultures.

The Westerdijk Institute maintains the Centraalbureau voor Schimmelcultures (CBS) collection of yeasts and filamentous fungi that was established as a public collection in 1904 and at present holds a very broad coverage of culturable filamentous fungi, yeasts, and oomycetes. The CBS collection comprises a total of 100,000 strains, representing 5100 genera, 19,600 species, and 12,600 type strains. The institute also maintains the Netherlands Culture Collection of Bacteria (NCCB), including 10,000 strains of wild-type bacteria and *Escherichia coli* mutants, actinobacteria (accessioned under the CBS acronym), and more than 500 plasmids and phages. Scientific and other data associated with these strains (including DNA barcode sequences of most of the CBS and NCCB strains) are maintained in databases and the information of publicly available strains are visible online. CBS collection of yeasts and filamentous fungi, which was established as a public collection in 1904 and at present holds a very broad coverage of culturable filamentous fungi, yeasts, and oomycetes. Globally, the culture collection community is represented by the World Federation of Culture Collections (WFCC). The WFCC website has become a clearing house for information on resources around the world. The WFCC operates under the umbrella of the International Union of Biologic Sciences.

Specialized and working collections

The plant breeder needs to familiarize themselves with Specialized Collections and Working Collections. Specialized collections are those that focus on one pathogen, for example, the World *Phytophthora* Genetic Resource Collection (WPC) at the University of California—Riverside, USA, contains about 8000 isolates of more than 140 species collected from multiple hosts or aquatic environments and from worldwide locations. The Herbarium at the University of Reunion Island in collaboration with the French Agency for Food, Environmental and Occupational Health and Safety (ANSES), and the French Agricultural Research Centre for International Development (CIRAD) maintain a collection of more than 6000 plant-infecting bacterial strains of the genera *Ralstonia* and *Xanthomonas*. The specialized collections are useful because they serve as a repository of historical isolates from a wide geographic area. However, they differ from a working collection in several ways.

A working collection is normally a collection maintained by an individual or institution and is used primarily for inoculating hosts. The working collection is an excellent source of virulent pathogens and for strains from specific regions. The working collection should be a dynamic collection that will change over time in response to the pathogen population but should also maintain long term a few relevant strains to serve as checks. For example, a working collection might consist of a few strains of a pathogen that were recently collected from grower fields in the target area, but also have a highly virulent strain that was collected several years ago. It is known that pathogen populations are constantly evolving, but also tend to move towards higher levels of virulence. It is often necessary for the plant breeder to work with plant pathologists to isolate and characterize pathogens to conduct screenings. Despite how large the specialized collections are, it is impossible for them to have every isolate. Furthermore, as has been already established the pathogens are constantly evolving to overcome host resistance and these repositories of pathogen diversity cannot keep up with production-guided pathogen evolution-highlighting the importance of working collections maintained at the intuitional or laboratory level.

Pathogenicity/virulence

Pathogenicity is the ability of a pathogen to cause disease in the host organism. Pathogenicity is a qualitative measurement, either the organism can cause disease or not. The disease is the relationship between the virulence of the pathogen and the resistance of the host, in addition to the growing environment and length of exposure. The pathogen has various cellular structures, molecules, and regulatory systems that contribute to the disease, which are termed virulence factors. Virulence factors are involved in the colonization of host cells, evasion of host immune response, inhibition of the host immune system, intercellular movement, and nutrient uptake from the host. Some pathogens have a wide range of virulence factors with various functions. Virulence factors encoded on mobile genetic elements can spread through horizontal gene transfer and can cause virulence to develop in previously nonpathogenic organisms. There are two general categories of virulence factors, those that are used to assist in and promote host cell colonization and those that are involved in damaging the host cell.

For plant breeders, virulence is the most important trait of a pathogen. The evolution and change in virulence are what determine if the pathogen will overcome the host resistance. James E. Vanderplank proposed that virulence described the capacity of a pathogen to infect a particular host genotype, while aggressiveness is the quantitative negative effect of a pathogen on its host, which in evolutionary biology is normally termed infectivity. The American Phytopathological Society adopted the convention of defining pathogenicity as the ability of a pathogen to cause disease on a particular host (i.e., a qualitative property), and virulence as the degree of damage caused to the host (i.e., a quantitative property), assumed to be negatively correlated with host fitness. From the plant breeding perspective, virulence is the pathogen genotype that can overcome a resistance factor. A pathogen would need to overcome nonhost resistance to be pathogenic to a new host, which is rare but does happen. More often a pathogen will become increasingly aggressive, or more virulent, to an existing host.

The relationship between parasite fitness and virulence is complicated and is still being explored. Most plant pathogens do not cause an immediate increase in mortality of the host. Normally, virulence is estimated as the effect of pathogen infection on plant seed production or on one of its correlates, such as plant size or biomass. Pathogen fitness is usually measured as fecundity, which has two important components: within host multiplication and between host transmission. Within host multiplication, for example, it can be spore production per leaf area or viral accumulation in infected tissues. Within host multiplication, it is positively correlated with between host transmission, which is immediate for spore-producing microbes. For vector-transmitted plant viruses, it has been shown that transmission efficiency is positively correlated with virus accumulation in source tissues.

Genetic variation of pathogens

Plant breeders take for granted that new genetic variation can be created in plants. It is just as important to realize that pathogens can produce new variations within their populations. They have evolved several processes to generate new genetic variation, including spontaneous mutation, sexual recombination, somatic hybridization, and horizontal gene transfer, among others. It is also important to remember the selection pressure that can be imposed upon pathogens by the activities of the plant breeder. In agricultural plant populations that are typically dominated by a limited number of cultivars, the presence of one or a few specific resistance (*R*) genes exerts strong selective pressure on pathogens to lose their corresponding avirulence (*Avr*) genes and regain virulence by the expression of other effectors. For instance, the fungus *F. oxysporum* f. sp. *cubensis* causes Panama disease of banana (*Musa acuminata*). Panama disease threatens a large part of the world's banana (*M. acuminata*) crop due to a single virulence gene that facilitates infection of the banana (*M. acuminata*) cultivar clone Cavendish, which is the most widely grown commercial banana (*M. acuminata*) cultivar worldwide.

The *avrBs2* gene of *Xanthomonas campestris* that causes bacterial spot controls induction of the HR in pepper (*C. annuum*) containing the *Bs2* resistance gene. The *Bs2* encodes a resistance protein of the nucleotide binding site—leucine-rich repeat (NBS-LRR) class and has been widely deployed in the field, providing a high level of resistance for many years. However, mutations in *avrBs2* have resulted not only in loss of avirulence to pepper (*C. annuum*) with *Bs2*, but also in reduced virulence, as reflected by a reduced growth rate in susceptible pepper (*C. annuum*) plants. Genes with homology to *avrBs2* are present in several other *Xanthomonas* species, and in some cases, these genes also confer a fitness function. These examples highlight the careful consideration that must be made by plant breeders in developing resistant cultivars. In the following sections, we will discuss the different mechanisms of genetic variation that can occur among different plant pathogens.

Genetic variation of viroids and viruses

Viroids and viruses are smaller and simpler in construction than unicellular microorganisms, such as bacteria. They contain only one type of nucleic acid—either DNA or RNA—never both. Viroids differ from the virus in structure and form in that they consist of solely short strands of circular, and single-stranded RNA without the protein coats. Viroids range from 246 to 401 nucleotides in length and are known as the smallest plant pathogens. They do not encode any proteins in their genome sequences; hence, they autonomously replicate depending on host plants' transcriptional machinery Horticultural crops infected by viroids include potato (*S. tuberosum*), tomato (*S. lycopersicum*), cucumber (*Cucumis sativus*), chrysanthemum (*Chrysanthemum indicum*), coconut palm (*Cocos nucifera*), avocado (*Persea americana*), and many more.

In 1971 Theodor O. Diener, a US Department of Agriculture plant pathologist, first discovered viroids, when he examined the Potato spindle tuber disease (PSTVd), a type species of the genus *Pospiviroid* that was causing huge losses to the potato (*S. tuberosum*) industry. Potato spindle tuber viroid has a wide host range and generally infects Solanaceae and Asteraceae plants. Cultivated tomatoes (*S. lycopersicum*) are one of the most prominent host plants and the Potato spindle tuber disease isolates are classified into four strains (mild, intermediate, severe, and lethal) depending on their virulence as indicated by the degree of disease symptoms on the cultivar, Rutgers tomato (*S. lycopersicum*). This difference in virulence on the same host indicates that the Potato spindle tuber disease genome sequence itself is one of the virulence determinants. For example, mutations of three or four nucleotides transformed the intermediate Potato spindle tuber disease isolate into lethal isolates.

As viruses and viroids have no ribosomes, mitochondria, or other organelles, they are completely dependent on their cellular hosts for energy production and protein synthesis. They replicate only within cells of the host that they infect. In simpler viruses, the virion consists of a single molecule of nucleic acid surrounded by a protein coat, the capsid; the capsid and its enclosed nucleic acid together constitute the nucleocapsid. Resistance based on denying the virus access to the host's DNA is a common form of resistance.

The different and unique host phenotypes produced by virus infection are one of the most important ways to access the variation of a virus and are the most important to the plant breeder. Viral-infected phenotypes range from mild to severe symptoms and vary depending on the host. Plants can be "infected" with virus and produce no symptoms, known as a latent virus. Wild plants and cultivated crops are often infected with latent viruses showing no symptoms. Although seemingly harmless at least to the host, these latent viruses pose a threat to horticultural crops because they can be transmitted by vectors and cause disease in the cultivated horticultural crop.

Recently in New Zealand, it is reported that carnations (*Dianthus caryophyllus*) had virus symptoms including leaf chlorotic spots and distortion. Further analysis with artificially inoculated host differential and direct sequencing revealed the presence of Grapevine Algerian latent virus (GALV, *Tombusvirus*). Grapevine Algerian latent virus was first reported in Italy from a symptomless Algerian grapevine (*Vitis vinifera*). Since that report Grapevine Algerian latent virus has spread and is causing disease in *Alstroemeria* species, *Gypsophila paniculata*, *Limonium sinuatum*, and *Solanum mammosum*. The infected ornamental host plants showed various types of foliar virus symptoms. This illustrates how a latent virus can appear innocuous in one crop but be a serious disease in other crops.

Plant virologists are not consistent with terminology, for example, isolate, variant, biotype, mutant, or strain are concepts that have been used with different meanings. An isolate, based on the most common usage in plant pathology, is the pure culture of a virus derived from an infected host plant. Isolates of the same virus that differ in some properties are called variants. Strains are sets of isolates that share some properties, such as host range, transmission, serology, or nucleotide sequence similarity, that clearly differentiate them from other isolates. The term strain is also used for the isolate that typifies the strain, a practice that can lead to confusion. Variants are called mutants if it is known that they derive from a particular isolate, and, ideally, which mutational event resulted in their generation. Differences among mutants will be smaller than among strains, which in fact arise by genetic divergence through the accumulation of mutations with time. The specific genetic constitution of a virus is its genotype. For haploid organisms, haplotype has the same meaning as genotype. Thus in a heterogeneous virus population, different variants can occur with different genotypes or haplotypes.

As early as 1926 evidence for genetic variation of plant viruses was reported. These variants were first obtained by isolation of symptom mutants from areas that showed atypical symptoms in systemically infected plants. It was also observed that serial passaging under different conditions could alter viral properties. Most often these experiments involved a host shift so that a virus adapted to a particular host was selected for passage into a different one. The resulting change in virus traits is called host adaptation.

Genetic variation is generated by errors occurring during the replication of genomes. For viruses, the two main types of errors so far described are mutation and recombination.

Recombination is the process by which segments of genetic information are switched between the nucleotide strands of different genetic variants during the process of replication. Thus recombination results in genetic exchange. Sequence analyses of populations of various RNA and DNA plant viruses provide evidence that recombination may be a major source of variation.

Genetic exchange can also result from the reassortment of genomic segments in viruses with a segmented genome, a process called pseudo-recombination by plant virologists. There is evidence that reassortment occurs in natural populations of plant viruses and may play an important role in virus evolution. Acquisition of new nucleic acid molecules may change the virus pathogenicity and be another source of genetic variation. This may result from associations between viruses, and between viruses and DNA satellites, which are common in plant viruses.

The distribution in the virus population of the genetic variants generated by mutation or genetic exchange will depend on two major evolutionary processes: genetic drift and selection. In Vietnam, Turnip mosaic virus (TuMV; *Potyvirus*), which infects a wide range of plant species in the Brassicaceae family, was collected and analyzed for genetic variation. The 30 isolates collected were screened, and based on host reaction, many of the isolates belonged to *Brassica/Raphanus* (BR) host-infecting type. Using sequence-based phylogenetic and population genetic analyses made from the complete polyprotein gene sequences and of four nonrecombinogenic regions of those sequences (i.e., genes of the helper-component proteinase protein, protein 3, nuclear inclusion b protein, and coat protein), it has been found that the virus had nine inter- and intralineage recombination type patterns, of which seven were novel. All the Vietnamese nonrecombinant isolates fell into the world-B group of TuMV and clustered with Chinese isolates. The estimates of genetic differentiation and gene flow revealed that the TuMV populations of Vietnam, China, and Japan are genetically linked but have clear local founder effects. This type of information helps the plant breeder select the resistance that is best suited for the region where the crop is grown.

Genetic variation of bacteria

As with viruses, mutation is the basic process by which new variation is created in bacteria. A mutation is heritable and passed on to the progeny of the variant cell to produce a subclone with characteristics different from the original parent, which is termed vertical inheritance. The large sizes of bacterial populations ensure that extremely rare genetic events are likely to occur. This genetic variation makes it possible for individual members of huge populations of bacteria to quickly evolve new traits, for example, new virulence factors.

Most bacterial cells contain a single circular chromosome. Because there is only one chromosome, each gene (with the occasional exception) is present in only one copy, and thus, bacteria are haploid. One important consequence of having a haploid genome is that genetic changes have an immediate effect on the phenotype or properties of the bacterial cell. In nature, these properties mean that evolution is rapid.

Other spontaneous events have greater consequences for the structure of the chromosome. Some bacterial mutants have large insertions, deletions, or inversions in the chromosomal DNA. One of these types of mutations is transposable genetic elements known as Insertion Sequences or IS elements. Scattered throughout the chromosome are active sequences of DNA with the remarkable ability to move into other regions of the chromosome. Transposition is spontaneous and occurs at a frequency comparable to that of point mutations. Most insertion sequences have extremely low target specificity and insert virtually anywhere in the genome. After insertion of the transposable element into a new location, depending on the element, a copy may be left behind in the original position (replicative transposition), or the original copy may be excised and transposed to the new location (conservative transposition). Insertion of an element into a gene can cause that gene to lose function and can have drastic consequences for the expression of other genes in the same transcriptional unit. These rearrangements can provide the raw material for new genes. The spontaneous and random formation of transposable genes and their subsequent insertion into plasmids or bacteriophages generate the potential for rapid dissemination of these genes to other bacteria.

Researchers at Viçosa Federal University, Brazil examined the extensive genetic diversity of *Ralstonia solanacearum*, the causal agent of vascular wilt disease. *R. solanacearum* is one of the most devastating plant pathogenic bacteria found worldwide. This soilborne pathogen is composed of a large-scale group of strains varying in geographical distribution and pathogenic behavior, known as the *R. solanacearum* species complex (RSSC). The genome of *R. solanacearum* is organized into two circular replicons, a chromosome and a megaplasmid. In investigating the repertoire of insertion sequences, an abundant amount of transposable elements diversity was found. Insertion sequences play an important role in the genome evolution of this pathogen. After analyzing 106 *R. solanacearum* and 15 *Ralstonia* species, they found 10,259 insertion sequences. A unique set of 20 insertion sequence families was widespread across the strains. In addition, internal rearrangement events associated with insertion sequences were found in *Ralstonia pseudosolanacearum* strains. They also found insertion sequence elements interrupting avirulence genes, providing evidence that insertion sequences play an important role in the virulence evolution of *R. solanacearum*. An aside note is that although the wilt disease caused by *R. solanacearum* is not managed with antibiotics, their results showed the acquisition of antibiotic resistance in this phytopathogen. Antibiotic-resistance genes are transferred by mobile elements that can potentially be acquired by other bacteria in the environment via horizontal gene transfer. The researchers demonstrated the potential impact of these elements on *Ralstonia* host range. In this study, many avirulence (*avr*) genes interrupted by insertion sequences were found. Therefore the inactivation of avirulence (*avr*) genes in this bacterium can lead to virulence in a resistant host plant. Similarly, insertion sequences have been found to interrupt avirulence (*avr*) genes in *Pseudomonas syringae*.

Bacterial variation can also occur by the horizontal transfer of genetic material from one cell to another. Horizontal gene transfer is nonsexual movement of genetic information between genomes. In many instances, genes acquired by horizontal gene transfer have clear functional or ecological implications for their new host. Genes responsible for antibiotic resistance in one species of bacteria can be transferred to another species of bacteria, resulting in the antibiotic-resistant genes' recipient against antibiotics. Effector and *Avr* genes have also been found to be transferred horizontally, and once acquired through horizontal gene transfer, they become fixed in the bacterial genome because they confer a selective advantage in terms of pathogenicity and can result in significant changes in the race structure of the pathogen.

At the University of Florida, researchers compared the bacterial pathogens, *Xanthomonas citri* pv. *citri* and *X. citri* pv. *aurantifolii* that cause citrus canker disease. These two phylogenetically distinct clonal groups of *X. citri* cause identical disease symptoms in susceptible citrus. *X. citri* pv. *citri* appears to have originated in Asia and is now present in more than 30 countries. *X. citri* pv. *aurantifolii* arose more recently in South America and causes economic losses in Brazil and Argentina. To investigate how these two phylogenetically distinct groups cause identical symptoms in susceptible citrus (*Citrus* species), the role of pathogenicity gene *pthA* homologs was investigated. Both pathovars elicit canker symptoms and encode a citrus-specific effector protein. They found that *X. citri* pv. *aurantifolii* strains carry two DNA fragments that hybridize to the pathogenicity gene, *pthA*. They concluded that the pathogenicity gene at some point was transferred from one pathovar to the other, illustrating that a single pathogenicity effector can confer a distinct selective advantage in the pathogen following horizontal gene transfer and account for the origination of phylogenetically distinct groups of strains causing identical disease symptoms.

Transformation, transduction, and conjugation

There are three other mechanisms for bacteria to transfer a trait from one cell to another, transformation, transduction, and conjugation. The new genetic information can be transferred from one cell to another; however, this is not a true exchange, because only one partner receives the new information. For all three processes, the transferred DNA must be incorporated into the genetic material of the recipient bacterium. This can occur in two ways: (1) recombination, or integration of the transferred DNA into the bacterial chromosome; or (2) establishment of a plasmid, that is, the transferred material essentially forms a minichromosome capable of autonomous replication. There are several mechanisms by which this takes place.

In transformation, the bacteria uptake naked DNA molecules (not associated with proteins, lipids, or any other molecule to help protect it) and maintain them in their cell. To take up the DNA efficiently, bacterial cells must be in a "competent state" that is defined by the capability of bacteria to bind free fragments of DNA and is formed naturally only in a limited number of bacteria. Plant bacteria causing the disease in horticultural crops belonging to species of *Pseudomonas*, *Ralstonia*, and *Xylella* have been found to be naturally transformable. These bacteria have developed highly specialized functions that will bind DNA fragments and transport them into the cell. In nature, the DNA to be taken up is thought to be released into the environment by the lysis of bacterial cells. Transformation is the least efficient mechanism of gene transfer because naked DNA is sensitive to nucleases in the environment.

Xanthomonas bacteria are responsible for substantial yield losses worldwide and infect many horticultural crops including *Citrus* species, tomato (*S. lycopersicum*), pepper (*C. annuum*), and cabbage (*Brassica oleracea* var. *capitata*). The bacteria inject transcription-activator-like effector (TALE) proteins into plant host cells to promote disease. In the plant cell nucleus, these transcription-activator-like effector proteins bind to matching DNA sequences, termed effector binding elements (EBEs), and transcriptionally activate downstream host target genes that are termed susceptibility (S) genes if their expression promotes disease. The transcription-activator-like effector-mediated activation of host target genes requires matching effector binding elements as well as accessible host helper proteins like the general transcription factor TFIIA.

During the plant and pathogen coevolution, plants evolved sequence variation in effector binding elements upstream of the susceptibility (S) gene coding sequences, as well as variations within genes encoding transcription-activator-like effector–helper proteins, that both can inhibit exploitation by transcription-activator-like effector proteins and that genetically are defined as recessively inherited plant resistance (r) genes. In addition, plants have evolved a unique type of dominantly inherited, transcriptionally controlled resistance R-gene. Members of this resistance gene type are composed of a promoter-embedded effector binding element and a downstream-encoded executor resistance protein that upon translation triggers resistance. Pepper (C. annuum) has evolved so-called executor resistance (R) genes, which upon transcriptional activation by transcription-activator-like effectors lead to immediate cell death and restrict bacterial growth. Bacterial spot 3 (Bs3), an executor resistance gene from pepper (C. annuum), causes cell death upon transcriptional activation by the corresponding transcription-activator-like effector from *Xanthomonas euvesicatoria*, that is, the avirulence gene, AvrBs3.

A simple correlation, known as the transcription-activator-like effector code, was discovered between certain transcription-activator-like effector residues and corresponding EBEs. Transcription-activator-like effector code–assisted effector binding elements prediction in combination with transcriptome profiling has become a robust method for the identification of transcription-activator-like effector host target genes, already leading to the molecular isolation of several transcription-activator-like effector-specific susceptible and resistance genes. The susceptible and resistance proteins have a high level of sequence diversity, suggesting that transcription-activator-like effectors interfere with a variety of distinct cellular functions to promote disease or to trigger defense. Knowledge of transcription-activator-like effector biology and recently CRISPR approaches for precision genome editing enables horticultural crops to be breed resistant to pathogens delivering transcription-activator-like effectors or transcription-activator-like effector-like proteins.

Transduction is the transfer of DNA from one bacterium to another by means of a bacteria-infecting virus called a bacteriophage. Bacteriophages represent a phenomenally successful strategy for survival in nature. They are ubiquitous—probably all bacteria have phages that can infect and replicate within them. They can mediate the efficient transfer of genes between bacteria, including genes for virulence. Some bacteriophages can convert harmless bacteria into pathogens. On the other hand, bacteriophages have received increased research interest as a realistic environmentally friendly means of controlling bacterial diseases. Their use presents a viable control measure for several destructive bacterial crop diseases, with some phage-based products already becoming available on the market.

Many varieties of bacteriophages have been identified. The nucleic acid can be DNA or RNA, double-stranded or single-stranded, circular, or linear. The genomes may be small, encoding as few as five or six genes, or large enough to encode more than 200 genes. The complexity of the genome is usually reflected in the protein coat of the virus particle. All bacteriophages have the same basic life cycle, which is known as the lytic cycle. They infect the bacterial cell, subvert the cell's machinery to replicate themselves, then lyse the cell to release hundreds of new bacteriophage particles into the environment. If other sensitive bacteria are nearby and they happen to encounter a newly released particle, the lytic cycle will repeat. Transduction is an efficient means of transferring DNA between bacteria because DNA enclosed in the bacteriophage is protected from physical decay and from attack by enzymes in the environment and is injected directly into cells by the bacteriophage. However, widespread gene transfer by means of transduction is of limited significance because the packaging of bacterial DNA into a virus is inefficient and the bacteriophages are usually highly restricted in the range of bacterial species that they can infect. Thus interspecies transfer of DNA by transduction is rare.

Conjugation is the transfer of DNA by direct cell-to-cell contact that is mediated by plasmids (nonchromosomal DNA molecules). Conjugative plasmids encode an extremely efficient mechanism that mediates their own transfer from a donor cell to a recipient cell. Plasmids are small, double-stranded DNA molecules that are maintained in the cell in addition to the bacterial chromosome. Usually, they are circular, but some linear plasmids also exist. These extrachromosomal elements are ubiquitous in the bacterial world. The process takes place in one direction because only the donor cells contain the conjugative plasmid. In gram-negative bacteria, donor cells produce a specific plasmid-coded pilus, called the sex pilus, which attaches the donor cell to the recipient cell. Once connected, the two cells are brought into direct contact, and a conjugal bridge forms through which the DNA is transferred from the donor to the recipient. Many conjugative plasmids can be transferred between, and reproduce in, many different gram-negative bacterial species. Plasmids vary in size, from a few thousand to more than 100,000 base pairs; the latter are sometimes called mega-plasmids. The bacterial chromosome can also be transferred during conjugation, although this happens less frequently than plasmid transfer. Conjugation allows the inheritance of substantial portions of genes and may be responsible for the existence of bacteria with traits of several different species. All known plasmids are not necessary for the basic growth and division of the bacterial cell. Nevertheless, they are extremely valuable to the success of the bacteria in nature because they are known to encode a wide variety of genes that confer a competitive advantage in certain environments. For example, plasmids have been found to encode metabolic pathways that allow a cell to use exotic compounds like the herbicide 2,4-D (2,4-dichlorophenoxyacetic acid) as a carbon source and resistance to nearly all known antibiotics. Plasmids also encode pathogenicity factors. The reason for the plasmid's success in nature is the ability to promote efficient transfer between bacteria by conjugation. This feature has important ramifications with respect to the development, spread, and control of plant disease-producing bacteria.

The use of antibiotics to control bacterial diseases in plants has limited use, and unfortunately, the efficacy of any antibiotic is undermined by the development of bacterial strains that are resistant to it. Plasmids are responsible for the rapid dissemination of antibiotic resistance to a wide variety of bacteria. It has been documented that plasmid can encode resistance to tetracycline, streptomycin, sulfonamides, chloramphenicol, kanamycin, spectinomycin, trimethoprim, gentamicin, and ampicillin.

Genetic variation of oomycetes

Like fungi, oomycetes are a distinct lineage of eukaryotic microorganisms that can reproduce both sexually and asexually. Asexual reproduction results in the production of deciduous sporangia that can release motile zoospores. The zoospores of plant pathogenic oomycetes move within the field when soil moisture is high and can be a source of widespread dispersal. When different mating types are in proximity, oomycetes can also reproduce sexually to produce thick-walled oospores capable of surviving winter or fallow periods. Sexual reproduction results in genetic recombination and the potential development of new or additional virulence factors to overcome host resistance. In 1961 Eva Sansome at the University College of Ghana provided evidence that oomycetes can also be polyploids. Since then, evidence of polyploidy in oomycetes has increased. Notably, it has been found that sexual, asexual, and polyploidy all contribute to genetic variation within the important plant pathogenic genus *Phytophthora*. In *P. infestans*, *P. capsici*, and *P. colocasiae*, there is evidence that polyploidization may contribute to adaptation, particularly where the populations are predominantly clonal. In populations that reproduce sexually, the isolates are often diploid, although there can be shifts from diploid to polyploid, and back to diploid, depending on when in the life cycle the karyotyping or sequencing was done. Intra- and intergenomic variations in ploidy in some isolates being diploid, triploid, tetraploid, and higher levels of ploidy have been reported. It has also been found that in some predominant diploid populations with higher rates of sexual reproduction, the virulence can be higher, and more resistance genes are overcome. In clonal populations where polyploidy is more common, the virulence is lower, and resistance is less likely to be overcome although it is hypothesized that polyploidy may be a strategy for the pathogen to develop new virulence factors when genetic recombination via sexual reproduction is possible.

Genetic variation of fungus

Fungi have ancient origins, with evidence indicating they first appeared about 1 billion years ago. Fungal hyphae being evident within the tissues of the oldest plant fossils suggests that they are an extremely ancient plant pathogen. As with viruses and bacteria, plant pathogenic fungi can evolve new virulence factors to overcome disease resistance genes. Fungi have evolved several mechanisms to assist in generating this new genetic diversity. As with the other pathogens discussed, mutation provides the fundamental basis underlying most of the observed variation in the fungi. Mutations affect traits such as host range, virulence, fitness, tolerance to chemicals, and blocks in sexual or asexual reproduction. Mutation provides for an extension of host range or virulence, increased fitness, and factors encouraging outcrossing. Mutation can also have a deleterious effect; for example, *Verticillium dahliae* forms microsclerotium that allows for long-term survival in soils, but then it can mutate to types that produce no microsclerotium. Mutations in single effector genes of the pathogens enable them to avoid recognition by the host plant. When one considers the explosive reproductive potential of fungi through spore production, it would seem reasonable that mutation could provide adequate variation to allow for the adaptation and survival of advantageous genotypes.

Fungi can reproduce both sexually and asexually. Even though both types of spores are produced by the same mycelium, they are very different. The asexual phase usually precedes the sexual phase in the life cycle and may be repeated frequently before the sexual phase appears. Some fungi may lack one or the other of the reproductive stages. Several fungi exhibit the phenomenon of parasexuality, in which processes comparable to sexual recombination, plasmogamy, karyogamy, and meiosis, take place.

Parasexual cycle

The parasexual cycle is a process peculiar to fungi and single-celled organisms. It is a nonsexual mechanism for transferring genetic material without meiosis or the development of sexual structures and, was first described by Italian geneticist Guido Pontecorvo in 1956. A parasexual cycle is initiated by the fusion of hyphae (anastomosis) during which nuclei and other cytoplasmic components occupy the same cell (heterokaryosis and plasmogamy). Fusion of the unlike nuclei in the cell of the heterokaryon results in the formation of a diploid nucleus (karyogamy) that is unstable and can produce segregants by recombination involving mitotic crossing-over and haploidization. Mitotic crossing-over can lead to the exchange of genes on chromosomes. Like a sexual cycle, parasexuality gives the species the opportunity to recombine the genome and produce new genotypes in their offspring. Both heterokaryosis and the parasexual cycle are very important for those fungi that have no sexual reproduction. This is a mechanism the plant pathogens, *Fusarium* and *Verticillium*, use to create new genetic variations. J.E. Puhalla with the US Dept. of Agriculture demonstrated that heterokaryons occurred between compatibility strains from wide geographic regions. The designation of genetically related populations within *V. dahliae* permitted a process to determine the origin of new pathotypes or the spread of known pathotypes. For example, two tomato (*S. lycopersicum*) isolates had different virulence reactions on tomatoes (*S. lycopersicum*) with *Verticillium* resistance, and both were in the same population. Because the two isolates can form heterokaryons with each other, a parasexual cycle could occur making the avirulent isolate virulent on tomato (*S. lycopersicum*).

This horizontal gene transfer and horizontal chromosome transfer provide a way for pathogens to broaden their host range. The literature cites hybridization between plant pathogenic fungi that affected their host range, including species of *Stagonospora/Pyrenophora*, *Fusarium*, and *Alternaria*. Li-Jun Ma, at the University of Massachusetts, USA, demonstrated that horizontal chromosome transfer between a pathogenic *F. oxysporum* f.sp. *lycopersici* and a nonpathogenic species occurred, enabling the latter one to become pathogenic. Horizontal chromosome transfer provides a powerful mechanism of genetic exchange between fungi, enabling them to become pathogenic on new host plants. Similarly, *Alternaria* species can broaden their host range by horizontal chromosome transfer of a single chromosome carrying a cluster of genes encoding host-specific toxins that enabled them to become pathogenic on new hosts such as apple (*Malus domestica*), Japanese pear (*Pyrus pyrifolia*), strawberry (*Fragaria × ananassa*), and tomato (*S. lycopersicum*).

Sexual reproduction

Sexual reproduction in fungi is an important source of genetic variability, allowing fungi to adapt to new environments and the resistance genes of their host. It is estimated that sexual recombination is 500 times greater in creating variability than mitotic recombination, which is about the same rate as mutation. The process of sexual reproduction among fungi is in many ways unique. Whereas nuclear division in other eukaryotes, such as animals and plants, involves the dissolution and reformation of the nuclear membrane, in fungi the nuclear membrane remains intact throughout the process. Sexual reproduction in fungi consists of three sequential stages: plasmogamy, karyogamy, and meiosis. Plasmogamy, the fusion of two protoplasts brings together two compatible haploid nuclei. At this point, two nuclear types are present in the same cell, but the nuclei have not yet fused. Karyogamy results in the fusion of these haploid nuclei and the formation of a diploid nucleus (i.e., a nucleus containing two sets of chromosomes) one from each parent. The cell formed by karyogamy is called the zygote. In most fungi, the zygote is the only cell in the entire life cycle that is diploid. The dikaryotic state that results from plasmogamy is often a prominent condition in fungi and may be prolonged over several generations. In the lower fungi, karyogamy usually follows plasmogamy almost immediately. Once karyogamy has occurred, meiosis generally follows and restores the haploid phase. Some produce specialized sex cells (gametes) that are released from differentiated sex organs called gametangia. In other fungi, two gametangia come in contact, and nuclei pass from the male gametangium into the female, thus assuming the function of gametes. In still other fungi the gametangia themselves may fuse to bring their nuclei together. Finally, some of the most advanced fungi produce no gametangia at all; the somatic (vegetative) hyphae take over the sexual function, come in contact, fuse, and exchange nuclei.

Sexual incompatibility

Many of the simpler fungi produce differentiated male and female organs on the same thallus but do not undergo self-fertilization because their sex organs are incompatible. Such fungi require the presence of thalli of different mating types for sexual fusion to take place. The simplest form of this mechanism occurs in fungi in which there are two mating types, often designated A_1 and A_2. Gametes produced by one type of thallus are compatible only with gametes produced by the other type. Such fungi are said to be heterothallic. Many fungi, however, are homothallic (i.e., sex organs produced by a single thallus), such as with *Gibberella zeae* that causes Fusarium head blight on maize (*Zea mays*). Compatibility, therefore, refers to a physiological differentiation, and sex refers to a morphological (structural) one; the two phenomena, although related, are not synonymous.

Horizontal chromosome transfer

Several species of filamentous fungi contain so-called dispensable or supernumerary chromosomes. These chromosomes are dispensable for the survival of the fungus but may carry genes required for specialized functions, such as infection of a host plant. It has been shown that some dispensable chromosomes are able to transfer horizontally (i.e., in the absence of a sexual cycle) from one fungal strain to another. There is evidence that accessory chromosomes are present in a "mosaic" pattern between races of *F. oxysporum*.

A landmark discovery by Li-Jun Ma and her colleagues demonstrated that accessory chromosomes could be horizontally transferred between strains of *F. oxysporum*, an important plant pathogen, causing blights, root rots, and wilts. By simply mixing two strains on a standard growth medium, the transfer of two whole chromosomes from *F. oxysporum* f.sp. *lycopersici*, a tomato (*S. lycopersicum*) pathogen, turns a nonpathogenic strain into a pathogenic one. This finding gave insight into a pathogen's evolution of host range and pathogenicity. The exchange of DNA and genetic exchange can occur via horizontal chromosome transfer. This discovery implies that isolates of fungi can produce new host specificities and that *F. oxysporum* can acquire new combinations of accessory chromosomes to evolve new pathogenic genotypes. Peter Henry at the US Department of Agriculture and colleagues from around the world collected 31 isolates of *F. oxysporum* f.sp. *fragariae* obtained from four continents and examined their pathogenicity. *F. oxysporum* f.sp. *fragariae* causes two distinct syndromes, yellows and wilt on strawberries (*Fragaria* × *ananassa*). The yellows syndrome causes greater disease severity, while the wilt syndrome is more widespread. They found that the pathogenicity in Australian and Spanish wilt isolates evolved independently from the yellows isolates. Furthermore, among isolates classified as causing the wilt syndrome, pathogenicity on strawberries (*Fragaria* × *ananassa*) appears to have evolved independently in both Spain and Australia. Their results confirmed that disease phenotyping can facilitate the identification of evolutionarily distinct groups within a forma specialis. Most importantly, this is the first time that the yellows and the wilt syndromes were shown to be caused by independently evolved pathogen genotypes that do not share a pathogenicity chromosome. As host resistance is a critical tool for breeding disease resistance in many Fusarium wilt pathosystems, differentiating among pathogen genotypes that emerged from the transfer of a common pathogenicity chromosome versus a different pathogenicity chromosome has important implications for identifying and deploying host resistance. They revealed that horizontal chromosome transfer promotes the diversification of *F. oxysporum* f.sp. *fragariae*, but pathogenic genotypes can also emerge independently, without receiving the same pathogenicity chromosome. Thus the plant breeder will need to be cognizant of the origin of the pathogenicity/virulence.

Host jump (species jump/new hosts)

Pathogens can transgress host species barriers and emerge as new pathogens and consequent epidemics in a "host jump." Recently, this has been an extremely important topic for human viruses, that is, coronavirus, Ebola, hantavirus, monkeypox, etc. Host jumps are common for plant pathogenic fungi, such as *Puccinia psidii*, that jumped from native Myrtaceae to introduced

Eucalyptus trees in South America. Similarly, *Cronartium ribicola* jumped to new *Pinus* species in Europe and North America and caused an epidemic that is still underway more than a decade after its introduction. *Fusarium circinatum* caused a pitch canker disease epidemic on *Pinus radiata* in California following its introduction into the area from native Mexican pines. Based on current trends, fungi are likely to undergo increasing numbers of plant host jumps due to the increasing spread of fungi worldwide because of human travel as well as global weather changes that negatively affect host plant communities. The connection between host jumps and human introduction gives greater significance to the need for quarantine measures to prevent the accidental movement of fungi into new areas.

An understanding of the importance of the different mechanisms, mutation, asexual recombination, and sexual recombination that contribute to the origin and maintenance of variation in pathogen populations is important to plant breeders. It is necessary to realize that the genomes of plant pathogens are highly variable, dynamic, and elastic. Pathogen gene repertoires can change resulting in a rapid loss of plant resistance. Plants "lose" resistance when plant pathogens change their genetic constitution under resistance selection. Thus the rapid evolution of pathogens is a serious threat to agriculture, and plant breeders must be vigilant to the adaptation of plant pathogens to resistant host plants.

Bibliography

Amil-Ruiz, F., Blanco-Portales, R., Muñoz-Blanco, J., Caballero, J.L., 2011. The strawberry plant defense mechanism: a molecular review. Plant and Cell Physiology 52, 1873–1903. Available from: https://doi.org/10.1093/pcp/pcr136.

APS, 1981. Microbial Collection of Major Importance to Agriculture. American Phytopathology Society St. Paul, MN.

Barchenger, D.W., Lamour, K.H., Sheu, Z.M., Shrestha, S., Kumar, S., Lin, S.W., et al., 2017. Intra- and intergenomic variation of ploidy and clonality characterize *Phytophthora capsici* on *Capsicum* in Taiwan. Mycological Progress 16, 955–963. Available from: https://doi.org/10.1007/s11557-017-1330-0.

Barchenger, D.W., Sheu, Z.M., Kumar, S., Lin, S.W., Burlakoti, R.R., Bosland, P.W., 2018. Race characterization of Phytophthora root-rot on *Capsicum* in Taiwan as a basis for anticipatory resistance breeding. Phytopathology 108 (8), 964–971. Available from: https://doi.org/10.1094/PHYTO-08-17-0289-R.

Bertolla, F., Frostegård, Å., Brito, B., Nesme, X., Simonet, P., 1999. During infection of its host, the plant pathogen *Ralstonia solanacearum* naturally develops a state of competence and exchanges genetic material. Molecular

Plant-Microbe Interactions 12, 467–472. Available from: https://doi.org/10.1094/MPMI.1999.12.5.467.

Boch, J., Bonas, U., Lahaye, T., 2014. TAL effectors – pathogen strategies and plant resistance engineering. New Phytologist 204, 823–832. Available from: https://doi.org/10.1111/nph.13015.

Boddy, L., 2016. Chapter 4: variation, sexuality, and evolution. In: Watkinson, S.C., Boddy, L., Money, N. (Eds.), The Fungi, 3rd Academic Press, pp. 99–139. ISBN-13: 978-0123820341.

Bosland, P.W., Williams, P.H., 1987. An evaluation of *Fusarium oxysporum* from crucifers based on pathogenicity, isozyme polymorphism, vegetative compatibility, and geographic origin. Canadian Journal of Botany 65, 2067–2073. Available from: https://doi.org/10.1139/b87-282.

Boller, T., Felix, G., 2009. A renaissance of elicitors: perception of microbe-associated molecular patterns and danger signals by pattern-recognition receptors. Annual Review of Plant Biology 60, 379–406. Available from: https://doi.org/10.1146/annurev.arplant.57.032905.105346.

Burdon, J.J., Zhan, J., Barrett, L.G., Papaïx, J., Thrall, P.H., 2016. Addressing the challenges of pathogen evolution on the world's arable crops. Phytopathology 106, 1117–1127. Available from: https://doi.org/10.1094/PHYTO-01-16-0036-FI.

Burnett, J.H., 1975. Mycogenetics. John Wiley & Sons, London, p. 375.

Buttimer, C., McAuliffe, O., Ross, R.P., Hill, C., O'Mahony, J., Coffey, A., 2017. Bacteriophages and bacterial plant diseases. Frontiers in Microbiology 8, 34. Available from: https://doi.org/10.3389/fmicb.2017.00034.

Castañeda, A., Reddy, J.D., El-Yacoubi, B., Gabriel, D.W., 2005. Mutagenesis of all eight avr genes in *Xanthomonas campestris* pv. *campestris* had no detected effect on pathogenicity, but one avr gene affected race specificity. Molecular Plant-Microbe Interaction 18 (12), 1306–1317. Available from: https://doi.org/10.1094/MPMI-18-1306.

Chitwood-Brown, J., Vallad, G.E., Lee, T.G., Hutton, S.F., 2021. Characterization and elimination of linkage-drag associated with fusarium wilt race 3 resistance genes. Theoretical and Applied Genetics 134, 2129–2140. Available from: https://doi.org/10.1007/s00122-021-03810-5.

Clark, W.A., Loegering, W.Q., 1967. Functions and maintenance of a type culture collection. Annual Review of Phytopathology 5, 319–342. Available from: https://doi.org/10.1146/annurev.py.05.090167.001535.

Coplin, D.C., 1989. Plasmids and their role in the evolution of plant pathogenic bacteria. Annual Review of Phytopathology 27, 187–212. Available from: https://doi.org/10.1146/annurev.py.27.090189.001155.

Cui, H., Tsuda, K., Parker, J.E., 2015. Effector-triggered immunity: from pathogen perception to robust defense. Annual Review of Plant Biology 66, 487–511. Available from: https://doi.org/10.1146/annurev-arplant-050213-040012.

Culver, J.N., Lindbeck, A.G.C., Dawson, W.O., 1991. Virus-host interactions: induction of chlorotic and necrotic responses in plants by tobamoviruses. Annual Review of Phytopathology 29, 193–217. Available from: https://doi.org/10.1146/annurev.py.29.090191.001205.

Diener, T.O., 1971. Potato spindle tuber "virus" IV. A replicating, low molecular weight RNA. Virology 45, 411–428. Available from: https://doi.org/10.1016/0042-6822(71)90342-4.

Domazakis, E., Lin, X., Aguilera-Galvez, C., Wouters, D., Bijsterbosch, G., Vleeshouwers, V.G.A.A., 2017. Effectoromics-based identification of cell surface receptors in potato. pp. 337–353. In: Shan, L., He, P. (Eds.), Plant Pattern Recognition Receptors. Methods in Molecular Biology, 1578. Humana Press, New York, NY. Available from: https://doi.org/10.1007/978-1-4939-6859-6_29.

Du, J., Vleeshouwers, V.G.A.A., 2014. The do's and don'ts of effectoromics. In: Birch, P., Jones, J., Bos, J. (Eds.), Plant-Pathogen Interactions. Methods in Molecular Biology (Methods and Protocols), 1127. Humana Press, Totowa, NJ. Available from: https://doi.org/10.1007/978-1-62703-986-4_19.

El Yacoubi, B., Brunings, A.M., Yuan, Q., Shankar, S., Gabriel, D.W., 2007. In planta horizontal transfer of a major pathogenicity effector gene. Applied Environmental Microbiology 73, 1612–1621.

Farnham, G., Baulcombe, D.C., 2006. Artificial evolution extends the spectrum of viruses that are targeted by a disease-resistance gene from potato. Proceeding of the National Academy of Sciences 103, 18828–18833. Available from: https://doi.org/10.1073/pnas.0605777103.

Gandon, S., Van Baalen, M., Jansen, V.A.A., 2002. The evolution of parasite virulence, superinfection, and host resistance. The American Naturalist 159, 658–669. Available from: https://doi.org/10.1086/339993.

Garcia-Arenal, F., Fraile, A., Malpica, J.M., 2001. Variability and genetic structure of plant virus populations. Annual Review of Phytopathology 39, 157–186. Available from: https://doi.org/10.1146/annurev.phyto.39.1.157.

Gassmann, W., Dahlbeck, D., Chesnokova, O., Minsavage, G.V., Jones, J.B., Staskawicz, B.J., 2000. Molecular evolution of virulence in natural field strains of *Xanthomonas campestris* pv. *vesicatoria*. Journal of Bacteriology 182, 7053–7059. Available from: https://doi.org/10.1128/JB.182.24.7053-7059.2000.

Gonçalves, O.S., Campos, K.F., Silva de Assis, J.C., et al., 2020. Transposable elements contribute to the genome plasticity of *Ralstonia solanacearum* species complex. Microbial Genomics 6. Available from: https://doi.org/10.1099/mgen.0.000374.

Goodwin, S.B., Cohen, B.A., Deahl, K.L., Fry, W.E., 1994. Migration from northern Mexico was the probable cause of recent genetic changes in populations of *Phytophthora infestans* in the United States and Canada. Phytopathology 84, 553–558. Available from: https://doi.org/10.1094/Phyto-84-553.

Grunwald, N.J., Flier, W.G., 2005. The biology of *Phytophthora infestans* at its center of origin. Annual Review of Phytopathology 43, 171–190. Available from: https://doi.org/10.1146/annurev.phyto.43.040204.135906.

Gu, B., Cao, X., Zhou, X., Chen, Z., Wang, Q., Liu, W., et al., 2020. The histological, effectoromic, and transcriptomic analyses of *Solanum pinnatisectum* reveal an upregulation of multiple *NBS-LRR* genes suppressing *Phytophthora infestans* infection. International Journal of Molecular Sciences i21 (9), 3211. Available from: https://doi.org/10.3390/ijms21093211.

Hansen, H.N., Smith, R.E., 1932. The mechanism of variation in imperfect fungi *Botrytis cinerea*. Phytopathology 22, 953–964.

Harrison, B.D., Robinson, D.J., 1999. Natural genomic and antigenic variation in whitefly-transmitted geminiviruses (Begomoviruses). Annual Review of Phytopathology 37, 369–398. Available from: https://doi.org/10.1146/annurev.phyto.37.1.369.

Haueisen, J., Stukenbrock, E.H., 2016. Life cycle specialization of filamentous pathogens—colonization and reproduction in plant tissues. Current Opinion in Microbiology 32, 31–37. Available from: https://doi.org/10.1016/j.mib.2016.04.015.

Henry, P.M., Pincot, D.D.A., Jenner, B.N., Borrero, C., Aviles, M., Nam, M.-H., et al., 2021. Horizontal chromosome transfer and independent evolution drive diversification in *Fusarium oxysporum* f. sp. *fragariae*. New Phytologist 230, 327–340. Available from: https://doi.org/10.1111/nph.17141.

Hooker, A.L., 1974. Cytoplasmic susceptibility in plant tissue. Annual Review of Phytopathology 12, 167–179. Available from: https://doi.org/10.1146/annurev.py.12.090174.001123.

Hu, J., Shrestha, S., Zhou, Y., Mudge, J., Liu, Z., Lamour, K., 2020. Dynamic Extreme Aneuploidy (DEA) in the vegetable pathogen *Phytophthora capsici* and the potential for rapid asexual evolution. PLOS ONE 15 (1), e0227250. Available from: https://doi.org/10.1371/journal.pone.0227250.

Hull, R., 1989. Movement of viruses in plants. Annual Review of Phytopathology 27, 213–240. Available from: https://doi.org/10.1146/annurev.py.27.090189.001241.

Jangir, P., Mehra, N., Sharma, K., Singh, N., Rani, M., Kapoor, R., 2021. Secreted in Xylem Genes: drivers of host adaptation in *Fusarium oxysporum*. Frontiers in Plant Science. Available from: https://doi.org/10.3389/fpls.2021.628611.

Jones, J.B., Stall, R.E., Bouzar, H., 1998. Diversity among Xanthomonads pathogenic on pepper and tomato. Annual Reviewof Phytopathology 36, 41–58. Available from: https://doi.org/10.1146/annurev.phyto.36.1.41.

Kamoun, S., Furzer, O., Jones, J.D.G., Judelson, H.S., Ali, G.S., Dalio, R.J.D., et al., 2015. The top 10 oomycete pathogens in molecular plant pathology. Molecular Plant Pathology 16, 413–434. Available from: https://doi.org/10.1111/mpp.12190.

Kandel, P.P., Almeida, R.P.P., Cobine, P.A., De La Fuente, L., 2017. Natural competence rates are variable among *Xylella fastidiosa* strains and homologous recombination occurs in vitro between subspecies *fastidiosa* and multiplex. Molecular Plant-Microbe Interactions 30. Available from: https://doi.org/10.1094/MPMI-02-17-0053-R.

Kang, S., Blair, J.E., Geiser, D.M., Khang, C.-H., Park, S.-Y., Gahegan, M., et al., 2006. Plant pathogen culture collections: it takes a village to preserve these resources vital to the advancement of agricultural security and plant pathology. Phytopathology 96, 920–925. Available from: https://doi.org/10.1094/PHYTO-96-0920.

Kearney, B., Staskawicz, B.J., 1990. Widespread distribution and fitness contribution of *Xanthomonas campestris* avirulence gene *avrBs2*. Nature 346, 385–386. Available from: https://doi.org/10.1038/346385a0.

Kikuchi, T., Eves-van den Akker, S., Jones, J.T., 2017. Genome evolution of plant-parasitic nematodes. Annual Review of Phytopathology 55, 333–354. Available from: https://doi.org/10.1146/annurev-phyto-080516-035434.

Kim, H., 2020. Effector-omics Approaches for Identifying *Phytophthora capsici* Effectors Inducing Hypersensitive Cell Death in *Nicotiana benthamiana*. (Ph. D. Diss). Seoul National University, Seoul, South Korea.

Kim, J.F., Charkowski, A.O., Alfano, J.R., Collmer, A., Beer, S.V., 1998. Sequences related to transposable elements and bacteriophages flank avirulence genes of *Pseudomonas syringae*. Molecular Plant-Microbe Interactions 11, 1247–1252. Available from: https://doi.org/10.1094/MPMI.1998.11.12.1247.

Kohn, L.M., 2005. Mechanisms of fungal speciation. Annual Review of Phytopathology 43, 279–308. Available from: https://doi.org/10.1146/annurev.phyto.43.040204.135958.

Kunkel, L.O., 1947. Variation in phytopathogenic viruses. Annual Review of Microbiology 1, 85–100. Available from: https://doi.org/10.1146/annurev.mi.01.100147.000505.

Lacy, G.H., Leary, J.V., 1979. Genetic systems in phytopathogenicity bacteria. Annual Review of Phytopathology 17, 181–202. Available from: https://doi.org/10.1146/annurev.py.17.090179.001145.

Lawson, W.R., Jan, C.C., Shatte, T., Smith, L., Kong, G.A., Kochman, J.K., 2011. DNA markers linked to the *R2* rust resistance gene in sunflower (*Helianthus annuus* L.) facilitate anticipatory breeding for this disease variant. Molecular Breeding 28, 569–576. Available from: https://doi.org/10.1007/s11032-010-9506-1.

Li, Y., Shen, H., Zhou, Q., van der Lee, T., Huang, S., 2017. Changing ploidy as a strategy; the Irish potato famine pathogen shifts ploidy in relation to its sexuality. Molecular Plant-Microbe Interactions 30, 45–52. Available from: https://doi.org/10.1094/MPMI-08-16-0156-R.

Ma, L.-J., van der Does, H.C., Borkovich, K.A., Coleman, J.J., Daboussi, M.-J., Di Pietro, A., et al., 2010. Comparative genomics reveals mobile pathogenicity chromosomes in *Fusarium*. Nature 464, 367–373. Available from: https://doi.org/10.1038/nature08850.

McKinney, H.H., 1935. Evidence of virus mutation in the common mosaic of tobacco. Journal of Agriculture Research 51, 951–981.

Mehrabi, R., Bahkali, A.H., Abd-Elsalam, K.A., Moslem, M., M'Barek, S.B., Gohari, A.M., et al., 2011. Horizontal gene and chromosome transfer in plant pathogenic fungi affecting host range. FEMS Microbiology Reviews 35, 542–554. Available from: https://doi.org/10.1111/j.1574-6976.2010.00263.x.

Menardo, F., Praz, C.R., Wyder, S., Ben-David, R., Bourras, S., Matsumae, H., et al., 2016. Hybridization of powdery mildew strains gives rise to pathogens on novel agricultural crop species. Nature Genetics 48, 201–205. Available from: https://doi.org/10.1038/ng.3485.

Milgroom, M.G., Del, M., Jiménez-Gasco, M., Olivares García, C., Drott, M.T., Jiménez-Díaz, R.M., 2014. Recombination between clonal lineages of the asexual fungus *Verticillium dahliae* detected by genotyping by sequencing. PLoS One 0106740. Available from: https://doi.org/10.1371/journal.pone.

Minsavage, G.V., Dahlbeck, D., Whalen, M.C., Kearney, B., Bonas, U., Staskawicz, B.J., et al., 1990. Gene-for-gene relationships specifying disease resistance in *Xanthomonas campestris* pv. *vesicatoria*-pepper interactions. Molecular Plant-Microbe Interactions 3, 41–47. Available from: https://doi.org/10.1094/MPMI-3-041.

Moseman, J.G., 1966. Genetics of powdery mildews. Annual Review of Phytopathology 4, 269–290. Available from: https://doi.org/10.1146/annurev.py.04.090166.001413.

Nguyen, H.D., Thi, H., Tran, N., Ohshima, K., 2013. Genetic variation of the Turnip mosaic virus population of Vietnam: a case study of founder, regional and local influences. Virus Research 171, 138–149. Available from: https://doi.org/10.1016/j.virusres.2012.11.008.

O'Brien, H.E., Thakur, S., Guttman, D.S., 2011. Evolution of plant pathogenesis in *Pseudomonas syringae*: a genomics perspective. Annual Review of Phytopathology 49, 269–289. Available from: https://doi.org/10.1146/annurev-phyto-072910-095242.

Ordonez, N., Seidl, M.F., Waalwijk, C., Drenth, A., Kilian, A., Thomma, B.P.H.J., et al., 2015. Worse comes to worst: bananas and Panama disease—when plant and pathogen clones meet. PLoS Pathogens 11, e1005197. Available from: https://doi.org/10.1371/journal.ppat.1005197.

Parker, I.M., Gilbert, G.S., 2004. The evolutionary ecology of novel plant-pathogen interactions. Annual Review of Ecology, Evolution and Systematics 35, 675–700. Available from: https://doi.org/10.1146/annurev.ecolsys.34.011802.132339.

Parmeter, J.R., Snyder, W.C., Reichle, R.E., 1963. Heterokaryosis and variability in plant-pathogenic fungi. Annual Review of Phytopathology 1, 51–76. Available from: https://doi.org/10.1146/annurev.py.01.090163.000411.

Pontecorvo, G., 1956. The parasexual cycle in fungi. Annual Review of Microbiology 10, 393–400. Available from: https://doi.org/10.1146/annurev.mi.10.100156.002141.

Puhalla, J.E., 1979. Classification of isolates of *Verticillium dahliae* based on heterokaryon incompatibility. Phytopathology 69, 1186–1189.

Roossinck, M.J., 1997. Mechanisms of plant virus evolution. Annual Review of Phytopathology 35, 191–209. Available from: https://doi.org/10.1146/annurev.phyto.35.1.191.

Sacristan, S., Garcia Arenal, F., 2008. The evolution of virulence and pathogenicity in plant pathogen populations. Molecular Plant Pathology 9, 369–384. Available from: https://doi.org/10.1111/j.1364-3703.2007.00460.x.

Sansome, E., 1961. Meiosis in the oogonium and antheridium of *Pythium debaryanum* Hesse. Nature 191, 927–928. Available from: https://doi.org/10.1038/191827a0.

Sansome, S., 1965. Meiosis in diploid and polyploid sex organs of *Phytophthora* and *Achlya*. Cytologia 30, 103–117. Available from: https://doi.org/10.1508/cytologia.30.103.

Schornack, S., Moscou, M.J., Ward, E.R., Horvath, D.M., 2013. Engineering plant disease resistance based on TAL effectors. Annual Review of Phytopathology 51, 383–406. Available from: https://doi.org/10.1146/annurev-phyto-082712-102255.

Seitz, P., Blokesch, M., 2013. Cues and regulatory pathways involved in natural competence and transformation in pathogenic and environmental Gram-negative bacteria. FEMS Microbiology Reviews 37, 336–363. Available from: https://doi.org/10.1111/j.1574-6976.2012.00353.x.

Shivas, R., Beasley, D., Thomas, J., Geering, A., Riley, I., 2005. Management of plant pathogen collections. Dept. Agric., Fisheries, and Forestry. Commonw. Aust. Available from: http://www.daff.gov.au/planthealth.

Shrestha, S.K., Miyasaka, S.C., Shintaku, M., Kelly, H., Lamour, K., 2017. *Phytophthora colocasiae* from Vietnam, China, Hawaii, and Nepal: intra–and intergenomic variations in ploidy and a long–lived, diploid Hawaiian lineage. Mycological Progress 16, 983-904. Available from: https://doi.org/10.1007/s11557-017-1323-z.

Sidhu, G.S., 1988. Genetics of plant pathogenic fungi; Advances in plant pathology, 6. Academic Press, San Diego, CA. p. 566. Available from: https://www.sciencedirect.com/bookseries/advances-in-plant-pathology/vol/6/suppl/C.

Soanes, D., Richards, T.A., 2014. Horizontal gene transfer in eukaryotic plant pathogens. Annual Review of Phytopathology 52, 583–614. Available from: https://doi.org/10.1146/annurev-phyto-102313-050127.

Stakman, E.C., 1914. A study in cereal rusts. Physiological races. Minn. Agriculture Exp. Sation Bull. 138.

Stukenbrock, E.H., 2016. The role of hybridization in the evolution and emergence of new fungal plant pathogens. Phytopathology 106, 104–112. Available from: https://doi.org/10.1094/PHYTO-08-15-0184-RVW.

Sullivan, M.J., Melton, T.A., Shew, H.D., 2005. Fitness of races 0 and 1 of *Phytophthora parasitica* var. *nicotianae*. Plant Disease 89, 1220–1228. Available from: https://doi.org/10.1094/PD-89-1220.

Swords, K.M.M., Dahlbeck, D., Kearney, B., Roy, M., Staskawicz, B.J., 1996. Spontaneous and induced mutations in a single open reading frame alter both virulence and avirulence in *Xanthomonas campestris* pv. *vesicatoria* avrBs2. Journal of Bacteriology 178, 4661–4669. Available from: https://doi.org/10.1128/jb.178.15.4661-4669.1996.

Sztuba-Solińska, J., Urbanowicz, A., Figlerowicz, M., Bujarski, J.J., 2011. RNA-RNA recombination in plant virus replication and evolution. Annual Review of Phytopathology 49, 415–443. Available from: https://doi.org/10.1146/annurev-phyto-072910-095351.

Tai, T.H., Dahlbeck, D., Clark, E.T., Gajiwala, P., Pasion, R., Whalen, M.C., et al., 1999. Expression of the *Bs2* pepper gene confers resistance to bacterial spot disease in tomato. Proceedings of the National Academy of Sciences of the United States of America 96, 14153–14158. Available from: https://doi.org/10.1073/pnas.96.24.14153.

Tang, J., Lilly, S., Veerakone, S., Kanchiraopally, D., Kelly, M., Delmiglio, C., et al., 2022. First report of grapevine Algerian latent virus in carnation in New Zealand. Plant Disease . Available from: https://doi.org/10.1094/PDIS-03-22-0597-PDN.

Tinline, R.D., MacNeill, B.H., 1969. Parasexuality in plant pathogenic fungi. Annual Review of Phytopathology 7, 147–170. Available from: https://doi.org/10.1146/annurev.py.07.090169.001051.

Van der Does, H.C., Rep, M., 2012. Horizontal transfer of supernumerary chromosomes in fungi. In: Bolton, M., Thomma, B. (Eds.), Plant Fungal Pathogens. Methods in Molecular Biology, 835. Humana Press. Available from: https://doi.org/10.1007/978-1-61779-501-5_26.

Van Schie, C.C.N., Takken, F.L.W., 2014. Susceptibility genes 101: how to be a good host. Annual Review of Phytopathology 52, 551–581. Available from: https://doi.org/10.1146/annurev-phyto-102313-045854.

Whitaker, V.W., Debener, T., Roberts, A.V., Hokanson, S.C., 2010. A standard set of host differentials and unified nomenclature for an international collection of *Diplocarpon rosae* races. Plant Pathology 59, 745–752. Available from: https://doi.org/10.1111/j.1365-3059.2010.02281.x.

Yarwood, C.E., 1979. Host passage effects with plant viruses. Advances in Virus Research 25, 169–190. Available from: https://doi.org/10.1016/S0065-3527(08)60570-9.

Zaitlin, M., Palukaitis, P., 2000. Advances in understanding plant viruses and virus diseases. Annual Review of Phytopathology 38, 117–143. Available from: https://doi.org/10.1146/annurev.phyto.38.1.117.

Zhang, X.-F., Qu, F., 2015. Multi-component plant viruses. eLS. John Wiley & Sons, Ltd, Chichester. Available from: http://doi.org/10.1002/9780470015902.a0024783.

5

Resistance: the environmental interaction

Introduction

The environment is the third member of the triangle for disease to develop, and a key component for a reliable and reproducible disease screen. Screening a set of accessions for resistance, the pathogen will reveal diversity in quality and quantity of infection. Some plants are not infected at all (immunity), others show at most some flecks but no reproduction of pathogen (resistance), and again others show various levels of infections and pathogen reproduction (partial resistance to susceptibility). For disease to occur, there must be a susceptible host, a virulent pathogen, and a favorable environment. Whether whole plant, detached leaves, or molecular techniques are used, the resistance found and selected must be functional in a grower's production system. It is essential that each breeding generation, when screened for disease resistance, be done under controlled conditions. It is imperative that the plant breeder correlates the controlled laboratory performance with the actual performance under production conditions. Grower production systems can change over time, for example, bell pepper (*Capsicum annuum*) in China was historically an open field crop, but recently production is increasingly moving to protected cultivation, resulting in new diseases and pests causing losses. Plant breeders must now switch from breeding for resistance to typically open-field biotic stresses to greenhouse stresses.

When cropping systems intensify, the microenvironment changes and can give pathogens a better environment to reproduce. For example, row spacing that creates higher plant populations in the field to achieve higher yields may lead to a more humid environment, which in turn is more favorable for fungal and bacterial diseases. A good example of this is the growth of lettuce (*Lactuca sativa*) for the "Spring mix" packaged salad product. Spring mix is a combination of baby (horticultural term used to market small immature leaves) leaf lettuce (*L. sativa*), radicchio (*Cichorium intybus*), baby spinach (*Spinacia oleracea*), baby arugula (*Eruca vesicaria sativa*), baby beet tops (*Beta vulgaris*), baby chard (*B. vulgaris*), baby kale (*Brassica oleracea*), and other assorted baby greens. Plants used to produce the "baby leaf lettuce" are grown at extremely high densities that enhance the occurrence of bacterial leaf spot (*Xanthomonas hortorum* pv. *vitians*), a disease that can make the crop unmarketable. Because there are no "baby leaf" cultivars on the market. Growing the plants very close together is the only way to achieve a small leaf size.

The environment can make any cultivar appear susceptible or resistant whether the cultivar is genetically resistant or not. One widely reported example of the environmental influence on host resistance is for bacterial wilt (*Ralstonia solanacearum*) of tomato (*Solanum lycopersicum*). This environmental response appears to be strain specific, with strains originating in temperate areas having higher virulence levels under cooler temperatures, while tropical strains are more virulent under hotter temperatures. In fact, the environmental influence on virulence is so profound in bacterial wilt that it affects quantitative trait loci (QTL) identification in tomato (*S. lycopersicum*) lines segregating for resistance.

Some pathogens can cause disease throughout the world, and other pathogens are less tolerant of environmental variations and are likely to be restricted in their geographical distribution. The fungal pathogen *Botryosphaeria dothidea* infects and causes disease in hundreds of woody plant species. The pathogen has a prolonged latent period and therefore can pass undetected by quarantine systems in commercial or personal traded living plants, fruits, and other plant parts, and as such, the pathogen now has a broad global distribution. Confoundingly, disease expression from *B. dothidea* infection seems to be promoted by environmental variation and is often associated with abiotic stresses, such as drought, physical damage, waterlogging, frost, and unsuitable growing environments.

Most often, environmental conditions such as free moisture on leaf surfaces, or air and soil temperatures are key important factors that can determine the outcome of a host–pathogen interaction. In the 1950s, for example, farmers in Kenya adopted a pruning strategy for their coffee (*Coffea arabica*) that resulted in an extension in the cropping season for less intense harvesting and more stable income; however, this also resulted in fruit setting that coincided with the rainy season. The continuous cropping in combination of exposure to intense rainfall resulted in a severe outbreak of coffee berry disease (*Colletotrichum kahawae*) across east Africa.

Some environmental conditions, however, can influence the outcome by changing the natural state (physiology) of the plant. Cold acclimation turfgrasses can result in a state of induced resistance to infection by snow mold pathogens (*Microdochium nivale* [formerly *Fusarium nivale*], *Typhula incarnata* and *Typhula ishikariensis*, *Coprinus psychrombidus*, *Myriosclerotinia borealis*) that are most aggressive at lower temperatures.

In addition to the physical environment, the biological environment that surrounds a plant can directly impact the success of a pathogen. Plant roots grow into and through an extraordinary array of "indigenous" soil microorganisms. Community characterization is not always genotypic in nature but may occur at different scales ranging from functional diversity to broader taxonomic diversity to simple abundance. Functional diversity can also be estimated by measuring functional genes that play a role in ecosystem processes. Root-microbial interactions encompass a range of specificity from "highly evolved" symbioses (legume rhizobium) to fewer specific associations (arbuscular mycorrhizas). Apparent symbioses are the most likely to develop host specificity. Plant roots exude a large amount and a complex assortment of organic compounds into the nearby soil. A variety of biotic interactions occur in the rhizosphere that can affect the diversity and composition of the microbial community associated with roots. Thus the biotic soil environment surrounding the roots of a plant may have an impact on the ability of pathogens to attack. It is important to appreciate that the environment can be above ground (aerial), below (soil), and both together.

Protected cultivation

The most basic method for the plant breeder to conduct effective disease screens is using greenhouses or polyhouses to manipulate the growing environment to ensure infection and disease symptoms. Most greenhouses are covered with a plastic glazing. Low-cost polyethylene film or covering applied as an air-inflated double cover can last up to 4 years. Semirigid structured sheets of polycarbonate or acrylic are more permanent and have a life of at least 15 years. Tempered glass is used for crops requiring high light levels and better environmental control. The closed environment of a greenhouse has its own unique requirements, compared with typical outdoor production. Diseases, and extremes of temperature and humidity, must be controlled, and frequent irrigation is necessary. Significant inputs of energy may be required, particularly in cooler environments, which maintain temperatures that are optimal for plant pathogens. These management inputs require extensive amounts of electricity and often use fossil fuels that are costly and contribute to pollution. Furthermore, while greenhouses can provide an optimal condition for the target disease, they can also provide an ideal environment for nontarget diseases under protected cultivation. Therefore the plant breeder must be diligent in scouting, monitoring, and controlling diseases in the protected cultivation setting. Alternatively, the plant breeder can use a simple polyhouse or hoop house without climate control to protect the plants from rain and maintain stable temperatures and humidity. For example, to conduct a disease screen in the tropics, a plant breeder may plant the trial during the rainy season with the expectation that the environment will be sufficiently stable to conduct an effective bioassay. However, in both greenhouses and polyhouses, the level of environmental control or the variability of temperature or humidity may be too great to obtain high-quality data. In such instances, a plant breeder may need to find alternative strategies to conduct their bioassay.

Growth chamber

Plant growth chambers provide a controlled environment, including temperature, light, humidity, and other factors for disease screening. Plant growth chambers can provide a particular environment, reducing confounding factors that might be present in a greenhouse setting and increasing the reproducibility of an experiment. While this might seem like an ideal situation to screen for disease resistance, there are limitations to using growth chambers. From a plant breeder's perspective, we must always consider the cost of things to be cost-efficient in our programs. Plant growth chambers are often extremely costly to operate and consume high amounts of electricity. Additionally, the size of growth chambers is often small, limiting the population size, replication number, and the number of entries that can be screened. Despite this small size, it has been shown that a "chamber effect" exists whereby results observed are not due to an experimental treatment but to inconspicuous differences in the growth chamber. The plant breeder must be aware that a growth chamber is not uniform and can lead to considerable degrees of variability in plant response to screening. If a chamber effect is strong, it could result in false interpretations and incorrect conclusions about the true resistance of a given plant. An appropriate experimental design and sufficient replication must always be used. Over time, the growth chamber will have light decay as the lighting source ages, and changes in temperature, humidity, and gas concentration because of sensor drift. Sensor drift is the term used by the environmental monitoring industry to refer to changes in equipment over time

Chamber effect is not only dependent on the duration of an experiment but also on the type of experimental setup or design. Normally, the disease screening experiment is contained within a single growth chamber, and each individual plant/pot is a unit of replication. Statisticians will state that each plant/pot is a pseudo-replicate and must be considered in the analysis. With this experimental setup, a chamber effect has been shown to be present. This chamber effect is caused by spatial nonuniformity within a growth chamber and is dependent on the positioning of plants within the chamber. The suggestion has been made that each day; each plant/pot should be moved to one position within the chamber to substantially reduce this bias. Thus at the end of the experiment, each plant has been exposed to the microclimate at each location within the chamber. Another fact to consider is that plants grown in the same chamber but during different time periods can exhibit the chamber effect. As a result, experiments should not be replicated in the same chamber twice. Therefore it is essential to establish if chamber effects exist in one's own growth chambers by running a pilot study before screening.

Phytotron

To validate a plant's responses in the production setting, experiments under realistic and reproducible conditions are essential. One alternative to using a growth chamber to conduct disease screenings is a phytotron, which is an enclosed greenhouse that allows researchers to control the entire growing environment, but on a larger scale. Phytotrons are used primarily to investigate how the environment affects plant growth and development, but they are used also to complement and supplement field and greenhouse research in areas like plant breeding and provide an opportunity to study plant response to biotic stress under optimal conditions for infection and disease. They often range in size from 100 m^2 to more than 600 m^2, allowing plant breeders to screen many more plants with greater replication as compared to growth chambers. Furthermore, unlike growth chambers, phytotrons have much less variability in environmental conditions within the growing area. Phytotrons are distinguished from the installation of a few plant growth chambers by the fact that phytotrons are operated in such a way that a wide range of environmental factors can be studied simultaneously. However, one important commonality between growth chambers and phytotrons is the cost of operation, that is, considerably higher as compared to a greenhouse or polyhouse. Furthermore, phytotrons are much rarer than growth chambers, and only a handful exist on each continent, so access is certainly limited.

Vertical farms

Vertical farming represents a novel approach to food production, building on methodological and technical innovations of protected horizontal farming growth systems. Proponents of the vertical farming claim that vertical farming will provide greater access to fresh vegetables and the ability to optimize land use to feed a growing world. Proponents also claim that it will prevent all pathogen access and eliminate any disease control requirements for crops in these protective structures, a dubious claim. Protected cultivation does restrict the entry of diseases, but they cannot realistically be expected to entirely prevent the occurrence of diseases in a crop. Thus plant breeders will need to realize that their new cultivar may be planted in one of these climate control units and need specialized disease resistance.

Professor Joe E. Roberts at Keele University, Staffordshire, United Kingdom and colleagues critiqued vertical farming and warned that the optimal growing conditions for the crop will also make them more conducive for disease development. Indeed, it is almost impossible to exclude pathogens from these facilities. Vertical farms would be expected to encounter the same disease pressure as conventional protected horticulture. Thus plant breeders will need to test their material in an environment that mimics the vertical farm environment.

The ability to introduce plant pathogens into protected horticulture systems can occur through several mechanisms, including accidental contamination via employees or seed; inadequate phytosanitation protocols; or poorly maintained structures. The most likely mechanism of introduction is through ventilation systems and doorways. Air filters and airlock-based systems with decontamination protocols such as the use of air showers can help to minimize pathogen entry but may provide difficulties when removing products for sale as large entry/exit spaces are normally required.

Even so, the small size of microorganisms, such as fungal spores, for example, the conidia of *Bremia lactucae*, the causal agent of downy mildew in lettuce (*L. sativa*) or insects such as western flower thrips (*Frankliniella occidentalis*) that vector viruses, facilitates their access into even the most well-maintained protected growing systems. Vertical farm operators will therefore need to be prepared for the eventuality of pathogen access and consider the factors that can influence their proliferation and control in such systems, such as using resistant cultivars.

Many vertical farming systems use stacked horizontal growing surfaces contained within a high-sided controlled environment facility, providing the possibility of vertical as well as horizontal spread of diseases. There will also be vertical temperature gradients. The increased height of vertical farming growth systems compared to conventional facilities could present large gradients of temperature, humidity, and light availability from the top to the bottom of the facility. Air circulation is essential in providing uniform temperatures, humidity, and carbon dioxide concentrations for plant growth and to aid control of many diseases, air circulation may also facilitate the spread of diseases within the crop. Spores of many plant pathogenic fungi, such as gray mold (*Botrytis cinerea*) are dispersed by air currents. The different temperature optima of different pathogens could mean that tailored cultivars may be required for each growing level contained within the system. Stress from nonoptimal high or low temperatures can lower the resistance of plants to bacterial, viral, and fungal pathogens.

In vertical farming, transpiration from the crop and evaporation from exposed hydroponic nutrient solution causes an increase in humidity that aids crop growth, but also provides suitable conditions for the proliferation of pathogens again, for example, powdery mildews like *B. cinerea*. In stacked vertical farming systems, humidity build-up in the restricted airspace between shelves may provide conditions very conducive to disease development. Proper control of humidity is therefore a key to minimizing diseases in vertical farms. Condensation forming on the undersides of stacked growing levels could generate water droplets that may fall back onto the surface of plants growing on the level below. Such droplets could promote the spread of disease through dispersal of fungal spores or bacteria. It is commonly recommended that overhead irrigation be discouraged to prevent spread of *Botrytis* and *Peronospora* spores. Therefore water droplets falling between levels in vertical farming systems due to the condensation of humidity, from irrigation or growing medium could act as a route for encouraging disease spread. Similarly, fungal spores could fall from higher to lower shelves under the influence of gravity alone, acting to encourage the spread of infection or damage from upper to lower shelves even without the aid of water droplets.

Many vertical farming approaches utilize hydroponic growing systems. Such systems bring further considerations for disease management. Many microorganism species have been found in recirculating hydroponic systems, where it is normal for fungi such as *Pythium* to multiply and spread. While this issue is relevant to hydroponic culture in general, they could be exacerbated by the large and complex hydroponic systems required in some vertical farming units.

Shading of the crop from levels of the growth system arranged above is an issue that must be addressed in the design of vertical farming systems. Adequate illumination is required not only for optimal growth of the crop, but the quality and quantity of available light also influences the response of plants to pathogens, with crops grown in low light often being more susceptible to disease. To offset decreased light levels found in the lower growing levels, many vertical farming systems use artificial lighting to provide either supplementary or the entire illumination for the crop. High-efficiency light-emitting diode (LED) provides a relatively low energy use requirement, the output spectrum can be tailored to the needs of the crop species being produced and their low heat output allows them to be placed close to the crop. The LED illumination wavelength could, however, affect pathogen growth and development and consequently alter approaches to their management. Light quality has been shown to affect disease development. In the case of fungi, the inhibition of sporulation and germ tube growth by light is strongly wavelength-dependent, for example, in *B. cinerea* near-ultraviolet light induces and blue light inhibits sporulation.

One of the main aims of vertical farming is to enable the production of higher yields of crops per unit area of land used. In optimizing the number of plants that can be grown on any given building footprint, plant density is an important factor in disease management due to the effect it has on the surrounding plant microclimate and therefore to disease development and spread. To prevent the spread of disease entirely, the spacing of plants would need to be unrealistically and prohibitively large. Therefore the aim of producing as much crop per unit area must be balanced against plant overcrowding.

In conventional protected horticulture, knowledge of disease control is well established; however, vertical farms bring additional considerations that are specific to the optimal operation of such systems. It is likely that challenges have been underestimated, particularly in claiming that vertical farming has near zero disease risk. Growers will need to consider the control requirements specific to such growth systems and be prepared to act appropriately in the event of a disease outbreak, one course would be to plant disease-resistant crops.

Vertical farming systems have vulnerabilities to pathogens, but the potential exists to enhance disease control through the adoption of Integrated Pest Management (IPM)-based strategies encompassing artificial light-based manipulation of disease behavior, sophisticated nutrient solution treatment, control and isolation systems, and importantly resistant cultivars.

Environmental variables

Plants are exposed to numerous environmental variables, including soil fertility, soil moisture, soil salinity, light quality (wavelength and intensity) and quantity (duration), and agrochemicals (plant growth regulators, herbicides, fungicides, and insecticides), among others. In general, the major variables that one must be cognizant of for a successful disease screen are temperature, light quantity and quality, and relative humidity (RH). Temperature is undoubtedly one of the most crucial factors influencing the occurrence and development of many diseases. Some diseases are most severe at low temperatures, others at elevated temperatures, although in laboratory culture the pathogen can grow over a wide temperature range. This is because the effects of temperature on disease, like those of some other environmental factors, may be attributed to effects on the pathogen, on the host, or on the interaction between host and pathogen. The plant breeder should be aware that when attempting to relate the results of laboratory studies to field conditions the temperature of the plant itself in the field may be higher than that of the surrounding air in the field.

The soil temperature is the most important when breeding resistance to soilborne diseases. A classic example is cabbage yellows (*Fusarium oxysporum* f. sp. *conglutinans*) of cabbages (*B. oleracea* var. *capitata*). Two types of resistance exist, a qualitative/monogene known as "Type A," and a polygenic resistance known as "Type B." Soil temperature has a significant effect on the expression of these two types of resistance. Type A resistance is effective in soil temperatures below 28°C. Type B begins to lose effectiveness at a lower soil temperature beginning to become ineffective at 22°C–24°C. Other examples of temperature affecting the resistance phenotype are cucumber scab (*Cladosporium cucumerinum*) where at a constant temperature of 22°C or above, cucumber (*Cucumis sativus*) plants become phenotypically resistant even though genetically susceptible. Resistance to bean yellow mosaic virus (BYMV, *Potyvirus*) of garden pea (*Pisum sativum*) is a monogenic recessively controlled trait. By maintaining the air temperature at 18°C or below during the assay, symptoms appeared only on homozygous susceptible plants and if the assay is conducted at 27°C, only homozygous resistant plants are free from symptoms. Thus the two homozygous classes could be distinguished from heterozygotes by manipulating the temperature. In *Capsicum*, resistance to tobacco mosaic virus (TMV, *Tobamovirus*) is effective up to 20°C, while at 32°C and above the plants are susceptible.

Both soil salinity and soil pH affect the outcome of a disease screen. The effects of soil salinity have been examined in connection with plant infection by a wide array of plant pathogens, including species of *Phytophthora*. Salinity has been reported to increase plant susceptibility and promote *Phytophthora* root rot of *Chrysanthemum*, *Citrus*, and tomato (*S. lycopersicum*). Salts of all kinds are found in both soils and water of the southwestern United States. Root rot and wilt diseases caused by *Phytophthora capsici* are major constraints in chile pepper (*C. annuum*) production. Because chile peppers (*C. annuum*) are considered a salt-sensitive crop and the irrigation water in the southwestern United States is considered salty; Soumaila Sanogo at New Mexico State University studied the effect of salinity on Phytophthora wilt. He found that salinity increases the mycelial growth of *P. capsici* and increases disease severity in susceptible cultivars. Fortunately, the resistance being bred into cultivars of chile pepper (*C. annuum*) is still effective against *P. capsici* even under increased salinity.

Soil pH markedly influences some diseases, such as the common scab of potato (*Spongospora subterranea*) and clubroot (*Plasmodiophora brassicae*) of crucifers. Potato scab is suppressed at a pH of 5.2 or slightly below. Scab is not normally a problem when the soil pH is about 5.2. Clubroot of crucifers, on the other hand, can usually be controlled by monitoring the soil until the pH becomes 7.2 or higher. Under both very acidic (pH of 3) and basic soil (pH >9) conditions, the growth and pathogen population of bacterial wilt (*R. solanacearum*) has been shown to be significantly reduced. However, it has been shown that in slightly acidic soils (pH of 4.5–5.5), the growth of the pathogen is favored, and bacterial wilt disease developed more quickly and severely. Soil amendments that increase the soil pH to become more neutral has been shown to decrease the survival of the pathogen in the soil.

Critical in bacterial infection and fungal spore germination is RH. High humidity favors the development of most leaf and fruit diseases caused by fungi, water molds, and bacteria. Moisture is generally needed for spore germination, the multiplication, and penetration of bacteria, and the initiation of infection. Spore germination of powdery mildew, caused by many different fungal species in the order Erysiphales, occurs best at 80%–90% RH, and of course, there is also a temperature effect with temperatures between 22 and 27°C favoring spore germination. Diseases in greenhouse crops—such as leaf mold (*Cladosporium fulvum*) of tomato (*S. lycopersicum*) and decay of flowers, leaves, stems, and seedlings of flowering plants, caused by *Botrytis* species—can be managed by lowering air humidity or by avoiding spraying plants directly with water. Similarly, moisture is more important than the temperature for apple scabs (*Venturia inaequalis*) to develop.

High soil-moisture levels favor disease development of water mold fungi (Oomycetes), such as species of *Aphanomyces*, *Pythium*, and *Phytophthora*. Over-saturated soil, by decreasing oxygen and raising carbon dioxide levels in the soil, makes genetically resistant plants more susceptible to root-rotting organisms. Recently, it has been reported that across different environmental gradients and infection histories between populations, an area of juniper (*Juniperus sp.*) symptomatic for *Phytophthora austrocedri* increased with waterlogging, increasing with soil moisture in sites where soils had higher peat or clay contents, and decreasing with proximity to watercourses where sites had shallower, sandier soils. In contrast, diseases such as the common scab of potato (*Streptomyces scabies*); and onion white rot (*Sclerotium cepivorum*) are most severe under low soil-moisture levels.

It is important for the plant breeder to consider all aspects of the environment when screening for resistance in your program. While temperature and RH are particularly important in conducting a disease assay, considerations such as soil moisture and pH can also play an important role in identifying host resistance.

Monitoring equipment

A range of equipment is available to measure and monitor environmental factors. Technology advances in the field of temperature measurement have led to a vast variety of sensors and measuring instruments available for making accurate data collection at relatively low costs. When selecting a temperature-measuring device, consider what is being measured. Is it the soil for a soilborne pathogen or air for a foliar pathogen? An example that seems simple at first is measuring room temperature to ±1°C accuracy. The problem here is that room temperature is not one temperature but many microtemperatures. Sensors need to be placed near and at the height of the experiment, not on the wall across the room. As has been pointed out earlier, a discrepancy of as little as 4°C can give a false indication of resistance. High-precision temperature measurement is possible using well-specified and suitably calibrated sensors and instrumentation. However, the accuracy of these measurements will be meaningless unless the equipment and sensors are used correctly.

Relative humidity

Monitoring and measuring RH are important for screening foliar pathogens. A humidity gauge, or RH meter, is a crucial tool for making quick, accurate measurements of RH conditions. There are several different RH sensors available on the market. One of the most crucial factors to consider when selecting the most appropriate RH sensor for a given area or bioassay is sensor tolerance; every humidity gauge has a built-in sensor tolerance—an amount by which the measurement provided by the meter will differ from the actual RH of the area. A very high-quality gauge might have a sensor tolerance of ±2%, while lower-quality devices might have a tolerance closer to ±5%–6%. The smaller this number, the better, because it indicates a more accurate device. Secondly, dew point range: dew point, or the temperature at which water will condense, is another way to monitor humidity. For powdery mildew (*Ascomycota phylum*), a high RH is best, but free water will impair infection by the pathogen. Similarly, when screening for resistance to anthracnose fruit rot (*Colletotrichum* species) of pepper (*C. annuum*), it is necessary to maintain 95%–98% RH for 10 days; however, if the water condenses on the surface of the fruit, it can wash away the inoculum and result in an inaccurate bioassay. Humidity gauges with dew point measurement ranges can make getting this information easier. Thirdly, temperature range and corrections; because the RH is a measure of how much water is needed to be added to the air to achieve saturation, temperatures can affect a RH reading. Basically, warmer air needs more moisture to reach saturation, while colder air needs less. Humidity gauges with built-in temperature measurements, or thermo-hygrometers, can automatically adjust RH measurements to take the current temperature into account. Finding the right humidity gauge means finding a device that has the right humidity measurement options and level of accuracy to meet the specific needs of the disease screen.

Soil moisture

Measuring soil moisture can greatly aid in having an accurate and dependable disease screen, especially for soilborne pathogens. A wide range of tools are available for determining soil moisture. They are not much more expensive than simple soil probes, but are much more accurate, and are straightforward to operate. Tensiometers are devices that measure soil moisture tension. Tensiometers are sealed, water-filled tubes with a porous ceramic tip at the bottom and a vacuum gauge at the top that are inserted in the soil to plants' root zone depth. Water moves between the tensiometer tip and surrounding soil until equilibrium is reached, and moisture tension registers on the gauge at the top of the unit, and the readings indicate water availability in the soil. Tensiometers operate best at soil moisture tensions near field capacity and need to be serviced before reuse if they dry out.

Electrical resistance blocks, also known as gypsum blocks, measure soil water tension. They consist of two electrodes embedded in a block of porous material, usually gypsum; the electrodes are connected to lead wires that extend to the soil surface for reading by a portable meter. As water moves in or out of the porous block in equilibrium with the surrounding soil, changes in the electrical resistance between the two electrodes occur. Resistance meter readings are converted to water tension using a calibration curve. Gypsum blocks operate across a wider range of soil moisture tensions than tensiometers but tend to deteriorate over time and may even need to be replaced yearly. Granular matrix sensors are newer devices that are like gypsum blocks but are less susceptible to degradation.

Time domain reflectometry (TDR) is a newer tool that sends an electrical signal through steel rods placed in the soil and measures the signal return to estimate soil water content. Wet soil returns the signal more slowly than dry soil. This type of sensor gives fast, accurate readings of soil water content and requires little to no maintenance. However, it does require more work in interpreting data and may require special calibration depending on soil characteristics.

Light

Light is one of the most important environmental factors regulating plant growth, development, and photosynthesis. Having a healthy plant before subjecting it to the pathogen is paramount for a successful and meaningful screening. A plant that is stressed due to the lack of appropriate light will not provide an accurate result, and the plant breeder will have a challenging time determining if symptoms are due to susceptibility to the pathogen or other stresses. Light quality will affect disease development. The spectral composition of LED light influences disease development arising from virus, fungal, and bacterial sources. In the case of fungi, the inhibition of sporulation and germ tube growth by light is strongly wavelength-dependent, for example, near ultraviolet light induces and blue light inhibits sporulation in *B. cinerea*. Enhancing relative blue light levels or reducing ultraviolet irradiation through screening can help reduce disease in some cases. In contrast, red light has been found to improve resistance, for example, to the leaf spot fungus *Alternaria tenuissima* in broad bean (*Vicia faba*) and powdery mildew (*Sphaerotheca fuliginea*) in cucumber (*C. sativus*). The effect of light on disease screening could occur by affecting leaf physical properties such as water content, mechanical toughness and trichome density, leaf chemical content, quality of the host as a food resource, and host defense responses.

In the last decade or so, LEDs have become one of the most effective light sources, and are being developed to provide powerful, effective, and environmental emission spectra covering the entire photosynthetically active radiation range to precisely regulate numerous types of light combinations. When light-emitting diodes arrived on the market, their tremendous efficiency and money-saving potential changed the playing field. Lumens, lux, and foot-candles finally became obsolete metrics for determining light requirements for plants. When measuring light in growing environments, the terms photosynthetic active radiation (PAR), photosynthetic photon flux (PPF), and photosynthetic photon flux density (PPFD) are now used. The PAR can often be misunderstood because it is not a measurement or "metric" like centimeters, meters, or kilograms. Rather, PAR defines the type of light (electromagnetic radiation) needed to support photosynthesis in plant life. Interestingly, plants use roughly the same part of the spectrum that is visible to the human eye, but the wavelengths humans perceive to be the brightest, that is, green light are not the most efficient wavelengths for photosynthesis. The PPF measures the total amount of light that is produced by a light source each second and is expressed as μmol/second. The PPFD is the light that arrives at the plant and is measured in micromoles per square meter per second (μmol/m^2/sec). One last term used for measuring light for plant growth is daily light integral (DLI), which is the total amount of light that is delivered to a plant every day. It can be thought of as the plant's daily "dose" of light. The DLI measures the number of "moles" of photons per square meter per day and is expressed as mol/m^2/d.

There are numerous factors that affect the total amount of light that is delivered by a light device. While "lumens" was easy, it really had no consistent link to the amount of light being delivered to plants. The PAR, PPF, PPFD, and DLI are precise and consistent terms and measurements used by researchers around the world to make comparisons among experiments more precise.

Finally, it is important to always check the condition of the sensors before using them. If a meter's sensor system is too irreparably damaged, it will need to be replaced before use. The accuracy of an environmental monitor needs to be at the highest level otherwise, the disease screen can be compromised. Other tips include taking multiple measurements throughout the screening, including throughout the day. If a colleague has an environmental monitoring device, one can use it to check the accuracy of your device. By using the right equipment getting accurate environmental measurements does not have to be difficult.

As plant breeders, we are aware of the genotype by environment interaction; this is even more imperative when breeding for disease-resistant horticultural plants. Plant breeding programs will vary in the resources allocated to control environmental variation. The practicality of the situation dictates what a plant breeder can do to control the environmental components. However, when possible, a protected environment will be the ideal situation to control external abiotic and biotic factors.

Bibliography

Berry, S.Z., Thomas, C.A., 1961. Influence of soil temperature, isolates, and method of inoculation on resistance of mint to verticillium wilt. Phytopathology 51, 169–174.

Bhatia, A., Munkvold, G.P., 2002. Relationships of environmental and cultural factors with severity of gray leaf spot in maize. Plant Disease 86, 1127–1133. Available from: https://doi.org/10.1094/PDIS.2002.86.10.1127.

Blaker, N.S., MacDonald, J.D., 1986. The role of salinity in the development of Phytophthora root rot of citrus. Phytopathology 76, 970–975. <https://www.apsnet.org/publications/phytopathology/backissues/Documents/1986Articles/Phyto76n10_970.PDF>.

Bosland, P.W., Williams, P.H., Morrison, R.H., 1988. Influence of soil temperature on the expression of yellows and wilt of crucifers by *Fusarium oxysporum*. Plant Disease 72, 777–780.

Carmeille, A., Caranta, C., Dintinger, J., Prior, P., Luisetti, J., Besse, P., 2006. Identification of QTLs for *Ralstonia solanacearum* race 3-phylotype II resistance in tomato. Theoretical and Applied Genetics 113, 110–121. Available from: https://doi.org/10.1007/s00122-006-0277-3.

Cerrudo, I., Keller, M.M., Cargnel, M.D., Demkura, P.V., deWit, M., Patitucci, M.S., et al., 2012. Low red/far-red ratios reduce Arabidopsis resistance to *Botrytis cinerea* and jasmonate responses via a COI1-JAZ10-dependent, salicylic acid-independent mechanism. Plant Physiology 158, 2042–2052. Available from: https://doi.org/10.1104/pp.112.193359.

Chakrabortya, S., Tiedemann, A.V., Teng, P.S., 2000. Climate change: potential impact on plant diseases. Environmental Pollution 108, 317–326. Available from: https://doi.org/10.1016/S0269-7491(99)00210-9.

Chaloner, T.M., Gurr, S.J., Bebber, D.P., 2021. Plant pathogen infection risk tracks global crop yields under climate change. Nature Climate Change 11, 710–715. Available from: https://doi.org/10.1038/s41558-021-01104-8.

Colhoun, J., 1973. Effects of environmental factors on plant disease. Annual Review of Phytopathology 11, 343–364. Available from: https://doi.org/10.1146/annurev.py.11.090173.002015.

Donald, F., Green, S., Searle, K., Cunniffe, N.J., Purse, B.V., 2020. Small scale variability in soil moisture drives infection of vulnerable juniper populations by invasive forest pathogen. Forest Ecology and Management 473, 118324. Available from: https://doi.org/10.1016/j.foreco.2020.118324.

Downs, R.J., 1975. Controlled Environments for Plant Research. Columbia Univ. Press, N.Y., p. 175.

Downs, R.J., 1980. Phytotrons. The Botanical Review 46, 447–489. Available from: https://doi.org/10.1007/BF02860534.

Elad, Y., Pertot, I., 2014. Climate change impacts on plant pathogens and plant diseases. Journal of Crop Improvement 28, 99–139. Available from: https://doi.org/10.1080/15427528.2014.865412.

Fraser, R.S.S., Loughlin, S.A.R., 1982. Effects of temperature on the TM-1 gene for resistance to tobacco mosaic virus in tomato. Physiological. Plant Pathology 20, 109–115.

Gautam, H.R., Bhardwaj, M.L., Kumar, R., 2013. Climate change and its impact on plant diseases. Current Science 105, 1685–1691. <http://www.jstor.org/stable/24099750>.

Griffiths, E., Waller, J.M., 1971. Rainfall and cropping patterns in relations to coffee berry disease. Annals of Applied Biology 67, 75–91. Available from: https://doi.org/10.1111/j.1744-7348.1971.tb02908.x.

Howard, A., 1921. The influence of soil factors on disease resistance. Annals of Applied Biology 7, 373–389. Available from: https://doi.org/10.1111/j.1744-7348.1921.tb05525.x.

Kandel, J.S., Valentin, G., Miranda, S., Zhou, W., Read, Q.D., Mou, B., et al., 2022. Identification of quantitative trait loci associated with bacterial leaf spot resistance in baby leaf lettuce. Plant Disease. Available from: https://doi.org/10.1094/PDIS-09-21-2087-RE.

Kim, J.H., Hilleary, R., Seroka, A., He, S.Y., 2021. Crops of the future: building a climate-resilient plant immune system. Current Opinion in Plant Biology 60, 101997. Available from: https://doi.org/10.1016/j.pbi.2020.101997.

Kuwabara, C., Imai, R., 2009. Molecular basis of disease resistance acquired through cold accumulation in overwintering plants. Journal of Plant Biology 52, 19–26. Available from: https://doi.org/10.1007/s12374-008-9006-6.

Li, S., Liu, Y., Wang, J., Yang, L., Zhang, S., Xu, C., et al., 2017. Soil acidification aggravates the occurrence of bacterial wilt in South China. Frontiers in Plant Microbiology 8, 703. Available from: https://doi.org/10.3389/fmicb.2017.00703.

MacDonald, J.D., 1982. Effect of salinity stress on the development of Phytophthora root rot of Chrysanthemum. Phytopathology 72, 214–219. <https://www.apsnet.org/publications/phytopathology/backissues/Documents/1982Articles/Phyto72n02_214.pdf>.

Marsberg, A., Kemler, M., Jami, F., Nagel, J.H., Postma-Smidt, A., Naidoo, S., et al., 2017. Botryosphaeria dothidea: a latent pathogen of global importance to woody plant health. Molecular Plant Pathology 18, 477–488. Available from: https://doi.org/10.1111/mpp.12495.

Michel, V.V., Mew, T.W., 1998. Effect of soil amendment on the survival of *Ralstonia solanacearum* in different soils. Phytopathology 88, 300–305. Available from: https://doi.org/10.1094/PHYTO.1998.88.4.300.

Porter, A.S., Evans-Fitz Gerald, C., McElwain, J.C., Yiotis, C., Elliott-Kingston, C., 2015. How well do you know your growth chambers? Testing for chamber effect using plant traits. Plant Methods 11, 44–47. Available from: https://doi.org/10.1186/s13007-015-0088-0.

Roberts, J.M., Bruce, T.J.A., Monaghan, J.M., Pope, T.W., Leather, S.R., Beacham, A.M., 2020. Vertical farming systems bring new considerations for pest and disease management. Annals of Applied Biology 176, 226–232. Available from: https://doi.org/10.1111/aab.12587.

Romero, A.M., Kousik, C.S., Ritchie, D.F., 2002. Temperature sensitivity of the hypersensitive response of bell pepper to *Xanthomonas axonopodis* pv. *vesicatoria*. Phytopathology 92, 197–203. Available from: https://doi.org/10.1094/PHYTO.2002.92.2.197.

Sanogo, S., 2004. Response of chile pepper to *Phytophthora capsici* in relation to soil salinity. Plant Disease 88, 205–209. Available from: https://doi.org/10.1094/PDIS.2004.88.2.205.

Schuerger, A.C., Brown, C.S., 1997. Spectral quality affects disease development of three pathogens on hydroponically grown plants. HortScience 32, 96–100. Available from: https://doi.org/10.21273/HORTSCI.32.1.96.

Shin, I.S., Hsu, J.C., Huang, S.M., Chen, J.R., Wang, J.F., Hanson, P., et al., 2020. Construction of a single nucleotide polymorphism marker-based QTL map and validation of resistance loci to bacterial wilt caused by *Ralstonia solanacearum* species complex in tomato. Euphytica 216, 54. Available from: https://doi.org/10.1007/s10681-020-2576-1.

Strangeways, I., 2000. Measuring the Natural Environment. Cambridge University Press, New York, p. 365.

Tibbitts, T.W., Kozlowski, T.T. (Eds.), 1979. Controlled Environment Guidelines for Plant Research. Academic Press, New York, p. 432.

Virtuoso, M.C.S., Valente, T.S., Costa Silva, E.H., Braz, L.T., de Cassia Panizzi, R., Vargas, P.F., 2022. Implications of the inoculation method and environment in the selection of melon genotypes resistant to *Didymella bryoniae*. Scientia Horticulturae (Amsterdam) 300, 111066. Available from: https://doi.org/10.1016/j.scienta.2022.111066.

Walker, J.C., 1965. Use of environmental factors in screening for disease resistance. Annual Review of Phytopathology 3, 197–208. Available from: https://doi.org/10.1146/annurev.py.03.090165.001213.

Wang, Y., Bao, Z., Zhu, Y., Hua, J., 2009. Analysis of temperature modulation of plant defense against biotrophic microbes. Molecular Plant Microbe Interactions 22, 498–506. Available from: https://doi.org/10.1094/MPMI-22-5-0498.

Yasin, M., Rehman, A., 2021. Impact of climate change on pests and disease incidence on agricultural crops: a global prospective. Academia Letters. Available from: https://doi.org/10.20935/AL3667. Article 3667.

6

Resistance: evaluating the interaction phenotype

Introduction

Accurate measurement of the "Interaction Phenotype" is of utmost importance in a breeding program for developing disease-resistant horticultural cultivars. In natural epiphytotic diseases, the level of infection is often light or irregular making it impossible to truly distinguish between resistant and susceptible individuals. Resistance does occur naturally but is enhanced by selection within a plant breeding program. It is the plant breeder, who decides what the resistance interaction phenotype will be for their crop. For example, a small amount of leaf spotting on a crop where the fruit is harvested may be tolerated and considered resistant. If the leaves are the harvested plant part, then no blemishes may be accepted. Once the plant breeder has decided on the phenotype of resistance, it is important to have accurate assessment methods to evaluate germplasm. A single assessment method is not the same or appropriate in all situations. As mentioned in previous chapters, many factors can alter the disease resistance rating, for example, age of plants, inoculum level, temperature, humidity, and so on.

Disease assessment scales normally use disease phenotypic symptoms to classify the level of resistance in the host. Physicians are accustomed to classifying human diseases by their effects on the body. Physicians speak of fevers, colds, boils, gangrene, measles, jaundice, and so on as diseases that are recognizable by visible symptoms. Plant diseases likewise can be classified by their visible symptoms and are named accordingly, for example, spots, wilts, blights, rots, canker, rusts, and so forth. It must be remembered that the same symptoms may be caused by entirely different pathogens and require entirely different R-gene(s) to provide resistance. Wilting of plants may be the result of bacterial or fungal invasion, as well as a lack of water in the soil.

Spots on the foliage and stem are common evidence of disease. They are caused by various fungi and bacteria, the size, shape, and color of the spot being generally rather constant for the causal agent. Spots are often called "zonate," when marked with concentric zones of different appearance, like zonate leaf spot on cabbage (*Brassica oleracea* var. *capitata*), where brown, water-soaked, roughly circular, zonate spots develop on the inner leaves of the cabbage (*B. oleracea* var. *capitata*). Other times, the dead tissue in the disease spot may fall out, leaving a hole. When this happens to a number of small spots, the resulting appearance is often known as "shothole." Blotch diseases differ from spot disease because the diseased areas of a leaf have irregular shapes or blotch look. Anthracnose is the term originally associated with a disease caused by *Colletotrichum*. A well-known example is anthracnose (*Colletotrichum lindemuthianum*) of green bean (*Phaseolus* species) recognized by rusty spots on the leaves and pods. Ornamental species of *Ficus* grown as house plants often develop anthracnose (*Glomerella cingulata*, *Colletotrichum* species) areas on the leaves.

Blight is similar to blotch, but normally affects young growing tissues, especially leaves and twigs. Fire blight (*Erwinia amylovora*) of pear (*Pyrus communis*) is a well-known disease. Others are tomato blight, pepper blight, and potato blight caused by *Phytophthora* species.

Cankers are more or less localized disease, particularly of woody plants, but can be found on herbaceous plants. The causal agents can be either bacteria or fungi. Infection results in a shrinking and dying of the tissues that later crack open. Brown canker (*Coniothyrium* species) of roses, citrus canker (*Xanthomonas axonopodis*), and tomato canker (*Clavibacter michiganensis*) are examples.

Wilting is due to a deficiency of water in the leaves and stems. This may be due to the effects of pathogens, lack of water in the soil, or mechanical injury to the plant's roots. Both fungi and bacteria cause this symptom, and it can be difficult to distinguish the cause. Wilt of dahlias (*Dahlia pinnata*) is caused by both bacteria and fungi. Three major fungi that cause wilting disease are *Fusarium*, *Phytophthora*, and *Verticillium*.

Damping-off is most common with seedlings. The pathogen kills the tissues of the stem and root near the ground line causing the plant to fall over. *Pythium* and *Rhizoctonia* are the two major fungi causing this disease; however, *Aphanomyces*, *Phytophthora*, *Botrytis*, *Fusarium*, *Cylindrocladium*, *Diplodia*, *Phoma*, and *Alternaria* can also cause damping-off. Given the diversity of the pathogens, damping-off can affect a wide range of plant species and can cause losses for a number of economically important horticultural crops. There are two types of damping-off: preemergence, in which sprouting seeds decay in the soil and young seedlings rot before emergence; and postemergence, in which newly emerged seedlings suddenly wilt, collapse, and die from a soft rot at the soil line. Woody seedlings wilt and wither but remain upright; root decay often follows.

Rot disease is when pathogens cause the disintegration of living cells of plants in large numbers. Normally, they are grouped by the plant organ attached, that is, basal rot, heart rot, and root rot. Familiar examples of rot disease are heart rot (*Rhizoctonia solani*) of celery (*Apium graveolens* var. *dulce*), root rot (*Aphanomyces euteiches*) of English pea (*Pisum sativum*), and basal rot that often starts at the bulb base (root plate), progressing upward and outward.

Rusts may refer to any disease that causes reddish-brown spotting; hollyhock (*Alcea rosea*) rust (*Puccinia malvacearum*), snapdragon (*Antirrhinum majus*) rust (*Puccinia antirrhini*), and carnation (*Dianthus caryophyllus*) rust (*Uromyces caryophyllinus*) are among the most common rusts of ornamentals. Smuts are black pustules, one of the most common is sweet corn smut (*Ustilago maydis*).

Powdery mildew is the name given to a group of diseases caused by several closely related fungi. Their common symptom is a grayish-white, powdery mat visible on the surface of leaves, stems, and flower petals. Downy mildews are distinctly different from powdery mildews. Downy mildew colonies often appear first on the underside of leaves, and they sometimes have a bluish tinge. In many cases, they can grow systemically throughout the plant. If growing abundantly on a leaf, downy mildew colonies can be confused with gray mold (*Botrytis*) or with powdery mildew.

Galls are seen as swellings or an abnormal, localized outgrowth of plant tissue. Galls can be caused by bacteria, fungi, viruses, and nematodes. Nematode root galls are often associated with *Meloidogyne incognita*. Club root is one of the important diseases affecting crucifers, like cabbage (*B. oleracea* var. *capitata*), Chinese cabbage (*Brassica rapa*), and some species of candytuft (*Iberis sempervirens*).

Witches' Broom is caused by phytoplasmas (mycoplasma-like organisms) that are obligate intracellular parasites of plant phloem tissue and of the insect vectors that are involved in their plant-to-plant transmission. Besides, witches' broom—proliferation of shoots or branches, they cause a wide variety of symptoms ranging from leaf stunting (little leaf), yellow discoloration of the foliage (yellows), greening of flower petals, precocious or suppressed flowering, precocious shoot growth, loss of apical dominance of the shoots, leading to deliquescent branching, branch dieback, suppressed root development, and eventual plant death.

Leaf mosaic and chlorosis are normally symptoms of viruses. The mosaic pattern is formed with a pattern of light and dark green areas, while chlorosis is associated with a yellowish or whitish discoloration. Other symptoms of virus infection include necrotic spots, mottling of leaves, growth distortion, stunting, ring patterns, and abnormal flower coloration and formation. Plants may also be infected with more than one virus or viral strain causing a combination of symptoms or more severe symptoms as a result of multiple infections.

Traditional methods assessing the resistance phenotype, such as the use of pictorial keys derived from standard area diagrams to evaluate disease severity on a 0%–100% scale, have now been joined by several new approaches made possible by rapid advances in computer technology. In addition, modern assays using immunological and molecular techniques for the identification, detection, and quantification of plant pathogenic organisms are exploited. Other new approaches include remote sensing, image analysis, and for field studies the detection of crop stress caused by disease using changes in chlorophyll fluorescence and foliage temperature.

Disease screen/index

Normally when evaluating plants for their disease resistance to a pathogen, the term "disease screen" is used when the resistant plants are saved, while "disease index" is most often used when the plants are scored for resistance and susceptibility and then discarded. It is worth repeating that for disease resistance evaluations, reliable and reproducible inoculation protocols are essential. Screening must be reliable, meaning that one can trust that a plant recorded as resistant will be resistant in production and that a plant scored susceptible would not provide protection for a grower. Reproducible means that year in and year out the test gives the same results. Furthermore, if another laboratory does the disease screening, they must feel confident that their screening technique is giving similar results. It is essential that for each breeding generation, the disease screen is done under controlled conditions. Crucial to the screening technique is that the test must not produce escapes, that is,

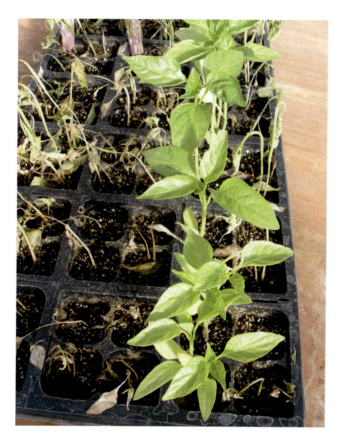

Figure 6.1 A tray of chile peppers (*Capsicum annuum*) that were screened for resistance to Phytophthora root rot. The "healthy" looking plants are in fact susceptible but are escapes because they were not inoculated with the pathogen, producing pseudoresistance.

plants having the phenotype resistance, but are genetically susceptible plants (pseudoresistant). The test should also not be so severe as to cause disease symptoms in resistant plants. Therefore the interaction phenotype must correlate with the genotype. This is critical because all entries are indistinguishable in the absence of the pathogen (Fig. 6.1).

Evaluation of disease resistance

Critical information needed from the screening is the amount of disease that is present. This can be measured as the proportion of a plant community that is diseased (disease incidence) or as the proportion of plant area that is affected (disease severity). Disease severity is normally what plant breeders are measuring. Screening done in the field, such as grower's fields or research plots, adds a layer of complexity to the test, through the introduction of confounding factors (uncontrolled conditions that result in the unclear expression of the disease or affect the phenotypes of the plants). For example, "sick plots" or a disease nursery, which are field plots where the soil is heavily infested with the pathogen of interest, are a common tool for field screening for resistance. Researchers at Michigan State University, United States use a disease nursery to screen for potato common scab (*Streptomyces scabies*) a major disease of potato (*Solanum tuberosum*). The Michigan State University field scab nursery was developed to promote a high incidence of potato common scab (*S. scabies*) disease by planting susceptible potato (*S. tuberosum*) varieties, inoculating with a pathogenic strain of *S. scabies*, and incorporating spring and fall manure applications for 3 years before field evaluation. This site has been planted continuously in potatoes (*S. tuberosum*) with periodic inoculations to maintain potato common scab (*S. scabies*) disease pressure. To account for the variability usually found in a field nursery, their trials are planted as a randomized complete block design with five-hill plots and four replications.

At the University of Illinois, United States, researchers in 1984 established a disease nursery to evaluate sweet corn (*Zea mays*) accessions disease reactions to four diseases that consistently were prevalent on sweet corn grown in North America, including common rust (*Puccinia sorghi*), northern corn leaf blight (*Exserohilum turcicum*), Stewart's wilt (*Pantoea stewartia/* syn. *Erwinia stewartii*), and maize dwarf mosaic (MDM, *Potyviridae*). In some years, sweet corn (*Z. mays*) accessions were also evaluated for reactions to diseases that occurred more sporadically on sweet corn (*Z. mays*), including southern corn leaf blight (*Bipolaris maydis*), anthracnose leaf blight (*Colletotrichum graminicola*), gray leaf spot (*Cercospora zeae-maydis*), and Goss's wilt (*C. michiganensis* subsp. *nebraskensis*). The researchers state that it is extremely difficult to develop an elite, superior inbred, but it is very easy to lose that superiority when attempting to improve an elite inbred for a specific trait, such as disease resistance. Thus sweet corn (*Z. mays*) breeders have relied heavily on simply inherited resistances when they are effective because simply inherited resistance can be backcrossed into elite materials with less risk of losing the superiority of the recurrent parent. Improvement in polygenic resistance has been more difficult but may occur more frequently in the future as the marker-assisted selection is used to improve elite sweet corn (*Z. mays*) lines by incorporating quantitative trait loci with major effects for disease resistance. As new, improved inbreds are used in hybrid combinations, field trials will continue to be necessary to confirm the phenotypic performance of these new hybrids. Trials like the Illinois disease nursery will continue to provide the sweet corn industry with documentation of the relative levels of resistance to economically important diseases among new sweet corn (*Z. mays*) hybrids.

It is well documented that neighboring plants influence the level of disease observed in a screening test. It is easy to see how a plant that is very susceptible to powdery mildew could produce more inoculum and cause its neighbor to have a phenotype that is less resistant than a plant next to a partially resistant plant. Whether neighbor plants differ in their levels of plant resistance is of particular interest and is poorly understood. The mechanism driving this neighbor effect can be broadly categorized as plant trait–mediated indirect effects. Plant trait–mediated indirect effects occur when neighbors interact directly with local plants and alter the phenotypic traits involved in plant resistance.

The role of neighbor identity has been relatively overlooked, especially in those studies looking at how competition influences plant resistance. This is perhaps because the effects of competition on resistance have been viewed generically in terms of resource availability, and although it is known that species vary in how they alter resource availability, few competition studies have specifically tested whether neighbor plant differs in their effects on plant resistance.

This concept of neighboring plants influencing the resistance phenotype leads to the use of multiline cultivars and cultivar mixtures for disease management of rusts and powdery mildews. Such mixtures are more useful under some epidemiological conditions than under others, and experimental methodology, especially problems of scale, may be crucial in evaluating the potential efficacy of mixtures on disease. There are now examples of mixtures providing both low and high degrees of disease control for a wide range of pathosystems, including crops with large plants, and pathogens that demonstrate low host specificity, or are splash dispersed, soilborne, or insect vectored. Though most analyses of pathogen evolution in mixtures consider static costs of virulence to be the main mechanism countering selection for pathogen complexity, many other potential mechanisms need to be investigated. Horticultural quality and marketing considerations must be carefully evaluated when implementing mixture approaches to crop management.

In the presence of drought stress, one cannot accurately phenotype for a wilting disease in a disease nursery. These confounding factors can be identified through the use of check lines that are entries with a known response to the pathogen, and usually include a highly resistant and a highly susceptible line. If the resistant check is wilting in the sick plot, one can deduce that there is likely another factor involved, and the results of the disease screen cannot be trusted. Therefore in most instances, the testing is done under a laboratory, growth chamber, or greenhouse environment, where greater control over the test can be administered.

Plant diseases bear names such as leaf blights, root rots, sheath blights, tuber scabs, and stem cankers, indicating that symptoms occur preferentially on specific parts of host plants. Accordingly, many plant pathogens are specialized to infect and cause disease in specific tissues and organs. Conversely, others can infect a range of tissues, albeit often disease symptoms fluctuate in different organs infected by the same pathogen. Depending on the disease, the plant breeder has choices to make when deciding what part of the plant to inoculate, for example, whether to use whole seedlings, mature whole plants, excised tissues, cultured tissues and cells, meristem, cotyledons, leaves, stems, roots, fruits, seeds, storage organs, flowers, detached organs, and so on. In some instances, the pathogen can cause different and independent disease syndromes on different plant organs as with Phytophthora stem blight, Phytophthora root rot, and Phytophthora foliar blight caused by *Phytophthora capsici* on pepper (*Capsicum annuum*). The key is for the inoculation to be representative of the infection process faced by the grower.

Nathan Cobb in 1892 developed the first standard area diagram for wheat leaf rust (*Puccinia triticina*), the Cobb scale. The scale was devised for estimating, by means of diagrams, the proportion of the area of a leaf or stem occupied by rust pustules. He divided rust severity into five grades representing 0%, 5%, 10%, 20%, and 50% of leaf area occupied by the visible or sporulating rust pustules. The highest grade (50%) represented the maximum possible cover.

After the Cobb scale, researchers devised many more assessments of disease scales. Many assessment measurements use a rating scale. A standard style is the "0–9 Scale" for nonparametric quantification, where 0 = immune (noninoculated control); 1 = very high resistance; 2 = high resistance; 3 = resistant; 4 = moderate resistance (weakly susceptible); 5 = intermediate resistance–susceptibility; 6 = moderate susceptibility (weakly resistant); 7 = susceptible; 8 = high susceptibility; 9 = very high susceptibility (death). The 0–9 system was developed in the era of computer cards where each integral had to be between 0 and

9, otherwise another column on the computer card needed to be used. Today, a scale could theoretically have more divisions. The plant breeder decides on the amount of disease severity for each category. For example, symptoms could be a hypersensitive response, necrosis, chlorosis, wilting, tissue maceration, tissue collapse, stunting, malformations, yield reduction, loss of flowering, loss of fruit, delay in development, and so on.

One of the first steps in developing the disease screen is choosing the right controls for the disease screen. Different cultivars can vary in their resistance and susceptibility. For the susceptible control, it is best to choose a cultivar that growers agree is susceptible in their growing operation. Knowing that resistance is a continuum, it may be appropriate to include a partial resistant and an immune control.

Next it is important to screen with the correct pathogen. This seems obvious, but there is an enlightening story about a plant breeder who spent years developing a powdery mildew (*Podosphaera xanthii*)-resistant cucurbit, but once it was planted in the field it succumbed to disease. The disease in the field was in fact downy mildew (*Pseudoperonospora cubensis*) not powdery mildew; unfortunately, the breeder had misidentified the pathogen and spent several years breeding resistance to the wrong pathogen.

A breeder needs to be aware of pathogenic variants (e.g., races, strains, pathotypes, etc.) and which one to use in the screening. A successful cultivar need not be resistant to all races or strains, but only to the prevalent one in the geographic region where the cultivar will be grown. Another aspect of most breeding programs is screening for multiple disease resistance. When undertaking multiple disease screening, factors that need to be considered are simultaneous and sequential inoculation of different pathogens or different races of the same pathogen, and the interactions caused by multiple inoculations. This topic will be examined in detail in Chapter 9.

Quantifying host resistance

The first step to quantify disease is to develop a key that describes the disease on the plant. Detail drawings, photographs, or descriptions of the various stages of the disease are needed. Standardized disease assessment keys have been developed for several horticultural crop plants enabling comparison between programs. The Horsfall–Barratt scale is a classic way to quantify host resistance. The Horsfall–Barratt scale assigns each plant a numerical value according to the percentage of leaf area showing disease symptoms. It was designed in 1945 by James G. Horsfall and R.W. Barratt to compensate for human error in estimating the amount of disease present. They stumbled onto two principles: (1) that the human eye is a photocell that reads in logarithms according to the Weber–Fechner law of human acuity and (2) that the eye reads the amount of diseased tissue below 50% and the amount of healthy tissue above 50% best.

The researchers at the Department of Plant Pathology at Viçosa Federal University in Brazil with help from the Department of Plant Pathology at the Ohio State University, United States, used standard area diagrams to assess the severity of potato early blight (*Alternaria grandis*) on leaves of potato (*S. tuberosum*). The proposed standard area diagrams include images of leaves with 10 distinct disease severities (0.1%, 1%, 3%, 5%, 10%, 20%, 40%, 60%, 80%, and 100% infection). The diagrams were validated by 12 raters who had no previous experience in evaluating plant disease. Lin's concordance correlation analysis of estimated versus actual disease severity (based on image analysis) showed that precision and accuracy improved for most raters using the diagrams as compared to assessments made without the diagrams. The diagrams improved raters' ability to accurately, precisely, and reliably estimate potato early blight severity, and as such will be beneficial when breeding for resistance (Fig. 6.2).

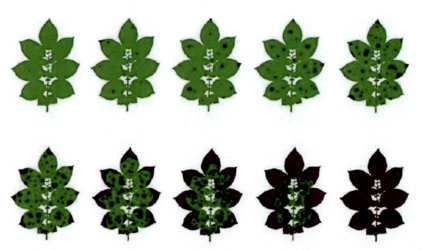

Figure 6.2 Standard area diagrams for early blight (*Alternaria grandis*) severity on potato (*Solanum tuberosum*) leaves. The numbers represent the percentage (%) of leaf area showing symptoms of the disease. Courtesy: European Journal of Plant Pathology, https://doi.org/10.1007/s10658-013-0234-3.

Identifying resistant genotypes in pepper (*Capsicum* species) to anthracnose (*Colletotrichum* species) has challenged plant breeders. Researchers at Darcy Ribeiro North Fluminense State University, Brazil, developed a quantitative ordinal 0–9 scale for quantifying anthracnose disease on detached pepper (*Capsicum* species) fruits. Their rating scale is based on the presence/absence of acervuli (small asexual fruiting body that erupts through the epidermis of host plants) and lesion diameter. They confirmed that inoculation and disease assessment techniques play an important role in finding anthracnose resistance in pepper (*C. annuum*) fruits, especially when considering different *Capsicum* species. Their scale had superior agreement, accuracy, and precision for assessing the anthracnose severity in four species of *Capsicum* fruits. Anthracnose assessments based on this scale produced more reliable results for discriminating resistant from susceptible genotypes, which directly impacts *Capsicum* breeding aimed at resistance to this disease. Unripe and ripe fruits from 11 genotypes were inoculated with 10 μL of conidial suspension of 1×10^6 conidia/mL by a microinjector. Five raters daily assessed anthracnose severity in 79 fruits, using three different methods, (1) lesion area by image analysis; (2) lesion area by caliper measure, and (3) two rating scales. On the ninth day after inoculation, the severity was estimated by seven raters using the two scales and measurement of lesion diameters. From the data collected, they defined nine severity levels on the new proposed susceptibility scale based on the presence/absence of acervuli/hyphae and the lesion diameter.

Disease assessment methods need to provide objective measurements for a specific growth stage of a crop so that data from different sources are comparable and provide an adequate sample of the crop for assessment. Whether it is disease incidence, or disease severity, or both, that are measured, depends on the nature of the disease. An "all or nothing" disease, for example, that inevitably kills any plant it infects could be measured just by counting the number of plants that are infected (disease incidence), for example, *Phytophthora*. However, in the case of a disease that causes varying degrees of damage to plants throughout the crop, a more complex measurement is needed that assesses disease severity. The best one is the simplest one that gives results that transfer to the growing condition of the crop.

To produce a disease assessment key, the development of disease over the whole disease cycle and at different stages of plant growth must be studied to make prototype standard diagrams and descriptions. The accuracy of the key then needs to be tested, by assessing disease severity in the field using the key and then assessing the same samples using accurate measurement techniques in the laboratory. There are also computer programs designed to train observers in disease severity assessment, by presenting images of diseased leaves, which the observer assesses, and comparing their result with the known level of disease in the diagram. This aims to reduce variation in results caused by different observers.

The US Department of Agriculture researchers have developed automated imaging and analysis methods for powdery mildew (*Erysiphe necator*) severity on grape (*Vitis vinifera*) leaf disks. Powdery mildews present specific challenges to phenotyping systems that are based on imaging because, in the earliest stages of development, the hyphae appear transparent and are closely appressed to a leaf surface overlain by a topographically complex and highly reflective wax cuticle prone to emit glare when live specimens are illuminated for microscopy and photomicrography. With appropriate lighting or staining, nascent colonies originating from conidia or ascospores of *E. necator* can be resolved using 3–10 magnifications within 48 hours after inoculation. They used low-throughput, quantitative microscopy to phenotype thousands of grape leaf disk samples for genetic analysis of resistance. The system captured 78% of the area of a 1-cm diameter leaf disk in 3–10 focus-stacked images within 13.5–26 seconds. The system agreed with human experts 89%–92% of the time. This live-imaging approach was nondestructive and a repeated measures time course of infection showed differentiation among susceptible, moderate, and resistant samples. Processing more than 1000 samples per day with good accuracy, the system can assess grape resistance to powdery mildew.

Scoring fatigue

Intrapersonal variability refers to differences taking place within one individual, while interpersonal variability refers to differences taking place between people. General fatigue affects a person's ability to perform a task. Being in a hot field or greenhouse for hours can easily bring about fatigue. Because evaluating plants for resistance involves heavy reliance on visual input, special attention needs to be given to the more specific problem of visual fatigue.

The term visual fatigue is imprecise, and it implies some form of discomfort or complaint associated with the eyes and has often been referred to as "eyestrain." Visual fatigue may be influenced by both environmental factors and individual factors. Visual fatigue is influenced by more than visual activity alone; environmental factors, such as pollen, wind, dust, and even one's perspiration getting into the eyes can accelerate visual fatigue, as well as an individual's own genetic make-up can influence susceptibility to visual fatigue. Visual fatigue is a real phenomenon and has been documented in such tasks as reading, and so-called "close work" such as sewing, proofreading, and visual inspection tasks in manufacturing settings. Closely examining plant organs or whole seedlings can fit into this "close work" category. It is interesting to note that in the 1980s through the 1990s, concern focused on office work, particularly work involving computers and the use of video. More recently, visual fatigue has also surfaced as a problem with 3D stereoscopic displays meaning that as we transition to more video and computer imaging for the resistance rating of plants, fatigue will still be with us.

Visual fatigue also occurs when examining a multitude of similar items consecutively. In the realm of breeding for disease-resistant horticultural plants, fatigue often strikes during the afternoon taking a toll on one's ability to distinguish between the different classes of resistance. The individual could be recuperating from a large lunch, hot temperatures, loss of sleep the night before, and so on. Many believe that visual fatigue occurs when eyes are simply overworked; however, researchers believe otherwise. The theory is that your brain, not the light receptors in your eye, becomes fatigued with similar sensory information. This is a more solid theory because our brains function like computers. When one experiences something with our senses, it sends a data signal to the brain. The brain then decodes the data into a sensory profile one can then experience. When multiple similar data signals are sent in rapid succession, the brain begins to mix up the signals and creates false readings like visual fatigue.

How does one prevail against visual fatigue? The simple answer is to take a break from scoring plants and give the brain a chance to clear its cache. Scoring fatigue is natural, thus the key is to stop it before it happens. However, there are more sophisticated and costly approaches for handling inter- and intrapersonal variability during scoring.

Automated data collection

To eliminate, or greatly reduce, the role of human error during phenotyping, as well as collecting a large amount of data in a more high-throughput manner, there has been a recent shift towards the use of automated data collection of the plant phenome. In 1949, the term phenome was first used in bacterium by Bernard Davis of Cornell University, United States, but recently has been adopted by plant scientists. Complementary to the genome, a phenome is the sum of a set of phenotypes expressed by a plant. Breeding disease-resistant horticulture crops and precision agriculture are key strategies to reduce yield losses due to plant disease in a sustainable way. Both rely on the detection, identification, and quantification of plant disease on various scales. In disease resistance breeding host–pathogen interactions are examined at the cell, tissue, whole plant, and field plot levels. Focusing on the cell or tissue level can uncover the distinct mechanisms that determine plant resistance or susceptibility, and precise quantification of disease or resistance levels in whole plants or field plots aids the selection of the best genotypes. The challenge to detect and quantify plant disease in an unbiased and precise way initiated the field of plant disease phenotyping. In general, a plant's phenotype is the manifestation of a genotype under specific environmental conditions. In the context of the host–pathogen interaction, the phenotype consists of changes that can be described as contrasting indications of disease: signs and symptoms. Whereas these terms were originally used for changes that are visible to the human eye, they can also be used for changes that can be detected by noninvasive sensors.

Manually obtaining a plant's phenome is tedious or nearly impossible, especially over the multiple weeks required to conduct a typically disease bioassay. To overcome this, several precise and sophisticated tools have been developed to capture the phenome in a nondestructive way over long periods of time. For automated data collection, sensors are typically placed above the plants either in a fixed position where plants are on a moving conveyor belt or on a gantry that moves across the entire growing area. The most common forms of the sensor for automated data collection are those that measure reflected red, blue, green, and infrared wavelengths, although other more costly and elaborate sensors utilize thermal imaging or hyperspectral imaging. No matter the form of data collected, the fundamental principle is that light reflectance from the interaction between the natural light spectrum with plant components can provide accurate information on the morphological and physiological status of plants. The light reflectance captured by specially designed optical instruments can then generate vegetation indices and digital plant objects.

Visual estimates are based only on the perception of wavelengths of the electromagnetic spectrum in the human visible range (380–750 nm), while hyperspectral and multispectral systems use wavelengths in the range 250–2500 nm. Some of the first methods to standardize plant disease evaluations was the use of image capture in the visible spectrum followed by processing using image analysis software to determine disease severity. More recently, the use of image capture in the invisible (hyperspectral and multispectral) ranges and chlorophyll fluorescence has been adopted to determine the amount of disease. Using these systems researchers can capture the plant phenome over time after inoculation with a particular pathogen. It is possible to have much more accurate data over a time course and be able to assess host resistance in a highly accurate manner. However, these systems are costly, and specialists are needed to manage the complex software and handle the large data sets. Furthermore, there are highly accurate ways to quantify disease resistance over a time course using manual measurements.

A new area of automated data collecting that may assist the plant breeder in increasing the efficiency of scoring resistance in the field is with the soilborne plant pathogens and the seedling, vascular, and root rot diseases they cause. It is laborious and time consuming to manually score and record the interaction phenotype of individual plants in a large field planting. Inexpensive and reliable disease quantification would optimize plant breeding programs.

Sensor technologies are a promising tool for automated plant disease quantification, which may assist the plant breeder in scoring large numbers of individuals. This is a rapidly expanding area of research. Sensors that can potentially be used to quantify plant disease severity for the plant breeder are grouped into two general categories: optical and nonoptic. Various types of optical sensors have been used to quantify plant disease. These include RGB (red–green–blue), multispectral and hyperspectral reflectance, thermal, fluorescence, and light detection and ranging (LiDAR) sensors. Among these sensors, spectral reflectance and infrared thermography are of particular interest in quantifying plant disease and plant phenotyping because they can be utilized with ground-based, airborne, and satellite-based platforms.

Among the nonoptical type sensors, those that can detect volatile organic compounds (VOCs) emitted by the plant and/or pathogen during disease development have been utilized the most for plant disease detection. These include but are not limited to VOC-trapping devices coupled with gas chromatography–mass spectrometry (GC–MS), electronic noses (e-nose), and other novel VOC sensors. Researchers at North Carolina State University, United States, used a VOC fingerprinting platform that allows noninvasive diagnosis of late blight (*Phytophthora infestans*) on tomato (*Solanum lycopersicum*) by monitoring characteristic leaf volatile emissions in the field. Their handheld device integrates a disposable colorimetric sensor array consisting of plasmonic nanocolorants and chemoresponsive organic dyes to detect key plant volatiles at the part-per-million (ppm) level within one minute of reaction. The field-portable VOC-sensing platform allowed for early detection of tomato late blight 2 days after inoculation, and differentiation from other pathogens of tomato (*S. lycopersicum*) that lead to similar symptoms on tomato (*S. lycopersicum*) foliage. Their detection accuracy was greater than 95% in the diagnosis of *P. infestans* in both laboratory-inoculated and field-collected tomato (*S. lycopersicum*) leaves in blind pilot tests.

Another example of using VOCs is with Aphanomyces root rot (*A. euteiches*), an important soilborne disease of peas (*P. sativum*). The typical symptoms include lesions on the root tissue, reduced root size/function, yellowing/wilting of lower leaves, and sometime premature plant death. Potential loss of up to 80% can be reached with this pathogen. Resistance in pea (*P. sativum*), to Aphanomyces root rot is quantitative with very few cultivars with high levels of partial resistance. In a proof-of-concept study, researchers at the Washington State University, United States, investigated whether VOCs and other semiochemicals can be utilized to phenotype resistance to Aphanomyces root rot in pea (*P. sativum*). They used a susceptible cultivar, Ariel, and a cultivar with high levels of partial resistance, Hampton. Both nondestructive (whole plant) and destructive (root and shoot) sampling of emitted volatiles using gas chromatography–flame ionization detector and GC–MS systems quantified the VOCs. In addition, the pyrolysis GC–MS system quantified the VOCs in the destructive sampling of shoot and root tissues. Plants were monitored nondestructively for VOC emission at three time points, 15, 20, and 30 days after inoculation using dynamic headspace sampling with gas chromatography–flame ionization detection (GC-FID) system, as well as destructively at the end of the experiments, using solvent extraction and pyrolysis of both shoot and root tissues. A noninoculated control (mock-inoculated with distilled water) was utilized to compare the plant responses within a cultivar. Unique chemical peaks present in inoculated samples, but not in control samples were also identified and their relative peak intensities were compared. Among the released green leaf volatiles, the normalized relative peak intensity of hexanal emission, at

20 days postinoculation, was higher in the susceptible cultivar as compared to the resistant cultivar. Based on the differences in putative chemical peaks between cultivars, their initial study supports the concept of utilization of biogenic biomarker–based phenotyping in distinguishing levels of resistance in pea (*P. sativum*). They concluded that the VOC profile integrated with high-throughput VOCs sensing techniques can serve as a novel mechanism for phenotyping disease responses in peas (*P. sativum*).

Although there has recently been an exponential increase in research aimed at utilizing various sensor technologies for quantifying plant disease, additional studies and chronological improvements aimed at identifying and detecting disease-specific signatures are needed before they can be used as a practical tool for the plant breeder. The sensitivity and specificity of sensor-based methods, which is highly dependent on spatial resolution, that is, the minimum size of a pixel in image-based optical sensors, rely on the distance between the sensor and the object. Proximal sensing platforms are suitable for quantifying disease at leaf and plant scale, whereas remote sensing with airborne platforms is useful for detecting soilborne disease patches in the field or in later stages of disease epidemics. Currently, one of the major limitations to using sensors for plant disease quantification is the lack of an efficient method to analyze and interpret the great amount of complex data generated with sensor measurements. Machine learning algorithms may offer a very promising approach that can be used to collate and statistically evaluate large amounts of sensor data more efficiently and without explicit programing.

Area under the disease progress curve

The area under the disease progress curve (AUDPC) is a quantitative measure of disease resistance and compares levels of resistance among accessions. The AUDPC is the progression of the disease level across time. The trapezoid method is the most common way to calculate AUDPC. It is performed by using a formula devised by C. Lee Campbell and Laurence V. Campbell in 1990 or by plotting a graph of the percentage of infection against time and summing the trapezoids between time intervals. A common method for estimating the AUDPC is to discretize (discretization is the process of transferring continuous functions into discrete counterparts) the time variable (hours, days, etc.) and calculate the average disease intensity between each pair of adjacent time points. This process will combine multiple observations of disease progress into a single value. A common formula for AUDPC is provided below, where t = time points with an interval (i) that can be consistent or vary, and y = the measurement of the disease level:

$$\text{AUDPC} = \sum_{i=1}^{N_i-1} \frac{(y_i + y_{i+1})}{2}(t_{i+1} - t_i)$$

Researchers at Clemson University compared 14 cucurbit species for susceptibility to gummy stem blight (*Stagonosporopsis citrulli*) with the AUDPC. The 14 cucurbit species of unknown susceptibility represented twelve genera, four taxonomic tribes, and four geographic origins. An additional species, *Cucumis melo*, was included as a control because of its known high susceptibility. Using the AUDPC, they found the cucurbit species *Apodanthera sagittifolia*, *Ecballium elaterium*, and *Kedrostis leloja* were as least as susceptible to gummy stem blight as the control reference *C. melo*. More importantly, they discovered that *Coccinia grandis* was highly resistant to gummy stem blight, and *Sicana odorifera* and *Zehneria pallidinervia* were grouped with the most resistant species. The AUDPC detected that the most susceptible species had the fastest disease progression.

Malaysian researchers used the AUDPC screen for resistance to black pod (*Phytophthora palmivora*) in cocoa (*Theobroma cacao*). The detached pod test has been regarded as the most economical and effective screening method as compared to selection of resistant genotypes in the field. They evaluated the accuracy of the assessment technique used in the detached pod test between the estimation of the AUDPC and the standard assessment of diameter lesion recorded on the sixth day after inoculation of four genotypes. The four genotypes were KKM4 (susceptible), KKM5 (moderate susceptible), BR25 (moderate resistant), and QH1003 (resistant) at two development pod stages, young and mature pods. The researchers found that the assessment of the mature cocoa (*T. cacao*) genotypes for resistance to black pod using AUDPC gave the best accuracy (100%) of resistant level as compared to standard assessment (50%) meanwhile both assessment techniques on young pods gave similar percentage (50%) of accuracy.

Detached leaf screening

Detached leaf screening has successfully tested for resistance and susceptibility for several crops. As with any screening technique, the detached leaf screen requires that the disease response be assessed with accurate and reproducible techniques. Detached leaf inoculation assays determined plant germplasm resistance to late blight (*P. infestans*) in tomato (*S. lycopersicum*), Alternaria blotch (*Alternaria mali*) in apple (*Malus domestica*), and American chestnut (*Castanea dentata*) for resistance to chestnut blight (*Cryphonectria parasitica*). For clonally propagated crops, detached leaf screening can reduce the time of screening for disease resistance benefiting the plant breeder. For example, inoculating detached strawberry (*Fragaria × ananassa*) leaves with anthracnose pathogens (*Colletotrichum* sp.) allows assessment for anthracnose resistance without destroying whole plants and lessens the time between inoculation and disease assessment. Whole strawberry (*Fragaria × ananassa*) plant inoculations to screen for anthracnose resistance are accurate and reproducible, but they are time consuming, and plants are often killed by the disease, which can present a problem for the breeder because the germplasm may have possessed other desirable horticultural traits.

Melinda A. Miller-Butler and her colleagues found that screening for anthracnose resistance using detached strawberry (*Fragaria × ananassa*) leaves is an acceptable alternative to inoculating whole plants and can eliminate the destruction of desirable germplasm. The detached leaf assay provided a rapid, nondestructive method of reliably identifying anthracnose-resistant germplasm, thus allowing the screening process to move forward with enhanced efficiency.

Richard Craig and colleagues at Pennsylvania State University, United States found that screening detached leaves of *Pelargonium* for *Botrytis* resistance was successful. They were able to differentiate levels of resistance among 45 different cultivars. They further determined that no trends in resistance when comparing diploid and tetraploid pelargoniums or when comparing ivy, zonal, and floribunda types was evident. Interestingly, they found cultivars introduced since 1990 have greater susceptibility than older genotypes. This implies that plant breeders were not selecting for resistance because fungicide applications were working well.

Another successful detached leaf screening is for downy mildew (*Peronospora effusa*) on spinach (*Spinacia oleracea*). The standard inoculation method was labor and resource-intensive test of whole plants, in a large tray format, in a temperature-controlled growth chamber and dew chamber. Researchers at the University of Arkansas, United States, evaluated the detached leaf inoculation method for disease incidence and disease severity on detached leaves and cotyledons and the same cultivars in the standard whole plant assay. They found 100% correlation between the disease reaction on whole plants and the disease reaction on detached leaves.

When powdery mildew (*P. xanthii*) resistance on cucumbers (*Cucumis sativus*) was tested using either a seedling spray inoculation in the field or a leaf disk infection in the laboratory, both gave the same results.

Unfortunately, not all detached leaf screening techniques are successful. When three methods, mycelial plug inoculations of cotyledons, cut stems, and detached leaves, were used to identify levels of resistance to *Sclerotinia sclerotiorum* in green beans (*Phaseolus vulgaris*), the detached leaf did not accurately identify susceptible and partially resistant cultivars. For the three resistance screening methods under controlled environmental conditions, the cut stem method was statistically better than the cotyledon and detached leaf methods for evaluating resistance in green bean cultivars.

A key objective for many *Capsicum* breeding programs is the development of cultivars resistant to Phytophthora foliar blight (*P. capsici*). A detached leaf technique that reflects the whole plant genotype could reduce the assay time and require only a leaf instead of the whole plant. At New Mexico State University, United States, a detached leaf technique was compared to the whole plant method; unfortunately, the detached leaf method could not produce results matching the existing whole plant screening method. Therefore the detached leaf method was not a suitable way to screen for foliar blight resistance in *Capsicum*.

Rating scales

In assessing disease resistance there are two major approaches, ranking versus rating scales. Ranking, theoretically, is the best because humans can place the plants in ascending or descending order of resistance. After the plants have been placed in order, one can make a demarcation choosing one side as resistant and the other side as susceptible. The drawback to ranking is that it is time consuming. Scoring the same plant material can take 2–3 times longer with ranking than with a rating scale.

The Horsfall–Barratt scale is considered a classic rating system. It is a visual rating system based on a semiquantitative scale to assess plant disease where each plant is assigned a numerical value according to the percentage of leaf area showing disease symptoms. This provided the rationale for their new system of grading in which the grades were placed logarithmically, not arithmetically. Thus Horsfall and Barratt proposed a $\log_{10}$-based scale to assign the percent foliage affected into 1 of 11 severity classes. They stated that humans can best separate disease on plants at above 50% and below 50%. As greater differentiation is made, it becomes more difficult to tell the difference by human eyes, and thus they believed this compensated for human error in the interpretation of the percentage of foliage infected. Small differences are easier to discriminate at the extremes of the scale, so the range of values for low infection and high infection percentages are narrow (Table 6.1).

In the middle of the scale, where it is more difficult to assess small differences, the range is larger for human error (and logarithmic laws of perception) in estimating the amount of disease present. A drawback to the Horsfall–Barratt scale is that there are overlaps for the components of the scale. For example, a rating of 5 is equal to 12%–25% infection, and a rating of 6 is equal to 25%–50% infection. A better demarcation would be 12%–25% and 26%–50%.

Rating scales have been modified since the introduction of the Horsfall–Barratt scale. Some researchers believe the nearest percent estimates (NPEs) of disease severity are better than the Horsfall–Barratt scale. US Department of Agriculture compared the NPEs with Horsfall–Barratt scale data using citrus canker

Table 6.1 The Horsfall–Barratt Scale.

Rating	% Infection	Range
1	0	0
2	0–3	3
3	3–6	3
4	6–12	6
5	12–25	13
6	25–50	25
7	50–75	25
8	75–87	12
9	87–94	7
10	94–97	3
11	97–100	3
12	100	0

(*Xanthomonas citri* subsp. *citri*) infected grapefruit (*Citrus* × *paradisi*) leaves. Results of their simulation showed standard deviations of mean NPEs were consistently like the original rater standard deviation from the field-collected data; however, the standard deviations of the Horsfall–Barratt scale data deviated from that of the original rater standard deviation, particularly at 20%–50% severity, over which Horsfall–Barratt scale grade intervals are widest; thus it is over this range that differences in scoring resistance and susceptibility are most likely to occur. Accurate raters had, on average, better resolving power for estimating disease compared with that offered by the Horsfall–Barratt scale. They concluded that there are various circumstances under which Horsfall–Barratt scale data have a greater risk of failing to differentiate resistance from susceptibility, but accurate raters always give a better result.

Clive H. Bock of the US Department of Agriculture and his international colleagues considered the accuracy and reliability of severity estimates using the Horsfall–Barratt rating estimates and the NPEs for pecan scab (*Fusicladium effusum*) infection on pecan (*Carya illinoinensis*). Raters assessed two cohorts of images with the actual area (0%–6%, 7%–25%, and 26%–75%) diseased. The mean estimated disease within each actual disease severity range varied substantially. The means estimated by the NPEs within each actual disease severity range were not necessarily good predictors of the Horsfall–Barratt scale estimate at less than 25% severity. Horsfall–Barratt estimates by raters most often placed severity in the wrong category compared with the actual disease level. Bootstrap analysis indicated that the NPEs provided either equally good or more accurate and precise estimates of disease as compared to the Horsfall–Barratt scale at disease severities of greater than 25%–75%. Interrater reliability using NPEs was greater at 25%–75% actual disease severity compared with using the Horsfall–Barratt scale. Using NPEs as compared to the Horsfall–Barrat scale will more often result in more precise and accurate estimates of pecan scab severity, particularly when estimating actual disease severities between 25 and 75%.

Similarly, researchers at the University of California at Davis, United States, compared two different scoring methods and the Horsfall–Barratt scale disease assessment scales for corky root (*Rhizomonas suberifaciens*) of lettuce (*Lactuca sativa*). The two qualitative interval scales, one a 7-level scale developed for assessing corky root severity of mature lettuce plants and the other a 10-level scale developed for screening seedlings for resistance 1 month after inoculation, were compared with a 12-level Horsfall–Barratt scale based on the percentage of the taproot area with corky root symptoms. To estimate accuracy and precision, six taproots in each of three severity classes (0%–20%, 20%–80%, and 80%–100% of taproots showing corkiness) were rated by four plant pathologists who had experience assessing corky root disease, three general plant pathologists, and three novices using each of the scales. No single scale was identified as the best for all situations. The qualitative scale for mature plants was generally the most accurate and most precise, but the Horsfall–Barratt scale was most accurate for roots in the 20%–80% severity class. Severity scores using the Horsfall–Barratt scale correlated best with yield loss. The qualitative scale for seedlings was inferior to the other scales except for early season yield loss prediction. Novices assessed disease severity with equally high bias regardless of the scale used, whereas plant pathologists (with or without experience with corky roots) were less biased when using two of the three scales. Correlations between disease severity and yield loss varied with lettuce phenological stage and severity scale used. Again, this illustrates the benefit of having trained evaluators.

So how does one make a rating scale to quicken the scoring? Suppose one wants to develop a 0–9 rating for resistance to a disease in the horticultural crop they are breeding. With most rating scales, zero is used for the uninoculated control. From the screening population, the first step is to select one plant to serve as the high resistant/immune plant, which becomes the #1 rating. Next select a plant that is highly susceptible/dead, which becomes the #9 rating. Now the scale has end points and the selection of a plant that is between those two limits turns out to be easy, which is the #5 rating. Next find a plant that is in between the #1 and #5 rating, which becomes the #3 rating. For the #7 rating, one finds a plant with symptoms between the #5 and #9 rating. The disease scale can now use the #2, #4, #6, and #8 as intermediates between the odd classes. Once the disease classes are set, one only must observe a plant and place it in the appropriate class.

Statistics used for assessing disease resistance

There are several statistics that are applicable when analyzing the results of a disease screen. The choice of the most appropriate statistic depends on whether a "rating" or "ranking" test is done. For rating, mean separation is the major statistic used. This is because it is assumed that the variances are homogeneous, and the data are normally distributed. For ranking, nonparametric statistics are needed. There are several nonparametric statistics available. Some of the most popular for breeding disease-resistant plants are χ^2 (chi-squared) test of goodness-of-fit, Kolmogorov–Smirnov one-sample (and two-sample) test, the sign test, Wilcoxon's signed rank test, Wilcoxon–Mann–Whitney two-sample test, the Median test, Kruskal–Wallis k-sample test, the median test for k samples, Friedman's test for the two-way classification, a median test for the two-way classification, Chebyshev' inequality, Spearman's coefficient of rank correlation, and the Olmstead–Tukey corner test of association. There are also many applications of using regression analysis in its many forms to assess whether resistance is statistically significant.

Martha A. Mutschler-Chu and her colleagues at Cornell University, United States, used regression and half-normal probability plot to differentiate the response of multigenic resistance and susceptibility in tomato (*S. lycopersicum*) to late blight (*P. infestans*). Late blight (*P. infestans*) resistant tomato (*S. lycopersicum*) lines were created using a wild relative of the domesticated tomato, *Solanum pimpinellifolium*, as the source of the resistance. They observed that late blight resistance differed in the different lines tested in the field. They hypothesized that possible causes could include a partial transfer of the late blight resistance derived from *S. pimpinellifolium* or the possibility of race specificity of this resistance. A crucial issue was determining the most appropriate and robust analytical method to use with data from laboratory analyses of the responses of nine tomato (*S. lycopersicum*) lines against five *P. infestans* isolates. Prior analysis by standard analysis of variance (ANOVA) revealed significant differences across (*S. lycopersicum*) lines but could not determine whether the disease responses in the resistant lines were different from those of the heterozygous F_1 hybrids, created by hybridizing susceptible tomatoes (*S. lycopersicum*) with the fixed resistant lines. Therefore a different analytical method was tested, a half-normal probability plot with regression analysis. The results of the analysis confirmed the results obtained by using a standard ANOVA but provided a clearer demonstration of the distributions of the individuals within the populations.

For some disease evaluation data, the underlying distribution is not easily specified, so to analyze such data, a statistic that is distribution-free is needed, that is, one that is not dependent on a specific parent distribution. For example, when data are categorized because of the lack of an adequate scale measurement then a rank is performed. When plants are scored for pathogen resistance and many locations are used, the accompanying variances may be heterogeneous. This is a violation of the usual assumption for a valid ANOVA test, and ranking is the best measure. Use of medians is preferable to means when data are not normally distributed, because medians are less sensitive to extremes. However, when data are normal, the true mean equals the true median and statements about the medians apply to the means.

For rating data, the most common statistical methods are those based on ANOVA, regression, and correlation. The valid use of these methods requires that the data have (1) normally distributed responses, (2) constant error variance, (3) independently distributed errors, and (4) a correctly specified model. However, many disease screening experiments yield data that do not adhere to these standard assumptions. For example, in an experiment involving population levels of a pathogen, rarely will population levels be normally distributed. Field counts of the number of healthy individuals in a plot many times will have different variances for various treatments.

Seeking the help of a statistician to select and use the best methods for obtaining and analyzing data is always recommended. The statistician has expertise and experience in designing experiments including sampling methods that are extremely helpful in statistical analysis and interpretation. The statistician's specialized knowledge can supplement your own expertise to enhance the integrity and validity of your study. It is important to consult with a statistician early in the project to assist in designing a study that will give an unequivocal answer to which plants are resistant. Of course, a statistician can determine appropriate methods of analysis when different types of data are analyzed in different ways too. Many times, when working with living plants and pathogens, experiments do not always go as planned, so instead of improvising and hoping for the best, a statistician can help to weigh the merits and drawbacks of different possible actions.

Bibliography

Abe, K., Iwanami, H., Kotoda, N., Moriya, S., Takahashi, S., 2010. Evaluation of apple genotypes and Malus species for resistance to Alternaria blotch caused by *Alternaria alternata* apple pathotype using detached-leaf method. Plant Breeding 129, 208–218. Available from: https://doi.org/10.1111/j.1439-0523.2009.01672.x.

Araújo, M.d.S.B., Sudré, C.P., Graça, G.A., da Silva Alencar, A.A., da Costa Geronimo, I.G., Rodrigues, R., 2022. A new approach to quantify anthracnose symptoms in inoculated *Capsicum* spp. fruits. Tropical Plant Pathology 47, 386–401. Available from: https://doi.org/10.1007/s40858-022-00499-9.

Baral, J.B.O.Sy, Bosland, P.W., 2004. A comparison between a detached leaf and a whole plant method for screening phytophthora foliar blight in chile (*Capsicum annuum*). Capsicum and Eggplant Newsletter 23, 125–128. Available from: https://cpi.nmsu.edu/_assets/documents/capegg23.pdf.

Barbedo, J.G.A., 2016. A novel algorithm for semi-automatic segmentation of plant leaf disease symptoms using digital image processing. Tropical Plant Pathology 41, 210–224. Available from: https://doi.org/10.1007/s40858-016-0090-8.

Bartley, S.H., Chute, E., 1945. A preliminary clarification of the concept of fatigue. Psychological Reviews 52, 169–174.

Bhattarai, G., Feng, C., Dhillon, B., Shi, A., Villarroel-Zeballos, M., Klosterman, S.J., et al., 2020. Detached leaf inoculation assay for evaluating resistance to the spinach downy mildew pathogen. European Journal of Plant Pathology 158, 511–520. Available from: https://doi.org/10.1007/s10658-020-02096-5.

Bierman, A., LaPlumm, T., Cadle-Davidson, L., Gadoury, D., Martinez, D., Sapkota, S., et al., 2019. A high-throughput phenotyping system using machine vision to quantify severity of grapevine powdery mildew. Plant Phenomics. Available from: https://doi.org/10.34133/2019/9209727. Article ID 9209727.

Bock, C.H., Gottwald, T.R., Parker, P.E., Ferrandino, F., Welham, S., van den Bosch, F., et al., 2010. Some consequences of using the Horsfall-Barratt scale for hypothesis testing. Phytopathology 100, 1030–1041. Available from: https://doi.org/10.1094/PHYTO-08-09-0220.

Bock, C.H., Wood, B.W., van den Bosch, F., Parnell, S., Gottwald, T.R., 2013. The effect of Horsfall-Barratt category size on the accuracy and reliability of estimates of pecan scab severity. Plant Disease 97, 797–806. Available from: https://doi.org/10.1094/PDIS-08-12-0781-RE.

Bock, C.H., Barbedo, J.G.A., Del Ponte, E.M., Bohnenkamp, D., Mahlein, A.K., 2020. From visual estimates to fully automated sensor-based measurements of plant disease severity: status and challenges for improving accuracy. Phytopathology Research 2, 9. Available from: https://doi.org/10.1186/s42483-020-00049-8.

Bosland, P.W., Lindsey, D.L., 1991. A seedling screen for Phytophthora root rot of pepper *Capsicum annuum*. Plant Disease 75, 1048–1050.

Brozek, J., 1948. Visual fatigue – a critical comment. American Journal Psychology 61, 420–424.

Campbell, C.L., Madden, L.V., 1990. Introduction to Plant Disease Epidemiology. Wiley, p. 560.

Chiang, K.-S., Bock, C.H., Lee, I.-H., El Jarroudi, M., Delfosse, P., 2016. Plant disease severity assessment—how rater bias, assessment method, and experimental design affect hypothesis testing and resource use efficiency. Phytopathology 106, 1451–1464. Available from: https://doi.org/10.1094/PHYTO-12-15-0315-R.

Chiang, K.-S., Liu, S.-C., Bock, C.H., Gottwald, T.R., 2014. What interval characteristics make a good categorical disease assessment scale? Phytopathology 104, 575–585. Available from: https://doi.org/10.1094/PHYTO-10-13-0279-R.

Cooke, B., 2006. Disease assessment and yield loss. In: Cooke B, B., Jones, D., Kaye, D. (Eds.), The Epidemiology of Plant Diseases. Springer, Dordrecht. Available from: https://doi.org/10.1007/1-4020-4581-6_2.

Davis, B.D., 1949. The isolation of biochemically deficient mutants of bacteria by means of penicillin. Proceedings of the National Academy of Sciences of the United States of America 35, 1–10. Available from: https://doi.org/10.10732/Fpnas.35.1.1.

Deery, D.M., Jones, H.G., 2021. Field phenomics: will it enable crop improvement? Plant. Phenomics . Available from: https://doi.org/10.34133/2021/9871989.

Dolinski, M.A., Duarte, H.D.S., da Silva, J.B., de Mio, L.L.M., 2017. Development and validation of a standard area diagram set for assessment of peach rust. European Journal of Plant Pathology 148, 817–824. Available from: https://doi.org/10.1007/s10658-016-1138-9.

Driscoll, J., Coombs, J., Hammerschmidt, R., Kirk, W., Wanner, L., Douches, D., 2009. Greenhouse and field nursery evaluation for potato common scab tolerance in a tetraploid population. American Journal of Potato Research 86, 96. Available from: https://doi.org/10.1007/s12230-008-9065-8.

Du, J., Vleeshouwers, V.G.A.A., 2014. The do's and don'ts of effectoromics. In: Birch, P., Jones, J., Bos, J. (Eds.), Plant–Pathogen Interactions. Methods in Molecular Biology (Methods and Protocols), 1127. Humana Press, Totowa, NJ. Available from: https://doi.org/10.1007/978-1-62703-986-4_19.

Duarte, H.S.S., Zambolim, L., Capucho, A.S., Júnior, A.F.N., Rosado, A.W.C., Cardoso, C.R., et al., 2013. Development and validation of a set of standard area diagrams to estimate severity of potato early blight. European Journal of Plant Pathology 137, 249–257. Available from: https://doi.org/10.1007/s10658-013-0234-3.

Eskridge, K.M., 1995. Statistical analysis of disease reaction data using nonparametric methods. HortScience 30, 478–481. Available from: https://doi.org/10.21273/HORTSCI.30.3.478.

Foolad, M.R., Sullenberger, M.T., Ashrafi, H., 2015. Detached-leaflet evaluation of tomato germplasm for late blight resistance and its correspondence to field and greenhouse screenings. Plant Disease 99, 718–722. Available from: https://doi.org/10.1094/PDIS-08-14-0794-RE.

Garrett, K., Madden, L., Hughes, G., Pfender, W., 2004. New applications of statistical tools in plant pathology. Phytopathology 94, 999–1003. Available from: https://doi.org/10.1094/PHYTO.2004.94.9.999.

Groth, J.V., Davis, D.W., Zeyen, R.J., Mogen, B.D., 1983. Ranking of partial resistance to common rust (*Puccinia sorghi* Schr.) in 30 sweet corn (*Zea mays*) hybrids. Crop Protection 2, 219–224. Available from: https://doi.org/10.1016/0261-2194(83)90047-9.

Guan, J., Nutter Jr, F.W., 2003. Quantifying the intrarater repeatability and interrater reliability of visual and remote-sensing disease-assessment methods in the alfalfa foliar pathosystem. Canadian Journal of Plant Pathology 25, 143–149. Available from: https://doi.org/10.1080/07060660309507062.

Haynes, K.G., Weingartner, D.P., 2004. The use of area under the disease progress curve to assess resistance to late blight in potato germplasm. American Journal of Potato Research 81, 137–141. Available from: https://doi.org/10.1007/BF02853611.

Holder-John, A.W.B., Elibox, W., Umaharan, P., 2021. A rapid leaf-disc vacuum-infiltration screening for assessing resistance to bacterial leaf spot disease in anthurium. Science Horticulturae 288, 110344. Available from: https://doi.org/10.1016/j.scienta.2021.110344.

Holland, J.B., Nyquist, W.E., Cervantes-Martínez, C.T., 2003. Estimating and interpreting heritability for plant breeding: an update. Plant Breeding Reviews 22, 9–112. Available from: https://doi.org/10.1002/9780470650202.ch2.

Horsfall, J.G., Barratt, R.W., 1945. An improved grading system for measuring plant disease. Phytopathology 35, 655.

James, W.C., 1974. Assessment of plant diseases and losses. Annual Review of Phytopathology 12, 27–48. Available from: https://doi.org/10.1146/annurev.py.12.090174.000331.

Johnson, R., Taylor, A.J., 1976. Spore yield of pathogens in investigations of the race specificity of host resistance. Annual Reviews of Phytopathology 14, 97–119. Available from: https://doi.org/10.1146/annurev.py.14.090176.000525.

Johnson, L.E.B., Bushnell, W.R., Zeyen, R.J., 1979. Binary pathways for analysis of primary infection and host response in populations of powdery mildew fungi. Canadian Journal of Botany 57, 497–511. Available from: https://doi.org/10.1139/b79-065.

Kim, M.-J., Federer, W., Mutschler, M.A., 2005. Using half-normal probability plot and regression analysis to differentiate complex traits: differentiating disease response of multigenic resistance and susceptibility in tomatoes to multiple pathogen isolates. Theoretical and Applied Genetics 112, 21–29. Available from: https://doi.org/10.1007/s00122-005-0084-2.

Kull, L.S., Vuong, T.D., Powers, K.S., Eskridge, K.M., Steadman, J.R., Hartman, G.L., 2003. Evaluation of resistance screening methods for sclerotinia stem rot of soybean and dry bean. Plant Disease 87, 1471–1476. Available from: https://doi.org/10.1094/PDIS.2003.87.12.1471.

Lacaze, A., Joly, D.L., 2020. Structural specificity in plant–filamentous pathogen interactions. Molecular Plant Pathology 21, 1513–1525. Available from: https://doi.org/10.1111/mpp.12983.

Li, Z., Paul, R., Tis, T.B., Saville, A.C., Hansel, J.C., Yu, T., et al., 2019. Non-invasive plant disease diagnostics enabled by smartphone-based fingerprinting of leaf volatiles. Nature Plants 5, 856–866. Available from: https://doi.org/10.1038/s41477-019-0476-y.

Lillemo, M., Singh, R.P., van Ginkel, M., 2010. Identification of stable resistance to powdery mildew in wheat based on parametric and nonparametric methods. Crop Science 50, 478–485. Available from: https://doi.org/10.2135/cropsci2009.03.0116.

Lind, A.S.H.C.H., Kamil, M.J.A., Chong, K.P.H., Ho., C.M., 2017. Assessing the cocoa genotypes for resistance to black pod using the area under the disease-progress curve (AUDPC). Bulgarian. Journal of Agricultural Science 23, 972–979. Available from: https://agrojournal.org/23/06-13.pdf.

Little, T.M., Hills, F.J., 1978. Agricultural Experimentation: Design and Analysis. John Wiley, & Sons, N.Y, p. 350.

Liu, J., Wang, X., 2021. Plant diseases and pest detection based on deep learning: a review. Plant Methods 17, 22. Available from: https://doi.org/10.1186/s13007-021-00722-9.

Liu, H.I., Tsai, J.R., Chung, W.H., Bock, C.H., Chiang, K.S., 2019. Effects of quantitative ordinal scale design on the accuracy of estimates of mean disease severity. Agronomy 9, 565. Available from: https://doi.org/10.3390/agronomy.9090565.

Loegering, W.Q., Sleper, D.A., Johnson, J.M., Asay, K.H., 1976. Rating general resistance on a single-plant basis. Phytopathology 66, 1445–1448.

Longzhou, L., Xiaojun, Y., Run, C., Junsong, P., Huanle, H., Lihua, Y., et al., 2008. Quantitative trait loci for resistance to powdery mildew in cucumber under seedling spray inoculation and leaf disc infection. Journal of Phytopathology 156, 691–697. Available from: https://doi.org/10.1111/j.1439-0434.2008.01427.x.

Madden, L.V., Paul, P.A., Lipps, P.E., 2007. Consideration of nonparametric approaches for assessing genotype-by-environment (G × E) interaction with disease severity data. Plant Disease 91, 891–900. Available from: https://doi.org/10.1094/PDIS-91-7-0891.

Mahlein, A.K., Kuska, M.T., Behmann, J., Polder, G., Walter, A., 2018. Hyperspectral sensors and imaging technologies in phytopathology: state of the art. Annual Review of Phytopathology 56, 535–558. Available from: https://doi.org/10.1146/annurev-phyto-080417-050100.

Martin, R.R., James, D., Lévesque, C.A., 2000. Impacts of molecular diagnostic technologies on plant disease management. Annual Review of Phytopathology 38, 207–239. Available from: https://doi.org/10.1146/annurev.phyto.38.1.207.

Marzougui, A., Rajendran, A., Mattinson, D.S., Ma, Y., McGee, R.J., Garcia-Pereza, M., et al., 2022. Evaluation of biogenic markers-based phenotyping for resistance to Aphanomyces root rot in field pea. Information Processing in Agriculture 9, 1–10. Available from: https://doi.org/10.1016/j.inpa.2021.01.007.

Megaw, E.D., 1995. The definition and measurement of visual fatigue. In: Wilson, J.R., Corlett, E.N. (Eds.), Evaluation of Human Work: A Practical Ergonomics Methodology, second ed. Taylor & Francis, Philadelphia, PA, pp. 840–863.

Miller-Butler, M.A., Smith, B.J., Babiker, E.M., Kreiser, B.R., Blythe, E.K., 2018. Comparison of whole plant and detached leaf screening techniques for identifying anthracnose resistance in strawberry plants. Plant Disease 102, 2112–2119. Available from: https://doi.org/10.1094/PDIS-08-17-1138-RE.

Mutka, A.M., Bart, R.S., 2015. Image-based phenotyping of plant disease symptoms. Frontiers in Plant Science. Available from: https://doi.org/10.3389/fpls.2014.00734.

Newhouse, A.E., Spitzer, J.E., Maynard, C.A., Powell, W.A., 2014. Chestnut leaf inoculation assay as a rapid predictor of blight susceptibility. Plant Disease 98, 4–9. Available from: https://doi.org/10.1094/PDIS-01-13-0047-RE.

Nutter, F.W., Esker, P.D., Netto, R.A.C., 2006. Disease assessment concepts and the advancements made in improving the accuracy and precision of plant disease data. European Journal of Plant Pathology 115, 95–103. Available from: https://doi.org/10.1007/s10658-005-1230-z.

Nutter Jr., F.W., Eggenberger, S.K., Streit, A.J., 2017. Intrarater and interrater agreement in disease assessment. In: Stevenson, K.L., Jeger, M.J. (Eds.), Exercises in Plant Disease Epidemiology, Second Edition ACS Publication (Chapter 25). Available from: https://doi.org/10.1094/9780890544426.

O'Brien, R.D., van Bruggen, A.H.C., 1992. Accuracy, precision, and correlation to yield loss of disease severity scales for corky root of lettuce. Phytopathology 82, 91–96. Available from: https://doi.org/10.1094/Phyto-82-91.

Oerke, E.C., 2020. Remote sensing of diseases. Annual Review of Phytopathology 58, 225–252. Available from: https://doi.org/10.1146/annurev-phyto-010820-012832.

Pataky, J.K., Williams II, M.M., Headrick, J.M., Nankam, C., du Toit, L.J., Michener, P.M., 2011. Observations from a quarter century of evaluating reactions of sweet corn hybrids in disease nurseries. Plant Disease 95, 1492–1506. Available from: https://doi.org/10.1094/PDIS-03-11-0236.

Rennberger, G., Keinath, A.P., 2018. Susceptibility of fourteen new cucurbit species to gummy stem blight caused by *Stagonosporopsis citrulli* under field conditions. Plant Disease 102, 1365–1375. Available from: https://doi.org/10.1094/pdis-12-17-1953-re.

Rideout, S.L., Brenneman, T.B., Stevenson, K.L., 2002. A comparison of disease assessment methods for southern stem rot of peanut. Peanut Science 29, 66–71. Available from: https://doi.org/10.3146/pnut.29.1.0012.

Simko, I., Piepho, H.-P., 2012. The area under the disease progress stairs: calculation, advantage, and application. Phytopathology 102, 381–389. Available from: https://doi.org/10.1094/PHYTO-07-11-0216.

Simko, I., Jimenez-Berni, J.A., Sirault, X.R.R., 2017. Phenomic approaches and tools for phytopathologists. Phytopathology 107, 6–17. Available from: https://doi.org/10.1094/PHYTO-02-16-0082-RVW.

Steel, R.G.D., Torrie, J.H., 1980. Principles and Procedures of Statistics: a biometrical approach. McGraw-Hill Book Publishing Company, New York.

Stern, J.A., Boyer, D., Schroeder, D., 1994. Blink rate – a possible measure of fatigue. Human Factors 36, 285–297. Available from: https://doi.org/10.11772/F001872089403600209.

Tanner, F., Tonn, S., de Wit, J., Van den Ackerveken, G., Berger, B., Plettl, D., 2022. Sensor-based phenotyping of above-ground plant-pathogen interactions. Plant Methods 18, 35. Available from: https://doi.org/10.1186/s13007-022-00853-7.

Uchneat, M.S.A., Zhigilei, Craig, R., 1999. Differential response to foliar infection with Botrytis cinerea within the genus *Pelargonium*. Journal of the American Society for Horticultural Science 124, 76–80. Available from: https://doi.org/10.21273/JASHS.124.1.76.

Veturi, Y., Kump, K., Walsh, E., Ott, O., Poland, J., Kolkman, J.M., et al., 2012. Multivariate mixed linear model analysis of longitudinal data: an information-rich statistical technique for analyzing plant disease resistance. Phytopathology 102, 1016–1025. Available from: https://doi.org/10.1094/PHYTO-10-11-0268.

Vidal, G.S., de Souza, B.L., De Mio, L.L.M., da Silva Silveira Duarte, H., 2019. Development and validation of a standard area diagram set for assessment of plum rust severity. Australasian Plant Pathology 48, 603–606. Available from: https://doi.org/10.1007/s13313-019-00662-y.

Wei, X., Aguilera, M., Walcheck, R., Tholl, D., Li, S., Langston Jr., D.B., et al., 2021. Detection of soilborne disease utilizing sensor technologies: lessons learned from studies on stem rot of peanut. Plant Health Progress 22, 436–444. Available from: https://doi.org/10.1094/PHP-03-21-0055-SYN.

West, J.S., Bravo, C., Oberti, R., Lemaire, D., Moshou, D., McCartney, H.A., 2003. The potential of optical canopy measurement for targeted control of field crop diseases. Annual Review of Phytopathology 41, 593–614. Available from: https://doi.org/10.1146/annurev.phyto.41.121702.103726.

Yadav, N.V.S., de Vos, S.M., Bock, C.H., Wood, B.W., 2013. Development and validation of standard area diagrams to aid assessment of pecan scab symptoms on fruit. Plant Pathology 62, 325–335. Available from: https://doi.org/10.1111/j.1365-3059.2012.02641.x.

7

Resistance sources

Natural sources of resistance

In the selection of parents, in addition to disease resistance, numerous horticultural traits must be considered. The objective of the plant breeder is to produce disease-resistant cultivars of high quality combined with other desirable traits. The selection level for economically important traits needs to be established early in the breeding program. For each trait, knowledge of the genetic variability of the traits should be a prime determinant of the population size needed to have resistant and horticultural acceptable offspring recovered. The population size will depend on balancing the resources allocated to the project, and the independence and correlations among the traits.

It would be fortuitous if traits are independent of or even positively correlated with disease resistance. Genetic linkage of desirable levels of horticultural characteristics with susceptibility to disease would severely limit overall progress. Horticultural traits in potential parents are commonly combined with resistance in wild species that have many undesirable traits. Several generations of backcrossing to genotypes with improved horticultural characteristics are necessary before that resistance is available in a genotype with acceptable commercial characteristics.

When a plant breeder needs to find a disease-resistant gene, where does one look? The first and may not be the most obvious place is other commercial cultivars. The resistance gene may be right in front of one's eyes. The current high-yielding cultivars have high yield potential and uniformity as compared to other sources of resistance like landraces and heirlooms. Many modern cultivars have "cryptic resistance" because not all resistance genes are reported for a given cultivar because companies like to keep this information as a "trade secret" or proprietary information. Modern cultivars constitute a major part of working collections and are extensively used as parents in breeding programs for further genetic improvement for various characters.

Taking a commercial F_1 hybrid, and saving seeds, is called "dehybridizing" in the vernacular. In her book, *Breed Your*

Own Vegetables, Carol Deppe writes about dehybridizing vegetable hybrids. Amateur plant breeders and seed savers do this often. It is important to realize that when the seed is planted in subsequent generations, the progeny will segregate for many traits, some good and some not so good. Commercial plant breeders deliberately insert deleterious alleles in the cultivar to discourage individuals from dehybridizing the hybrid. Nevertheless, if the segregating progeny has individual plants with disease resistance, they can be used in the breeding program. Alternatively, the hybrid itself can be used as a parent in the hybridization.

If after screening, no commercial cultivar has the resistance needed, then scrutinizing old or "obsolete" cultivars is the best bet. These cultivars also known as heirloom varieties were popular in the past but have been replaced by higher yielding cultivars with better quality. These cultivars still have desirable characteristics and constitute an important part of the primary genepool.

The next level to delve into is landraces (primitive cultivars) of the species. Landraces are considered a local variety of domesticated plant species that have developed adaptation to the natural and cultural environment in which it lives. It differs from a cultivar that has been selectively bred to conform to a particular standard of characteristics. Landrace populations are often variable in appearance, but they can be identified by their appearance and have a certain genetic similarity. Landraces have continuity with improved cultivars. The relatively high level of genetic variation of landraces is one of the advantages that these can have over improved cultivars. Although yields may not be as high, the stability of landraces in face of adverse conditions is typically high. As a result, new diseases may affect some, but not all, the individuals in the population. Modern cultivars, heirloom varieties, and landraces of the same species constitute the primary genepool of a breeding program, and typically there are no genetic barriers to successful hybridization among accessions within the primary genepool.

An example of screening cultivated and wild material for resistance is of the work in India by Venkataravanapp and colleagues, where they screened 147 advanced okra (*Abelmoschus esculentus*) breeding lines, 31 popular cultivars, and 146 accessions from 14 wild species acquired from different national institutes for resistance to okra yellow vein mosaic virus (OYVMV, *Begomovirus*) and okra enation leaf curl virus (OELCuV, *Begomovirus*) diseases. Depending on the crop's growth stage and time of the virus infection, the yield losses range from

50% to 94%. The resistance levels of both cultivated and wild species were assessed by visual scoring of symptoms in the field under natural conditions for two consecutive years. None of the cultivated genotypes and wild species tested was found to be disease free except *Abelmoschus enbeepeegeearnse*, a species found at low elevations in the Western Ghats of India. Nevertheless, of the 178 cultivated/advanced lines screened against OYVMV and OELCuV, seven genotypes showed high resistance, and of the 146 accessions from the wild species, 17 accessions had a highly resistant reaction. With OELCuV, 52 okra genotypes had high resistance. They concluded that the highly resistant cultivated/advanced lines could be used directly as cultivars to manage both viruses. Furthermore, the resistance in the wild accessions could be used in future breeding programs to develop okra cultivars resistant against both OYVMV and OELCuV.

Another example is melon (*Cucumis melo*) in India where feral and cultivated melons are found. Narinder P. Dhillon of the World Vegetable Center, East and Southeast Asia Regional Center in Thailand, and colleagues state that Indian melon germplasm provides resistance to Alternaria leaf blight (*Alternaria cucumerina*), downy mildew (*Pseudoperonospora cubensis*) Fusarium wilt (*Fusarium oxysporum* f. sp. *melonis*), monosporascus root rot and vine decline (*Monosporascus cannonballus*) powdery mildew (*Podosphaera xanthii*), cucumber mosaic virus (CMV, *Bromoviridae*), cucurbit aphid-borne yellows virus (CABYV, *Luteoviridae*), cucurbit leaf crumple virus (CuLCrV, *Begomovirus*), Kyuri green mottle mosaic virus, (KGMMV, *Orthornavirae*); lettuce infectious yellows virus (LIYV, *Closteroviridae*), Moroccan watermelon mosaic virus (MWMV, *Potyviridae*), papaya ringspot virus (PRSV, *Potyviridae*), squash mosaic virus (SqMV, *Secoviridae*), watermelon chlorotic stunt virus (WmCSV, *Geminiviridae*), watermelon mosaic virus (WMV, *Potyviridae*), and zucchini yellow mosaic virus (ZYMV, *Potyviridae*).

The next source to explore is within the secondary genepool that constitutes wild accessions of the same species or progenitor species. Wild forms of cultivated species have generally a high degree of disease resistance and can be utilized in breeding programs for genetic improvement. Normally, they hybridize easily with cultivated species because these naturally occurring plant species have common ancestry with crops. Among the most important examples of the use of crop wild relatives is in tomato (*Solanum lycopersicum*), with sources to most of the most devastating pests and diseases facing producers originating in wild accessions (Fig. 7.1).

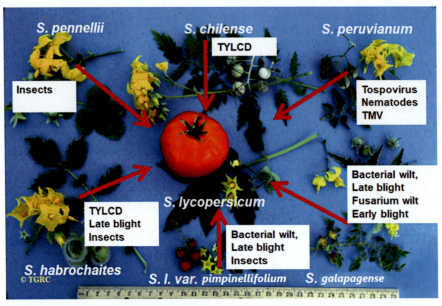

Figure 7.1 Sources of resistance to tomato (*Solanum lycopersicum*) diseases. Courtesy: the Tomato Genetics Resource Center, U.C. Davis, U.S.A. Photograph taken by Charles M. Rick.

For example, it is estimated that nearly one-quarter of the tomato (*S. lycopersicum*) genome is made of the introgressed genome from wild relatives into cultivated tomato (*S. lycopersicum*), including a 50 Mb introgression on chromosome nine, associated with a *Tm2a* resistance to the tomato mosaic virus (ToMV), originating from *Solanum peruvianum*.

If a source of resistance is not found within the wild relatives of the same species, then looking at closely related species is appropriate, which constitutes the tertiary genepool. Most of the time, interspecific hybridization is the last resort in breeding, because introgressing genes from the hybridization can lead to hybrid sterility, hybrid inviability, and the transfer of undesirable genes to the cultivated species along with desirable alleles (linkage drag).

In 1990 Van der Meer and de Vries at Wageningen University and Research, the Netherlands reported that a complete resistance to downy mildew (*Peronospora destructor*) was found in *Allium roylei*, a wild relative to onion (*Allium cepa*). They were able to successfully hybridize *A. cepa* to *A. roylei* yielding partial fertile interspecific hybrids. With continued backcrossing to onion (*A. cepa*), they succeeded in transferring resistance from the wild species to the cultivated species.

However, it took 20 years from the discovery of an *A. roylei* plant that was resistant to downy mildew to the release of a commercial cultivar with resistance to downy mildew (*P. destructor*) derived from this source. For this reason, the plant breeder should start the primary genepool when looking for resistance to a particular disease. However, when resistance is rare or easily overcome by the pathogen, the use of secondary and tertiary genepools serves as important sources of resistance.

Species bridge

The plant breeder must be cognizant that there are often prezygotic and postzygotic barriers to fertilization success when hybridizing members of tertiary genepools. The use of "bridge crosses" can sometimes be utilized to overcome these issues. For example, in cucurbits, the wild species *Cucurbita argyrosperma* (pipiana squash; cushaw pumpkin; or silverseed gourd), which is consumed primarily for its seeds instead of its flesh, has been widely used as a bridge species for successful hybridizations among the various domesticated species with *Cucurbita*.

In the *Capsicum* genus, species bridges have been used to introduce disease resistance from *Capsicum baccatum*, commonly known as ají, to improve pepper (*Capsicum annuum*). Strong interspecific hybridization barriers exist between the two species. Researchers at the Instituto de Conservación y Mejora de la Agrodiversidad Valenciana, Universitat Politècnica de València, Spain formulated a species bridge to introgress *C. baccatum* genes into *C. annuum* using *Capsicum chinense* and *Capsicum frutescens* as bridge species. They concluded that *C. chinense* functioned as a good bridge species between *C. annuum* and *C. baccatum*, with the best results being obtained with the hybridization combination *C. baccatum* as the female hybridized to *C. chinense* as the male, then using the F_1 as female hybridized to *C. annuum* as the male. While *C. frutescens* gave poor results as bridge species due to strong prezygotic and postzygotic barriers. Virus-like-syndrome or dwarfism was observed in F_1 progeny when both *C. chinense* and *C. frutescens* were used as female parents. These results provide plant breeders with useful hybridization information for the regular utilization of the *C. baccatum* genepool in *C. annuum* breeding.

Embryo rescue

In some interspecific hybridizations, a technique known as "embryo rescue" must be accomplished. Embryo rescue is an in vitro culture technique to assist in the development of an immature or weak embryo into a viable plant. It has been used successfully to produce interspecific and intergeneric hybrids. Embryo culture is the most used method for embryo rescue. Generally, seeds from controlled pollination plants are collected before the expected embryo abortion occurrence, followed by isolation and excision of embryos, which are then placed directly onto a culture medium for the generation of plants. Besides embryo culture, ovule, and ovary culture, which are more suitable for small-seeded species or very young embryos, are also utilized for embryo rescue. This requires laboratory facilities to excise the embryo from the developing seed and grow it on artificial media. The resulting interspecific plant can then be backcrossed to the recurrent parent species.

An example of interspecific hybridization with embryo rescue is with seedless grape cultivars (*Vitis vinifera*). Seedless table and raisin grapes are obtained either by parthenocarpy or an unusual path called stenospermocarpy. In the stenospermocarpic grapes, fertilization occurs but seed development stops, resulting in no seeds or only seed traces. Conventional breeding methods to produce new seedless grape cultivars in the past used seeded grapes as female parents, while seedless cultivars were used only as pollen parents. The breeding efficiency of these traditional methods was greatly limited due to the low percentage of seedless progenies in the F_1 generation. Once seedlings using in vitro culture of stenospermic grape ovules with embryo rescue became widely adopted for the hybridization of seedless grapes, breeding seedless grapes proceeded rapidly. The usage of embryo rescue for hybridizing stenospermic grapes has resulted in a significantly high frequency of seedlessness in offspring compared to the traditional methods.

Researchers at the Key Laboratory of Horticultural Plant Germplasm Resources & Genetic Improvement in Northwest China, P.R. China used in vitro embryo rescue to incorporate resistance from several wild Chinese *Vitis* species. They exploited *Vitis amurensis* for anthracnose (*Sphaceloma ampelinum*), ripe rot (*Gloeosporium fructigenum*), and white rot (*Coniothyrium diplodiella*) resistance. With *Vitis yanshanensis*, resistance to downy mildew (*Plasmopara viticola*) anthracnose, ripe rot, and white rot was introduced. The species *Vitis qinlingensis* provided resistance to powdery mildew (*Uncinula necator*), anthracnose, ripe rot, and white rot. *V. hancockii* provided

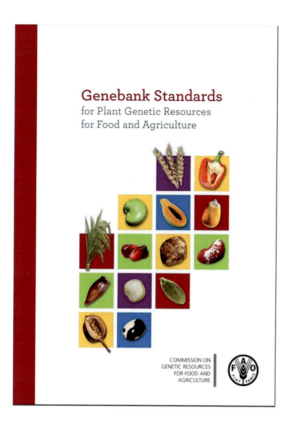

Figure 7.2 One of several books that can be found at https://colostate.pressbooks.pub/cropwildrelatives/chapter/published-best-practices. Cover photo, courtesy: the Commission on Genetic Resources for Food and Agriculture, FAO.

downy mildew and anthracnose, while *Vitis romanetii* provided anthracnose resistance. *V. vinifera* as the female parent and the wild Chinese *Vitis* spp. as the pollen donors. In ovulo embryo rescue developed interspecific hybrid plants from the seedless females. In vitro embryo rescue allowed for the successful development of hybrids with fungal disease-resistant genes using Chinese wild *Vitis* spp.

Germplasm repositories

At the global level, an organization called the Alliance has the mission to curb the loss of biodiversity and support systems that contribute to more diversity. This area of work encompasses the design of integrated conservation strategies at global and national scales for priority crop genetic resources, and the preparation of action plans to implement these strategies. They identify incentives for farmers and natural resource managers to conserve, share, and use genetic resources (Fig. 7.2).

The Alliance was formed through collaborations between Bioversity International and the International Center for Tropical Agriculture (CIAT). Bioversity International was originally established by the Consultative Group for International Agricultural Research (CGIAR) as the International Board for Plant Genetic Resources (IBPGR) in 1974. In October 1993, IBPGR became the International Plant Genetic Resources Institute (IPGRI) and in 1994 IPGRI began independent operation as one of the centers of the CGIAR. At the request of the CGIAR, in 1994 IPGRI took over the governance and administration of the International Network for the Improvement of Banana and Plantain (INIBAP).

IPGRI network promotes collection, conservation, documentation, evaluation, and utilization of plant genetic resources. The IPGRI is an autonomous international scientific organization, supported by the CGIAR. The IPGRI's mandate is to advance the conservation and use of genetic diversity for the well-being of present and future generations. The IPGRI's headquarters are based in Rome, Italy, with offices in another 19 countries worldwide. It operates through three programs: (1) the Plant Genetic Resources Program, (2) the CGIAR Genetic Resources Support Program, and (3) the INIBAP.

In 1996 150 countries adopted the first Global Plan of Action (GPA) for conserving and using crop diversity. The GPA called for a rational global conservation system, based on the principles of effectiveness, efficiency, and transparency. In 2011 the Second GPA reiterated that call. The International Treaty on Plant Genetic Resources for Food and Agriculture, which came into force in 2004, placed an effective and efficient global system at the core of its efforts to conserve and use crop diversity for food security. Bioversity International established the Crop Trust on behalf of the CGIAR and the UN Food and Agriculture Organization (FAO) to help support this global system in a sustainable way, through a Crop Diversity Endowment Fund. This fund provides long-term grants to safeguard collections of unique and valuable crop diversity held in genebanks around the world. Priority is given to 25 crops the International Treaty has determined to be of particular importance to the food security of least developed countries.

National seed banks play a vital role in preserving genetic diversity. One of the largest seed banks in terms of crop diversity is the US National Plant Germplasm System (NPGS). It is an effort to safeguard the genetic diversity of agriculturally important plants. The mission of the US NPGS is to support agricultural production by acquiring, conserving, evaluating, documenting, and distributing crop germplasm. The Germplasm

Resources Information Network (GRIN)-global database maintains electronic information on more than 570,000 unique plant accessions at 20 NPGS locations. Distribution of available germplasm and information is free to researchers and educators worldwide. In return, recipients are asked to provide information regarding the utility of the germplasm for crop improvement, direct use, and scientific research. This information helps curators understand germplasm users' needs and better target the use of plant genetic resources. Thus if one screens the germplasm for resistance to a pathogen, it is then expected that the results will be sent to GRIN for inclusion in its database.

In addition to national genebanks, there are several international genebanks. Typically, these international genebanks focus on one or a few crops and are managed by the international research institute working on those crops. The vast majority of international research institutes work exclusively on grain or pulse crops, although there are a few focusing on horticultural crops. The International Institute of Tropical Agriculture (IITA), based in Nigeria, houses germplasm for important horticultural crops such as plantain (*Plantago* species), banana (*Musa acuminata*) species, yam (*Dioscorea* species), cassava (*Manihot esculenta*), among other crops. The International Potato Center (CIP) in Lima, Peru manages potato (*Solanum tuberosum*) and sweet potato (*Ipomoea batatas*) germplasm collections. In Cali, Colombia, International CIAT preserves the world's largest and most diverse collection of beans (*Phaseolus* species) as well as cassava. The World Vegetable Center (WorldVeg) operates two international genebanks for vegetable crops. The primary genebank is based in Shanhua, Tainan, Taiwan, and houses more than 72,000 accessions of more than 50 genera collected from 155 countries. Additionally, the World Vegetable Center has a genebank in Tanzania that focuses on conserving traditional African vegetable crops and in total, the World Vegetable Center has about 12,000 accessions of indigenous vegetables, a few examples are African nightshade (*Solanum scabrum*), scarlet wisteria, (*Sesbania grandiflora*), Sweet leaf bush (*Sauropus androgynus*), and Madeira vine (*Anredera cordifolia*).

These genebanks, both national and international, provide genetic material to the public for free or for a nominal fee, and the diversity conserved provides an important resource for plant breeders. Sources of disease resistance can be accessed from genebank and used directly in the plant breeding program. The limitation is knowing where to start when screening exceptionally large collections for sources of disease-resistance traits.

One feasible way is to access accessions collected in the region where the target pathogen originated. It is possible that the center of diversity for the pathogen may also be where host resistance evolved. Alternately, plant breeders can work, at least initially, with representative collections managed by genebanks.

Core collections

Plant germplasm denotes the available genetic resources for plant breeding. Many germplasm accessions are collected in genebanks all over the world, but methods for managing and utilizing such a diverse collection efficiently remain a challenging task for plant breeders. In 1984 Sir Otto Herzberg Frankel first proposed sampling the collections to yield a manageable sample or so-called "core collection." Core collections play a significant role in screening for disease resistance. The idea is that a core collection contains 10% of an entire collection. Because some collections have literally thousands of accessions, an added concept is a mini-core collection that contains 10% of the core or 1% of the entire collection. These collections preserve maximum genetic diversity within the smallest number of accessions. The core collection or mini-core has identified disease resistance sources in an efficient and cost-effective manner. The composition of the core is perfected as new material is included, or better data are obtained. The remaining accessions in the collection form the reserve that is conserved as a secondary source. There is an adage in breeding for disease resistance that says, "resistance is where you find it." The core collection assists the plant breeder to narrow the search. For example, a few sources of resistance to white mold disease (*Sclerotinia sclerotiorum*) in common bean (*Phaseolus vulgaris*) were known and used by plant breeders. Phillip N. Miklas with US Department of Agriculture, Agricultural Research Service (ARS) screened a mini-core of the active US Department of Agriculture NPGS collection of 1698 accessions of common bean (*P. vulgaris*) and found that a mini-core collection was useful for identifying resistance to white mold.

In another germplasm screening, Yariv Ben-Naim and colleagues at Bar-Ilan University, Israel evaluated 113 accessions of *Ocimum* (sweet basil) species including 83 US Department Agriculture Plant Introduction entries and 30 commercial entries for resistance against downy mildew (*Peronospora belbahrii*), at the seedling stage in growth chambers, and during three seasons, in the field. In this study, most entries belonged to *Ocimum basilicum* and were highly susceptible whereas most entries belonging to *Ocimum americanum, Ocimum kilimanadascharicum, Ocimum gratissimum, Ocimum campechianum,* or *Ocimum tenuiflorum* were highly resistant at both the seedling stage and in the field.

Developing a core collection is not a simple or inexpensive endeavor, and if done improperly there is the risk of not being representative of the diversity contained within the genebank, limiting effectiveness. As one might expect, the available core collections are much more numerous for agronomic crops as compared to horticultural crops, although the availability of core collections is increasing. For the four major vegetable crops in Solanaceae [tomato (*S. lycopersicum*), potato (*S. tuberosum*), eggplant (*Solanum melongena*), and pepper (*C. annuum*)] core collections are publicly available and have been phenotyped for numerous traits. Genome-wide association studies are often conducted using core collections that help a plant breeder identify small effects, in addition to major loci contributing to host resistance, and facilitate pyramiding or stacking of resistance genes. When finding a core collection for the crop of interest, a good approach is to contact the major genebanks that conserve that crop to see if they have a core collection available.

Roses (*Rosa* species) are one of the most prized flowers in the world, and breeding disease-resistant cultivars is one of the most important goals for plant breeders. Resistant accessions are a prerequisite to improve the narrow gene pool of modern roses. Rose black spot (*Diplocarpon rosae*) is one of the most devastating diseases of field-grown roses. A novel source of resistance can be public gardens; for example, Dietmar Schulz and colleagues at the University of Hannover, Germany make observations of black spots at the Sangerhausen rose garden containing 486 accessions over 2 years. They discovered that 289 accessions were resistant to black spot.

Another example is the New Mexico State University Chile Pepper Institute Teaching Garden where more than 150 different accessions of *Capsicum* consisting of six species are grown each year. During natural field epidemics in 1999 and in 2017, the plants in the Chile Pepper Institute Teaching Garden were evaluated for resistance to beet curly top virus (BCTV, *Curtovirus*) and powdery mildew (*Leveillula taurica*), respectively. The epidemics provided a unique opportunity to identify sources of resistance in *Capsicum*. It was observed for curly top virus that resistance could be found in three accessions each of *C. annuum* and *C. frutescens* and one accession each of *Capsicum chacoense* and *C. chinense*. For powdery mildew, major differences in disease severity and incidence were observed among the accessions. There were 53 rated as resistant, included in 16 *C. annuum* accessions, 8 *C. baccatum*, 21 *C. chinense*, 5 *C. frutescens*, 1 *C. chacoense*, and 1 *Capsicum rhomboideum* accession. These results provide several accessions with resistance that can be used in breeding for disease-resistant peppers (*Capsicum* species). Especially important are the *C. annuum* resistant accessions, as this resistance can be quickly incorporated into commercially important *C. annuum* cultivars as compared with interspecific hybridization.

Mutation

Improving crops through induced mutations was initiated more than 90 years ago with the discovery of mutagenic effects of X-rays on barley (*Hordeum vulgare*) and maize (*Zea mays*) by Stadler in 1928. A wide range of traits have been changed through mutation breeding including disease resistance. Recently, induced mutagenesis has gained importance in plant molecular biology as a tool to identify and isolate genes and to study their structure and function in plant resistance. The findings have an impact on the future of breeding disease-resistant crops.

When no natural source of resistance is found, mutation may be a way to create resistance. Irradiation, chemicals, and somaclonal variation have created a variation that produced new disease resistance horticultural crops. A classic example of inducing resistance with irradiation is the use of cobalt-60 gamma irradiation on peppermint (*Mentha × piperita*) for Verticillium wilt (*Verticillium dahlia*) resistance by the Todd Mint Co. in Wisconsin. Peppermint is asexually reproduced, and the company irradiated 100,000 clones and placed them in an infected field. One clone appeared resistant and was released as the cultivar Todd's Mitcham.

Another example of using Ethyl methanesulfonate (EMS)-induced mutagenesis is the development of the banana cultivar ReFen 1 (*Musa* species ABB, Pisang Awak subgroup) by the Hainan Banana Healthy Seedling Propagation Engineering Research Center at the Haikou Experimental Station, Chinese Academy of Tropical Agricultural Sciences, China. When compared with local banana cultivars, (*Musa* species) ReFen1 had significantly improved horticultural traits and resistance to Sigatoka leaf spot disease (*Mycosphaerella fijiensis*).

There was a lull in the interest of using mutation to breed for disease resistance because with mutation breeding the product is normally a recessive allele, a loss of function change. With resistance being perceived as an active function, the loss of function would not be practical, and therefore mutation breeding would not provide resistance. Recently, the advent of the loss-of-susceptible concept has renewed interest in mutation breeding. Many powdery mildew pathogens and virus infections need genes in the host to complete a successful infection, and when these genes are made nonfunctioning resistance occurs. The antiviral genes, *eIF4E* and *eIFiso4E*, are the most common recessive resistance genes whose absence inhibits infection by plant viruses in *Potyvirus*, *Carmovirus*, and *Cucumovirus* genera.

It will be interesting to see in the future whether the clustered regularly interspaced short palindromic repeats (CRISPR)/CRISPR-associated protein 9 (Cas9) will be considered a form of mutation breeding and non-genetic modified organism (non-GMO). Currently, the European Union and New Zealand classify the technique as genetic modified organism (GMO), while the United States of America does not. It may be possible with the CRISPR-Cas9 system to genome edit the various components of the plant immune system to acquire durable resistance in plants against pathogens. The modification of susceptible host genes (target genes, receptors involved in disease development, etc.) can be a practical and alternative approach to improve resistance. Also, loss of function mutation in the susceptibility gene(s) does not impact the overall plant health and developmental process. Therefore resistance developed by this method may provide an effective and durable resistance.

Globally, *Citrus* production faces a serious disease challenge with citrus canker a bacterial disease (*Xanthomonas citri* subsp. *citri*) that causes lesions on leaves, stems, and fruit; in addition, it affects the vitality of the trees, causing leaves and fruit to drop prematurely. Breeding cultivars resistant to this disease is the most efficient and sustainable approach. Classical breeding of *Citrus* and other perennial fruit trees is challenging due to extended juvenility and long hybridization cycles. Targeted genome editing technology using CRISPR/Cas 9 has the potential to shorten cultivar development for some traits, including disease resistance.

University of Florida researchers using CRISPR/Cas9 technology modified the canker susceptibility gene, *CsLOB1*, in a grapefruit (*Citrus x paradisi*) cultivar because grapefruit is one of the most canker-susceptible citrus varieties. They identified the *CsLOB1* gene as a critical citrus disease susceptibility gene for citrus canker. When inoculated with the pathogen, no canker symptoms were observed on the two lines they developed. No phenotypic changes were detected in the "mutated" plants. This study indicates that genome editing using CRISPR technology provides a promising pathway to generate disease-resistant citrus varieties. More importantly, this recessive resistance due to mutation of the gene, *CsLOB*1, is expected to be durable and efficient against all *Xanthomonas* pathotypes causing citrus canker because they all rely on the induction of the susceptibility gene *CsLOB1* to induce canker symptoms. Using the CRISPR technique, a mutation of the coding region for two alleles of the susceptibility gene, *CsLOB1*, generated citrus canker-resistant plants. Importantly, this study illustrated that disease-resistant citrus cultivars can be developed using CRISPR technology.

Somaclonal variation

The genetic variations found within in vitro cultured cells are collectively referred to as somaclonal variation. The plants derived from such cells are referred to as somaclones. The growth of plant cells in vitro is an asexual process involving only the mitotic division of cells. Thus culturing of cells is the method to clone a particular genotype. It is therefore expected that plants arising from a given tissue culture should be the exact copies of the parental plant.

The occurrence of phenotypic variants among regenerated plants from tissue cultures has been known for decades. These variations were earlier dismissed as tissue culture artifacts. The term "somaclonal variation" was first used by Philip J. Larkin of the Division of Plant Industry, The Commonwealth Scientific and Industrial Research Organization, Canberra, Australia and William R. Scowcroft of Research and Development, Biotechnica Canada Inc, in 1981 for variations arising due to culture of cells, that is, variability generated by tissue culture, which is now universally accepted. The explant used in tissue culture may come from any part of the plant. These include leaves, roots, protoplasts, microspores, and embryos, and somaclonal variations are reported in all these plant tissues. In recent years, the term gametoclonal variations describes variations observed in the regenerated plants from gametic cells, for example, anther culture.

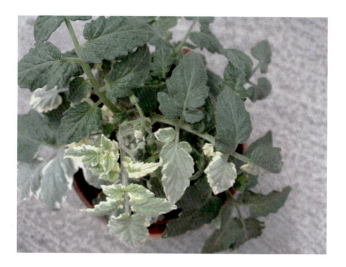

Figure 7.3 A somaclonal mutation (sport) on a tomato (*Solanum lycopersicum*) branch.

The genetic changes associated with somaclonal variations in addition to mutation include polyploidy, aneuploidy, chromosomal breakage, deletion, translocation, and gene amplifications. The occurrence of mutations in cultures is relatively low. The variation may be due to varied nutrients, culture conditions, and mutagenic effects of metabolic products that accumulate in the medium. Somaclonal variations due to transposable elements, mitotic crossing over, and changes in the cytoplasmic genome have also been reported (Fig. 7.3).

Disease-resistant plants have been obtained from somaclonal variations including potato (*S. tuberosum*) with resistance to scab (*Streptomyces scabie*), early blight (*Alternaria solani*), late blight (*Phytophthora infestans*), and potato virus X (PVX; *Potyvirus*) and potato virus Y (PVY; *Potyvirus*). Somaclonal resistance was developed in tomato (*S. lycopersicum*) against bacterial wilt (*Ralstonia solanacearum*) and Fusarium wilt (*F. oxysporum*).

Despite several applications of somaclonal variation, there are limitations to this approach. The limitation of in vitro selection approach is that it is not directed. As with any mutation experiment, most of the somaclonal variations will not be useful because the variation is unpredictable. Consequently, the appearance of a desired trait is purely by chance. A genetic trait obtained by somaclonal variation may not be stable and heritable. Somaclonal variation can be cultivar-dependent, which is frequently a time-consuming process. Finally, and most importantly, somaclones can only be produced in those species that regenerate to complete plants. Furthermore, this procedure is time-consuming and requires the screening of many regenerated plants.

Genetic transformation

In the late 20th century, and now in the 21st century, genetic transformation (i.e., GMOs) have become important in disease-resistance breeding. Virus resistance using virus coat proteins has made promising advancements. With increased access to the diverse genetic variation found in crops and natural populations of wild relatives, the opportunity to recover disease-resistance traits is more promising; many of these are encoded by genes for pattern recognition and leucine-rich repeat receptors that were lost during domestication or that have evolved independently in different plant lineages. Advances in genome sequencing and assembly technologies, coupled with new methods for capturing near-complete immune-receptor gene panels from complex genomes, hold promise for attaining sustainable disease resistance. Merging these approaches with genome-wide association studies taps into immune-receptor gene variants that have adapted to local environments and achieved a more durable disease resistance. The use of molecular tools and genetic modification is covered in more detail in Chapter 9.

Bibliography

Altieri, M.A., Merrick, L.C., 1987. In situ conservation of crops. Genetic resources through maintenance of traditional farming systems. Economic Botany 41, 86–96. Available from: https://doi.org/10.1007/BF02859354.

Anderson, P.A., Okubara, P.A., Arroyo-Garcia, R., Meyers, B.C., Michelmore, R.W., 1996. Molecular analysis of irradiation-induced and spontaneous deletion mutants at a disease resistance locus in *Lactuca sativa*. Molecular and General Genetics 251, 316–325. Available from: https://doi.org/10.1007/BF02172522.

Ben-Naim, Y., Falach, L., Cohen, Y., 2015. Resistance against basil downy mildew in *Ocimum* species. Phytopathology 105, 778–785. Available from: https://doi.org/10.1094/PHYTO-11-14-0295-R.

Bonneuil, C., 2019. Seeing nature as a 'universal store of genes': how biological diversity became 'genetic resources', 1890–1940. Studies in History and Philosophy of Science Part C: Studies in History and Philosophy of Biological and Biomedical Sciences 75, 1–14. Available from: https://doi.org/10.1016/j.shpsc.2018.12.002.

Borrelli, V.M.G., Brambilla, V., Rogowsky, P., Marocco, A., Lanubile, A., 2018. The Enhancement of plant disease resistance using CRISPR/Cas9 technology. Frontiers in Plant Science 9, 1245. Available from: https://doi.org/10.3389/fpls.2018.01245.

Bosland, P.W., 2000. Sources of curly top virus resistance in Capsicum. HortScience 35, 1321–1322. Available from: https://doi.org/10.21273/HORTSCI.35.7.1321.

Brown, A.H.D., 1989. Core collections: a practical approach to genetic resources management. Genome/National Research Council Canada = Genome/Conseil National De Recherches Canada 31, 818–824. Available from: https://doi.org/10.1139/g89-144.

Brush, S.B., 2004. Farmers' Bounty: Locating Crop Diversity in the Contemporary World. Yale University Press, p. 327. Available from: https://doi.org/10.12987/yale/9780300100495.001.0001.

Chikh-Rouhou, H., Gómez-Guillamón, M.L., González, V., Sta-Baba, R., Garcés-Claver, A., 2021. *Cucumis melo* L. Germplasm in Tunisia: unexploited sources of resistance to Fusarium wilt. Horticulturae 7, 208. Available from: https://doi.org/10.3390/horticulturae7080208.

Cooper, C., Crowther, T., Smith, B.M., Isaac, S., Collin, H.A., 2006. Assessment of the response of carrot somaclones to *Pythium violae*, the causal agent of cavity spot. Plant Pathology 55, 427–432. Available from: https://doi.org/10.1111/j.1365-3059.2006.01355.x.

Curry, H.A., 2019. From bean collection to seed bank: transformations in heirloom vegetable conservation, 1970–1985. BJHS Themes 4, 149–167. Available from: https://doi.org/10.1017/bjt.2019.2.

Deppe, C., 2000. Breed Your Own Vegetable Varieties: The Gardener's and Farmer's Guide to Plant Breeding and Seed Saving, second edition Chelsea Green Publishing, p. 384, ISBN-13: 978-1890132729.

Dhillon, N.P.S., Monforte, A.J., Pitrat, M., et al., 2011. Chapter 3 — Melon landraces of India: contributions and importance. In: Janick, Jules (Ed.), Plant Breeding Reviews, vol. 35. Wiley Press, pp. 85–150. 407 pages. Available from: https://doi.org/10.1002/9781118100509.ch3.

Dugdale, L.J., Mortimer, A.M., Isaac, S., Collin, H.A., 2000. Disease response of carrot and carrot somaclones to *Alternaria dauci*. Plant Pathology 49, 57–67. Available from: https://doi.org/10.1046/j.1365-3059.2000.00389.x.

Dutfield, G., 2004. Intellectual Property, Biogenetic Resources, and Traditional Knowledge. Earthscan, VA, p. 258.

Engels, J.M.M., Ramanatha Rao, V., Brown, A.H.D., Jackson, M.T., 2002. Managing Plant Genetic Diversity. CABI Publishing, p. 487.

Erpen-Dalla Corte, L., Mahmoud, L.M., Moraes, T.S., Mou, Z., Grosser, J.W., Dutt, M.J., 2019. Development of improved fruit, vegetable, and ornamental crops using the CRISPR/Cas9 genome editing technique. Plants 8, 601. Available from: https://doi.org/10.3390/plants8120601.

Fowler, C., Mooney, P., 1990. Shattering. The University of Arizona Press, Tucson, p. 278.

Fowler, C., Lower, R.L., 2005. Politics of plant breeding. In: Janick, J. (Ed.), Plant Breeding Reviews, vol. 25. pp. 21–56.

Frankel, O.H., 1977. Genetic resources. In: Day, P.R. (Ed.). The Genetic Basis of Epidemics in Agriculture. New York Academy of Sciences, N.Y., pp. 332–344.

Frankel, O.H., 1984. Genetic perspectives of germplasm conservation. In: Arber, W., Illmensee, K., Peacock, W.J., Starlingeret, P. (Eds.), Genetic Manipulation: Impact on Man and Society. Cambridge University Press, Cambridge, UK, pp. 161–170.

Garrett, K.A., Andersen, K.F., Asche, F., Bowden, R.L., Forbes, G.A., Kulakow, P.A., et al., 2017. Resistance genes in global crop breeding networks. Phytopathology 107, 1268–1278. Available from: https://doi.org/10.1094/PHYTO-03-17-0082-FI.

Gray, T.S., Stenson, A.J., 1999. The Politics of Genetic Resource Control. St. Martin's Press, p. 175.

Guerrant Jr., E.O., Havens, K., Maunder, M., 2004. Ex situ Plant Conservation: Supporting Species Survival in the Wild. Island Press, Washington D.C., p. 536.

Harlan, J.R., 1977. Sources of genetic defense. In: Day, P.R. (Ed.), The Genetic Basis of Epidemics in Agricultural. N.Y. Acad. Sci., NY, pp. 345–356.

I.A.E.A., 1971. Induced mutations against plant disease. In: Proceedings of a Symposium. Int. Atomic Energy Agency, Vienna. 580 pages.

Jia, H., Zhang, Y., Orbović, V., Xu, J., White, F.F., Jones, J.B., et al., 2016. Genome editing of the disease susceptibility gene CsLOB1 in citrus confers resistance to citrus canker. Plant Biotechnology Journal 15, 817–823. Available from: https://doi.org/10.1111/pbi.12677.

Harmeet Kaur, H., Pandey, D.K., Goutam, U., Kumar, V., 2021. CRISPR/Cas9-mediated genome editing is revolutionizing the improvement of horticultural crops: recent advances and future prospects. Scientia Horticulturae 289, 110476. Available from: https://doi.org/10.1016/j.scienta.2021.110476.

Kloppenburg, J.R. (Ed.), 1988. Seeds and Sovereignty. The Use and Control of Plant Genetic Resources. Duke University Press, Durham, NC, p. 368.

Kellerhals, M., Szalatnay, D., Hunziker, K., Duffy, B., Nybom, H., Ahmadi-Afzadi, M., et al., 2012. European pome fruit genetic resources evaluated for disease resistance. Trees 26, 179–189. Available from: https://doi.org/10.1007/s00468-011-0660-9.

Knott, D.R., Dvorak, J., 1976. Alien germplasm as a source of resistance to disease. Annual Review of Phytopathology 14, 211–235. Available from: https://doi.org/10.1146/annurev.py.14.090176.001235.

Kong, C., Chen, G., Yang, L., Zhuang, M., Zhang, Y., Wang, Y., et al., 2021. Germplasm screening and inheritance analysis of resistance to cabbage black rot in a worldwide collection of cabbage (*Brassica oleracea* var. *capitata*) resources. Scientia Horticulturae 288, 110234. Available from: https://doi.org/10.1016/j.scienta.2021.110234.

Lenné, J.M., Wood, D., 1991. Plant diseases and the use of wild germplasm. Annual Review of Phytopathology 29, 35–63. Available from: https://doi.org/10.1146/annurev.py.29.090191.000343.

Leppik, E.E., 1970. Gene centers of plants as sources of disease resistance. Annual Review of Phytopathology 8, 323–344. Available from: https://doi.org/10.1146/annurev.py.08.090170.001543.

Lin, T., Zhu, G., Zhang, J., Xu, X., Yu, Q., Zheng, Z., et al., 2014. Genomic analyses provide insights into the history of tomato breeding. Nature Genetics 46, 1220–1226.

Manzur, J.P., Fita, A., Prohens, J., Rodríguez-Burruezo, A., 2015. Successful wide hybridization and introgression breeding in a diverse set of common peppers (*Capsicum annuum*) using different cultivated ají (C. baccatum) accessions as donor parents. PLoS ONE. Available from: https://doi.org/10.1371/journal.pone.0144142.

McCoy, J.E., Bosland, P.W., 2019. Identification of resistance to powdery mildew in chile pepper. HortScience 54, 4–7. Available from: https://doi.org/10.21273/HORTSCI13596-18.

Miklas, P.N., Delorme, R., Hannan, R., Dickson, M.H., 1999. Using a subsample of the core collection to identify new sources of resistance to white mold in common bean. Crop Science 39, 569–573. Available from: https://doi.org/10.2135/cropsci1999.0011183X003900020044x.

Murray, M.J., Todd, W.A., 1972. Registration of Todd's Mitcham peppermint. Crop Science 12, 128. Available from: https://doi.org/10.2135/cropsci1972.0011183X001200010056x.

Plucknett, D.L., Smith, N.J.H., Williams, J.T., Anishetty, N.M., 1987. Gene Banks and the World's Food. Princeton Univ. Press, p. 247.

Barrera-Redondo, J., Sánchez-de la Vega, G., Aguirre-Liguori, J.A., Castellanos-Morales, G., Gutiérrez-Guerrero, Y.T., Aguirre-Dugua, X., et al., 2021. The domestication of *Cucurbita argyrosperma* as revealed by the genome of its wild relative. Horticulture Research 8, 109. Available from: https://doi.org/10.1038/s41438-021-00544-9.

Rodgers, P.C., Smith, D., Bosland, P.W., 1997. A novel statistical approach to analyze genetic resources evaluations, using Capsicum as an example. Crop Science 37, 1000–1002. Available from: https://doi.org/10.2135/cropsci1997.0011183X003700030050x.

Schulz, D.F., Linde, M., Blechert, O., Debener, T., 2009. Evaluation of *Genus Rosa* germplasm for resistance to black spot, downy mildew, and powdery mildew. European Journal of Horticultural Science 74, 1–9. Available from: http://www.jstor.org/stable/24126486.

Shepard, J.F., 1983. Somatic modification of germplasm and the potential for genetic engineering. In: Kommedahl, T., Williams, P.H. (Eds.), Challenging Problems in Plant Health. American Phytopathology Society, St. Paul, MN, pp. 145–153. 538 pages.

Shepard, J.F., Bidney, D., Shakin, E., 1980. Potato protoplasts in crop improvement. Science 208, 17–24. Available from: https://doi.org/10.1126/science.208.4439.17.

Shulman, S., 1986. Seeds of controversy: nations square off over who will control plant genetic resources. Bioscience 36, 647–651. Available from: https://doi.org/10.2307/1310382.

Simon, M.D., 1979. Modification of host–parasite interactions through artificial mutagenesis. Annual Review of Phytopathology 17, 75–96. Available from: https://doi.org/10.1146/annurev.py.17.090179.000451.

Song, S., Hong, J.-E., Hossain, M.R., Jung, H.-J., Nou, I.-S., 2022. Development of clubroot resistant cabbage line through introgressing six CR loci from Chinese cabbage via interspecific hybridization and embryo rescue. Scientia Horticulturae 300, 111036. Available from: https://doi.org/10.1016/j.scienta.2022.111036.

Sprague, G.F., 1980. Germplasm resources of plants: their preservation and use. Annual Review of Phytopathology 18, 147–165. Available from: https://doi.org/10.1146/annurev.py.18.090180.001051.

Taylor, J.D., Conway, J., Roberts, S.J., Astley, D., Vicente, J.G., 2002. Sources and origin of resistance to *Xanthomonas campestris* pv. campestris in Brassica genomes. Phytopathology 92, 105–111. Available from: https://doi.org/10.1094/PHYTO.2002.92.1.105.

Tian, L., Wang, Y., Niu, L., Tang, D., 2008. Breeding of disease-resistant seedless grapes using Chinese wild *Vitis* spp.: I. In vitro embryo rescue and plant development. Scientia Horticulturae 117, 136–141. Available from: https://doi.org/10.1016/j.scienta.2008.03.024.

Tyagia, S., Kumarb, R., Kumarc, V., Wona, S.Y., Shuklad, P., 2020. Engineering disease resistant plants through CRISPR-Cas9 technology. GM Crops & Food 12, 125–144. Available from: https://doi.org/10.1080/21645698.2020.1831729.

van der Meer, Q.P., de Vries, J.N., 1990. An interspecific cross between *Allium roylei* Stearn and *Allium cepa* L., and its backcross to *A. cepa*. Euphytica 47, 29–31. Available from: https://doi.org/10.1007/BF00040359.

van Hintum, T.J.L., Brown, A.H.D., Spillane, C., 2000. Core Collections of Plant Genetic resources. IPGRI Technical Bulletin No.3. International Plant Genetic Resources Institute, Rome Italy.

Veley, K.M., K. Elliott, K., Jensen, G., Zhong, Z., Feng, S., Yoder, M., et al., 2023. Improving cassava bacterial blight resistance by editing the epigenome. Nature Communications 14, 85. Available from: https://doi.org/10.1038/s41467-022-35675-7.

Venkataravanappa, V., Sanwal, S.K., Lakshminarayana Reddy, C.N., Singh, B., Umare, S.N., Krishna Reddy, M., 2022. Phenotypic screening of cultivated and wild okra germplasm against yellow vein mosaic and enation leaf curl diseases of okra in India. Crop Protection 156. Available from: https://doi.org/10.1016/j.cropro.2022.105955.

Volk, G., Byrne, P., 2022. Crop wild relatives and their use in plant breeding. https://colostate.pressbooks.pub/cropwildrelatives/.

Volk, G., 2022. Links to some published best practices for genebanking. https://colostate.pressbooks.pub/cropwildrelatives/chapter/published-best-practices/.

Wang, X., Wang, A., Li, Y., Xu, Y., Wei, Q., Wang, J., et al., 2021. A novel banana mutant 'RF-1' (*Musa* spp. ABB, Pisang Awak subgroup) for improved agronomic traits and enhanced cold tolerance and disease resistance. Frontiers in Plant Science 12, 730718. Available from: https://doi.org/10.3389/fpls.2021.730718.

Williams, P.H., 1983. Conservation of plant and symbiont germplasm. In: Kommendahl, T., Williams, P.H. (Eds.), Challenging Problems in Plant Health. American Phytopathology Society, St. Paul, MN, pp. 131–144. 538 pages.

Zewdie, Y., Tong, N., Bosland, P., 2004. Establishing a core collection of Capsicum using a cluster analysis with enlightened selection of accessions. Genetic Resources and Crop Evolution 51, 147–151. Available from: https://doi.org/10.1023/B:GRES.0000020858.96226.38.

Zhang, Q., Yu, E., Medina, A., 2012. Development of advanced interspecific-bridge lines among *Cucurbita pepo*, *C. maxima*, and *C. moschata*. HortScience 47 (4), 452–458. Available from: https://doi.org/10.21273/HORTSCI.47.4.452.

8

Resistance: Classical Breeding Methods

Introduction

When breeding for disease-resistant horticultural plants, there are two classical approaches: (1) selection and (2) hybridization. First, plants of a given population can show segregation for resistance and susceptibility, and the resistant plants can be selected within the population. If the plants are self-pollinating, the seeds from a single plant can be collected, a process called pure line selection. This is one of the earliest and basic breeding methods and was developed using common bean (*Phaseolus vulgaris*), a self-pollinated crop.

Pure line selection

In the early 20th century, Wilhelm Johannsen of the University of Copenhagen, Denmark, proposed the pure line theory and the genotype versus the phenotype distinction. This theory is one of the most important foundational theory to genetics and Mendelian plant breeding. Most historians concluded that pure line theory did not change breeding practices directly. Instead, breeding became more orderly because of pure line theory, which structured breeding programs.

The effectiveness of selection largely depends on two main factors: (1) extent of genetic variability present in the base population in which selection is to be practiced, and (2) heritability of the character. Selection is more effective when sufficient genetic variation is present in the base population. Similarly, selection is more effective for those characters having high heritability than those having low heritability. Selection leads to the depletion of genetic variability in a population. An interesting footnote is that variation within a pure line is entirely due to environmental factors and an excellent way to measure the effect of environment on the disease screen. A caveat to this is that spontaneous mutations do occur changing the genetic constitution of the cultivar.

Single plant selection

Single plant selection is similar to pure line selection. While pure line selection may contain seeds from more than one plant of a given phenotype, single plant selection is based on a single plant. A good example of single plant selection is with potatoes (*Solanum tuberosum*). Potatoes are asexually reproduced; thus, a single plant of potato with tubers can reproduce many offspring. A hybridization is made between two parents, and the seed of the hybridization is planted. The progeny is then subjected to single plant selection. In the first year, single plant observations for traits like tuber shape, appearance, and plant maturity are selected and are good predictors of the clone performance. Single plants are not reliable for evaluating yield or any other quantitative traits.

Mass selection

If the plants are cross-pollinating, then many individuals need to be combined to reduce the chance of inbreeding depression. Inbreeding of cross-pollinating crops leads to a strong reduction of vigor in the early generations. Normally, a group of 60–90 plants are needed to be selected to be statistically safe not to initiate the process of inbreeding. This "mass selection" is one of the earliest breeding methods for cross-pollinated crops. A mass-selected cultivar is a mixture of heterozygotes and homozygotes plants. Thus it is a heterozygous and heterogeneous population. When domestication of crops began, selection for disease resistance was probably one of the traits selected or at least selection against susceptibility.

Hybridization

Hybridizations between resistant sources and a plant with the coveted horticultural traits are the most frequently employed plant breeding technique (Fig. 8.1). The aim of hybridization is to bring together desired traits found in different plant lines into one cultivar. This is a more sophisticated approach than pure line, single plant selection, or mass selection. There are many breeding methods based on hybridization and selection. There can be multiple hybridizations and cycles of selection. If resistance is from a wild relative of the crop, a large quantity of undesired traits like low yield, bad palpability, and low

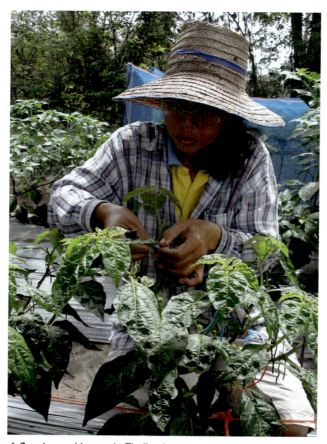

Figure 8.1 Hybridization of *Capsicum chinense* in Thailand. Courtesy of the authors.

nutritional value are also transferred to the crop. These unfavorable traits must be removed before the cultivar can be released.

Backcross method

One of the most common approaches is to backcross to a well-adapted parent. The backcross breeding approach can be employed to introduce a specific trait, such as disease resistance, from one line, often an unimproved line, to another line that is typically an elite breeding line. The parent with the desired trait, for example, disease resistance, is called the donor parent and normally will not perform as well as the recurrent parent that usually performs well and has been accepted by growers. Because the established cultivar has already been bred intensively for maximum performance, the resulting backcross cultivar should be acceptable to growers.

Backcrossing involves making an initial hybridization between the donor and recurrent parent (Fig. 8.2). The resultant F_1 progeny have 50% of their genetic material from each parent. The F_1 individuals are backcrossed to the recurrent parent to develop a backcross one (BC_1) population. Individuals from the BC_1 population are once again backcrossed to the recurrent parent. Each generation of backcrossing reduces the proportion of the donor parent present in the population by half. This cycle of backcrossing progeny to the recurrent parent continues until a new line that is identical to the recurrent parent, but with the desired resistance from the donor parent is created. By the BC_4 generation, the lines are greater than 96% identical to the recurrent parent. The backcrossing process can often be accelerated using marker-assisted backcrossing.

The backcross method has been used to develop multilines, and isogenic lines. The method is more effective in transferring one to a few characters than polygenic traits. The product of backcross method is very much like the parent variety except for the disease resistance that has been transferred from the donor source.

Some plant breeders criticize the backcross breeding method as being conservative. This criticism is related to backcross-derived cultivars being superior to their recurrent parent for only the trait from the donor parent. During the development period of a backcross-derived cultivar, a new cultivar that is superior in performance to the recurrent parent may become available, resulting in diminished importance of the backcross-derived cultivar. However, a backcross-derived cultivar must be compared with the best cultivar in production. A standard two-parent or multiparent backcross-derived cultivar can be

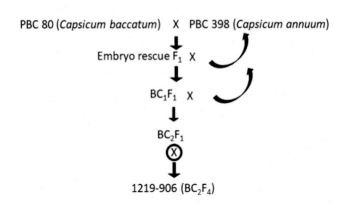

Figure 8.2 Diagram illustrates Backcross method.

available to growers in 3 years after the first hybridization to the recurrent parent.

Pedigree method

The pedigree method is applicable to both self-pollinated and cross-pollinated species and is the most prevalent breeding method in countless programs. The pedigree keeps information of the ancestry of an individual selected plant or population. Proper record of the ancestry of each selected plant or plant progeny is maintained for all generations of selection. Important characters of each selected plant and progeny are recorded. The pedigree method is laborious because of the comprehensive recording of the relationship of individual plants and the population they are derived, plus their resistance phenotype. The amount of extra work by the pedigree method varies by the individual breeder. It is extensively used for developing disease-resistant cultivars.

Recurrent selection

Recurrent selection is a term coined by Fred H. Hull of the Florida Agricultural Experiment Station, Gainesville, Florida, USA, in 1945 for a cyclical improvement method aimed at concentrating desirable alleles in a population through a process of detecting better individuals of a population. Recurrent selection is used in cross-pollinating crops and self-pollinating crops, but principally for cross-pollinating crops, but has a place in clonally propagated plants. For example, the cultivated rose (*Rosa* sp.) is affected by several diseases like black spot (*Diplocarpon rosae*), powdery mildew (*Sphaerotheca pannosa*), botrytis (*Botrytis cinerea*), downy mildew (*Peronospora sparsa*), and Rose rosette disease (RRD, *Emaravirus*). Currently, rose breeders use a recurrent phenotypic selection approach and perform selection for disease resistance for most pathogens in a 2–3-year field trial.

Somatic hybridization

As discussed in Chapter 4, Resistance: the pathogen, somatic hybridization is a natural way for plant pathogens to generate new virulence. For plants, it was introduced more than 35 years ago as a technological aid to classical breeding to overcome the failure of wide hybridization. Somatic hybrids have been used to create new sources of cytoplasmic male sterility (CMS), for example, the Ogura CMS a naturally occurring mutation found in radish (*Raphanus sativus*) that has been transferred into *Brassica* crops. Clubroot disease (*Plasmodiophora brassicae*), a major plant root disease of cruciferous vegetables is controlled in a few clubroot-resistant cabbage (*Brassica oleracea* var. *capitata*) cultivars by using the Ogura cytoplasmic male sterile as the source of resistance. Plant breeders at Syngenta Seeds B.V. produced interspecific hybridizations between a broccoli (*B. oleracea* var. *italica*) inbred line and Chinese cabbage (*Brassica rapa*), and then conducted a backcross program with cauliflower (*B. oleracea* var. *botrytis*), cabbage, (*B. oleracea* var. *capitata*), and Brussels sprouts (*B. oleracea* var. *gemmifer*) to transfer clubroot (*P. brassicae*) resistance genes from the Chinese cabbage clubroot resistance sources. The project entailed several years of backcrosses, selections, line developments, and test crosses. Therefore transfer of a clubroot (*P. brassicae*) resistance by wide hybridization typically requires several years of successive backcrosses to reduce the background genes of the donor parent. Although a few clubroot (*P. brassicae*)-resistant varieties of cabbage (*B. oleracea* var. *capitata*) are available on the market, almost all are Ogura cytoplasmic male sterile cultivars and thus cannot be self-pollinated.

Another application of breeding for disease resistance in horticulture crops is to increase resistance in *Citrus* rootstocks. A major strategy of the University of Florida Citrus Research and Education Center is rootstock improvement using protoplast fusion to produce allotetraploid somatic hybrids that combine complementary rootstock germplasm. A trifoliate orange (*Poncirus trifoliata*) rootstock "50–7" has superior resistance to *Phytophthora nicotianae*. It was hybridized with sour orange (*Citrus aurantium*), 'Changsha' mandarin (*Citrus reticulata*), navel orange (*Citrus sinensis*), and a seedy white Duncan type grapefruit (*Citrus paradisi*). A high-yielding 'Benton' citrange, a hybrid of 'Ruby Blood' sweet orange (*C. sinensis*), is *Phytophthora citrophthora* and Citrus tristeza virus (CTV, *Closterovirus*) resistance and *P. trifoliata* was hybridized with 'Changsha' mandarin and sour orange. More than 200 plants of each of these six new somatic hybrids were propagated via tissue culture and rooted cuttings.

Progress with somatic hybridization will be the consequence of improvements in several areas: new fusion methods, better heterokaryon selection strategies, better protoplast culture methods, and more powerful molecular tools for analyzing the hybrids.

Doubled haploids

Doubled haploids are a very efficient tool to produce completely homozygous lines from heterozygous donor plants in a single step. The discovery of haploids in higher plants led to the use of doubled haploid technology in plant breeding. Doubled haploids are created by doubling the chromosomes of a haploid. A haploid plant contains the same number of chromosomes in their somatic cells as the normal gametes, pollen, and eggs of the species. The term "haploid sporophyte" normally designates such sporophytes having the gametic chromosome number. Spontaneous haploids have been discovered, generally by their small stature as plants. Fortunately, many methods have been developed for the in vitro induction of haploids from either male or female gametophytes. Haploids expedient plant breeding because selection can be markedly improved by using homozygous progenies. Doubled haploids achieve homozygosity in one generation. Thus the plant breeder can eliminate numerous cycles of inbreeding necessary to achieve practical levels of homozygosity by conventional methods. Theoretically, absolute homozygosity for all traits is not achievable by conventional breeding methods. Consequently, an efficient doubled haploid technology enables plant breeders to reduce the time and the cost of cultivar development relative to conventional breeding practices.

Researchers at Chiang Mai University, Thailand, used doubled haploids to develop cucumbers (*Cucumis sativus*) resistant to Cucumber mosaic virus (CMV, *Cucumovirus*). They screened 100 varieties of cucumber (*C. sativus*) from China, India, Japan, Malaysia, Pakistan, Philippines, Thailand, and the United States. The lines showed an assortment of different symptoms ranging from severe to mild mosaic and no symptoms. Of the 100 lines tested 42 were selected for their resistance and were self-pollinated. The S_1 generation was retested for resistance to CMV, and of those lines, five showing no symptoms were subjected to doubled haploid plant production. The doubled haploid resistant lines produced were selfed and seed harvested. Therefore doubled haploid cucumber (*C. sativus*) production and screening for resistance to CMV accelerated the breeding program.

Breeding symbols

Communicating among plant breeders is important, and having a system understood by everyone eliminates ambiguity.

There are plant breeding symbols that are sometimes used incorrectly, so a short description on these symbols related to breeding generations is needed. They are the symbols for hybridization, filial generation, self-pollinated, and backcrossing. Normally, a capital "X" designates the hybridization; for example, A X B refers to parent "A" being hybridized by parent "B." There is an adage in plant breeding that states "ladies first," so the "A" parent is the female seed parent, while "B" is the male pollen parent. It is easy to see how the word "cross" became the verb for making a hybridization, when X is the symbol used. The next symbol is "F" that refers to the word "filial" coming from Latin *filius*, meaning "son," and *filia*, "daughter," in English it applies to any gender, and the subscript associated with the "F" is the reference to the generation in the sequence of generations following a hybridization. For example, the F_1 symbolizes the first generation after the hybridization or selection. The F_2 (Fig. 8.3) symbolizes the second generation after the hybridization or selection, and the numbering system continues until the end of selection. There are examples where the F_8 or larger are recorded. The $\otimes$ is the symbol used for a plant that is self-pollinated. The next symbol is the "S" that signifies an individual that is self-pollinated. The "S_0" is used to designate the starting or base population of the self-pollinated generation. As with the filial (F) generational designations, many generations can be self-pollinated to generate a cultivar. The symbol for backcrossing is "BC." The F_1 individual to a recurrent parent would be designated as BC_1F_1 and a second backcross as BC_2F_1. Another example is to take a plant selected in the F_2 generation, and then start the backcrossing protocol, which is written as BC_1F_2. A symbol that is not used often in horticultural crops because not many horticultural crops are "synthetic cultivars" is the "syn." This symbol designates generations in developing a synthetic cultivar, the generations are annotated as syn-0, syn-1, syn-2, etc. The synthetic method of breeding is suitable for improving cross-pollinating crops. The synthetic cultivar is produced from cross-pollinating crops with planned matings involving selected genotypes. This method differs from mass selection because the synthetic variety is developed by intercrossing several genotypes of known superior combining ability, while the mass selection cultivar is made up of genotypes bulked together without having undergone preliminary testing to determine their performance in hybrid combination. Synthetic cultivars are only maintained for a specific set of generations. Lastly, there is the "M" symbol denoting generations in mutation breeding. The generation where treatment,

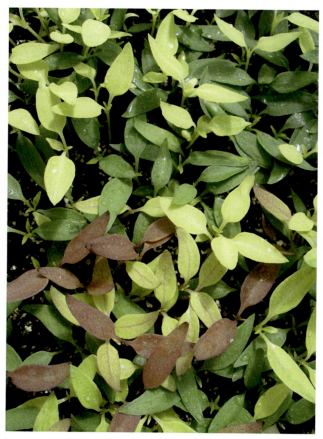

Figure 8.3 Pepper (*Capsicum annuum*) F_2 seedlings segregating for cotyledon colors. Courtesy of the authors.

whether it is radiation or chemical, is applied to the plant material, normally seeds, are the M_0 generation. The M_1 generation is the grow-out stage where the treated seeds are planted, and the seeds harvested from the parents. The M_2 generation is plants that are self-pollinated and begin to show changes from the mutation treatment. Because most mutants are recessive, the homozygous loci are now in greater number. The numbering continues in each generation normally until the M_5 generation. At this point, quantitative differences will be manifested, and selection can occur.

Bibliography

Acquaah, G., 2020. Principles of Plant Genetics and Breeding, third ed. Wiley-Blackwell, 848 pages, ISBN-13:978–1119626329.

Baenziger, P.S., Erayman, M., Budak, H., Campbell, B.T., 2004. Breeding pure line cultivars. In: Goodman, R.M. (Ed.), Encyclopedia of Plant and Crop Science. Marcel Dekker, New York, pp. 196–201.

Berry, D., 2014. The plant breeding industry after pure line theory: lessons from the National Institute of Agricultural Botany. Studies in History and Philosophy of Science Part C: Studies in History and Philosophy of Biological and Biomedical Sciences 46, 25–37. Available from: https://doi.org/10.1016/j.shpsc.2014.02.006.

Blakeslee, A.F., Belling, J., Farnham, M.E., Bergner, A.D., 1922. A haploid mutant in the Jimson weed, "*Datura stramonium*.". Science (New York, N.Y.) 55, 646–647. Available from: https://doi.org/10.1126/science.55.1433.646.

Brown, J.P., Caligari, Campos, H., 2014. Plant Breeding, second ed. Wiley-Blackwell, 256 pages, ISBN-13:978-0470658307.

Deppe, C., 2000. Breed Your Own Vegetable Varieties: The Gardener's and Farmer's Guide to Plant Breeding and Seed Saving, second ed. Chelsea Green Publishing, 384 pages, ISBN-13:978-1890132729.

Diederichsen, E., Frauen, M., Linders, E.G.A., Hatakeyama, K., Hirai, M., 2009. Status and perspectives of clubroot resistance breeding in crucifer crops. Journal of Plant Growth Regulation 28, 265–281. Available from: https://doi.org/10.1007/s00344-009-9100-0.

Grosser, J.W., Chandler, J.L., 2000. Somatic hybridization of high yield, cold-hardy and disease resistant parents for citrus rootstock improvement. The Journal of Horticultural Science and Biotechnology 75, 641–644. Available from: https://doi.org/10.1080/14620316.2000.11511300.

Kang, M.S., 2020. Quantitative Genetics, Genomics and Plant Breeding, second ed. CABI, 416 pages, ISBN-13:978–1789240214.

Kingsbury, N., 2011. Hybrid: The History and Science of Plant Breeding. University of Chicago Press, 493 pages, ISBN-13:978–0226437132.

Li, Y.G., Stoutjestijk, P.A., Larkin, P.J., 1999. Somatic hybridization for plant improvement. In: Soh, W.Y., Bhojwani, S.S. (Eds.), Morphogenesis in Plant Tissue Cultures. Springer, Dordrecht. Available from: https://doi.org/10.1007/978-94-015-9253-6_13.

Orton, T.J., 2020. Horticultural Plant Breeding. Academic Press, 410 pages, ISBN-13:978-0128153963.

Plapung, P., Khumsukdee, J., Smitamana, P., 2014. Development of cucumber lines resistant to cucumber mosaic virus by ovule culture. Journal of Agricultural Technology 10 (3), 733–741. Available from: http://www.ijat-aatsea.com/.

Tychonievich, J., 2013. Plant Breeding for the Home Gardener: How to Create Unique Vegetables and Flowers. Timber Press, 216 pages, ISBN-13:978-1604693645.

Weyen, J., 2021. Applications of doubled haploids in plant breeding and applied research. In: Segui-Simarro, J.M. (Ed.), Doubled Haploid Technology. Methods in Molecular Biology, vol. 2287. Humana, New York, NY. Available from: https://doi.org/10.1007/978-1-0716-1315-3_2.

9

Breeding for multiple disease resistance

Introduction

Most breeding programs have an active multiple disease resistance component. Breeding for multiple disease resistance can mean several species of pathogens or multiple races of one pathogen species. Multiple disease–resistant cultivars are common, and often companies indicate the resistances present using a special naming system. For example, tomatoes (*Solanum lycopersicum*) labeled VFFFNTA, indicates that the cultivar has resistance to Verticillium wilt (*Verticillium albo-atrum*), three races of Fusarium wilt (*Fusarium oxysporum* f. sp. *lycopersici*), nematodes (*Meloidogyne*), tomato mosaic virus (ToMV; *Tobamovirus*), and *Alternaria* species. In addition, gray leafspot (*Stemphylium solani*) and Cladosporium leaf mold (*Cladosporium fulvum*) resistance has been bred into commercial tomato (*S. lycopersicum*) cultivars, while a few varieties have resistance to races of late blight (*Phytophthora infestans*). Other examples would include garden pea (*Pisum sativum*), which may possess resistance to powdery mildew (*Erysiphe pisi*), Fusarium wilt (*F. oxysporum*), pea enation mosaic virus (PEMV; *Umbravirus*), pea seedborne mosaic virus (PSbMV; *Potyvirus*), and *bean leafroll virus* (BLRV; *Luteovirus*). A multiple disease–resistant slicing cucumber (*Cucumis Cucumis sativus*) cultivar, Marketmore 97, has resistance to cucumber mosaic virus (CMV; *Cucumovirus*), cucumber scab (*Cladosporium cucumerinum*), downy mildew (*Pseudoperonospora cubensis*), powdery mildew (*Podosphaera xanthii*), Alternaria leaf spot (*Alternaria alternata* f. sp. *cucurbitae*), Ulocladium leaf spot (*Ulocladium cucurbitae*), target spot (*Corynespora cassiicola*), watermelon mosaic virus (WMV; *Potyvirus*), papaya ringspot virus (PRSV; *Potyvirus*), and zucchini yellow mosaic virus (ZYMV; *Potyvirus*) (Fig. 9.1).

Historically, William Allen Orton, a plant pathologist at the US Department of Agriculture, in 1909 is credited with the first multiple disease–resistant cultivars when he bred for Fusarium wilt (*F. oxysporum* f. sp. *tracheiphilum*) and root-knot nematode (*Meloidogyne* spp.) resistance in cowpea (*Vigna unguiculata*)

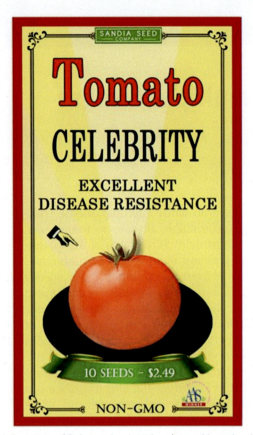

Figure 9.1 Seed packet of Celebrity tomato (*Solanum lycopersicum*), a cultivar that has multiple disease resistance. Courtesy of Sandia Seed Company, USA

and cotton (*Gossypium hirsutum*). Nowadays, most new cultivars need to be multiple disease–resistant to ensure they are adopted and grown. Although it varies by crop, it is quite common that resistance to certain diseases is a prerequisite for release. Growers have come to expect certain "disease packages," as they have come to be known, in new cultivars and without these a cultivar will not be widely grown. Even though it is obvious, it is easy to forget that a single cultivar or breeding line can provide more than one resistance gene to the progeny.

Interactions

With screening for multiple disease resistance, one must be aware of interactions. Some pathogens can enhance the defensive capacity of their host and activate responses against subsequent pathogen inoculations; conversely, some pathogens can suppress the defensive mechanism and allow pathogens to survive on a resistant host.

When screening for multiple diseases, an interaction among the pathogens can occur. Table 9.1 lists hypothetical reactions when cultivars are challenged with five pathogens.

When each hypothetical cultivar is examined, it is obvious that the multiple screening caused different interaction phenotypes. The phenotype of Cultivar 1 aligns with the genotype, meaning that if the plant has genetic resistance, it is phenotypically resistant, and if genetically susceptible, it is phenotypically susceptible. However, Cultivar 2 has an interaction with the pathogens that do not allow the genetic resistance to manifest itself, causing the plant to appear susceptible even though it has the genes for resistance. For Cultivar 3, the interaction of the pathogens causes pseudoresistance, that is, where genetically susceptible plants appear phenotypically resistant. This phenomenon has been shown to occur with multiple inoculations of fungi, bacteria, viruses, and nematodes.

Breeding approaches for multiple disease resistance follow one of two methods: (1) combine resistance genes by hybridization and screen segregating populations (F_2, recurrent selection, etc.) or (2) create an F_1 hybrid to combine resistance genes. Breeding approach #2 is sometimes called "Divide and Conquer" where each parent carries different resistance genes and when combined creates a cultivar with greater resistance (Fig. 9.2). For this approach to work, the resistance must be dominant; otherwise, both parents need to be homozygous for the recessive resistance gene.

W. Alan Erb and Randall C. Rowe at The Ohio State University, Wooster, Ohio, USA, used two different procedures to screen

Table 9.1 Hypothetical cultivar interactions with five different pathogens.

Pathogens:	A	B	C	D	E
Cultivar 1	R	S	R	R	S
Cultivar 2	S*	S	S*	S*	S
Cultivar 3	R	R*	R	R	R*

Interactions:
Cultivar (1) genotype R = phenotype R
Cultivar (2) genotype R = phenotype S*
Cultivar (1) genotype S = phenotype S
Cultivar (3) genotype S = phenotype R*

	Host	A		B		F_1	
Pathogen		1		2		1	4
		4	X	3	=	2	5
		5		6		3	6

Figure 9.2 The F_1 hybrids created by hybridizing parents A and B, each with different resistance genes. The F_1 hybrid has the resistance of both parents.

tomato (*S. lycopersicum*) seedlings for resistance to three pathogens. In one scheme, seeds were sprayed with a spore suspension of *F. oxysporum* f. sp. *radicis-lycopersici* that causes Fusarium crown and root rot. Resistant seedling survivors were root-dipped 17 days later in a spore suspension of *Verticillium dahliae*, and then 1 week after the root dip, leaves were rubbed with tobacco mosaic virus (TMV; *Tobamovirus*) suspension.

In another screening, 2-week-old seedlings were dipped in a spore suspension of *F. oxysporum* f. sp. *lycopersici* races 1 and 2 that causes tomato wilt. *F. oxysporum* f. sp. *lycopersici* is a different pathogen than *F. oxysporum* f. sp. *radicis-lycopersici*. Resistant seedlings were root-drenched 10 days later with a suspension of root-knot nematode (*Meloidogyne incognita*), and then 1 week later, the leaves were rubbed with a Tobacco mosaic virus (TMV; *Tobamovius*) suspension. These screening procedures identified multiple disease–resistant individuals and reduced the time required for the development of two multiple disease–resistant populations. Inbred lines from each population could be hybridized to produce F_1 hybrids resistant to five diseases. One caveat is that because Tobacco mosaic virus resistance is recessive, each parent needed to be homozygous for virus resistance.

It is also common to conduct disease screenings for different generations. For example, a plant breeder can make a population that combines resistance to four different pathogens. After the hybridization, the F_1 is self-pollinated to produce a segregating population, the plant breeder can then screen for disease resistance. Single-plant selections can be made among the segregating F_2 plants to develop multiple F_3 families to be screened with the next pathogen. This procedure is continued until all the diseases have been screened and the plant breeder has several multiple disease–resistant F_5 families. However, like the simultaneous inoculation method developed by Erb and Rowe, this method works best when the resistance genes have a dominant effect, which highlights the major limitation of this method that is the plant breeder is also selecting for heterozygotes that will segregate in the subsequent generations. To resolve this, the fixed lines that result from this method should be screened again for all the diseases to ensure the resistance was not lost through self-pollination. Alternatively, the use of molecular markers eliminates the need for screening a second time or at all, depending on their efficacy, as discussed later in this chapter. The most common approach in this scheme is to screen for the most destructive disease first, to impose the highest level of selection pressure early on, allowing subsequent generations to be smaller and more manageable.

Inoculation of a single pathogen but with multiple races can have the same interactions as seen when inoculating with different pathogens. Screening with multiple races of the same pathogen has been both successful and a failure. When more than one physiological race or isolate of a pathogen species is inoculated on a single plant, researchers report synergistic effects resulting in increased disease symptoms or expression of induced resistance in the host. Thus multiple-race screening can make resistant materials appear susceptible, and susceptible plants appear resistant.

An important goal in breeding chile peppers (*Capsicum annuum*) for disease resistance is to screen plants for resistance to several physiological races of *Phytophthora capsici*. Generally, individual plants are inoculated with only one isolate, requiring many plants and additional resources. A screening method to test chile pepper (*C. annuum*) plants for Phytophthora foliar blight resistance with multiple physiological races of *P. capsici* was developed at New Mexico State University. The inoculation method was precise and accurate. Precision was based on whether the disease was confined to the foliar region and only the inoculated leaf showed disease symptoms; neither the stem nor the root had disease symptoms. For accuracy, susceptible and resistant plants had to be clearly distinguishable. For the multiple-race inoculation, plants resistant to one, two, or three physiological races should be clearly delineated. Thus each single leaf displayed an independent reaction toward the specific physiological race inoculated. The novel screening technique was successful in differentiating between susceptible and resistant plants for multiple races causing the Phytophthora foliar blight disease. The use of the paper disc infiltrated with zoospores prevented runoff of the inoculum toward the stems and the roots. Therefore root rot and stem blight disease symptoms did not confound the screening results, which was one of the main issues with the foliar blight screening techniques used in the past. An application of two thousand zoospores per leaf provided excellent differentiation between resistant and susceptible genotypes. When leaves of an individual plant were inoculated with different physiological races of *P. capsici*, no change in the expression of resistance or susceptibility was observed. Each leaf displayed the same reaction in the multiple-race inoculation as displayed using the single-race inoculation method (Fig. 9.3).

Marker-assisted selection

Selecting for multiple disease resistance is likely the area where marker-assisted selection (MAS) can be of the greatest assistance to a plant breeder. Molecular markers are developed based on differences in genomic sequences and are linked to genes of interest in a marker-assisted breeding program. Plant breeders always want to use breeding strategies that make selections more effective and reliable. The identification of molecular markers tightly linked to resistance genes allows indirect selection because the markers' expression is not masked by epistatic interactions and the environment, which reduces reliance on laborious and time-consuming screening procedures. Molecular markers do not necessarily represent the resistance gene but act as a flag or indicator because they are statistically associated with a phenotype that is controlled by a gene or

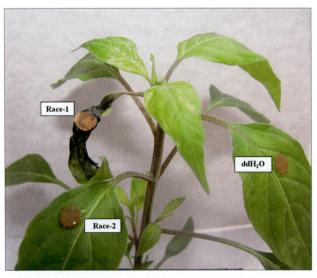

Figure 9.3 Phenotypic response of New Mexico Recombinant Inbred Line-S plant 3 days after inoculation with two *Phytophthora capsici* races 1 and 2 and distilled water (ddH2O) using the Phytophthora foliar blight multiple-race screening technique. Courtesy of the authors.

multiple genes. The markers have no effect on the phenotypes of the trait of interest and occupy a specific position in the genome within chromosomes called the locus.

(Over the past 2 decades, several genes conferring resistance to a diverse range of pathogens have been mapped. Having molecular markers associated with disease resistance genes expedites breeding for multiple disease resistance. Many types of molecular markers including isozyme, amplified fragment length polymorphisms (AFLP), sequence-related amplified polymorphism (SRAP), inter-simple sequence repeat (ISSR), restriction fragment length polymorphism (RFLP), random amplification of polymorphic DNA (RAPD), and single-nucleotide polymorphism (SNP)-based molecular markers such as cleaved amplified polymorphic sequences (CAPS), derived cleaved amplified polymorphic sequences (dCAPS), kompetitive allele-specific polymerase chain reaction (PCR) (KASP), and high resolution melting (HRM) markers have been found linked to disease-resistant genes.

Efficiency is based on "tightness" of the molecular marker and the resistant gene. In segregating populations, the molecular marker can be separated from the resistance gene because these markers are based on statistical associations between genetic polymorphisms and a phenotype. A centimorgan (cM) is a unit used to measure genetic linkage. The centimorgan is named after the American geneticist Thomas Hunt Morgan. One centimorgan equals a 1% chance that the marker will become separated from the resistance gene due to crossing over in a single generation. The closer the molecular marker and the resistance gene the better for the breeder. The "perfect marker" is a molecular marker that is inherently related to disease resistance, specifically to the defense mechanisms of the host. A perfect molecular marker could be based on a high-effect polymorphism, meaning the SNP, insertion, deletion, etc. cause a change in gene expression. The most common forms of high-impact polymorphisms result in frameshifts or premature stop codons. As molecular technologies improve, molecular markers are getting better and are often nearly perfect markers, making selection more accurate. Molecular markers make it possible to track the introgression of several resistant genes into a single cultivar from various sources during a hybridization program.

Genome-wide association study

One of the most serious chile pepper (*Capsicum* species) diseases worldwide is Phytophthora blight (*P. capsici*). It is crucial to assess the resistance of pepper (*Capsicum* species) genetic resources to Phytophthora blight, understand the genetic resistances, and develop markers for selecting resistant pepper (*Capsicum* species) materials in breeding programs. Professor Byoung-Cheorl Kang at the Seoul National University, Seoul, South Korea and colleagues evaluated the resistance of 342 pepper (*Capsicum* species) accessions to *P. capsici*. The disease severity score method evaluated the phenotypic responses of pepper accessions inoculated with the KCP7 isolate. A genome-wide association study (GWAS) was performed to identify SNPs linked to *P. capsici* (isolate KCP7) resistance. The pepper population was genotyped using the genotype-by-sequencing (GBS) method, and 45,481 SNPs were obtained. A GWAS analysis was performed using resistance evaluation data and SNP markers. Significantly associated SNPs for *P. capsici* resistance at 4 weeks after inoculation of the GWAS pepper (*C. annuum*) population were selected. These SNPs for Phytophthora blight resistance were found on all chromosomes except Chr.05, Chr.09, and Chr.11. One of the SNPs found on Chr.02 was converted into an HRM marker, and another marker (QTL5−1) from the previous study was applied to pepper accessions and breeding lines for validation and comparison. This SNP marker was selected because the resistance phenotype and the HRM marker genotype matched well. The selected SNP was named Chr02−1126 and was located at 112 Mb on Chr.02. The Chr02−1126 marker predicted *P. capsici* resistance with 78% accuracy, while the QTL5−1 marker predicted resistance with 80% accuracy. Along with the marker for major quantitative traits loci (QTLs) on Chr.05, this Chr02−1126 marker could be used to accurately predict Phytophthora blight resistance in pepper (*C. annuum*) genetic resources. Therefore this study will assist in the selection of resistant pepper (*C. annuum*) plants to breed new Phytophthora blight−resistant varieties.

It is extremely important that the nature and pattern of inheritance of the resistance gene(s) be known, before trying to find and identify linked molecular markers. Any "leakage" or weakness with the disease screen for precision and accuracy will reduce the efficiency of finding an effective molecular marker. Recently, molecular markers developed using the DNA sequence of the resistant gene of interest have aided in optimizing the process of making molecular markers.

After developing a mapping population and correctly phenotyping the resistant and susceptible individuals, polymorphic molecular markers among parental lines must be identified. After the identification of a set of polymorphic molecular markers, the next step is to carry out a cosegregation analysis for these markers. A simple strategy known as bulked-segregate analysis (BSA) can be used to identify markers quickly that cosegregate with a trait of interest. BSA is a rapid method to detect polymorphisms in specific genomic regions using segregating populations. However, BSA is only effective when the trait is controlled by a single gene. Race- or strain-specific resistance is often conferred by a single gene or a few tightly linked genes; however, as previously discussed, broad-spectrum resistance is almost always quantitative biologically.

As the availability of annotated reference genomes is becoming more common for a diverse range of crops, one can more accurately identify molecular markers based on the resistance genes themselves. Linkage maps are a "road map" indicating the position and relative genetic distances between molecular markers along the chromosomes. Based on the segregation pattern of molecular markers, linkage maps are constructed. Recombination frequency is calculated based on cosegregation patterns for each pair of markers in terms of centimorgans. Various statistical software packages such as "Mapmaker," "Mapmanager," "JoinMap," "Cartographer," and "Linkage" can be used to construct linkage maps.

The last and most important step in tagging and mapping the gene of interest is to validate the markers and their linkage distances in alternate populations. Alternate populations can be developed by selecting another donor line possessing the same resistance gene and hybridizing it with a susceptible parent. For example, Rebecca J. McGee and colleagues at the US Department of Agriculture developed kompetitive allele-specific PCR (KASP) markers for powdery mildew (*E. pisi*) of pea (*P. sativum*). To identify additional pea (*P. sativum*) germplasm with powdery mildew resistance, KASP markers for the *er1* gene conferring powdery mildew resistance genotyped a pea (*P. sativum*), collection derived from the US Department of Agriculture pea (*P. sativum*) single-plant collection. Simultaneously, a phenotypic screening and a genotypic validation were conducted on the pea single-plant collection. One pea (*P. sativum*) accession, Plant Introduction 142775, was identified by both phenotyping and genotyping to carry the allele *er1−1* for powdery mildew resistance, indicating that the KASP assay is an efficient and robust tool for breeding for powdery mildew resistance.

At the World Vegetable Center, a program was initiated to develop fresh market tomato (*S. lycopersicum*) lines resistant to tomato yellow leaf curl virus (TYLCV; *Begomovirus*), *P. infestans* causing late blight, *Ralstonia solanacearum* causing bacterial wilt, *Stemphyllium* species causing gray leaf spot, *F. oxysporum*

f. sp. *lycopersici* race 2, and TMV (*Tobomovirus*). They combined the use of laboratory, greenhouse, and field protocols to screen for disease resistance as well as the use of molecular markers in a stepwise manner to select for multiple disease resistance. The use of molecular markers was critically important in their breeding program because it allowed them to conduct background selection for resistance to diseases while screening against others. At the end of the project, five multiple disease-resistant fresh market tomato (*S. lycopersicum*) lines were selected. Resistance of the five lines to the abovementioned diseases was confirmed in subsequent evaluations.

Marker serendipity

Unexpected discoveries occur all the time, even with breeding disease-resistant plants. A serendipitous discovery is a fenthion and bacterial speck (*Pseudomonas syringae* pv. *tomato*) disease relationship within tomato (*S. lycopersicum*). The *Pto* locus in tomato (*S. lycopersicum*) confers resistance in a gene-for-gene interaction specifically to *P. syringae* pv. *tomato*. The *Pto* locus was originally identified in a wild species of tomato, *Solanum pimpinellifolium*, and has been introgressed into many tomato (*S. lycopersicum*) cultivars. In 1984, to control an infestation of leafminers (*Tuta absoluta*) in a greenhouse, fenthion an organophosphorous insecticide was applied to a population of greenhouse-grown tomatoes (*S. lycopersicum*). French plant breeders using the greenhouse observed an association between the presence of the *Pto* locus and sensitivity to fenthion, they observed that tomato (*S. lycopersicum*) lines containing the *Pto* locus were also sensitive to fenthion. Leaves of tomato (*S. lycopersicum*) cultivars that contain the *Pto* bacterial resistance gene develop small necrotic lesions within 24 hours after exposure to fenthion.

Further research ascertained that the *Pto* gene was a member of a clustered multigene family with similarity to various protein-serine/threonine kinases. The *Fen* gene is distinct from the *Pto* gene, but both are members of the same gene family. The *Fen* protein shares 87% similarity with *Pto* but does not confer resistance to *P. syringae* pv. *tomato*. The results suggest that one can select for *Pto* resistance, by spraying with fenthion.

Disease-resistant rootstock

Grafting horticultural crop scions on resistant rootstocks is an important tool for managing diseases in both conventionally and organically grown vegetable crops. Due to the ban of methyl bromide and the loss of other soil fumigants and nematicides, which had been used as the primary control for soilborne diseases and plant-parasitic nematodes. Historically, the grafting of plants was documented more than 2000 years ago in China, Greece, and Rome. It is estimated that 95% of watermelon (*Citrulus lanatus*), 95% of greenhouse-grown cucumbers (*C. sativus*), and 30% of field-grown cucumbers (*C. sativus*) in Japan and Korea are grafted primarily for the prevention of infection by *F. oxysporum*. In 2019 it is estimated that North American nurseries graft nearly 58 million plants per year. Approximately 60%–65% of Solanaceous crops such as tomato (*S. lycopersicum*) and eggplant (*Solanum melongena*), and 10%–15% of pepper (*C. annuum*) are grafted in East Asia.

Disease resistance genes are often linked to loss of quality or yield, which is a phenomenon termed linkage drag. An important example of linkage drag is *P. capsici* resistance derived from Criollos de Morelos 334 (CM-334), a Mexican landrace chile pepper (*C. annuum*), and fruit size. The Criollos de Morelos 334 is one of the best sources of resistance to *P. capsici*, and resistance seems to be controlled by a major QTL on chromosome 5; however, when Criollos de Morelos 334 is used as a parent fruit size in the resulting progeny is typically small. Recovery of the large fruit trait almost always results in a significant reduction in resistance in subsequent generations. For this reason, producers almost always prefer to grow susceptible cultivars that have higher fruit quality. Therefore plant breeders often look for alternative ways to develop host resistance. An old approach that is in resurgence is grafting. To control *P. capsici*, seed companies are using Criollos de Morelos 334 as a parent to create resistant F_1 rootstocks.

Grafting is accomplished by connecting two plant segments, the shoot piece known as "scion" and the root piece called "rootstock." Grafting has been practiced for many centuries with perennials, mainly fruit trees, but, in the early 20th century, vegetable crops, mainly Cucurbitaceae and Solanaceae species, were grafted to resistant rootstocks as an effective strategy to manage a variety of soilborne diseases and root-knot nematodes. Consequently, grafting is considered an important practice and an alternative to soil fumigants in horticultural crop production. This can be thought of as *sui generis* example of nonhost resistance. The ready availability of disease-resistant rootstocks and the development of highly efficient grafting techniques have led to expansion in the use of grafted plants worldwide. Research on herbaceous vegetable grafting began in the late 1920s when

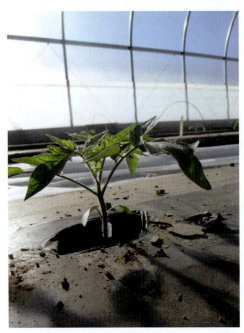

Figure 9.4 Grafted tomato (*Solanum lycopersicum*) plant growing in a high tunnel. Photograph courtesy of Dr. Wenjing Guan, Purdue University.

watermelon (*Citrullus lanatus*) was routinely grafted onto pumpkin (*Cucurbita maxima*) rootstocks in Asia for resistance to soilborne diseases. Grafting has also been reported to improve resistance to foliar fungal diseases such as powdery mildew (*P. xanthii*) and downy mildew (*P. cubensis*) on cucumbers (*C. sativus*) when certain rootstocks are used (Fig. 9.4).

Many genetic barriers to breeding disease–resistant crops can be circumvented when using rootstocks bred for resistance. If the rootstocks are compatible with the scion and provide the desired resistance without contributing negative traits to the scion, it can be a more efficient breeding approach.

The use of grafted tomato (*S. lycopersicum*) continues to expand. Pioneered in Asia, herbaceous grafting assists in managing many soilborne pathogens. Bacterial wilt (*R. solanacearum*) is an aggressive soilborne pathogen that affects tomatoes (*S. lycopersicum*) grown worldwide. Traditional fumigation methods using chloropicrin and methyl bromide have proven to have limited effectiveness in the management of this pathogen. Grafting of susceptible tomato (*S. lycopersicum*) cultivars onto resistant rootstocks is an effective cultural technique for managing bacterial wilt. This practice is widely used throughout many Asian and Mediterranean countries where intensive greenhouse production is prevalent.

In 2014 Matthew D. Kleinhenz, at The Ohio State University, USA, produced a table indicating which diseases tomato (*S. lycopersicum*) rootstocks were resistant. He points out that rating rootstock for disease resistance is complex because strains/races of pathogens differ and thus plant responses to pathogens are rarely "yes" or "no." Therefore many approaches are used to rate rootstock characteristics. His table is a compilation of publicly available information provided by seed companies in catalogs and at websites. He also included additional information from peer-reviewed technical and scientific reports. He reported that there were currently, at least 65 tomato (*S. lycopersicum*) resistant rootstocks have been developed by commercial breeders. In addition to bacterial wilt, corky root rot (*Pyrenochaeta lycopersici*), Fusarium wilt races 1 and 2 (*F. oxysporum* f. sp. *lycopersici*), Fusarium crown and root rot (*F. oxysporum* f. sp. *radicis-lycopersici*), southern blight (*Athelia rolfsii* = *Sclerotium rolfsii*), and Verticillium wilt (*V. dahliae*) have been developed.

Researchers at North Carolina State University, USA, compared the bacterial wilt resistance of three commercially available tomato (*S. lycopersicum*) rootstocks, Cheong Gang, RST-04–106-T, and Shield. A susceptible cultivar Red Mountain was the scion. All three resistant rootstocks provided protection, while the susceptible cultivar had between 30% and 80% disease incidence. They estimated the resistant rootstock improved marketable yields by 88%–125% when compared to the nongrafted plants (Fig. 9.5).

At the Olive Research Institute in Izmir, Turkey researchers screened 77 olive (*Olea europaea*) cultivars that included 71 domestic cultivars, 6 international cultivars, and 4 clonal rootstocks available in the olive gene bank for resistance to the wilt-causing pathogen, *V. dahliae*. Verticillium wilt is one of the most important pathogens of olives in Turkey and in the world as it has been reported in all important olive cultivation areas of the world. An issue with the disease is that propagation of symptomless but infected planting material is done by nurseries and distribution to uninfected areas occurs. Therefore research has been focused on resistant cultivar/rootstock selection as alternative procedures for the management of the disease.

V. dahliae isolates have two distinct pathotypes: defoliating and nondefoliating types. The defoliating pathotype is generally more aggressive than the nondefoliating pathotype and causes faster disease development. Olive (*O. europaea*) trees exhibit a high susceptibility to the defoliating pathotype of pathogen, even at very low inoculum levels. For this reason, the resistance

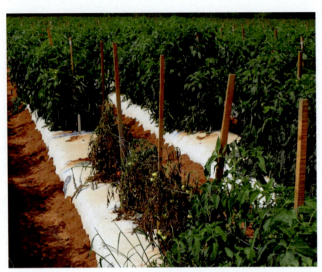

Figure 9.5 Nongrafted tomato (*Solanum lycopersicum*) plants showing severe bacterial wilt symptoms at the on-farm location in Salisbury, North Carolina in naturally infested soils. Citation: HortTechnology https://10.21273/HORTTECH04318-19.

of domestic cultivars to the defoliating pathotype of *V. dahliae* is of upmost importance in breeding for resistance.

Cuttings of the 81 cultivars and rootstocks were struck and propagated by rooting under moist conditions. To accelerate rooting, the cutting was dipped into 4000 parts-per-million solution of indolebutyric acid solution. Rooted cuttings were planted in pots and transferred to a lath house and watered sparingly. After a growing period of 8–12 months, the potted saplings were tested.

A spore suspension of 107 conidia mL/L from a highly virulent *V. dahliae* defoliating strain was obtained. A 500 μL spore was injected into the plant stems on two opposite sides at 5 cm above the soil layer. The tests were arranged in a randomized block design with four replicates, each consisting of 6–10 plants. Control plants were treated with the same amount of sterilized water only. Inoculated saplings were placed in a growth chamber, adjusted to 24°C and a 16-hour photoperiod, for a total of 4 months. Then all plants were transferred into a lath house. Observations of disease progression in the lath house were monitored for 1 year.

Disease progress recording began with the expression of the first wilt symptoms, the disease symptoms were evaluated at 1-month intervals using a 0–4 scale where 0 = healthy plant or plant without symptoms; 1 = affected plant in 1%–25% wilted leaves; 2 = 26%–50%; 3 = 51%–75%; 4 ≥ 75% wilted leaves. Disease severity index (DSI) was calculated by the McKinney index: DSI = [Σ (rating no. × no. of plants in rating) × 100]/(total no. of plants × highest disease rating). The results yielded the following resistance categories corresponding to the Disease Severity Index ranges: highly resistant (HR) = 0%–10%, resistant (R) = 11%–30%, moderately susceptible (Ms) = 31%–50%, susceptible (S) = 51%–70%, extremely susceptible (ES) = 71%–100%. Arcsine transformation was performed on the data before analysis. The normality test of transformed data was done with the Shapiro–Wilk test, and the results indicated that the data were distributed randomly and there were no violations of the analysis of variance (ANOVA) assumptions. Then, the ANOVA was followed by mean separation. Duncan's multiple comparison test ($P<.05$) was constructed using the general linear model (GLM) procedure of SAS (previously Statistical Analysis System).

Using this technique, the researchers found most accessions were ES to the disease; however, six cultivars were highly resistant, as their disease severities did not exceed 10%. Additionally, 11 cultivars were resistant, with disease severities less than 30%. Most of the highly resistant or resistant accessions were from the southeastern Anatolia region. A possible reason for this is the existing genetic diversity of olives in the region, which is one of the major olive gene centers in the world.

Maximum and final disease severity values differed and were not constant between 5 and 12 months on most cultivars. As is known, even in the case where Verticillium wilt causes serious damage, a recovery originating from various reasons may be observed later. If new root infections do not develop, some decrease may occur in disease severity.

In conclusion, the researchers concluded that the highly resistant cultivars revealed in their screening will be useful for inclusion in Verticillium wilt breeding programs. Furthermore, they established a national database including nearly all known domestic cultivars and clonal rootstocks of wild origin. Highly resistant cultivars found in this study may become resistant rootstocks and could be considered a new alternative solution in the management of Verticillium wilt in olive (*O. europaea*).

The main reasons for improved disease control in grafted horticultural crops are the inherent resistance within rootstocks, and improved plant nutrient uptake. However, increasing evidence indicated that systemic defense mechanisms may also play an important role in plant defense because of grafting. Many rootstocks developed for vegetable grafting are selected or bred from wild genotypes. In addition to specific disease resistance, they are characterized by large and vigorous root systems. Soilborne pathogens often infect and damage plant roots, and as a result, plant nutrient and water uptake can be affected. Therefore root system size and vigor may be associated with resistance to soilborne diseases. Moreover, vigorous roots help improve nutritional status and thus the overall health of plants, which may augment resistance against foliar diseases. Plant nutrients, in addition to their essential roles in plant growth and development, can be directly involved in plant defense pathways. For example, foliar application of phosphate salts can induce systemic protection against anthracnose (*Colletotrichum orbiculare*) in cucumbers (*C. sativus*).

Nitrogen deficiency can compromise elicitor-induced resistance to pathogen infection. In addition, many other mineral nutrients such as calcium, sulfur, and micronutrients also play significant roles in plant defense mechanisms. Research has demonstrated the influence of mineral nutrients on plant disease development. Several mineral elements, including silicon, have played critical roles in plant defense. The increase of susceptibility to target leaf spot (*C. cassiicola*) in grafted cucumbers (*C. sativus*) with a tested rootstock was related to reduced silicon uptake because grafted cucumber (*C. sativus*) plants using another rootstock demonstrated improved disease resistance and a higher level of silicon absorption.

Grafting-induced systemic acquired resistance to pathogen attack occurs at two levels. The first level involves the production of physical barriers, for example, trichomes, to prevent or restrict pathogen invasions. The second level is derived from systemic plant defense mechanisms. As reviewed in Chapter 2, systemic acquired resistance is activated by plant–pathogen recognition. Among these responses are accumulation of reactive oxygen species, production of antimicrobial compounds, expression of pathogenesis-related genes, synthesis of nitric oxide, and hypersensitive responses.

Does grafting with rootstocks induce systemic defense? Studies have shown that plants grafted on certain rootstocks generally exhibit a higher activity of defense-related enzymes compared with self-rooted plants under certain stressful conditions. Preconditioning, which can occur with grafting, can include plant growth–promoting rhizobacteria, which can reduce diseases in above-ground plant parts through the induction of systemic resistance. Moreover, systemic defense responses may be triggered by localized tissue damage in plants. A proteomics study of leaves from cucumber (*C. sativus*) plants grafted onto *Cucurbita moschata* and leaves from self-rooted cucumbers (*C. sativus*) showed that the expression of two types of proteins was significantly higher in grafted plants compared with self-rooted plants. The first protein type was related to plant defense responses, and the second type included photosynthesis-related proteins. Gene expressions of Gala apple trees (*Malus domestica*) grafted onto two rootstocks, one with moderate resistance to fire blight (*Erwinia amylovora*) and the other susceptible to fire blight, were examined using cDNA amplified fragment length polymorphism. Interestingly, scions grafted onto the resistant rootstock showed increased expression of stress-related genes, whereas scions grafted onto the susceptible rootstock did not. A similar study of eggplants (*S. melongena*) grafted onto tomato (*S. lycopersicum*) rootstocks indicated altered expression of diverse functional genes. Functions of these genes ranged from metabolism, signal transduction, and stress response to cell cycle and transcription/translation. Defense-related enzymes are often induced by a variety of abiotic and biotic stresses. It is important to distinguish between the effects of the grafting process and rootstock–scion interactions. Changes in both the roots and shoots of grafted plants need to be elucidated to gain a complete understanding of rootstock–scion interactions in induced systemic defense.

In some ways, grafting simplifies breeding for multiple disease resistance. For example, what if one wanted to breed a yellow bell pepper, an orange bell pepper, and a red bell pepper (*C. annuum*) with resistance to several soilborne diseases? The mature fruit color trait in pepper is known to be regulated by three independent loci ($C1$, $C2$, and Y). In this model, mature fruit color can be classified into eight groups according to their allelic combinations, ranging from white ($c1\ c2\ y$) to dark red ($C1\ C2\ Y$). Therefore breeding three cultivars with different fruit colors is a complex goal, not to mention combining different resistance loci to various soilborne diseases. Another approach is to breed one rootstock with soilborne disease resistance to all the soil pathogens and graft the colored bell peppers onto the rootstock.

There has been a resurgence in grafting vegetable crops because of the increase in growing them in greenhouses and/or for organic production. Both intraspecies and interspecies rootstocks are being developed. In unheated European and Mexico greenhouses where plants are grown directly in the soil, soilborne disease resistance is the primary reason for grafting. These low-input greenhouses are often not heated and have limited cooling ability, which may further increase the necessity for disease-resistant plants. The primary reason for grafting tomatoes (*S. lycopersicum*) in Asia under open field production is for control of bacterial wilt (*R. solanacearum*) and brown root rot (complex of *Colletotrichum coccodes* and *P. lycopersici*).

The environments for bacterial wilt and brown root diseases are quite different, as bacterial wilt prefers warm temperatures, such as occurs in the open field in summer, and brown root rot tends to occur in cooler conditions, such as found in winter greenhouse culture. This has required different rootstocks selected for each environment. Bacterial wilt–resistant rootstocks should have a certain level of heat tolerance, while brown root rot–resistant rootstocks need to be tolerant to cool temperatures. It appears from the literature that most bacterial wilt–resistant rootstocks were selected by screening tomato (*S. lycopersicum*) cultivars and wild species for resistance. The World Vegetable Center reports screening multiple solanaceous varieties and wild accessions for resistance to bacterial wilt. They recommend using the cultivar Hawaii 7996 as a rootstock for tomato (*S. lycopersicum*) to control bacterial wilt except where flooding or saturated soils are expected, in which case they recommend the eggplant (*S. melongena*) cultivar Surya. More recently, reports indicate that other eggplant rootstocks not only provide high levels of resistance to bacterial wilt, but also result in higher tomato (*S. lycopersicum*) yields.

There has also been an increase in the use of grafting for heirloom tomatoes (*S. lycopersicum*), especially in organic production. In these situations, disease-resistant plants are foremost. One major limitation to grafting tomato (*S. lycopersicum*) is that Tomato mosaic virus (ToMV, *Tobamovirus*) resistance in the rootstock and scion must be compatible. Resistance to ToMV can be derived from the *Tm-1* or *Tm-2* alleles; the *Tm-1* allele confers a tolerance, or symptomless response in the host, while the *Tm-2* alleles confer a hypersensitive response. If a rootstock carries *Tm-1* resistance and the scion carries *Tm-2* resistance, then the rootstock can transmit virus to the scion and induce systemic necrosis. Other examples of incompatible reactions have been noted where the scion may collapse, or the rootstock may lose specific disease resistance in certain rootstock/scion combinations, but the exact mechanisms are not known.

Developing transgenic rootstocks with specific disease resistances have been developed. For example, a cucumber green mottle mosaic virus (CGMMV, *Tobamovirus*) coat protein gene and a replicase gene were introduced into watermelon (*C. lanatus*) and cucumber (*C. sativus*) rootstocks, respectively. Susceptible scions grafted onto transgenic rootstocks exhibited high resistance against viral pathogens.

Grafting is an important strategy to manage soilborne pathogens. Rootstocks can include intraspecific selections that utilize specific major resistance genes and interspecific and intergeneric selections that exploit nonhost resistance mechanisms or multigenic resistance. Again, overreliance on specific rootstocks in production systems has led to the emergence of new pathogens or shifts in the host specificity of the pathogen population, emphasizing the need for the plant breeder to be aware of the complexity of disease resistance whether soilborne pathogens or foliar pathogens. The use of grafting to manage diseases will be most successful when carried out with increasing knowledge about the biology, diversity, and population dynamics of the pathogen and when complemented with sustainable farming system practices.

Breeding for multiple disease–resistant cultivars is complex and multidimensional, but a necessity for the modern plant breeder. The plant breeder may use many breeding approaches to accomplish that goal. With the inclusion of molecular markers linked to targeted resistance genes included into the breeding program, faster and more efficient selection can occur. The new cultivars will still need to be tested in production to see if the resistance is truly multiple disease.

Bibliography

Cavatorta, J., Moriarty, G., Henning, M., Glos, M., Kreitinger, M., Munger, H.M., et al., 2007. 'Marketmore 97': a monoecious slicing cucumber inbred with multiple disease and insect resistance. HortScience 42, 707–709. Available from: https://doi.org/10.21273/HORTSCI.42.3.707.

Dickson, M.H., Boettger, M.A., 1977. Breeding for multiple root rot resistance in snap beans. Journal of the American Society Horticultural Science 102, 373–377.

Erb, W.A., Rowe, R.C., 1992. Screening tomato seedlings for multiple disease resistance. Journal of the American Society Horticultural Science 117, 622–627. Available from: https://doi.org/10.21273/JASHS.117.4.622.

Erten, L., Yıldız, M., 2011. Screening for resistance of Turkish olive cultivars and clonal rootstocks to Verticillium wilt. Phytoparasitica 39, 83–92. Available from: https://doi.org/10.1007/s12600-010-0136-2.

Guan, W., Zhao, X., Hassell, R., Thies, J., 2012. Defense mechanisms involved in disease resistance of grafted vegetables. HortScience 47, 164–170. Available from: https://doi.org/10.21273/HORTSCI.47.2.164.

Hanson, P., Lu, S.-F., Wang, J.-F., Chen, W., Kenyon, L., Tan, C.-W., et al., 2016. Conventional and molecular marker-assisted selection and pyramiding of genes for multiple disease resistance in tomato. Scientia Horticulturae 201, 346–354. Available from: https://doi.org/10.1016/j.scienta.2016.02.020.

Hurtado-Hernandez, H., Smith, P.G., 1985. Inheritance of mature fruit color in *Capsicum annuum* L. Journal of Heredity 76, 211–213. Available from: https://doi.org/10.1093/oxfordjournals.jhered.a110070.

Kelly, J.D., Miklas, P.N., 1998. The role of RAPD markers in breeding for disease resistance in common bean. Molecular Breeding 4, 1–11. Available from: https://doi.org/10.1023/A:1009612002144.

Khan, A., Korban, S.S., 2022. Breeding and genetics of disease resistance in temperate fruit trees: challenges and new opportunities. Theoretical Applied Genetics . Available from: https://doi.org/10.1007/s00122-022-04093-0.

King, S.R., Davis, A.R., Zhang, X., Crosby, K., 2010. Genetics, breeding and selection of rootstocks for Solanaceae and Cucurbitaceae. Scientia Horticulturae 127, 106–111. Available from: https://doi.org/10.1016/j.scienta.2010.08.001.

Kleinhenza, M.D., 2014. Description of commercial tomato rootstocks. http://www.vegetablegrafting.org/wp/wp-content/uploads/2014/06/usda-scri-combined-rs-tables-feb-14.pdf

Kroon, B.A.M., Scheffer, R.J., Elgersma, D.M., 1991. Induced resistance in tomato plants against fusarium wilt invoked by *Fusarium oxysporum* f. sp. *dianthi*. Netherlands Journal of Plant Pathology 97, 401–408. Available from: https://doi.org/10.1007/BF03041387.

Loh, Y.T., Martin, G.B., 1995. The disease-resistance gene *Pto* and the fenthion-sensitivity gene fen encode closely related functional protein kinases. Proceedings of the National Academy of Sciences USA 92, 4181–4184. Available from: https://doi.org/10.1073/pnas.92.10.4181.

Louws, F.J., Rivard, C.L., Kubota, C., 2010. Grafting fruiting vegetables to manage soilborne pathogens, foliar pathogens, arthropods, and weeds. Scientia Horticulturae 127, 127–146. Available from: https://doi.org/10.1016/j.scienta.2010.09.023.

Ma, Y., Coyne, C.J., Main, D., Pavan, S., Sun, S., Zhu, Z., et al., 2017. Development and validation of breeder-friendly KASPar markers for *er1*, a powdery mildew resistance gene in pea (*Pisum sativum* L.). Molecular Breeding 37, 151. Available from: https://doi.org/10.1007/s11032-017-0740-7.

Manickam, R., Chen, J.R., Sotelo-Cardona, P., Kenyon, L., Srinivasan, R., 2021. Evaluation of different bacterial wilt resistant eggplant rootstocks for grafting tomato. Plants 10, 75. Available from: https://doi.org/10.3390/plants10010075.

Michelmore, R.W., Paran, I., Kenseli, R.V., 1991. Identification of markers linked to disease resistance genes by bulked segregant analysis: a rapid method to detect markers in specific genomic regions using segregating populations. Proceedings of the National Academy of Sciences USA 88, 9828–9832. Available from: https://doi.org/10.1073/pnas.88.21.9828.

Mishra, A.N., Prasad, S.N., Mishra, D.K., 2003. Multiple disease resistance screening of late maturing pigeon-pea. Annals of Plant Protection Sciences 11, 392–393.

Monroy-Barbosa, A., Bosland, P.W., 2010. A rapid technique for multiple-race disease screening of Phytophthora foliar blight on single *Capsicum* plant. HortScience 45, 1563–1566. Available from: https://doi.org/10.21273/HORTSCI.45.10.1563.

Murphy, A.M., De Jong, H., Proudfoot, K.G., 1999. A multiple disease resistant potato clone developed with classical breeding methodology. Canadian Journal of Plant Pathology 21, 207–212. Available from: https://doi.org/10.1080/07060669909501183.

Pan, R.S., More, T.A., 1996. Screening of melon (*Cucumis melo* L.) germplasm for multiple disease resistance. Euphytica 88, 125–128. Available from: https://doi.org/10.1007/BF00032443.

Pathania1, A., Rialch, N., Sharma, P.N., 2017. Marker-assisted selection in disease resistance breeding: A boon to enhance agriculture production. Current

Developments in Biotechnology and Bioengineering 187–213. Available from: https://doi.org/10.1016/B978-0-444-63661-4.00009-8. Chapter 9.

Rava, C.A., da Costa, J.G.C., Fonseca, J.R., Salgado, A., 2003. Identification of sources of resistance to anthracnose, common bacterial blight, and bacterial wilt in common bean. Revista Ceres 50, 797–802.

Ro, N., Haile, M., Hur, O., Geum, B., Rhee, J., Hwang, A., et al., 2022. Genome-wide association study of resistance to *Phytophthora capsici* in the pepper (*Capsicum* spp.) collection. Frontiers in Plant Science 13, 902464. Available from: https://doi.org/10.3389/fpls.2022.902464.

Roberto, S.R., Novello, V., Fazio, G. (Eds.), 2022. New Rootstocks for Fruit Crops: Breeding Programs, Current Use, Future Potential, Challenges and Alternative Strategies. Frontiers Media SA, Lausanne. Available from: https://doi.org/10.3389/978-2-88974-923-2.

Saleem, M.Y., Akhtar, P.K., Iqbal, Q., Asghar, M., Hameed, A., Shoaib, M., 2016. Development of tomato hybrids with multiple disease tolerance. Pakistan Journal of Botany 48, 771–778.

Sidhu, G.S., Webster, J.M., 1979. Genetics of tomato resistance to the *Fusarium-Verticillium* complex. Physiological Plant Pathology 15, 93–98.

Sidhu, G.S., Webster, J.M., 1983. Horizontal resistance in tomato against the *Meloidogyne-Fusarium* complex: an artifact of parasitic epistasis. Crop Protection 2, 205–210. Available from: https://doi.org/10.1016/0261-2194(83)90045-5.

Stavely, J.R., 1983. A rapid technique for inoculation of *Phaseolus vulgaris* with multiple pathotypes of *Uromyces phaseoli*. Phytopathology 73, 676–679.

Suchoff, D.H.F.J., Louws, Gunter, C.C., 2019. Yield and disease resistance for three bacterial wilt-resistant tomato rootstocks. HortTechnology 29, 330–337. Available from: https://doi.org/10.21273/HORTTECH04318-19.

Tarn, T.R., Murphy, A.M., Wilson, D.H., Burns, V.J., Proudfoot, K.G., 2003. Multiple resistance to diseases in a population of long-day adapted Andigena potatoes. Acta Horticulturae 619, 189–194. Available from: https://doi.org/10.17660/ActaHortic.2003.619.21.

Wiesner-Hanks, T., Nelson, R., 2016. Multiple disease resistance in plants. Annual Review of Phytopathology 54, 229–252. Available from: https://doi.org/10.1146/annurev-phyto-080615-100037.

Wyszogrodzka, A.J., Williams, P.H., Peterson, C.E., 1987. Multiple-pathogen inoculation of cucumber (*Cucumis sativus*) seedlings. Plant Disease 71, 275–280.

Resistance: biotechnology and molecular applications

Introduction

Plant breeders have not yet exhausted the genetic resources available for crop improvement through classical techniques; however, biotechnology can expand the genetic resources available to a plant breeder. Although having little impact on horticultural crops at present, transgenes (used to create genetically modified organisms or GMOs) have the potential, to provide a greater array of genetic resistance to pathogens. There is at present, a dichotomy in agriculture regarding GMOs. Creation of GMO cultivars for major agronomic crops, for example, cotton (*Gossypium hirsutum*), maize (*Zea mays*), and soybean (*Glycine soja*), actively continues, while research and development of GMO cultivars in the horticultural crops lag. The reasons for this are complex and have political and social, as well as technical reasons. Some GMO vegetables and fruits have been released. These include ripening-inhibitor tomatoes (*Solanum lycopersicum*), virus-resistant summer squash (*Cucurbit pepo*), earworm-resistant sweet corn (*Z. mays*), and virus-resistant papaya (*Carica papaya*).

A cultivar of potato (*Solanum tuberosum*) called NewLeaf developed by Monsanto that contains the *Bacillus thuringiensis* (*Bt*) toxin-producing genes from the bacterium *B. thuringiensis* allows the plant to resist attacks by the Colorado potato beetle (*Leptinotarsa decemlineata*), a major pest of potato production. The *Bt* gene is very valuable because it has been exceedingly difficult to achieve Colorado leaf beetle resistance through classical breeding. The *Bt* toxin-producing genes are widely used in breeding for insect-resistant crops. More recently was the development of a *Bt* eggplant (*Solanum melongena*) that was released in Bangladesh through funding from the US Agency for International Development (USAID). During the 2016−17 season, *Bt* eggplant resulted in 61% savings in pesticide costs by resource-poor farmers, which translated to sixfold higher economic returns-not to mention the dramatic reduction in exposure to pesticides. However, until the social and political aspects of GMOs are sorted out, few cultivars of horticultural crops are likely to be available to growers.

Tissue culture

Plant tissue culture represents an important technique in breeding for disease-resistant horticultural crops. Whether it is considered biotechnology depends on one's point of view. We will consider its application as one of the early steps with biotechnology to assist in breeding for disease-resistant horticultural crops.

Plant tissue culture can be traced back to Gottlieb Haberlandt, an Austrian botanist. He first pointed out the possibilities of the culture of isolated plant tissues. He suggested the potentialities of individual cells via tissue culture. His original idea presented in 1902 was called totipotentiality: "Theoretically all plant cells are able to give rise to a complete plant."

Almost any part of a plant can be used to generate callus cultures. A feature that makes callus cultures useful for plant breeders is that the callus can redifferentiate into entire plants. Plant tissue cultures form the basis of several techniques that have been developed to effect genetic changes in plants. The tissues of plant species that are propagated vegetatively are normally genetic mosaics regarding many characteristics, including resistance to disease. Thus some of the plants regenerated from cultured cells are more resistant to pathogens than the parent plants. Disease-resistant plants of a small number of species have been regenerated from cells selected in culture for their resistance to toxins produced by pathogens, both with and without prior exposure to mutagens. This procedure is not widely applicable because most pathogens do make a specific toxin to cause disease.

Nevertheless, progress has been made in the application of these techniques in breeding new, disease-resistant cultivars. Researchers at the Scottish Crop Research Institute working with the Agricultural Research and Training Institute in Tanzania used an in vitro protocol to screen *Coffea arabica* genotypes for resistance to coffee berry disease (*Colletotrichum kahawae*). Initially, cultural conditions that influenced the growth of isolates of *C. kahawae* on agar media suitable for callus growth were determined. The growth of the fungus on the callus derived from susceptible and resistant genotypes was then assessed. This ensured that no detrimental competition for nutrients between the pathogen and the callus occurred.

Optimization of the concentration of the phytohormones added to the media, the temperature and incubation period were found to be important in the expression of differential responses of callus to inoculation with the pathogen as detected by measurement of hyphal growth. The screening of callus of nine *C. arabica* genotypes showed that this method identified genotypes highly resistant or susceptible to the disease and was sufficiently sensitive to distinguish those genotypes with moderate or low resistance.

Another example comes from the Institut National de la Recherche Agronomique (INRA) in Guadeloupe. They evaluated the reactions of 60 water yam (*Dioscorea alata*) cultivars to three isolates of the yam anthracnose (*Colletotrichum gloeosporioides*) using tissue culture-derived whole-plant assay. A wide range of variations in resistance of the water yam cultivars, and significant effects of pathogen isolate and isolate–cultivar interactions were observed. The tissue culture-derived whole-plant assay to select resistance in their breeding program was confirmed.

In addition, researchers at Lucknow University in India were successful in creating resistance to leaf blight (*Alternaria alternata*) in rose-scented geranium (*Pelargonium graveolens*) using a culture filtrate of *A. alternata* to produce resistant callus. Rose-scented geranium yields an essential oil used in the cosmetic and perfume industry. The geranium crop in northern Indian plains is affected by severe leaf blight. Although the spread of disease is reduced with the use of copper fungicides, a long-term solution to the problem is the development of resistant cultivars. Because rose-scented geranium is a polyploid and highly sterile, classical breeding is not practical. Callus cultures were subjected to various concentrations of *A. alternata* filtrate. Callus cultures resistant to the filtrate were regenerated. The regenerants were confirmed resistant to *A. alternata* by challenging the leaves to the fungus, proving that the induction of disease resistance in rose-scented geranium plants did occur at the cellular level.

Pyramiding resistance genes

Pyramiding or stacking resistance genes involves combining multiple genes for resistance into a cultivar to develop durable resistance. In general, pyramiding describes the stacking of two or more genes controlling a single trait in a single cultivar. It is a relatively straightforward process when the same donor parent contributes all the genes. However, when two or more donor parents are to be used, a relatively different strategy is needed for gene pyramiding. Marker-assisted gene pyramiding can be employed to successfully introgress oligogenes into a single cultivar to achieve durable resistance against one or more diseases in an efficient and effective manner.

Gene pyramiding allows the incorporation of several resistance genes into one cultivar, making it more difficult for a pathogen to overcome them all. An elegant example in beans (*Phaseolus vulgaris*) is the use of protected *I* gene resistance, where a recessive bean common mosaic virus (BCMV; *Potyvirus*) resistance gene is combined with the dominant *I* gene to confer resistance to all know races of BCMV. Pyramiding is used successfully for resistance to rust (*Puccinaiales*) and anthracnose (*Colletotrichum* species) in several crops. The technique seems applicable to other diseases, such as late blight (*Phytophthora infestans*). Biotechnology can enhance the efficiency of resistance breeding by using DNA markers to pyramid genes and confirm the presence of resistance genes/alleles in the plant.

In a study conducted in Turkey, the genes that confer resistance to potato virus Y (PVY; *Potyvirus*), tomato spotted wilt virus (TSWV; *Tospovirus*), and pepper mild mottle virus (PMMoV; *Tobamovirus*) were successfully combined in superior pepper (*Capsicum annuum*) lines using molecular markers and virus resistance assays. As a result, a new pepper (*C. annuum*) line resistant to PVY, TSWV, and PMMoV was developed. The results show the applicability of a pyramiding strategy for breeding multiple disease resistance.

New molecular tools are allowing breeders to understand the underlying genetics of quantitatively inherited resistance and allow the efficient manipulation of those genes. Using molecular mapping and quantitative trait locus analysis in scarlet runner bean (*Phaseolus coccineus*), a species related to green bean (*P. vulgaris*), to characterize high levels of resistance to white mold (*Sclerotinia sclerotiorum*) are being done. Molecular tools will help to transfer resistance from scarlet runner beans (*P. coccineus*) into green beans (*P. vulgaris*). An especially important caveat to using DNA markers is that they must be accurate and repeatable across the breeder's germplasm, as discussed in the previous chapter.

Resistance gene analogs/comparative genetics/synteny

Plant disease-resistant genes have highly conserved genetic regions corresponding to characteristic amino acid domains.

These conservative structures make it possible to isolate resistance gene analogs. Most cloned resistant genes occur in clusters of related sequences. Resistance genes containing nucleotide-binding site (NBS) leucine-rich repeats (LRRs) are the most prevalent type of resistance gene in plants. Researchers at the University of Wisconsin used the Verticillium wilt-resistant *Ve* gene information in tomato (*S. lycopersicum*) to detect *Ve* orthologs in tetraploid potato (*S. tuberosum*) cultivars. Orthologs are genes in different species that evolved from a common ancestral gene by speciation, and, in general, orthologs retain the same function during evolution. Verticillium wilt resistance gene orthologs, showing high sequence identity with *Ve1* (83%−90%) and *Ve2* (74%−91%), were detected in resistant potato cultivars. Using this information, the introduction of resistance into potatoes was accelerated. At New Mexico State University, the utility of this method was further illustrated using the synteny information from tomato (*S. lycopersicum*) and potato (*S. tuberosum*) to find Verticillium wilt resistance gene orthologs in another Solanaceae crop, *Capsicum*, to accelerate breeding for Verticillium wilt resistance.

Pan-genomics

An approach to finding resistance gene analogs can be the pan-genomic approach. The availability of high-quality genomes of more and more species has led to the realization that a single genome may not be enough to reflect the genomic complexity of a species because of the large number of variations among accessions (Fig. 10.1). Therefore the pan-genome concept was conceived to represent all the genetic information of a species, including core genes that are present in all accessions and dispensable genes that are present only in a subset of strains. A sequence-based pan-genome could capture genic as well as nongenic sequences. Pan-genomic studies have been accomplished in the horticultural crops, maize (*Z. mays*), cucumber (*Cucumis sativus*), eggplant (*S. melongena*) sunflower (*Helianthus annuus*), strawberry (*Fragaria × ananassa*), cabbage (*Brassica oleracea* var. *capitata*) and tomato (*S. lycopersicum*). These pan-genomes have provided a basis for breeding programs. Horticultural crops have narrow genetic diversity because of domestication, so it is very important for plant breeders to obtain as much genetic variation information as possible for crop improvement. Lei Gao at Cornell University, USA, and an international group of collaborators constructed the first tomato (*S. lycopersicum*) pan-genome based on

232 Chapter 10 Resistance: biotechnology and molecular applications

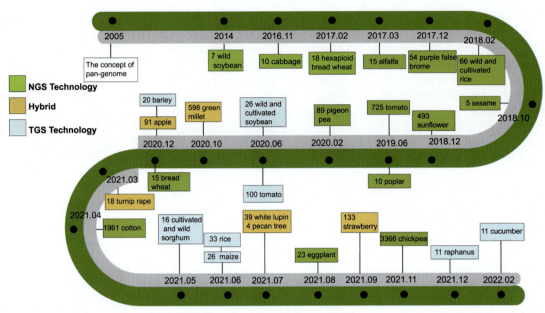

Figure 10.1 Timeline and basic information for the released plant pan-genomes. The different sequencing technologies used to construct the pan-genomes are indicated using different colors. Solid black circles indicate past events in plant pan-genomics. The technologies are indicated using colored rectangular boxes: light green (next-generation sequencing), dark orange (hybrid sequencing), and light blue (long-read sequencing). The sample size and species are indicated in the colored rectangular boxes. Courtesy of Journal of Genetics and Genomics, Li et al. (2020).

the resequencing data of 725 representative accessions using a map-to-pan strategy, and gene presence/absence variations (PAV) analyses detected substantial gene loss and intense negative selection of genes related to disease resistance during the domestication and improvement process.

Direct gene transfer/transformation

The term "direct gene transfer" is used to discriminate among methods of plant transformation that rely on methods that do not use *Agrobacterium* to genetically change a plant. Direct gene transfer methods deliver large amounts of "naked" DNA while the plant cell is temporary permeable. One type of direct gene transfer method is particle bombardment, biolistic method, or "shotgun method." Particle bombardment uses a gene gun to shoot the DNA directly in the cell. In this technique, tungsten or gold particles are coated with the DNA to transform the plant tissue. The particles are propelled at high speed into the target plant material, where the DNA is released within the cell and can integrate into the genome. The delivery of the DNA using this technology rarely has the DNA integrated into the cell's genome. To generate transgenic plants, the plant material, the tissue culture regime, and the transformation conditions must be optimized carefully. Developments to this technology led to the production of several systems, such as an electrostatic discharge device and others based on the gas flow. Of the latter type, a commercially produced, helium-driven, particle bombardment apparatus (PDS-1000 He) has become the most widely used. This method is found to be suitable for cereals, which are otherwise recalcitrant to *Agrobacterium*-mediated transformation. However, the major complication is the vector DNA is often rearranged and the transgene copy number can be very high.

Because lily (*Lilium longiflorum*) is recalcitrant to molecular genetic manipulation because of limitations that restrict utilization of *Agrobacterium tumefaciens* technologies that are routinely applied to dicotyledonous plants, researchers used microprojectile bombardment to introduce resistance to cucumber mosaic virus (CMV, *Bromoviridae*) into lily (*L. longiflorum*). Approximately, 5000 pieces of morphogenic calli, 3–4 mm in diameter, derived from segments of sterile bulblet scales of *L. longiflorum* cultivar Snow Queen were microprojectile bombarded. After several rounds of callus selection, plants were regenerated in vitro. The plants were resistant to CMV.

Another approach is the polyethylene glycol (PEG) mediated transformation method. Plant protoplasts can be transformed with naked DNA by treatment with PEG in the presence of divalent cations (usually calcium). The PEG and the divalent cations destabilize the plasma membrane of the plant protoplast and render it permeable to naked DNA. Once entered into the protoplast the DNA enters the nucleus and integrates into the genome. Plant protoplasts are not easy to work with, and the regeneration of fertile plants from protoplasts is problematic for some species, limiting the usefulness of the technique. The DNA used for transformation is also susceptible to degradation and rearrangement. Despite these limitations, the technique does have the advantages that protoplasts can be isolated and transformed in large numbers from a wide range of plant species.

The electroporation of cells can deliver DNA into plant cells and protoplasts. Electroporation utilizes short, high-voltage electric shocks to make cells permeable to exogenous molecules, for example, nucleic acids. In plants, electroporation is used to stimulate the uptake of plasmids for stable and transient genetic transformation. Protoplasts are normally utilized in plant electroporation because the cell wall is a major barrier to the diffusion of macromolecules. However, recent work indicates that plasmid DNAs can be introduced into walled plant cells by electroporation. Most of the instruments currently used for electroporation are capacitive-discharge instruments; a capacitor bank is charged by a high-voltage power supply and then discharged into a chamber containing the experimental material.

The vectors are simple plasmids. The genes of interest require plant regulatory sequences, but no specific sequences are required for integration. Material is incubated in a buffer solution containing DNA and subjected to the high-voltage electrical pulses. The DNA migrates then through high voltage induced pores in the plasma membrane and integrates into the genome. Initially, protoplasts were used for transformation, but one of the advantages of the system is that both intact cells and tissues, such as callus cultures, immature embryos and inflorescence material can be used.

To add a desired trait to a crop using direct gene transfer, a foreign gene (transgene) encoding the trait must be inserted into plant cells, along with a "cassette" of additional genetic material. The cassette includes a DNA sequence called a "promoter," that determines where and when the foreign gene is expressed in the host, and a "marker gene" that allows breeders to determine which plants contain the inserted gene by screening or selection. For example, marker genes may render plants resistant to antibiotics that are not used medically (e.g., agromycin or canamycin) or tolerant to certain herbicides.

One of the most common and important method is transformation with *A. tumefaciens* that causes crown gall disease in many species. This bacterium has a plasmid, or loop of non-chromosomal DNA, which contains tumor-inducing genes (T-DNA), along with additional genes that help the T-DNA integrate into the host genome. For genetic engineering purposes, *Agrobacterium* is first "disarmed" so that it does not cause the galling of the plant. This is done by removing most of the T-DNA while leaving the left and right border sequences, that integrate a foreign gene into the genome of cultured plant cells.

Cisgenesis

In 2006 the term cisgenes was defined as "a crop plant that has been genetically modified with one or more genes (containing introns and flanking regions such as native promoter and terminator regions in a sense orientation) isolated from a hybridizer donor plant." Cisgeneics represents a step toward a new generation and definition of GMO crops. The lack of selectable genes (e.g., antibiotic or herbicide resistance) in the final product and the fact that the inserted gene(s) derive from organisms sexually compatible with the target crop should raise less environmental concerns and increase consumer's acceptance. This concept implies that plants must only be transformed with genetic material derived from the species itself or from closely related species capable of sexual hybridization.

Thalia Vanblaere and her colleagues at the Institute of Integrative Biology in Switzerland reported generating a cisgenic apple (*Malus domestica*) plant by inserting the endogenous apple scab (*Venturia inaequalis*) resistance gene *HcrVf2* under the control of its own regulatory sequences into the scab susceptible apple cultivar Gala. A previously developed method based on *Agrobacterium*-mediated transformation combined with a positive and negative selection system and a chemically inducible recombination machinery allowed the generation of the apple cultivar Gala carrying the scab resistance gene *HcrVf2* under its native regulatory sequences and no foreign genes.

CRISPR-Cas 9 system

Clustered regularly interspaced palindromic repeats (CRISPR)/Cas9 is a new generation of a genome editing tool causing great excitement in plant breeding. The CRISPR technology, a microbial defense system, has been developed based on its remarkable ability to bring the endonuclease Cas9 to specific locations within complex genomes by a short RNA, to precisely edit the genome, to build toolkits for synthetic biology, and to monitor DNA in live cells.

The CRISPR/Cas9 system enables promising new opportunities to create genetic diversity for breeding in an unprecedented way. Unlike most other genetic modification tools, multiple targets can be modified simultaneously in an efficient way in the CRISPR/Cas9 system, enabling pyramiding of multiple resistance gene into elite backgrounds within a single generation. One important example of the use of the CRISPR-Cas9 system is in cucumber (*C. sativus*), where Israeli researchers introduced multiple sequence insertions/deletions (indels) affecting eukaryotic translation initiation factor 4E proteins (eIF4Es), which successfully induced resistance against multiple

RNA viruses. Homozygous T3 progeny following Cas9/sgRNA that had been targeted to both eIF4E sites exhibited immunity to cucumber vein yellowing virus (CVYV, *Ipomovirus*) infection and resistance to the zucchini yellow mosaic virus (ZYMV, *Potyvirus*) and papaya ring spot mosaic virus-W (PRSV-W, *Potyvirus*). In contrast, the heterozygous mutant and nonmutant plants were highly susceptible to these viruses. Unlike other genetic engineering techniques, the use of CRISPR-Cas9 is largely not considered a genetic modification technique by many because it simply edits the existing DNA as opposed to introducing new DNA from other species.

Fungus-resistant GMO plants

Genetic engineering enables new ways of managing fungal infections. Several approaches have been taken: (1) introducing genes from other plants or bacteria encoding enzymes like chitinase or glucanase. These enzymes degrade chitin or glucan, respectively, which are essential components of fungal cell walls. Chitinases are expressed at low levels in healthy plants but are increased when under pathogen attack. They are located primarily in the cell wall and vacuole. Extracts containing chitinases inhibit growth of fungi by degrading their cell walls. Chitinases have been cloned from several plants including bean (*Phaseolus vulgarus*). Bean chitinase was expressed in tobacco (*Nicotiana tabacum*) under the control of the CaMV 35 S promoter. Transformed plants showed two to threefold more chitinase activity in the roots and 20–40-fold more in the leaves. Transgenic tobacco (*N. tabacum*) plants exhibited resistance to infection by soil fungus, *Rhizoctonia solani*, that normally kills untransformed plants. Expression of bean chitinase also worked when introduced in canola (*Brassica napus*). In field conditions, transformed canola was more vigorous and showed decreased root rot and mortality.

Viral cross-protection

Protection of a plant by one strain of virus against infection with a second strain is called "cross-protection." In the book *Matthews' Plant Virology*, cross-protection is defined as the use of a viral strain to infect a plant that subsequently prevents superinfection of that plant by closely related strains of the virus. The mild strain of a virus protects against the economic damage by more virulent strains of the same virus.

Its application in controlling virus diseases has met with some success in cross-protecting tomatoes (*S. lycopersicum*) with mild strains of Tobacco mosaic virus (TMV, *Tobamovirus*), *Citrus* with mild strains of citrus tristeza virus (CTV; *Closterovirus*), and papaya (*C. papaya*) with mild strains of PRSV (*Potyvirus*). Cross-protection has not gained widespread use because appropriate mild strains of viruses are often not available, and mild strains are not effective against all severe strains present in different localities.

Nevertheless, it is possible to genetically transform with the complete virus coat protein gene, which forms the shell of the virus to protect the genetic material. Roger N. Beachy of Washington University in St. Louis Missouri, USA, found in the case of Tobacco mosaic virus that overexpression of the coat protein gene led to virus resistance because the excess coat protein interfered with the ability of the virus to complete its lifecycle and move systemically in the plant. All genetically modified virus-resistant plants on the market, for example, papaya (*C. papaya*) resistant to PRSV (*Potyvirus*), squash (*Cucurbita pepo*) resistant to ZYMV (*Potyvirus*), cucumbers (*C. sativus*) resistant to CMV (*Cucumovirus*), and watermelon (*Citrullus lanatus*) resistant to watermelon mosaic virus (WMV; *Potyvirus*) have coat protein-mediated resistance.

Metabolic engineering

It has been estimated that there are 40,000 natural products known in plants, and a majority are for defending against pathogens. Plants employ a diverse hierarchy of controls to regulate the biosynthesis of defense metabolites. In addition to transcriptional and posttranscriptional controls of biosynthetic genes, there are a variety of upstream signal and regulatory factors that regulate resistant genes. Resistance could be engineered by regulating an entire biosynthetic pathway. Known transcription factors associated with disease resistance include basic leucine zipper (bZIP), myeloblastosis (MYB), myelocytomatosis (MYC), WRKY, and ethylene-responsive factor (ERF) families. Transcription factors are not limited to the original source species.

Research is reporting that several genes from a single plant defense pathway are found clustered together. The plant kingdom produces a diverse array of chemicals, collectively making an estimated 1 million different metabolites. These compounds have important ecological functions, for example, in providing protection against pathogens. While it is well known that the genes for some well-characterized plant natural product pathways are dispersed throughout the genome, the last two decades have revealed a growing number of examples in which the genes for specific biosynthetic pathways are colocalized in plant genomes in biosynthetic gene clusters (BGCs). Doil Choi and colleagues at Seoul National University in Korea demonstrated that capsidiol BGCs specifically expanded in pepper (*C. annuum*) genomes contribute to nonhost resistance against *P. infestans*. The rapid accumulation of capsidiol by the multigene families is sufficient for pepper to resist the unadapted pathogen *P. infestans*, whereas the adapted *Phytophthora capsici* can overcome this chemical barrier.

Another example of defense-related gene family was accomplished by the Department of Biotechnology at Punjab University, India. In their research, they performed a genome-wide identification of defensive genes that are expressed during powdery mildew (*Uncinula necator*) and downy mildew (*Plasmopara viticola*) infections in grapevine (*Vitis vinifera*). They identified 6, 21, 2, 5, 3, and 48 genes of enhanced disease susceptibility-1 (EDS1), nonrace-specific disease resistance (NDR1), phytoalexin-deficient 4 (PAD4), nonexpressor of PR gene (NPR), required for Mla-specified resistance (RAR), and pathogenesis related (PR), respectively, that were activated by pathogen inoculation.

Although much progress has been made in our understanding of BGCs in plants, one notable question is the extent to which gene clustering occurs in plant chemical defense pathways. Many of the compounds produced by plant BGCs have been shown to provide protection against pathogens. Thus the discoveries of novel BGCs may provide new approaches to crop improvement and disease resistance.

Future of GMO and disease resistance

Though promising, to insert single genes for resistance, it should be kept in mind that the use of a single resistance gene is risky as pathogens mutate rapidly allowing for new virulence. The success of a GMO-resistant crop will be its sustained survival in the market. A GMO-resistant crop will have to provide a technical solution beyond the range of conventional breeding, and all strategies need to be developed from durable non-GMO technology. To substantiate the latter statement, the concept of pathogen-derived resistance, for example, the strategy of virus-resistant GMO crops showing proficiency is based on a non-GM technology that of cross-protection of plants, by which plants are purposely inoculated with a mild strain of a virus to establish protection against later infection by a more severe strain similar principle as that of vaccination. This technology has been applied particularly in fruit tree production and precisely this knowledge was the driving force behind the early research toward virus-resistant papaya (*C. papaya*).

Bibliography

Ali, Z., Mahfouz, M.M., 2021. CRISPR/Cas systems versus plant viruses: engineering plant immunity and beyond. Plant Physiology 186, 1770–1785. Available from: https://doi.org/10.1093/plphys/kiab220.

Ali, Q., Yu, C., Hussain, A., Ali, M., Ahmar, S., Sohail, M.A., et al., 2022. Genome engineering technology for durable disease resistance: recent progress and future outlooks for sustainable agriculture. Frontiers in Plant Science. Available from: https://doi.org/10.3389/fpls.2022.860281.

Andolfo, G., Iovieno, P., Frusciante, L., Ercolano, M.R., 2016. Genome-editing technologies for enhancing plant disease resistance. Frontiers in Plant Science 7, 1813–1815. Available from: https://doi.org/10.3389/fpls.2016.01813.

Bae, J.J., Halterman, D., Jansky, S., 2008. Development of a molecular marker associated with Verticillium wilt resistance in diploid interspecific potato hybrids. Molecular Breeding 22, 61–66. Available from: https://doi.org/10.1007/s11032-008-9156-8.

Baranski, R., Klimek-Chodacka, M., Lukasiewicz, A., 2019. Approved genetically modified (GM) horticultural plants: a 25-year perspective. Folia Horticulturae 3, 3–49. Available from: https://doi.org/10.2478/fhort-2019-0001.

Barchenger, D.W., Jiang, L., Rodriguez, K., Hanson, D.S., Bosland, P.W., 2017. Allele-specific CAPS marker in a Ve1 homolog of *Capsicum annuum* for improved selection of *Verticillium dahliae* resistance. Molecular Breeding 37. Available from: https://doi.org/10.1007/s11032-017-0735-4.

Bart, R.S., Taylor, N.J., 2017. New opportunities and challenges to engineer disease resistance in cassava, a staple food of African small-holder farmers. PLoS Pathology 13, e1006287. Available from: https://doi.org/10.1371/journal.ppat.100628.

Bates, G.W., 1995. Electroporation of plant protoplasts and tissues. In: Galbraith, D.W., Bourque, D.P., Bohnert, H.J. (Eds.), Methods in Cell Biology. Academic Press, pp. 363–373. Academic Press. Available from: https://doi.org/10.1016/S0091-679X(08)61043-2.

Baltes, N., Hummel, A., Konecna, E., Cegan, R., Bruns, A.N., Bisaro, D.M., et al., 2015. Conferring resistance to geminiviruses with the CRISPR–Cas prokaryotic immune system. Nature Plants 1. Available from: https://doi.org/10.1038/nplants.2015.145.

Beachy, R.N., 1999. Coat-protein-mediated resistance to tobacco mosaic virus: discovery mechanisms and exploitation. Philosophical Transactions of the Royal Society Biological Science 354, 659–664. Available from: https://doi.org/10.1098/rstb.1999.0418.

Belkhadir, Y., Subramaniam, R., Dangl, J.L., 2004. Plant disease resistance protein signaling: NBS–LRR proteins and their partners. Current Opinion in

Plant Biology 7, 391–399. Available from: https://doi.org/10.1016/j.pbi.2004.05.009.

Bortesia, L., Fischera, R., 2015. The CRISPR/Cas9 system for plant genome editing and beyond. Biotechnology Advances 33, 41–52. Available from: https://doi.org/10.1016/j.biotechadv.2014.12.006.

Brettel, R.I.S., Ingram, D.S., 1979. Tissue culture in the production of novel disease resistant crop plants. Biological Reviews 54, 329–345. Available from: https://doi.org/10.1111/j.1469-185X.1979.tb01015.x.

Cao, H.X., Wang, W., Le, H.T.T., Vu, G.T.H., 2016. The power of CRISPR-Cas9-induced genome editing to speed up plant breeding. International Journal of Genomics . Available from: https://doi.org/10.1155/2016/5078796.

Chandler, S.F., Sanchez, C., 2012. Genetic modification; the development of transgenic ornamental plant varieties. Plant Biotechnology Journal 10, 891–903. Available from: https://doi.org/10.1111/j.1467-7652.2012.00693.x.

Chandrasekaran, J., Brumin, M., Wolf, D., Leibman, D., Klap, C., Pearlsman, M., et al., 2016. Development of broad virus resistance in non-transgenic cucumber using CRISPR/Cas9 technology. Molecular Plant Pathology 17, 1140–1153. Available from: https://doi.org/10.1111/mpp.12375.

Collinge, D.B., Jørgensen, H.J.L., Lund, O.S., Lyngkjær, M.F., 2010. Engineering pathogen resistance in crop plants: current trends and future prospects. Annual Review of Phytopathology 48, 269–291. Available from: https://doi.org/10.1146/annurev-phyto-073009-114430.

Collinge, D.B., Sarrocco, S., 2022. Transgenic approaches for plant disease control: status and prospects 2021. Plant Pathology 71, 207–225. Available from: https://doi.org/10.1111/ppa.13443.

Cristopoulou, M., Wo, S.R.-C., Kozik, A., McHale, L.K., Truco, M.-J., Wroblewski, T., et al., 2015. Genome-wide architecture of disease resistance genes in lettuce. G3 Genes|Genomes|Genetics 5, 2655–2669. Available from: https://doi.org/10.1534/g3.115.020818.

Daub, M.E., 1986. Tissue culture and the selection of resistance to pathogens. Annual Review of Phytopathology 24, 159–186. Available from: https://doi.org/10.1146/annurev.py.24.090186.001111.

Debener, T., Byrne, D.H., 2014. Disease resistance breeding in rose: current status and potential of biotechnological tools. Plant Science 228, 107–117. Available from: https://doi.org/10.1016/j.plantsci.2014.04.005.

Dogimont, C., Palloix, A., Daubze, A., Marchoux, G., Selassie, K.G., Pochard, E., 1996. Genetic analysis of broad-spectrum resistance to potyviruses using doubled haploid lines of pepper (*Capsicum annuum* L.). Euphytica 88, 231–239. Available from: https://doi.org/10.1007/BF00023895.

Dong, O.X., Ronald, P.C., 2019. Genetic engineering for disease resistance in plants: recent progress and future perspectives. Plant Physiology 180, 26–38. Available from: https://doi.org/10.1104/pp.18.01224.

Efferth, T., 2019. Biotechnology applications of plant callus cultures. Engineering 5, 50–59. Available from: https://doi.org/10.1016/j.eng.2018.11.006.

Friedman, A.R., Baker, B.J., 2007. The evolution of resistance genes in multiprotein plant resistance systems. Current Opinion in Genetics & Development 17, 493–499. Available from: https://doi.org/10.1016/j.gde.2007.08.014.

Gao, C., 2021. Genome engineering for crop improvement and future agriculture. Cell 184, 1621–1635. Available from: https://10.1016/j.cell.2021.01.005.

Gao, L., Gonda, I., Sun, H., Ma, Q., Bao, K., Tieman, D.M., et al., 2019. The tomato pan-genome uncovers new genes and a rare allele regulating fruit flavor. Nature Genetics 51, 1044–1051. Available from: https://doi.org/10.1038/s41588-019-0410-2.

Georges, F., Ray, H., 2017. Genome editing of crops: a renewed opportunity for food security. GM Crops & Food 8, 1–12. Available from: https://doi.org/10.1080/21645698.2016.1270489.

Gonsalves, D., 1998. Control of papaya ringspot virus in papaya: a case study. Annual Review of Phytopathology 36, 415–437. Available from: https://doi.org/10.1146/annurev.phyto.36.1.415.

Gosal, S.S., Kang, M.S., 2012. Plant tissue culture and genetic transformation for crop improvement. In: Tuteja, N., Singh Gill, S., Tiburcio, A.F., Tuteja, R. (Eds.), Improving Crop Resistance to Abiotic Stress. Wiley-VCH Verlag GmbH & Co., pp. 357–397. 1466 pp. Available from: https://doi.org/10.1002/9783527632930.ch16.

Goyal, N., Bhatia, G., Garewal, N., Upadhyay, A., Singh, K., 2021. Identification of defense related gene families and their response against powdery and downy mildew infections in *Vitis vinifera*. BMC Genomics 22, 776. Available from: https://doi.org/10.1186/s12864-021-08081-4.

Grube, R.C., Radwanski, E.R., Jahn, M., 2000. Comparative genetics of disease resistance within the Solanaceae. Genetics 155, 873–887. Available from: https://doi.org/10.1093/genetics/155.2.873.

Guo, Q., Liu, Q., Smith, N.A., Liang, G., Wang, M.-B., 2016. RNA Silencing in Plants: mechanisms, technologies and applications in horticultural crops. Current Genomics 17, 476–489.

Gurr, S.J., Rushton, P.J., 2005. Engineering plant with increased disease resistance: what are we going to express? Trends in Biotechnology 23, 275–282. Available from: https://doi.org/10.1016/j.tibtech.2005.04.007.

Hammerschlag, F.A., 1984. In vitro approaches to disease resistance. In: Collins, G.B., Petolino, J.G. (Eds.), Application of Genetic Engineering to Crop Improvement. Martinus Nijohoff/Dr. W. Junk Publishers, pp. 453–490. 604 pp. Available from: https://doi.org/10.1007/978-94-009-6207-1_14.

Hofvander, P., Andreasson, E., Andersson, M., 2022. Potato trait development going fast-forward with genome editing. Trends in Genetics 38, 218–221. Available from: https://doi.org/10.1016/j.tig.2021.10.004.

Holdsworth, W.L., Mazourek, M., 2015. Development of user-friendly markers for the pvr1 and Bs3 disease resistance genes in pepper. Molecular Breeding 35, 28–32. Available from: https://doi.org/10.1007/s11032-015-0260-2.

Holme, I.B., Wendt, T., Holm, P.B., 2013. Intragenesis and cisgenesis as alternatives to transgenic crop development. Plant Biotechnology Journal 11, 395–407. Available from: https://doi.org/10.1111/pbi.12055.

Hsu, P.D., Lander, E.S., Zhang, F., 2014. Development and applications of CRISPR-Cas9 for genome engineering. Cell 157, 1262–1278. Available from: https://doi.org/10.1016/j.cell.2014.05.010.

Hübner, S., Bercovich, N., Todesco, M., Mandel, J.R., Odenheimer, J., Ziegler, E., et al., 2019. Sunflower pan-genome analysis shows that hybridization altered gene content and disease resistance. Nature Plants 5, 54–62. Available from: https://doi.org/10.1038/s41477-018-0329-0. 2019.

Jacobsen, E., Visser, R.G.F., 2022. Cisgenesis: enabling an innovative green agriculture by deploying genes from the breeders' gene pool. In: Chaurasia, A., Kole, C. (Eds.), Cisgenic Crops: Potential and Prospects. Concepts and Strategies in Plant Sciences. Springer, Cham. Available from: https://doi.org/10.1007/978-3-031-06628-3_2.

Jirschitzka, J., Mattern, D.J., Gershenzon, J., D'Auria, J.C., 2013. Learning from nature: new approaches to the metabolic engineering of plant defense pathways. Current Opinion in Biotechnology 24, 320–328. Available from: https://doi.org/10.1016/j.copbio.2012.10.014.

Joosten, M.H.A.J., De Wit, P.J.G.M., 1989. Identification of several pathogenesis-related proteins in tomato leaves inoculated with *Cladosporium fulvum* (syn. *Fulvia fulva*) as 1,3-β-glucanases and chitinases. Plant Physiology 89, 945–951. Available from: https://doi.org/10.1104/pp.89.3.945.

Karmakar, S., Das, P., Panda, D., Xie, K., Baig, M.J., Molla, K.A., 2022. A detailed landscape of CRISPR-Cas-mediated plant disease and pest management. Plant Science 323. Available from: https://doi.org/10.1016/j.plantsci.2022.111376.

Kim, J., Kang, W.-H., Hwang, J., Yang, H.-B., Dosun, K., Oh, C.-S., et al., 2014. Transgenic *Brassica rapa* plants over-expressing eIF(iso)4E variants show broad-spectrum Turnip mosaic virus (TuMV) resistance. Molecular Plant Pathology 15, 615–626. Available from: https://doi.org/10.1111/mpp.12120.

Kumar, P., Nagarajan, A., Uchil, P.D., 2019. DNA transfection by electroporation. Electroporation. Cold Spring Harbor Protocols. Available from: https://cshprotocols.cshlp.org/content/2019/7/pdb.top096271.

Kuoriwa, K., Thenault, C., Nogué, F., Perrot, L., Mazier, M., Gallo, J.-L., 2022. CRISPR-based knock-out of eIF4E2 in a cherry tomato background successfully recapitulates resistance to pepper veinal mottle virus. Plant Science 316. Available from: https://doi.org/10.1016/j.plantsci.2021.111160.

Kushalappa, A.C., Yogendra, K.N., Sarkar, K., Kage, U., Karre, S., 2016. Gene discovery and genome editing to develop cisgenic crops with improved resistance against pathogen infection. Canadian Journal of Plant Pathology 38, 279–295. Available from: https://doi.org/10.1080/07060661.2016.1199597.

Larkin, P.J., Scowcroft, W.R., 1981. Somaclonal variation–a novel source of variability from cell cultures for plant improvement. Theoretical and Applied Genetics 60, 197–214. Available from: https://doi.org/10.1007/bf02342540.

Lee, H.-A., Kim, S., Kim, S., Choi, D., 2017. Expansion of sesquiterpene biosynthetic gene clusters in pepper confers nonhost resistance to the Irish potato famine pathogen. New Phytologist 215, 1132–1143. Available from: https://doi.org/10.1111/nph.14637.

Li, W., Liu, J., Zhang, H., Liu, Z., Wang, Y., Xing, L., et al., 2022. Plant pan-genomics: recent advances, new challenges, and roads ahead. Journal of Genetics and Genomics. Available from: https://doi.org/10.1016/j.jgg.2022.06.004.

Lipsky, A., Cohen, A., Gaba, V., Kamo, K., Gera, A., Watad, A., 2002. Transformation of *Lilium longiflorum* plants for cucumber mosaic virus resistance by particle bombardment. Acta Horticulturae 568, 209–214. Available from: https://doi.org/10.17660/ActaHortic.2002.568.30.

Liu, X., Ao, K., Yao, J., Zhang, Y., Li, X., 2021. Engineering plant disease resistance against biotrophic pathogens. Current Opinion in Plant Biology 60, 1101987. Available from: https://doi.org/10.1016/j.pbi.2020.101987.

Magbanua, Z.V., Wilde, H.D., Roberts, J.K., 2000. Field resistance to tomato spotted wilt virus in transgenic peanut (*Arachis hypogaea* L.) expressing an antisense nucleocapsid gene sequence. Molecular Breeding 6, 227–236. Available from: https://doi.org/10.1023/A:1009649408157.

Matern, U., Strobel, G., Shepherd, J., 1978. Reactions to phytoalexins in a potato population derived from mesophyll protoplasts. Proceedings of the National Academy of Sciences USA 75, 4935–4939. Available from: https://doi.org/10.1126/science.7902614.

Mekapogu, M., Jung, J.-A., Kwon, O.-K., Ahn, M.-S., Song, H.-Y., Jang, S., 2021. Recent progress in enhancing fungal disease resistance in ornamental plants. International Journal of Molecular Sciences 22, 7956. Available from: https://doi.org/10.3390/ijms22157956-2.

Melchers, L.S., Stuiver, M.H., 2000. Novel genes for disease-resistance breeding. Current Opinion in Plant Biology 3, 147–152. Available from: https://doi.org/10.1016/S1369-5266(99)00055-2.

Melchinge, A.E., 1990. Use of molecular markers in breeding for oligogenic disease resistance. Plant Breeding 104, 1–19. Available from: https://doi.org/10.1111/j.1439-0523.1990.tb00396.x.

Nyange, N.E., Williamson, B., McNicol, R.J., Hacker, C.A., 1995. In vitro screening of coffee genotypes for resistance to coffee berry disease (*Colletotrichum kahawae*). Annals of Applied Biology 127, 251–261. Available from: https://doi.org/10.1111/j.1744-7348.1995.tb06670.x.

Onyeka, T.J., Pétro, D., Ano, G., Etienne, S., Rubens, S., 2006. Resistance in water yam (*Dioscorea alata*) cultivars in the French West Indies to anthracnose disease based on tissue culture-derived whole-plant assay. Plant Pathology 55, 671–678. Available from: https://doi.org/10.1111/j.1365-3059.2006.01436.x.

Özkaynak, E., Devran, Z., Kahveci, E., Doğanlar, S., Başköylü, B., Doğan, F., et al., 2014. Pyramiding multiple genes for resistance to PVY, TSWV and PMMoV in pepper using molecular markers. European Journal of Horticultural Science 79, 233–239. Available from: http://www.jstor.org/stable/24126862.

Pandolfi, V., Costa Ferreira Neto, J.R., da Silva, M.D., Barbosa Amorim, L.L., Wanderley-Nogueira, A.C., de Oliveira Silva, R.L., et al., 2017. Resistance (R) Genes: applications and prospects for plant biotechnology and breeding. Current Protein and Peptide Science 18, 323–334. Available from: https://doi.org/10.2174/1389203717666160724195248.

Park, T.-H., Vleeshouwers, V.G.A.A., Jacobsen, E., van der Vossen, E., Visser, R.G.F., 2009. Molecular breeding for resistance to *Phytophthora infestans* (Mont.) deBary in potato (*Solanum tuberosum L.*): a perspective of cisgenesis. Plant Breeding 128, 109–117. Available from: https://doi.org/10.1111/j.1439-0523.2008.01619.x.

Paul, N.C., Park, S.-W., Liu, H., Choi, S., Ma, J., MacCready, J.S., et al., 2021. Plant and fungal genome editing to enhance plant disease resistance using the CRISPR/Cas9 system. Frontiers in Plant Science 12, 700925. Available from: https://doi.org/10.3389/fpls.2021.700925.

Polturak, G., Osbourn, A., 2021. The emerging role of biosynthetic gene clusters in plant defense and plant interactions. PLoS Pathology 17, e1009698. Available from: https://doi.org/10.1371/journal.ppat.1009698.

Pramanik, D., Shelake, R.M., Park, J., Kim, M.J., Hwang, I., Park, Y., et al., 2021. CRISPR/Cas9-mediated generation of pathogen-resistant tomato against tomato yellow leaf curl virus and powdery mildew. International Journal of Molecular Science 22, 1–18. Available from: https://doi.org/10.3390/ijms22041878.

Prins, M., Laimer, M., Noris, E., Schubert, J., Wassenegger, M., Tepfer, M., 2008. Strategies for antiviral resistance in transgenic plants. Molecular Plant Pathology 9, 73–83. Available from: https://doi.org/10.1111/j.1364-3703.2007.00447.x.

Qiao, Q., Edger, P.P., Xue, L., Qiong, L., Lu, J., Zhang, Y., et al., 2021. Evolutionary history and pan-genome dynamics of strawberry (Fragaria spp.). Proceedings of the National Academy of Sciences USA 118 (45). Available from: https://doi.org/10.1073/pnas.210543111e2105431118.

Ragimekula, N., Varadarajula, N.N., Mallapuram, S.P., Gangimeni, G., Reddy, R.K., Kondreddy, H.R., 2013. Marker assisted selection in disease resistance breeding. Journal of Plant Breeding and Genetics 1, 90–109. Available from: http.escijournals.net/JPBG.

Sanchez, M.J., Bradeen, J.M., 2006. Towards efficient isolation of R gene orthologs from multiple genotypes: optimization of long range-PCR.

Molecular Breeding 17, 137–148. Available from: https://doi.org/10.1007/s11032-005-4475-5.

Saxena, G., Verma, P.C., Rahman, L., Banerjee, S., Shukla, R.S., Kumar, S., 2008. Selection of leaf blight-resistant *Pelargonium graveolens* plants regenerated from callus resistant to a culture filtrate of *Alternaria alternata*. Crop Protection 27, 558–565. Available from: https://doi.org/10.1016/j.cropro.2007.08.013.

Schaeffer, S.M., Nakata, P.A., 2015. CRISPR/Cas9-mediated genome editing and gene replacement in plants: transitioning from lab to field. Plant Science 240, 130–142. Available from: https://doi.org/10.1016/j.plantsci.2015.09.011.

Shahin, E.A., Spivey, R., 1986. A single dominant gene for Fusarium wilt resistance in protoplast-derived tomato plants. Theoretical and Applied Genetics 73, 164–169. Available from: https://doi.org/10.1007/BF00289270.

Shelton, A.M., Hossain, M.J., Paranjape, V., Azad, A.K., Rahman, M.L., Khan, A.S. M.M.R., et al., 2018. Bt eggplant project in Bangladesh: history, present status, and future direction. Frontiers Bioengineering Biotechnology 6, 106. Available from: https://doi.org/10.3389/fbioe.2018.00106.

Shepherd, J.F., Bidney, D., Shamin, E., 1980. Potato protoplasts in crop improvement. Science (New York, N.Y.) 208, 17–24. Available from: https://doi.org/10.1126/science.208.4439.17.

Simko, I., Jia, M., Venkatesh, J., Kang, B.-C., Weng, Y., Barcaccia, G., et al., 2021. Genomics and marker-assisted improvement of vegetable crops. Critical Reviews in Plant Sciences 40, 303–365. Available from: https://doi.org/10.1080/07352689.2021.1941605.

Takken, F.L.W., Albrecht, M., Tameling, W.I.L., 2006. Resistance proteins: molecular switches of plant defence. Current Opinion in Plant Biology 9, 383–390. Available from: https://doi.org/10.1016/j.pbi.2006.05.009.

Talakayalaa, A., Ankanagari, S., Garladinne, M., 2022. CRISPR-Cas genome editing system: a versatile tool for developing disease resistant crops. Plant Stress 3, 100056. Available from: https://doi.org/10.1016/j.stress.2022.100056.

Torres, A.M., 2010. Application of molecular markers for breeding disease resistant varieties in crop plants. In: Jain, S.M., Brar, D.S. (Eds.), Molecular Techniques in Crop Improvement. Springer, Netherlands, pp. 185–205.

Vanblaere, T., Szankowski, I., Schaart, J., Schouten, H., Flachowsky, H., Broggini, G.L., et al., 2011. The development of a cisgenic apple plant. Journal of Biotechnology 154, 304–311. Available from: https://doi.org/10.1016/j.jbiotec.2011.05.013.

Yin, K., Qiu, J.-L., 2019. Genome editing for plant disease resistance: applications and perspectives. Philosophical Transactions of the Royal Society Biological Science 374, 20180322. Available from: https:/doi.org/10.1098/rstb.2018.0322.

Young, R.A., Kelly, J.D., 1996. RAPD markers flanking the Are gene for anthracnose resistance in common bean. Journal of the American Society of Horticultural Science 121, 37–41. Available from: https://doi.org/10.21273/JASHS.121.1.37.

Zhao, Y., Yang, X., Zhou, G., Zhang, T., 2020. Engineering plant virus resistance: from RNA silencing to genome editing strategies. Plant Biotechnology Journal 18, 328–336. Available from: https://doi.org/10.1111/pbi.13278.

Zhou, J., Li, D., Wang, G., Wang, F., Kunjal, M., Joldersma, D., et al., 2020. Application and future perspective of CRISPR/Cas9 genome editing in fruit crops. Journal of Integrative Plant Biology 62, 269–286. Available from: https://doi:10.1111/jipb.12793.

11

Resistance: gene deployment—durable resistance

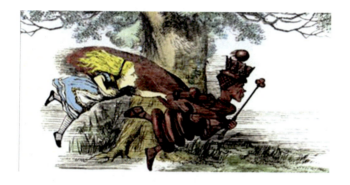

Through the Looking-Glass and What Alice Found There

by Lewis Carroll.

Chapter: The Garden of Live Flowers

Alice never could quite make out, in thinking it over afterward, now it was that they began; all she remembers is that they were running hand in hand, and the Queen went so fast that it was all she could do to keep up with her; and still the Queen kept crying, "Faster! Faster!" But Alice felt she could not go faster, though she had no breath left to say so. The most curious part of the thing was that the trees and other things around them never changed their places at all; however, fast they went they never seemed to pass anything. "I wonder if all the things move along with us?" thought poor puzzled Alice.

Introduction

Lewis Carroll's *Through the Looking-Glass and What Alice Found There*, is the source of the term "Red Queen" in the hypothesis in biology that states that species must constantly adapt, evolve, and proliferate to survive while pitted against ever-evolving opposing species. When breeding for disease-resistant horticultural crops, it is the hosts that must keep improving just to stay in place against the disease pathogen.

In nature, there is a never-ending "arms race" driving coevolution between pathogens and hosts. The major key to remember is there are heritable factors in the host; heritable factors in the pathogen; and the environment interacts with the host and pathogen to create disease. The success of a disease interaction, whether from the point of view of the surviving plant or of the victorious pathogen, depends on mechanisms of evolution

A good example of this principle is downy mildew (*Peronospora farinosa* f. sp. *spinaciae*) of spinach (*Spinacia oleracea*). Downy mildew (*P. farinosa* f. sp. *spinaciae*) is the most economically important spinach disease worldwide. *P. farinosa* f. sp. *spinaciae* infects only spinach (*S. oleracea*), but may possibly infect a few *Chenopodium* weed species, such as Lamb's quarters (*Chenopodium album*). The pathogen exists as distinct genetic races and shows an ability to adapt quickly to new resistant spinach cultivars. During the past 50 years, each outbreak of a new downy mildew race is controlled by the development of a resistant spinach line. There has been a rapid appearance of 10 new races in the past 10 years, creating substantial concern within the industry. Currently, 12 races have been identified. The use of resistant cultivars is the most effective means of controlling spinach downy mildew, and plant breeders are productive in developing resistant cultivars to most newly occurring races. However, a comprehensive deployment of effective management strategies to this disease needs to be addressed, which would greatly assist in managing this globally important disease of spinach.

Joy Bergelson and her colleagues at the Department of Ecology and Evolution, University of Chicago, USA, analyzed *R*-gene evolution and found that the most striking feature is the similarity in the patterns of evolved differences seen among alleles at individual loci and between genes belonging to evolutionary clusters (biosynthetic gene clusters). They were impressed by the presence of *R*-gene alleles and paralogs, representing a very wide range of evolutionary ages, undergoing rapid adaptive evolution. They found rates of adaptive evolution to appear greatest between closely related *R*-genes, suggesting that genetic exchange has contributed to the production of new adaptive alleles. Furthermore, selection plays a profound role in R-gene dynamics. They suggested that the classic arms race involving a succession of adaptive variants may be a poor metaphor for *R*-gene dynamics because alleles are not young, and loci are not monomorphic.

Theoretically, any breeding method can create a resistant cultivar, understanding the life cycle of both the host and the pathogen leads to a much more efficient breeding program. Every plant breeder hopes that the resistance in their new cultivar will be effective in a large geographic area and will remain effective for an extended period, the definition of DURABLE RESISTANCE. The obvious question is how to extend the duration of effectiveness of resistance genes. Technically, durable resistance is defined as a retrospective, empirical description of resistance that has remained effective during prolonged and widespread use in an environment conducive to the disease. An excellent example of durable resistance is fusarium yellows (*Fusarium oxysporum* f. sp. *conglutinans*) resistance in cabbage (*Brassica oleracea* var. *capitata*) that was bred into cultivars in the 1930s and is still effective today (Fig. 11.1).

In tomatoes (*Solanum lycopersicum*), the symbol "St" indicates resistance to tomato gray leaf spot disease (*Stemphylium solani* and *Stemphylium lycopersici*). Resistance is inherited via the gene *Sm*, a single dominant gene. The discovery of the gene in 1942 within the wild species, *Solanum pimpinellifolium*, became the source of resistance. The *Sm* gene is still effective today, more than 80 years later.

Nevertheless, some plant breeders perceive resistance genes as problematic because under certain growing environments, new virulent pathogens emerge making the resistance ineffective. Mostly the resistance that is not durable is the single gene resistance that is deployed singly. The issue is the mutation of

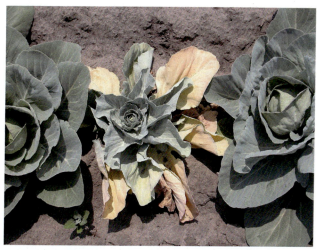

Figure 11.1 Fusarium yellows (*Fusarium oxysporum* f. sp. *conglutinans*) symptoms on a susceptible cabbage (*Brassica oleracea* var. *capitata*) plant. Courtesy: Ontario, Canada, Ministry of Agriculture, Food and Rural Affairs, http://www.omafra.gov.on.ca/IPM/english/brassicas/diseases-and-disorders/fusarium-wilt.html.

the pathogen's corresponding avirulence (*Avr*) gene. Many examples of so-called "boom-and-bust" cycles in agriculture can be cited where resistance genes were no longer effective against the pathogen.

As Eric Holub at Warwick University pointed out, disease is a major driving force of evolution, generating natural selection that acts both on host defenses and on genes enabling pathogens to overcome those defenses. He proposes that two types of polymorphism resulted from the coevolution of interacting host and pathogen loci. Long-term maintenance of polymorphism is predicted by the "trench warfare" hypothesis, resulting from balancing selection acting on both host and pathogen genes. Polymorphism at host and pathogen loci is predicted to be ancient with substantial phenotypic and molecular diversity within species at population and metapopulation levels. Alternatively, in the "arms race" scenario, there is the recurrent fixation of favorable alleles by selective sweeps. In this situation, alleles are short-lived, and transient polymorphism is only observable for a short period of time. An important topic in population genetics of host–pathogen interactions is to understand the ways in which natural selection interacts with the organisms' ecology to promote the occurrence of each scenario in natural populations.

Recent research at Warwick University using a systematic approach pioneered more than 4 decades ago at the National Vegetable Research Station, Wellesbourne, UK, for predictive breeding of durable resistance to downy mildew (*Bremia lactucae*) in lettuce (*Lactuca sativa*). Their approach was a success in identifying race nonspecific resistance to bacterial diseases of green bean (*Phaseolus vulgaris*) and pea (*Pisum sativum*) and identifying sources of resistance to black rot (*Xanthomonas campestris* pv. *campestris*), downy mildew (*Hyaloperonospora parasitica*) (syn. *Peronospora parasitica*), and white blister rust (*Albugo candida*) in a core collection of more than 400 *B. oleracea* accessions.

To explore durable resistance, this same approach was applied to downy mildew (*H. parasitica*) of *B. oleracea* in this host–pathogen interaction. The disease is distributed worldwide wherever brassica crops are grown and is favored by cool humid weather. Several sources of single major disease seedling resistance to *H. parasitica* in *B. oleracea* have been reported. The development and deployment of cultivars with the single major disease resistance genes have frequently failed to provide durable disease control due to the quick evolution of pathotypes virulent on resistant cultivars.

The researchers identified downy mildew resistance against two standard United Kingdom isolates of *H. parasitica* by screening a

B. oleracea collection. Sources of resistance were chosen from this material and developed further by generating doubled haploid and inbred lines. Seedlings from the new lines were tested for resistance to a larger collection of *H. parasitica* isolates collected from the main *B. oleracea* production regions of the United Kingdom. Three lines were broadly resistant to the pathogen isolates. Three of the remaining lines exhibited strong isolate-specific resistance, while several examples of weak or basal level resistance to some isolates were observed. A new *H. parasitica* variant collected was virulent in the broadly resistant lines but was avirulent in a line with narrow specificity of resistance. The F_2 and BC_1 seedlings derived from outcrossing each of the three broadly resistant lines to susceptible *Brassica* lines segregated in a manner indicating that the resistance was controlled by a single dominant gene. No susceptibility was observed among F_2 seedlings derived from intercrossing the three resistant lines, indicating that they all share the same or closely linked broad-spectrum resistance gene(s). They recommended that a combination of resistance from lines with broad and narrow specificity for controlling downy mildew be bred into brassica for the United Kingdom.

The gene-for-gene relationship is a model system for host–pathogen coevolution because the molecular biology of the interactions between host and pathogen genotypes is well understood. As stated in Chapter 2, Resistance: the phenotype, there is only one combination in the gene-for-gene system that allows the host to manifest resistance, this is when a host has a resistance gene that can recognize a specific avirulence gene. A pathogen is not detected by a host and resistance is not manifested if the host has a susceptibility allele or a resistance allele to a different pathogen's virulence allele. Thus even if the host has a resistance gene to the pathogen, it is ineffective unless the pathogen has the specific avirulence gene to match it. Coevolutionary dynamics are driven by indirect frequency-dependent selection, in which the strength of natural selection acting on resistance genes depends on the frequencies of pathogenic genes and vice versa. The resulting "boom-and-bust" phenomena cause unstable coevolutionary cycles, leading to the fixation of alleles in host and pathogen populations (the "arms race" scenario). In this case, there is a point at which there is balanced polymorphism at the host resistance and pathogen avirulence loci, but this equilibrium is unstable. Long-term maintenance of polymorphism in gene-for-gene systems (i.e., via stable equilibrium or cycling of host and parasite allele frequencies) generally requires the existence of a stable equilibrium point at which there is balanced polymorphism at resistant and avirulence loci. Unfortunately, with our current monoculture farming systems and the effects of climate change the risk and potential severity of disease increases, not only because genetic diversity is limited but also because agricultural environments are generally uniform.

An example, where the spread of the disease is predicated on the gene-for-gene system, is the population dynamics of bacterial leaf spot (*X. campestris* pv. *vitians*) on lettuce (*L. sativa*). Dr. Carolee T. Bull and colleagues at the US Department of Agriculture examined the effect of lettuce (*L. sativa*) genotype on its influence of colonization by *X. campestris* pv. *vitians* and its consequence on disease development. Understanding the differences in population dynamics of a pathogen on various cultivars is important because differences in population levels translate to differences in disease incidence and/or severity.

On lettuce (*L. sativa*), *X. campestris* pv. *vitians* causes small angular leaf spots that begin as water soaked and can later become necrotic. When the disease occurs, it can result in a reduction in the size of the lettuce (*L. sativa*) head and can increase the potential for postharvest loss. The pathogen remains viable in plant residue for several months and this infested residue serves as an inoculum source for subsequent crops. The best approach to controlling this disease is host resistance. A single dominant gene is responsible for conferring resistance in the cultivar, La Brillante. The same gene or a closely linked gene is also responsible for resistance in cultivars, Little Gem and Pavane, and all provide a hypersensitive response.

Their research established that the relationship between bacterial population levels, in a sense inoculum, and disease severity of other cultivars is influenced by neighboring host genotype, and the epidemiology of bacterial leaf spot on lettuce is dependent on the host to which *X. campestris* pv. *vitians* immigrates. The progression of bacterial leaf spot (*X. campestris* pv. *vitians*) in lettuce production fields is predicated on a succession of factors. First, *X. campestris* pv. *vitians* is deposited on the leaf surface. Once on the leaf surface, *X. campestris* pv. *vitians* may survive as epiphytes before colonization of natural openings or wounds in the leaf tissue. Internal colonization initiates direct interaction between the bacteria and plant's cells.

When differences in pathogen epidemiology in a compatible and an incompatible interaction were studied, significant differences in bacterial population were found. The population levels of *X. campestris* pv. *vitians* in Little Gem, the hypersensitive response cultivar, was consistently lower than any other cultivar. The population of *X. campestris* pv. *vitians* increased at an intermediate rate on the partial resistant cultivars, Iceberg and

Batavia Reine des Glaces. As one would expect, the bacterial population growth was greatest in the susceptible cultivars. The differences in the relationship between disease development for Little Gem and the other cultivars tested were due to the hypersensitive response in Little Gem. Their data indicated that both population growth rate and final population size are smaller in the incompatible interaction in Little Gem than in compatible interactions in other lettuce cultivars. They demonstrated that resistant and susceptible cultivars respond differently to increasing populations of pathogen. Lesion development in Little Gem, in particular, did not increase at the same rate as in the susceptible cultivars in response to higher inoculum levels.

Commercial production of lettuce in California has shown little to no bacterial leaf spot disease on susceptible cultivars when the inoculum level is low. Therefore for the plant breeder, the resistance is most clearly detected when the plants are inoculated with high levels of the pathogen. In their experiments, rates of multiplication and maximum bacterial populations are greater in the susceptible than in the resistant cultivars, and the population dynamics varied among resistant cultivars, which presumably had different mechanisms of resistance. This information can be used to improve screening methods to identify resistance.

In addition, these findings have implications for disease management and lettuce breeding because *X. campestris* pv. *vitians* interacts differently with cultivars that differ in their resistance mechanisms. The population level of *X. campestris* pv. *vitians* in Little Gem tissue did not change or increased very little. In contrast, population levels in susceptible cultivars and in the partial resistant cultivars increased significantly during the same period. Overall, this resulted in significantly lower levels *X. campestris* pv. *vitians* in Little Gem than in the other cultivars. Meaning that the hypersensitivity response reduces inoculum in the field decreasing the infection rate.

Emerging disease

When host and pathogen are geographically separated, disease does not occur. Unfortunately, when pathogen and host are brought together, disease epidemics can occur causing huge losses in yields as well as annihilate entire species such as was the case with Dutch Elm Disease (*Ophiostoma novo-ulmiin*) in North America and Europe. An epidemic of potato late blight (*Phytophthora infestans*), led to the Great Irish Famine and the loss of many lives and a massive migration.

With increased global trade and travel, pathogens have more opportunities to infect crops in new areas. Emerging diseases can cause tremendous crop losses. The economic and social impact in developing countries is often underestimated. Currently, examples of important emerging diseases are cassava mosaic virus disease (CMD; *Begomovirus*), caused by 11 different species of plant pathogenic virus in the genus, including the African cassava mosaic virus (ACMV; *Begomovirus*), East African cassava mosaic virus (EACMV; *Begomovirus*), and South African cassava mosaic virus (SACMV; *Begomovirus*), which are capable of reducing yields by 80%—90% and causing the suspension of cassava (*Manihot esculenta*) cultivation in many areas of Africa. Another devastating emerging disease is Xanthomonas wilt (*X. campestris* pv. *musacearum*) of banana (*Musa acuminata*), a bacterial disease that caused nearly 50% yield losses at the beginning of the 21st century in Uganda and is threatening the food security of 70 million people owing to its impact on an important staple crop. In the United States, *Phytophthora ramorum* (sudden oak death), a pathogen that infects more than 100 plant species causes economic damage to forests, ornamental nursery production, and home landscapes.

As stated in a previous chapter, the "disease triangle" consists of a susceptible host, virulent pathogen, and a conducive environment. For the disease to occur, all three must be present. There is a fourth element sometimes overlooked and that is the time that contributes to the development of an epidemic. If the susceptible host, virulent pathogen, and a conducive environment are present disease can initiate, however, an epidemic will only ensue if all three continue to be present through time. Controlling emerging diseases needs to have a sound strategy with breeding disease-resistant plants an important ingredient of that strategy. For this reason, some have updated the historical disease triangle and now refer to the "pyramid," accounting for time (Fig. 11.2).

Systems approach

A current approach to controlling epidemics is called a Systems Approach. The Systems Approach originated in the world of business, not agriculture. However, it is a concept that is compatible for plant disease control. In the 1960s an approach to management emerged that unified prior schools of thought. Its early contributors include Ludwing Von Bertalanfty, Lawrence J. Henderson, W.G. Scott, Deniel Katz, Robert L. Kahn, W. Buckley, and J.D. Thompson. The system is composed of several subsystems, and all the subsystems are related to each other.

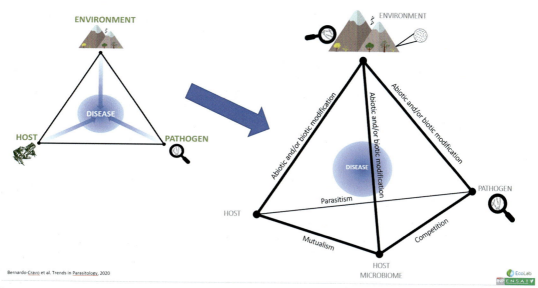

Figure 11.2 The disease triangle evolving into disease pyramid, a combination of host, environment, pathogen, and time are required for pathogens to be successful. Courtsey of Bernado-Cravo, et al., Trends in Parasitology, https://doi.org/10.1016/j.pt.2020.04.010.

The Systems Approach to plant disease management is a scenario that creates coordinative relations among all related entities (i.e., the grower, the plant breeder, government agencies, and society). Controlling the epidemic takes all the interacting and interdependent parts. The Systems Approach takes the epidemic, made up of subsystems into an orderly totality. Systems Approach is based on the generalization that everything is interrelated and interdependent. A system is composed of related and dependent elements that when interact forms a unitary whole.

If all the criteria are not met, such as a susceptible host with a virulent pathogen is present, but the environment is not conducive to the pathogen infecting and causing disease, a disease cannot occur. For example, if a grower plants chile pepper (*Capsicum annuum*) into a field with plant residue containing the oomycetes *Phytophthora capsici*, the causal agent of Phytophthora wilt, and the weather is too dry, the fungus in the residue cannot germinate and initiate infection. Likewise, it stands to reason if the host is susceptible and the environment favors the development of disease, but the pathogen is not present there is no disease. Taking the example above, if a chile pepper crop is rotated to a field that did not have chile pepper (*C. annuum*) planted, and *P. capsici* is not present but the weather is conducive to disease, no infection occurs. When a pathogen requires a vector to be spread, then for an epidemic to occur the vector must be plentiful and active.

Wise resistance management

Wise gene management minimizes the likelihood of epidemics and thus minimizes losses from endemic disease. The plant breeder chooses the type of resistant gene(s) for incorporation into their crop. They can choose from single dominant genes, oligogenes, or quantitative genes. The plant breeder should be aware of the "Vertifolia effect." The word "Vertifolia" refers to a potato (*Solanum tuberosum*) cultivar where this effect was first noticed for potato late blight resistance (*P. infestans*). This term was coined by James Edward Vanderplank to describe the loss of general (horizontal, minor gene, multigenic, polygenic) resistance in a cultivar after several generations of selection during which a major gene conferring resistance to the dominant race or biotype of the pathogen is introduced into a cultivar.

Researchers at Institut national de recherche pour l'agriculture, l'alimentation et l'environnement (INRAE) in France studied whether the Vertifolia effect would increase the potential for the durability of major resistance genes for the blackleg disease (*Leptosphaeria maculans*)/canola (*Brassica napus*) pathosystem. They found that the qualitative resistance gene *Rlm6* combined with quantitative resistance limited the population size of the virulent isolate. They took two cultivars, Eurol with a susceptible background and Darmor with quantitative resistance, and confirmed that the combination of qualitative and quantitative resistance is an effective approach for controlling the pathogen epidemics over time. This combination did not prevent isolates virulent against the major gene from amplifying in the long term, but the quantitative resistance significantly delayed for 5 years the loss of effectiveness of the qualitative resistance and disease severity was maintained at a low level on the genotype with both types of resistance after the fungus population had adapted to the major gene. They also showed that the diversity of *AvrLm6* virulence alleles was comparable in isolates recovered after the recurrent selection on lines carrying either the major gene alone or in combination with quantitative resistance: a single repeat-induced point mutation and deletion events were observed in both situations. They concluded that breeding cultivars with combined qualitative and quantitative resistance can effectively contribute to disease control by increasing the potential for the durability of major resistance genes.

Principles of disease control

A set of general principles of plant disease control that help to address the management of diseases on crops in any environment were first articulated by Herbert Hice Whetzel in 1929 and modified by others over the years. The traditional principles of disease control are:

1. *Avoidance:* prevent disease by selecting a time of the year or a site where there is no inoculum or where the environment is not favorable for infection.
2. *Exclusion:* prevent the introduction of inoculum.
3. *Eradication:* eliminate, destroy, or inactivate the inoculum.
4. *Protection:* prevent infection by means of a pesticide or some other barrier to infection.
5. *Resistance:* utilize cultivars that are resistant to infection.
6. *Therapy:* cure plants that are already infected.

While these principles are as valid today as they were in 1929, in the context of modern concepts of plant disease management, they have some critical shortcomings. First, these principles are stated in absolute terms (e.g., "exclude," "prevent," and "eliminate") that imply a goal of zero diseases. Plant disease "control" in this sense is not practical, and in most cases is not even possible. Indeed, the disease does not have to be eliminated, its progress needs to be reduced, and disease development needs to be at or below an economical acceptable level. Instead of plant disease control, plant disease management should be the goal. Finally, the traditional principles of plant disease control tend to emphasize tactics without fitting them into an adequate overall strategy. This does not mean that the traditional principles should be abandoned. The principles need to fit into an appropriate overall strategy based on epidemiological principles.

Any endeavor that requires a series of connected tasks for its completion also requires an overall plan. Each individual task, no matter how skillfully executed or how successful its outcome, for example a resistant cultivar, will not advance progress toward the final objective unless it has a coherent relationship with all the other necessary tasks. Even though the plant breeder is focused on developing resistant cultivars, breeding must be done in the context of the whole picture.

Multilines

Multilines could be thought of as a breeding method, while others might say it is a product that uses other breeding methods to achieve the goal. Nevertheless, multilines are one of several crop diversification strategies for disease control. The idea behind multilines is to grow mixtures of plants that differ in their reaction to a pathogen. The concept underlying the use of multiline cultivars, which are mixtures of lines bred for phenotypic uniformity of horticultural traits and diversity of resistance alleles, and cultivar mixtures that are mixtures of horticulturally compatible cultivars with no additional breeding for phenotypic uniformity is to present many resistance alleles to the pathogen. In the event of the occurrence of a new disease race, some plants may be susceptible, but not all. This mix of susceptible and resistant plants provides a buffering effect against rapid epidemic disease development and thus extends the life of resistance genes. The usefulness of multiline cultivars and cultivar mixtures for disease management has been well demonstrated for rusts and powdery mildews of small grain crops; however, they are used less in horticultural crops. An example where multilines were used successfully is with bean (*P. vulgaris*). Researchers at the Universidade Federal de Lavras (UFLA) in Minas Gerais, Brazil found that a multiline containing equal amounts of seven lines of Carioca-type bean (*P. vulgaris*), all horticulturally uniform but each presenting different patterns of resistance to anthracnose (*Colletotrichum lindemuthianum*), is less damaged by anthracnose than individual pure lines.

Such mixtures are more useful under some epidemiological conditions than under others, and experimental methodology, especially problems of scale, may be crucial in evaluating the potential efficacy of mixtures on disease. There are now examples of mixtures providing both low and high degrees of disease control for a wide range of pathosystems, including crops with large plants, and pathogens that demonstrate low host specificity, or are splash dispersed, soilborne, or insect vectored. Although most analyses of pathogen evolution in mixtures consider static costs of virulence to be the main mechanism countering selection for pathogen complexity, many other potential mechanisms need to be investigated. Horticultural and marketing considerations must be carefully evaluated when implementing mixture approaches to crop management.

It must be remembered that not all multilines will reduce disease if the components of the mixture are randomly selected. Rather, mixture components need to be relevant and functional to the pathogen population in question. The effects of mixtures on disease intensity as compared to their component pure line comparatives can range from a disease increase to nearly complete disease control. Intercropping, which is the mixture of different crop species, is not considered a multiline population.

For the multiline to be functional, there must be an appropriate match between the resistance genes incorporated in the multiline and the avirulence genes present in the target pathogen population. Thus a matrix of host and pathogen genotypes needs to be considered, to minimize the percentage of the host population that will be virulent. Such information needs to be used to construct, and alter over time, the resistance genes utilized in multiline cultivars.

One of the major reasons multiline cultivars are not widely adopted by growers is the advent of F_1 hybrid cultivars. Not only do hybrids have greater yields, but they are also highly uniform. Modern agriculture is based around uniformity-ranging from uniform growth, flowering, maturity, and harvests to uniform size, shape, and quality for the processor and consumer. While multilines should be uniform for all traits except resistance, it is next to impossible to develop F_1 hybrids in the multiline system, because the seed producer would need to develop many different lines to be sold.

Anticipatory breeding/preemptive breeding

Monitoring changes and shifts in a pathogen population's adaptation to resistance genes is essential for the long-term management of numerous plant diseases where host resistance is the primary means of managing a disease. Surveillance of the pathogen population composition has helped plant breeders respond to the appearance of new pathogen strains where changes in virulence are observed. For example, the annual monitoring of *Puccinia tritcina*, the cause of leaf rust on wheat (*Triticum aestivum*) in the United States, has documented shifts in pathogen virulence both within and among regions enables plant breeders to prepare for the movement of races to new regions that could otherwise threaten wheat production. The Australian plant breeder, Robert A. McIntosh, coined the phrase "Anticipatory Breeding," and the breeding strategy has been referred to as "Pre-emptive Breeding" for this approach of monitoring the pathogen population and changing resistant parents as needed.

Evolutionary forces

Bruce A. McDonald and Celeste Linde at the Federal Institute of Technology in Switzerland list five evolutionary forces that change the pathogen population that the plant breeder needs to be aware of when selecting the resistance source. They are (1) mutation, population size, and random genetic drift; (2) gene and genotype flow; (3) reproduction and mating system; (4) selection imposed by major gene resistance; and (5) quantitative resistance. Mutation is the ultimate source of genetic variation and can lead to the "breaking" of major gene resistance. Mutations can also erode quantitative resistance. Mutations are especially important for pathogens such as bacteria and viruses that exist as extremely large populations within individual plants.

Population size affects the probability of change occurring. Large population sizes of pathogens have greater evolutionary potential than pathogens with small population sizes. Populations that go through "bottlenecks," for example, because of crop rotation or breeding a new resistance gene into the crop are less diverse and slower to adapt than populations that maintain a high population size year-round. This is evident with tropical versus temperate climates.

With gene and genotype flow, the form of propagation is important. Asexually propagated crops will have much less genetic diversity than a sexually propagated crops. Gene and genotype flow will move virulent mutant alleles and genotypes among different field populations. A high degree of gene and genotype flow equals greater genetic diversity than pathogens with low degrees of gene/genotype flow. It also increases the effective population size by increasing the size of the genetic neighborhood. Human activities move many pathogens far beyond their natural dispersal limits through agricultural practices and intercontinental travel and commerce.

As mentioned in Chapter 4, Resistance: the pathogen, on pathogen variability, reproduction and mating system affect how gene diversity is distributed within and among individuals in a pathogen population. Reproduction can be sexual, asexual, or both. Resistance gene pyramids may not be an effective long-term breeding strategy against pathogens that undergo regular recombination. Pathogens that outcross pose a greater risk than inbreeding pathogens because more new genotypes are created through outcrossing.

The foundations of breeding for durable resistance are diverse germplasm with variation in partial resistance, field trial sites with high disease levels, where consistent selection can be applied, and an efficient breeding system. Selection for resistance must be done alongside selection for other important traits. This should lead to the steady accumulation of minor genes for resistance in cultivars that also have desirable yield, quality, and other horticulturally important characteristics.

Selection for partial resistance at several sites increases the probability but does not guarantee that resistance will be durable. Knowledge of genetics, resistance mechanisms, and epidemiology is indispensable. Using genes that are likely to be durable and avoiding extensive use of those likely to be ephemeral should increase the durability of resistance.

Because durable resistance does not have a set time limit, the longer the resistance is effective the better for the plant breeder, the grower, and society. Humans began to grow crops approximately 12,000 years ago, but scientific plant breeding commenced a mere 150 years ago, and only a very few genes have provided durable resistance for several decades. Plant breeders face the need to feed a growing human population. Pyramiding or stacking several resistance genes of diverse race specificity in the same cultivar has provided high and durable resistance to major diseases, such as potato late blight (*P. infestans*), especially when plant breeders combine highly efficient genes for broad-spectrum resistance that are novel to the intruding pathogens.

Plant breeders are in a unique position to help society by providing horticultural crops with durable disease resistance. Plant breeders will continue to improve existing plant varieties and create new ones to improve resistance to disease. Whether they work in a commercial, academic, or international centers, all will benefit society with their work.

Bibliography

Anderson, P.K., Cunningham, A.A., Patel, N.G., Morales, F.J., Epstein, P.R., Daszak, P., 2004. Emerging infectious diseases of plants: pathogen pollution, climate change and agrotechnological drivers. Trends in Ecology and Evolution 19, 535–544. Available from: https://doi.org/10.1016/j.tree.2004.07.021.

Andrus, C.F., Reynard, G.B., Wade, B.L., 1942. Relative Resistance of Tomato Varieties, Selections, and Crosses to Defoliation by Alternaria and Stemphylium. U.S. Department of Agriculture Circular, 652.

Armstrong, M.R., Vossen, J., Lim, T.Y., Hutten, R.C.B., Xu, J., Strachan, S.M., et al., 2018. Tracking disease resistance deployment in potato breeding by enrichment sequencing. Plant Biotechnology Journal 1, 540–549. Available from: https://doi.org/10.1111/pbi.12997.

Barka, G.D., Lee, J., 2020. Molecular marker development and gene cloning for diverse disease resistance in pepper (*Capsicum annuum L.*): current status and prospects. Plant Breeding and Biotechnology 8, 89–113. Available from: https://doi.org/10.9787/PBB.2020.8.2.89.

Bergelson, J., Kreitman, M., Stahl, E.A., Tian, D., 2001. Evolutionary dynamics of plant R-genes. Science (New York, N.Y.) 292, 2281–2285. Available from: https://doi.org/10.1126/science.1061337.

Bernardo-Cravo, A., Schmeller, D.S., Chatzinotas, A., Vredenburg, V.T., Loyau, A., 2020. Environmental factors and host microbiomes shape host–pathogen dynamics. Trends in Parasitology 36, 616–633. Available from: https://doi.org/10.1016/j.pt.2020.04.010.

Bousset, L., Chèvre, A.-M., 2013. Stable epidemic control in crops based on evolutionary principles: adjusting the metapopulation concept to agro-ecosystems. Agriculture, Ecosystems and Environment 165, 118–129. Available from: https://doi.org/10.1016/j.agee.2012.12.005.

Brown, J.K.M., 2015. Durable resistance of crops: a Darwinian perspective. Annual Review of Phytopathology 53, 513–539. Available from: https://doi.org/10.1146/annurev-phyto-102313-045914.

Bull, C.T., Gebben, S.J., Goldman, P.H., Trent, M., Hayes, R.J., 2015. Host genotype and hypersensitive reaction influence population levels of *Xanthomonas campestris* pv. vitians in lettuce. Phytopathology 105, 316–324. Available from: https://doi.org/10.1094/PHYTO-07-14-0185-R.

Chepsergon, J., Motaung, T., Moleleki, L., 2021. Core RxLR effectors in phytopathogenic oomycetes: a promising way to breeding for durable resistance in plants? Virulence 12, 1921–1935. Available from: https://doi.org/10.1080/21505594.2021.1948277.

Clay, K., Kover, P.X., 1996. The Red Queen hypothesis and plant/pathogen interactions. Annual Review of Phytopathology 34, 29–50. Available from: https://doi.org/10.1146/annurev.phyto.34.1.29.

Cowger, C., Brown, J.K.M., 2019. Durability of quantitative resistance in crops: greater than we know? Annual Review of Phytopathology 57, 253–277. Available from: https://doi.org/10.1146/annurev-phyto-082718-100016.

Crandall, S.G., Gold, K.M., del Mar Jiménez-Gasco, M., Filgueiras, C.C., Willett, D.S., 2020. A multi-omics approach to solving problems in plant disease ecology. PLoS One . Available from: https://doi.org/10.1371/journal.pone.0237975.

Dangl, J.L., Horvath, D.M., Staskawicz, B.J., 2013. Pivoting the plant immune system from dissection to deployment. Science (New York, N.Y.) 341, 746–751. Available from: https://doi.org/10.1126/science.1236011.

Delourme, R., Bousset, L., Ermel, M., Duffé, P., Besnard, A.L., Marquer, B., et al., 2014. Quantitative resistance affects the speed of frequency increase but not the diversity of the virulence alleles overcoming a major resistance gene to *Leptosphaeria maculans* in oilseed rape. Infection, Genetics and Evolution 27, 490–499. Available from: https://doi.org/10.1016/j.meegid.2013.12.019.

Holub, E.B., 2001. The arms race is ancient history in Arabidopsis, the wildflower. Nature Reviews. Genetics 2, 516–527. Available from: https://doi.org/10.1038/35080508.

Jacobs, T., Parlevliet, J.D., 1993. Durability of Disease Resistance. Kluwer Academic Publishers, Agricultural University, Wageningen, The Netherlands.

Johnson, R., 1981. Durable resistance: definition of, genetic control and attainment in plant breeding. Phytopathology 71, 567–568.

Karasov, T.L., Shirsekar, G., Schwab, R., Weigel, D., 2020. What natural variation can teach us about resistance durability. Current Opinion in Plant Biology 56, 89–98. Available from: https://doi.org/10.1016/j.pbi.2020.04.010.

Laine, A.-L., Burdon, J.J., Dodds, P.N., Thrall, P.H., 2011. Spatial variation in disease resistance: from molecules to metapopulations. Journal of Ecology 99, 96–112. Available from: https://doi.org/10.1111/j.1365-2745.2010.01738.x.

Li, W., Deng, Y., Ning, Y., He, Z., Wang, G.L., 2020. Exploiting broad-spectrum disease resistance in crops: from molecular dissection to breeding. Annual Review of Plant Biology 71, 575–603. Available from: https://doi.org/10.1146/annurev-arplant-010720-022215.

Louwaars, N.P., 2018. Plant breeding and diversity: a troubled relationship? Euphytica 214, 114. Available from: https://doi.org/10.1007/s10681-018-2192-5.

Luo, F., Evans, K., Norelli, J.L., Zhang, Z., Peace, C., 2020. Prospects for achieving durable disease resistance with elite fruit quality in apple breeding. Tree Genetics and Genomes 16, 21. Available from: https://doi.org/10.1007/s11295-020-1414-x.

McDonald, B.A., Linde, C., 2002. Pathogen population genetics, evolutionary potential, and durable resistance. Annual Review of Phytopathology 40, 349–379. Available from: https://doi.org/10.1146/annurev.phyto.40.120501.101443.

Mundt, C.C., 2014. Durable resistance: a key to sustainable management of pathogens and pests. Infection, Genetics and Evolution 27, 446–455. Available from: https://doi.org/10.1016/j.meegid.2014.01.011.

Parra, L.B., Simko, I., Michelmore, R., 2021. Identification of major quantitative trait loci controlling field resistance to downy mildew in cultivated lettuce (*Lactuca sativa* L.). Phytopathology. Available from: https://doi.org/10.1094/PHYTO-08-20-0367-R.

Pink, D.A.C., Lot, H., Johnson, R., 1992. Novel pathotypes of lettuce mosaic-virus—breakdown of a durable resistance. Euphytica 63, 169–174. Available from: https://doi.org/10.1007/BF00023921.

Rabbinge, R., Rossing, W.A.H., Vanderwerf, W., 1993. Systems approaches in epidemiology and plant disease management. Netherland Journal of Plant Pathology 99, 161–171.

Rimbaud, L., Fabre, F., Papaïx, J., Moury, B., Lannou, C., Barrett, L.G., et al., 2021. Models of plant resistance deployment. Annual Review of Phytopathology 59, 125–152. Available from: https://doi.org/10.1146/annurev-phyto-020620-122134.

Salvaudon, L., Giraud, T., Shykoff, J.A., 2008. Genetic diversity in natural populations: a fundamental component of plant–microbe interactions. Current Opinion in Plant Biology 11, 135–143. Available from: https://doi.org/10.1016/j.pbi.2008.02.002.

Silva Botelho, F.B., Patto Ramalho, M.A., Barbosa Abreu, Â.D.-F., Andrade Rosa, H.J., 2010. Multiline as a strategy to reduce damage caused by *Colletotrichum lindemuthianum* in common bean. Journal of Phytopathology 159, 175–180. Available from: https://doi.org/10.1111/j.1439-0434.2010.01743.x.

Soubeyrand, S., Laine, A.-L., Hanski, I., Penttinen, A., 2009. Spatial-temporal structure of interactions in a host–pathogen metapopulation. American Naturalist 174, 308–320. Available from: https://doi.org/10.1086/589451.

Stuthman, D.D., Leonard, K.J., Miller-Garvin, J., 2007. Breeding crops for durable resistance to disease. Advances in Agronomy 95, 319–367. Available from: https://doi.org/10.1016/S0065-2113(07)95004-X.

Tellier, A., Brown, J.K.M., 2011. Spatial heterogeneity, frequency-dependent selection and polymorphism in host–parasite interactions. BMC Evolutionary Biology 11, 319. Available from: https://doi.org/10.1186/1471-2148-11-319.

Thrall, P.H., Burdon, J.J., 2003. Evolution of virulence in a plant host–pathogen metapopulation. Science (New York, N.Y.) 299, 1735–1737. Available from: https://doi.org/10.1126/science.1080070.

van den Bosch, F., Gilligan, C.A., 2003. Measures of durability of resistance. Phytopathology 93, 616–625. Available from: https://doi.org/10.1094/PHYTO.2003.93.5.616.

Vicente, J.G., Gunn, N.D., Bailey, L., Pink, D.A.C., Holub, E.B., 2011. Genetics of resistance to downy mildew in *Brassica oleracea* and breeding towards durable disease control for UK vegetable production. Plant Pathology 61, 600–609. Available from: https://doi.org/10.1111/j.1365-3059.2011.02539.x.

Von Bertalanffy, L., 1950. An outline of general system theory. British Journal for the Philosophy of Science 1, 134–165. Available from: https://doi.org/10.1093/bjps/I.2.134.

Vurro, M., Bonciani, B., Vannacci, G., 2010. Emerging infectious diseases of crop plants in developing countries: impact on agriculture and socio-economic consequences. Food Security 2, 113–132. Available from: https://doi.org/10.1007/s12571-010-0062-7.

Wolfe, M.S., 1985. The current status and prospects of multiline cultivars and variety mixtures for disease resistance. Annual Review of Phytopathology 23, 251–273. Available from: https://doi.org/10.1146/annurev.py.23.090185.001343.

12

Resistance: plant-parasitic nematodes

Introduction

Currently, plant-parasitic nematodes comprise about 15% of the total number of nematode species known in the world. Plant-parasitic nematodes on horticultural crops are grouped into root-knot, cyst, and lesion types and are responsible annually for billions of dollars of losses to horticultural crops (Fig. 12.1). Plant breeders have developed improved cultivars of important horticultural crops with resistance to plant-parasitic nematodes. The earliest reports of selection for plant resistance to nematodes date back to the late 19th century and were based on phenotypic selection for plants that had fewer galls on roots when infected with root-knot nematodes. With a better understanding of plant-parasitic nematode and host interactions, host interactions are defined by the varying degrees of susceptibility and resistance they display when infected. When breeding for nematode resistance, the goal is to reduce nematode reproduction, optimistically to zero.

The effectiveness of breeding efforts depends on the availability of efficient screening procedures, identification of adequate sources of durable resistance, and knowledge of the inheritance of resistance. These factors determine, to a large degree, the breeding method and the potential success of the project. Studies to search for plant-parasitic nematode resistance have identified resistant germplasm within crop species or from closely related species. When the resistance gene is from a related species, issues with wide hybridization must be overcome. When related species are used, backcrossing to the cultivated species may be sufficient to incorporate the resistance gene and recover the desirable commercial traits of the horticultural crop. If the resistance gene is present within the crop species, the choice of breeding method depends on the inheritance of the resistance, type of screening procedure, and other important breeding objectives for the species.

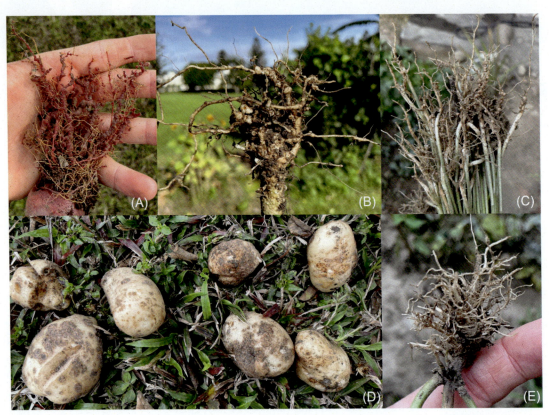

Figure 12.1 Various symptoms and degrees of severity of nematode damage on beet (*Beta vulgaris*) (A), okra (*Abelmoschus esculentus*) (B), mung bean (*Vigna radiata*) (C), potato (*Solanum tuberosum*) (D), and kangkong (*Ipomoea aquatica*) (E) from a single garden in Taiwan.

Plant resistance to plant-parasitic nematodes is one of several important components in nematode management required for efficient horticultural crop production. The development and utilization of nematode-resistant cultivars result in increased yield, enhanced grower profits, and lower costs for the consumer. Resistant cultivars provide specific advantages in a nematode management program including suppressed nematode reproduction, reduced length of crop rotations, lower risk of toxic residues in the environment and food chain, lack of a requirement for special application technology or equipment, and generally with similar seed cost as compared to the susceptible cultivars. However, major limitations in the use of nematode-resistant cultivars include the paucity of cultivars resistant to multiple nematode species, resistance to newly evolved pathotypes with the ability to overcome previously employed resistance, and crop species in which resistance has not been identified in the species or related wild relatives.

Standardized definitions for terms describing host–nematode relationships are important for the plant breeder to communicate their results. Resistance describes the ability of a host to suppress nematode development and reproduction. It can range from low resistance to intermediate resistance to high resistance. A highly resistant plant allows no nematode reproduction or only trace amounts. Intermediate-resistant plants, as one would expect, allow intermediate amounts of reproduction. Conversely, a susceptible host allows nematodes to reproduce freely. In practice, nematode resistance is a relative concept, derived through genotype comparisons, and it frequently includes an indication of levels of resistance within a continuum of host–nematode interactions. A highly resistant genotype supports little nematode reproduction, whereas a partially resistant genotype supports an intermediate level of reproduction relative to a susceptible genotype. Implicit in the suppression of nematode reproduction by the host is a corresponding cellular response in the host that adversely affects nematode parasitism. For the plant breeder, measuring nematode development or reproduction is more informative, for example, counting eggs produced than determining the host reaction in most cases. For example, root-knot nematodes may reproduce freely on a host, but no gall or knots are formed. The plant breeder may believe that no galls on the roots imply resistance, but that is incorrect. Resistance is distinctly different from tolerance. As with diseases, tolerance is a relative concept that describes the sensitivity of a host to parasitism or the amount of damage sustained and is measured in terms of yield suppression. A tolerant cultivar suffers little or no yield reduction, even when heavily infected with nematodes, whereas yield is greatly suppressed on a similarly infected susceptible cultivar.

Not all nematodes are pathogenic or have pathogenicity on horticultural plants. With more than 20,000 species of nematodes, most nematode species are not pathogenic. Nevertheless, one of the most pathogenic plant-parasitic nematodes is *Radopholus similis*. It is a devastating migratory endoparasitic plant-parasitic nematode that is known to infect more than 350 host plant species, including many horticultural crops such as fruits, ornamentals, and vegetable plants.

As with bacteria, fungi, bacterium, and viruses, virulence genes are present in plant-parasitic nematodes that correspond to resistance genes in the host plant—gene-for-gene situation. Virulence is defined according to the ability of a nematode to reproduce on a host plant that possesses one or more resistance genes. Virulent nematodes can reproduce, whereas avirulent nematodes are unable to reproduce in the presence of a specific resistance gene or genes. An important aspect of virulence is that a population of nematodes comprises a mixture of virulent and avirulent individuals. The frequency of each can range from all to none. The frequency of virulent individuals will determine the potential for the selection of virulence in the presence of resistant host plants. These genes encoding this trait are also called avirulence or *Avr* genes, similar to bacteria, fungi, and viruses.

Different terms are used to categorize the type of physiological variation based on host responses that are encountered with a nematode species. Terms to categorize these differences are confusing because of a largely indiscriminate use of them for different nematode types. The terms race or host-race has been used for categorizing variation with *Meloidogyne incognita*, and pathotype has been used for the potato cyst nematode (*Globodera pallida* and *Globodera rostochiensis*). The term biotype for variations within the stem and bulb nematode (*Ditylenchus dipsaci*). A common, but not universal interpretation of these terms has been that races of nematodes species are separated by differential reactions on hosts of widely different plant species, for example, *races* of root-knot nematode (*M. incognita*), differentiated on pepper (*Capsicum* species), tobacco (*Nicotiana tabacum*), cotton (*Gossypium hirsutum*), peanut (*Arachis hypogaea*), and tomato (*Solanum lycopersicum*), where *pathotypes* are differentiated by genes for resistance in different cultivars and of the same plant species, for example, *Globodera* species on potato (*Solanum tuberosum*).

Genetic variation for resistance

The mode of inheritance of plant-parasitic nematode resistance is important to the plant breeder in designing the most efficient breeding strategies to incorporate the resistance into cultivars. Resistance genes can be classified based on their effects on resistance expression, qualitative versus quantitative, race-specific or race-nonspecific, and mode of inheritance, that is, monogenic, oligogenic, and polygenic. Once the source of resistance is identified, the plant breeder is interested in the number of genes conditioning the resistance. Reviews on the genetic control of resistance to plant-parasitic nematodes found 52% were monogenic, 28% were oligogenic, and 20% were polygenic control. Monogenic and oligogenic resistance is desirable from the standpoint of the ease of introducing host resistance into advanced cultivars. However, the reported genetic studies of plant-parasitic nematode resistance may be biased toward monogenic resistance because of the genetic simplicity and high level of resistance expression, which could mask the effects of small effects or linked genes that contribute to resistance. Plant-parasitic nematodes are separated frequently into three general groups according to feeding habits, ectoparasites, migratory endoparasites, and sedentary endoparasites. The type of feeding relationship influences the potential availability of resistance genes and the protocol to identify resistant genotypes.

Ectoparasites remain outside host tissue and use their stylets to feed on epidermal or internal cells. There are several nematode genera that feed on plant stems and foliage, including *Aphelenchoides, Bursaphelenchus, Anguina, Ditylenchus,* and *Litylenchus*. While most members of *Aphelenchoides* feed on fungi, three species have populations that are facultative plant parasites and feed on live plant tissue. With the exception of a few ectoparasitic nematodes that elicit a specific cellular response, most nematodes with this feeding habit do not establish a lasting relationship with their host and therefore are unlikely to have exerted selection pressure on the host for the evolution of resistance genes.

Migratory endoparasites, for example, *Pratylenchus* species, enter and migrate within host tissue, feed on various tissues, and generally cause considerable tissue destruction. Most migratory endoparasites are also general feeders that do not require a specialized host-response for successful parasitism. The root-lesion nematode (*Pratylenchus brachyurus*) is a major pest on pineapple (*Ananas comosus*) cucumber (*Cucumis sativus*), okra (*Abelmoschus esculentus*), tomato (*S. lycopersicum*), and cantaloupe (*Cucumis melo*). Antagonistic host responses that suppress nematode development and reproduction have been identified in a limited number of crops for nematodes with this feeding habit.

Sedentary endoparasites, that is, root-knot nematodes (*Meloidogyne* species) and cyst nematodes (*Globodera* and *Heterodera* species), have evolved highly specialized feeding relationships with their hosts and depend on a few host cells modified by the nematode to provide nourishment for its development and reproduction. This intimate relationship between nematode and host is controlled by the genetic systems of both organisms and has resulted in the evolution of resistance genes in many crop species.

In general, as nematode parasitism becomes specialized with a concomitant restriction in the host range, the potential for identifying host resistance genes greatly increases. For host and nematode combinations where resistance genes have not been identified, the development of tolerant cultivars is an alternative approach for increasing yields on land infested with pathogenic nematodes. Numerous methods have been developed to identify resistant genotypes in a plant population. The method of choice will vary depending on the feeding habit of the target nematodes.

Evaluating the interaction phenotype

The screening protocol to identify individuals resistant to plant-parasitic nematodes must be repeatable and reliable. A climate-controlled environment permits tests to be conducted throughout the year. A climate-controlled environment may be a greenhouse, laboratory, growth chamber, and so on. Although breeding lines may be evaluated in naturally infested fields, the lack of uniformity of nematode infestations in fields, weather restrictions, and mixed nematode communities are disadvantages to this approach. Naturally, nematode-infested soil can be utilized in greenhouse tests; however, the lack of uniformity of inoculum concentration and the introduction of contaminating organisms that may include other nematode species in naturally infested soil are drawbacks. Cultured/propagated nematodes are the preferred inoculum. Additional benefits of propagated inoculum include standardization of inoculum levels, uniform distribution of inoculum, evaluation of resistance in localities where a specific nematode species or race is not indigenous, and the elimination of seasonal restrictions when evaluating genotypes.

Many laboratory assays for identifying resistant genotypes have been developed. Availability and type of nematode inoculum can be a limitation for screening plant germplasm. Sedentary endoparasitic nematodes are readily cultured and large quantities of inoculum, preferably eggs, can be obtained easily. The selection of a nematode isolate for inoculum is a critical part of any screening program. Utilization of an aggressive nematode isolate is important for detecting genotypes possessing the highest level of resistance. In addition, screening with a mixture of isolates from diverse geographical areas will permit the identification of breeding lines with broad resistance that should have usefulness over a wide geographic area.

Maintenance of the virulence and aggressiveness of the nematode isolate is also important and can be accomplished by culturing the nematode on a host that does not exert selection pressure. Even so, nematode aggressiveness and purity of nematode inoculum must be monitored regularly.

Environmental conditions can vary in a greenhouse and significantly influence the results of a screening test. When breeding for resistance, an important component to be considered with the nematode screen is the effect of soil temperature as it is with soilborne pathogens. A significant number of nematode resistance genes in plants are sensitive to low and high temperatures although not all nematode R-genes are temperature sensitive. Soil temperature can produce pseudoresistance or escapes when the soil temperature is too low, while if the soil temperature is above an optimum, resistance breeding material may appear susceptible when in fact, they are genetically resistant. The optimum temperature varies for different host–nematode combinations. Each root-knot nematode species has its own optimum temperature range requirement for development. For example, the minimum larva-to-larva life cycle of the root-knot nematode (*M. incognita*) on a tomato (*S. lycopersicum*) is 25 days at 27°C. At 16.5°C, the time from larva-to-larva life cycle is increased to 87 days. It has been reported that penetration and development of *M. incognita* in roots of resistant tomato (*S. lycopersicum*) cultivars increased at higher soil temperatures. With green beans (*Phaseolus vulgaris*), it has been shown that resistance to *M. incognita* decreased with an increase in soil temperature from 16°C to 28°C. When the effect of soil temperature on the *N* gene that confers resistance to the southern root-knot nematode (*M. incognita*) in pepper (*Capsicum annuum*) was investigated, it was shown that the eggs per gram of fresh root, a reproductive factor of *M. incognita*, number of second-stage juveniles in soil, egg mass production, and root galling increased as soil temperature increased.

Air temperature can also affect the screening of germplasm. When a tomato (*S. lycopersicum*) is subjected to heat stress, the resistance to *M. incognita* is reduced. In tomato (*S. lycopersicum*), resistance to root-knot nematodes is controlled by the gene *Mi-1*, but heat stress interferes with *Mi-1*-associated resistance. Under controlled day/night temperatures of 25°C/21°C, the cultivar Amelia that possesses the *Mi-1* gene was deemed resistant and the cultivar Rutgers, which does not possess the *Mi-1* gene, was susceptible to *M. incognita* infection. Exposure to a single 3-hour heat spike of 35°C was sufficient to increase the susceptibility of the cultivar Amelia but did not affect the cultivar Rutgers. Despite this change in resistance, *Mi-1* gene expression was not affected by heat treatment or nematode infection. The heat-induced breakdown of *Mi-1* resistance in the cultivar Amelia did recover with time regardless of additional heat exposures and *M. incognita* infection. These findings may aid in the development of management strategies to protect the tomato (*S. lycopersicum*) crop at times of heightened *M. incognita* susceptibility.

In each screening, the inclusion of susceptible and resistant genotypes as internal controls helps normalize variations in test conditions. Furthermore, having a susceptible and a resistant genotype can be utilized to develop a rating scale. Inclusion of a standard resistant genotype also will facilitate the identification of genotypes with superior levels of resistance. After the initial screening, selected breeding lines should be tested in nematode-infested fields in several environments.

Sources of resistance

The transfer of resistance into an acceptable commercial cultivar is greatly simplified if resistant germplasm can be found in adapted cultivars or in advanced breeding lines. As with bacteria, fungi, and virus resistance genes, the order of priority recommended for screening is first commercial cultivars, then plant introductions of the cultivated species, and if the search within the crop species is unsuccessful, the germplasm accessions of wild relatives of the crop species can be screened. Wild relatives have been used successfully to develop nematode-resistant potatoes (*S. tuberosum*), cucumbers (*C. sativus*), carrots (*Daucus carota*), and tomatoes (*S. lycopersicum*). Wild relatives are usually challenging to hybridize with the crop species and will normally contribute many unacceptable traits along with nematode resistance to the resulting progeny, through linkage drag.

A classic example of the use of wild relatives is the incorporation of *M. incognita* resistance into cultivated tomato (*S. lycopersicum*) from its wild relative, *Solanum peruvianum*. The gene *Mi* confers resistance to three major *Meloidogyne* species, *M. incognita*, *Meloidogyne javanica*, and *Meloidogyne arenaria*. *M. incognita* is where the gene (*Mi*) derives its name. The resistance was originally identified in *S. peruvianum*, a species that does not normally hybridize with cultivated tomatoes (*S. lycopersicum*). In the early 1940s, an interspecific hybrid was successfully produced using embryo rescue by Prof. Paul G. Smith at the University of California at Davis, USA. This one interspecific hybrid plant is the source of all root-knot nematode resistance in currently available fresh-market and processing tomato (*S. lycopersicum*) cultivars. The *Mi* gene has provided durable resistance to the three root-knot nematode species for many years. Serendipity plays a part with the *Mi* gene because a unique condition of the gene is that it also confers resistance to the potato aphid (*Macrosiphum euphorbiae*).

Another example of a source of resistance is the wild *Solanum* species. Tomato (*S. lycopersicum*) is highly susceptible to *Meloidogyne enterolobii*. Accessions of *Solanum acanthodes* and *Solanum lycocarpum* are highly resistant to immune to *M. enterolobii*. Some accessions of *Solanum subinerme* and *Solanum scuticum* are resistant, while others are susceptible. In other studies, entries of *Solanum sisymbriifolium* were highly resistant to *M. enterolobii* and *Meloidogyne haplanaria* but are extremely susceptible to *M. javanica*.

The treatment with mutagenic agents has created nematode resistance in very few horticultural crops. Somaclonal variation another form of mutagenesis has a paucity of examples where plant-parasitic nematode resistance was created. The random nature of somaclonal variation makes it a costly approach in horticultural crops.

Protoplast fusion is a procedure that combines the genomes of unrelated species by somatic hybridization, providing a method of gene transfer in otherwise sexually isolated species. Protoplast fusion between the root-knot nematode-resistant wild species, *S. sisymbriifolium*, and eggplant (*Solanum melongena*) was accomplished to move nematode resistance genes into cultivated eggplant. The resulting plants require backcrossing and selection after the desired trait is transferred to eggplant (*S. melongena*).

Biotechnology approaches to plant-parasitic nematode control

Earlier efforts of biotechnology focused on using marker-assisted breeding methods to identify sources of nematode resistance. Marker-assisted breeding assists the plant breeder in introducing plant-parasitic nematode resistance genes by providing an indirect method to identify and combine the best nematode resistance genes. Marker-assisted selection (MAS) is very useful in a nematode resistance breeding program. In tomato (*S. lycopersicum*), the *Mi* gene for resistance to

M. incognita, *M. javanica*, and *M. arenaria* was found to be tightly linked to the acid phosphatase-1 (*Aps-l*) locus, and resistant genotypes were identified by assaying for a variant allele of *Aps-1*. This approach eliminates the time-consuming propagation of nematodes for inoculum and permits analyses of young plant tissue. MAS may be especially useful for the rapid and efficient introgression of resistance genes from wild or uncultivated species into improved cultivars.

Molecular methods used for mapping of nematode populations include Restriction Amplified Length Polymorphisms (RFLPs), Amplified Fragment Length Polymorphisms, Random Amplified Polymorphic DNA, Sequenced Characterized Amplified Regions (SCAR), and Sequence Tagged Site—based methods and more recently deep sequencing technologies, such as genome-wide association study. MAS for nematode resistance is a major focus to make breeding nematode-resistant crops more efficient. Substantial breeding efforts are being undertaken to identify stable sources of resistance to the different species and pathotypes of nematodes. For example, both polygenic and monogenic genes for resistance to potato cyst nematodes (*G. rostochiensis*) have been identified, and markers closely linked to these alleles have since been developed for use in potato (*S. tuberosum*) resistance breeding programs. Similarly, different types of resistance genes have been identified, mapped, and/or cloned from host plants that confer near complete and partial resistances to the nematodes, *Heterodera glycines*, *Heterodera avenae*, and *Heterodera schachtii*.

A caveat to using MAS is that the marker developed for MAS may not be specific when interspecific and intergeneric hybridization is used. False positives produced by markers for *Mi 1.2* gene in hybrid tomato (*S. lycopersicum*) rootstocks explain why rootstocks such as Beaufort and Maxifort often vary in their resistance and susceptibility to populations of *M. incognita*, *M. javanica*, and *M. arenaria*, and such markers may not reliably predict the presence or absence of *Mi 1.2* in intergeneric tomato (*S. lycopersicum*) hybrids.

RNAi-based nematode resistance

An emerging breakthrough approach to breeding for plant-parasitic nematode resistance is the use of RNA interference (RNAi) technology. This natural mechanism for sequence-specific gene silencing may revolutionize nematode resistance in horticultural plants. Transgenic plants expressing double-stranded RNA (dsRNA) hairpin structures targeting root-knot nematode essential genes provide a highly effective resistance mechanism. Gene silencing can be achieved by the transformation of plants with constructs that express self-complementary (termed hairpin) RNA-containing sequences homologous to the target genes. The DNA sequences encoding the self-complementary regions of hairpin RNA constructs form an inverted repeat. The discovery that RNAi is a conserved biological response to dsRNA that facilitates resistance to both endogenous parasitic and exogenous pathogenic nucleic acids and regulates the expression of protein-coding genes. The dsRNA or small interfering RNAs (siRNAs) are taken up by establishing plant-parasitic nematodes, which elicit a systemic RNAi response and then induce a highly detrimental or lethal RNAi phenotype in the nematode. So, the transgenic plants obtain resistance to root-knot nematodes.

Having the plant delivery of dsRNA through host cells from a constitutive promoter is a way to have them continuously expressed. This mode of delivery of dsRNA appears to be an ideal and economical approach to control obligate parasites such as plant-parasitic nematodes. In host delivery of dsRNA of two target genes, an integrase and a pre-mRNA splicing factor, the reduction in replication of *M. incognita* on transgenic tobacco (*N. tabacum*) plants was first demonstrated. This was followed by the approach of expressing dsRNA to a *M. incognita* effector protein in transgenic plants and showed reduced nematode reproduction. Since then, a series of crop plants have been engineered to generate inverted repeats.

One of the attractions of developing transgenic resistance to plant nematodes using RNAi technology is the potential to confer broader resistance to several species in one construct, in contrast to the more specific resistance conferred by natural resistance genes. The principle is that hairpin dsRNA to a number of different target genes can be made either from the same or different species or to target different populations of the same nematode species. When *Pratylenchus thornei*, a nematode of many horticultural crops, for example, asparagus (*Asparagus acutifolius*), carrot (*Dacus carota*), celery (*Apium graveolens* var. *dulce*), globe artichoke (*Cynara cardunculus*), cole crops (*Brassica* species), onion (*Allium cepa*), papaya (*Carica papaya*), strawberry (*Fragaria × ananassa*), sweet pea (*Lathyrus odoratus*), tomato (*S. lycopersicum*), almond (*Prunus amygdalus*), and so on, was soaked in dsRNA sequences of two target genes, there was a reduction in subsequent reproduction on carrot (*D. carota*) disks irrespective of the target gene source.

However, so far there are no convincing reports from transgenic *in planta* experiments that two different nematode species can be controlled with one hybrid dsRNA construct. Perhaps the RNAi mechanism can be overwhelmed if too many siRNA are generated, and with more subtle expression or choice of target sequence, the potential for broad resistance to different nematode species may be achieved.

Since the discovery that reproduction of sedentary endoparasitic nematodes such as *Heterodera* species, *Gobodera* species, *Meloidogyne* species, *Rotylenchulus* species, *Nacobbus* species, and *Tylenchulus* species depends on the successful formation and function of giant cells, syncytia or similarly modified host cells, strategies to disrupt feeding site formation have been investigated. Success with this type of approach depends on identifying plant promoters that are specifically or highly upregulated in feeding cells, and that can be linked to the expression of a cytotoxic gene that when expressed in feeding cells results in cell death or impairment. *Barstar* is a small protein from the bacterium *Bacillus amyloliquefaciens*. Its function is to inhibit the ribonuclease activity of its binding partner *barnase*, with which it forms an extraordinarily tightly bound complex within the cell until *barnase* is secreted. Expression of *barstar* is necessary to counter the lethal effect of expressed active *barnase*. Even when combined with constitutive expression of the gene *barstar* that neutralizes the activity of *barnase*, unless it is highly upregulated there is a danger of unintended side effects on the plant. Although a series of genes highly upregulated or downregulated in nematode feeding cells have been identified, such as the heat shock promoter *Hahsp17.7G4*, it appears that none of these promoters alone is sufficiently tightly expressed in the feeding cells to link them to a cytotoxic gene without collateral damage elsewhere in the plant. An alternative approach, based on using two nematode-responsive promoters, both of which must be upregulated in nematode-feeding cells for the expression of a cytotoxic gene to occur, may overcome this issue of target cell specificity of expression.

As biotechnology advances, new strategies for nematode control are emerging, both for transgenic approaches and in genome editing that may be regarded as a form of mutation rather than "genetic modification." With such advances in biotechnology, the release of commercial cultivars of horticultural crops with new forms of nematode resistance is likely to become a commercial reality. To improve durability, transgenic traits could be based on resistance with different modes of action: for example, RNAi-based technology combined with the expression of peptides that disrupt sensory activities. Ideally, biogenic traits need to be introduced into existing horticultural crop genotypes that have the best natural nematode resistance, to increase the effectiveness and durability of the nematode resistance trait.

Breeding for multiple pest resistance

As discussed in Chapter 9, breeding for multiple disease and pest resistance is a cornerstone of most horticultural breeding programs. The development of disease in horticultural crops has long been known to depend on the complex interrelationship between host, pathogen, and environmental conditions. In the case of soilborne pathogens, further complications exist for interactions with nematodes. The significant role of nematodes in the development of diseases caused by soilborne pathogens has been demonstrated in many horticultural crops throughout the world. In many cases, such nematode–fungus disease complexes involve root-knot nematodes *Meloidogyne* species, although several other endoparasitic like *Globodera* species, *Heterodera* species, *Rotylenchulus* species, *Pratylenchus* species and ectoparasitic *Xiphinema* species, *Longidorus* species nematodes have been associated with diseases caused by soilborne fungal pathogens. As early as 1892, it was reported that root-knot nematodes (*Meloidogyne* species) interacted with the expression of Fusarium wilt resistance (*Fusarium oxysporum* f. sp. *vasinfectum*) of cotton (*G. hirsutum*), causing plants to be more susceptible to *Fusarium* than when nematodes are absent. A classic example in a horticultural crop is the biotic interaction of the predisposition of tomato (*S. lycopersicum*) to the wilt fungus *F. oxysporum* f.sp. *lycopersici* by the root-knot nematode *M. incognita*.

Since then, many more investigations on interactions between plant-parasitic nematodes and several fungi on different horticultural crops have been reported. The example of tomato (*S. lycopersicum*) affected by the complex *Fusarium-M. incognita* showed that tomato (*S. lycopersicum*) resistance to soilborne fungi differed when the nematode was present. This evidence is true also in other types of combinations: that is, *Meloidogyne* species and *F. oxysporum*. f. sp. *dianthi* on carnation (*Dianthus caryophyllus*); *Pratylenchus* species promote diseases induced by *Verticillium* and *Fusarium* on several hosts. In addition, interactions have been shown in coffee (*Coffea arabica*) with *Meloidogyne arabicida* and *Fusarium xylarioides*; and pea (*Pisum sativum*) with *Rotylenchulus reniformis* and *F. oxysporum* f. sp. *pisi*. It was no time at all before it was clear that nematodes "breakdown" genetic resistance to wilt-fungi. However, not all nematode and *Fusarium* interactions cause the breakdown of resistance. On watermelon (*Citrullus lanatus*), *M. incognita* and *F. oxysporum* f. sp. *niveum* do not interact, therefore the presence of one of these pathogens will not aggravate the disease caused by the other.

The reason plant cultivars that were ordinarily resistant to fungi then become infected by the fungi if previously attacked by nematodes is most probably related to morphological and physiological changes that occur in the nematode-infected plant, although it seems that mechanical wounding caused by nematodes to plants may also induce some host-response that lowers natural resistance to fungi.

Research using a split-root technique demonstrated that a portion of the root system not exposed to nematode damage was predisposed to Fusarium wilt as if it was part of the root inoculated with nematodes. This supported that root predisposition to fungal invasion is not restricted to the galled areas or sites of nematode activity. Similar relationships have been observed between other sedentary, endoparasitic nematodes, for example, *Heterodera* species, *Meloidogyne* species, and *Globodera* species. With some phytopathogenic fungi, the nematodes prevent the root invasion by fungi. It seems that antibiotic-like substances are involved.

Nematode-resistant rootstocks

As with soilborne diseases, grafting to a resistant rootstock has shown to improve resistance to plant-parasitic nematodes. Grafting cucurbits on resistant rootstocks is currently in use in several countries for managing root-knot nematodes. Rootstocks with resistance to plant-parasitic nematodes are available for cucumber (*C. sativus*), eggplant (*S. melongena*), muskmelons (*C. melo*), peach (*Prunus persica*), plum (*Prunus domestica*), tomato (*S. lycopersicum*), and watermelons (*C. lanatus*).

Again, organic growers often face nematode challenges with few effective control methods, making organic production more difficult and potentially less profitable than conventional production. With the use of appropriate rootstocks, grafting may be a useful technique for vegetable producers to overcome plant-parasitic nematodes.

Root-knot nematodes (*Meloidogyne* spp.) are devastating soilborne pests of tomato (*S. lycopersicum*) worldwide. Although a number of root-knot–resistant tomato (*S. lycopersicum*) cultivars have been developed, many resistant cultivars do not have all the other desirable horticultural traits including fruit type and quality, and resistance to diseases that are sought after by growers and consumers. Grafting tomato (*S. lycopersicum*) on nematode-resistant tomato rootstocks (such as the interspecific hybrid, *S. lycopersicum* × *Solanum habrochaites*) has been useful for reducing root galling and nematode reproduction that can result in significant yield increases over nongrafted nematode susceptible tomato (*S. lycopersicum*) cultivars. Two *Mi*-gene homozygous resistant tomato (*S. lycopersicum*) rootstock cultivars, Beaufort (*S. lycopersicum* × *S. habrochaites*) and Hypeel45 differed in their reactions to *M. incognita* populations. Although fruit yields of scions grafted on both rootstocks were significantly greater than on nongrafted plants, Beaufort was tolerant having significant root galling and nematode reproduction, while Hypeel45 was resistant having no significant galling or nematode reproduction.

Tomato (*S. lycopersicum*) hybrids and interspecific tomato hybrids (*S. lycopersicum* × *S. habrochaites*) are used to control plant-parasitic nematodes. The plant breeder needs to be aware that differences among resistant rootstocks exist and indicated that the plant breeder must test the new resistant rootstock in a production system before releasing it to the public. The inconsistent function of the *Mi* resistance gene in these rootstocks suggests the need to measure the rootstock performance in fields infested with nematodes to gauge the effectiveness of the rootstocks.

Cucumber (*C. sativus*) benefits from grafting because it is highly susceptible to *M. incognita* and *M. javanica* root-knot nematodes. Cucumber (*C. sativus*) grafted onto wax gourd (*Benincasa hispida*), squash (*Cucumis maxima*), and bottle gourd (*Lagenaria siceraria*) shows lower root galling and egg numbers than nongrafted plants regardless of the growing season. Cucumber (*C. sativus*) grafted onto wax gourd (*B. hispida*) increased growth and total yield and reduced nematode numbers in comparison to nongrafted cucumber (*C. sativus*). Melon (*C. melo*) is also highly susceptible to *M. incognita* and *M. javanica* causing considerable yield losses. Grafting melon (*C. melo*) onto pumpkin (*Cucumis moschata*) reduced root galling compared to nongrafted plants. *Cucumis metuliferus* has been proposed as a rootstock for melon (*C. melo*) because it effectively reduced root-knot nematode reproduction and disease severity and increased melon growth in comparison to nongrafted melon (*C. melo*). In some melon (*C. melo*), grafts with *C. metuliferus* fruit quality traits such as flesh firmness and total soluble solids were negatively affected.

Interspecific squash hybrids or intergeneric rootstocks have shown undesirable effects on fruit quality, thus grafting watermelon (*Citrulus lanatus*), onto resistant watermelon (*C. lanatus*), rootstocks would be a better option because of improved scion-rootstock compatibility and the elimination of the undesirable effect on fruit quality. On the other hand, some plant introduction lines of *Cucumis amarus* have shown simultaneous resistance to *F. oxysporum* f. sp. *niveum* race 2 and *M. incognita*, and, therefore, would be the preferred choice for fields infested with the fungus and nematode. A commercial rootstock *C. amarus*, Ojakkyo, is more effective in reducing root galling and root-knot nematode egg production than *L. siceraria*. The wild watermelon *Cucumis africanus* and wild cucumber *Cucumis myriocarpus* reduced *M. incognita* reproduction and root galling with no effect on watermelon (*C. lanatus*) yield components. The resistance of these wild *Cucumis* species is related to the failure of the J2 nematode stage to establish feeding sites, inhibition of J2 development, and conversion of J2 to males. *Cucumis pustulatus* is resistant to both *F. oxysporum* f. sp. *niveum* and *M. incognita* and is highly compatible with cucumber (*C. sativus*), melon (*C. melo*), and watermelon (*C. lanatus*). Grafted plants increased plant growth and yield with no adverse effect on fruit quality in comparison to nongrafted plants.

Recent advances now make it possible to exploit specific aspects of plant-parasitic nematode and host—plant interactions to design control strategies that include enabling plants to prevent nematode invasion, reduce the effectiveness of nematode migration through tissues, prevent successful establishment, and reduce feeding ability and nematode fecundity. Therefore when breeding resistant rootstocks, it is important to identify the *Meloidogyne* species that are present at moderate to high populations in each field where the rootstock will be used to achieve root-knot nematode control.

Conclusion

Plant-parasitic nematodes are among the most notoriously difficult crop pests to control. Historically, minimizing nematode-induced crop damage is achieved with the utilization of plant resistance, crop rotation, and cultural practices. In Chapter 1, we point out that the plant breeder must consider two distinct biological systems, the plant and the pathogen. When nematodes are introduced in the breeding equation, three biological systems must be considered. Collaborating with a nematologist can expedite the development of plant-parasitic nematode-resistant crop cultivars. Nematologists need to understand the nature and timeline of cultivar development. For an annual self-pollinating crop, normally 10 years or more are required to develop a new cultivar. Even with the use of climate-controlled facilities, it is a time-consuming undertaking. After the development of the initial plant-parasite nematode-resistant cultivar, there are additional improvements to be made in yield, quality, and other resistances.

One can expect the 21st century to be exciting and prolific in the development of nematode-, and disease-resistant horticultural crop cultivars. The heightened concerns for the environment will increase the importance of plant breeding, helping growers rely less result on pesticides as a control tactic. Fundamental studies in the plant sciences will generate new approaches to breeding plant-parasitic nematode resistance in horticultural crops. With the lowering costs associated with sequencing biological genomes, this technology will improve the efficiency of plant breeding by expediting the movement of desirable genes among genotypes within a species, allowing the transfer of novel genes from related wild species, and making possible the analysis of complex polygenic characters as ensembles of single genes. The ability to improve the efficiency of the integration of resistance genes from wild relatives by reducing the number of backcrosses is particularly important for the development of plant-parasitic nematode resistance.

The ability to introduce synthetic transgenes will increase the availability of genes that can contribute to desired resistances. Furthermore, an important feature of transgene technology is the necessity of a plant regeneration phase to recover transformed plants. Currently, certain genotypes of a plant species are more amenable to regeneration than others, for example, *Capsicum* is recalcitrant to genetic transformation. The opportunities and challenges for plant breeders are exciting. With the increased priority placed on breeding for resistance, one can hope that it will result in additional funding for this research area. The combination of new molecular tools with conventional breeding methodology should greatly enhance progress in the development of cultivars with multiple resistance to nematodes and diseases.

Bibliography

Aarts, J.M.M.J.G., Hontelez, J.G.J., Fischer, P., Verkerk, R., van Kammen, A., Zabel, R., 1991. Acid phosphatase-11, a tightly linked molecular marker for root-knot nematode resistance in tomato: from protein to gene using PCR and degenerate primers containing deoxyinosine. Plant Molecular Biology 16, 647–661. Available from: https://doi.org/10.1007/BF00023429.

Ayala-Doñas, A., de Cara-García, M., Talavera-Rubia, M., Verdejo-Lucas, S., 2020. Management of soil-borne fungi and root-knot nematodes in cucurbits through breeding for resistance and grafting. Agronomy 10 (11), 1641. Available from: https://doi.org/10.3390/agronomy10111641.

Back, M.A., Haydock, P.P.J., Jenkinson, P., 2002. Disease complexes involving plant parasitic nematodes and soilborne pathogens. Plant Pathology 51, 683–697. Available from: https://doi.org/10.1046/j.1365-3059.2002.00785.x.

Bingefors, S., 1982. Nature of inherited nematode resistance in plants. In: Harris, K.F., Maramorsch, K. (Eds.), Pathogens, Vectors, and Plant Disease. Academic Press, Orlando, FL, eBook ISBN: 9781483273488.

Chitwood, D.J., 2002. Phytochemical based strategies for nematode control. Annual Review of Phytopathology 40, 221–249. Available from: https://doi.org/10.1146/annurev.phyto.40.032602.130045.

de Almeida Engler, J.B., Favery, G., Engler, Abad, P., 2005. Loss of susceptibility as an alternative for nematode resistance. Current Opinion in Biotechnology 16, 112–117. Available from: https://doi.org/10.1016/j.copbio.2005.01.009.

Dunbar, K.B., Stephens, C.T., 1989. An in vitro screen for detecting resistance in Pelargonium somaclones to bacterial blight of geranium. Plant Disease 73, 910–912.

Fassuliotis, G., 1985. The role of the nematologist in the development of resistant cultivars. In: Sasser, J.N., Carter, C.C. (Eds.), An Advanced Treatise on Meloidogyne, Vol: 1: Biology and Control. North Carolina State University Graphics, Raleigh.

Fassuliotis, G., 1987. Genetic basis of plant resistance to nematodes. In: Veech, J.A., Dickson, D.W. (Eds.), Vistas on Nematology: A Commemoration of the Twenty-fifth Anniversary of the Society of Nematologists, Orlando, Florida, USA.

Fassuliotis, G., Deakin, J.R., Hoffman, J.C., 1970. Root-knot nematode resistance in snap beans: breeding and nature of resistance. Journal of the American Society for Horticultural Science 95, 640–645. Available from: https://doi.org/10.21273/JASHS.95.5.640.

Fosu-Nyarko, J., Jones, M.G.K., 2015. Chapter fourteen - application of biotechnology for nematode control in crop plants. Advances in Botanical Research 73, 339–376. Available from: https://doi.org/10.1016/bs.abr.2014.12.012.

France, R.A., Abawi, G.S., 1994. Interaction between *Meloidogyne incognita* and *Fusarium oxysporum* f. sp. *phaseoli* on selected bean genotypes. Journal of Nematology 26, 467–474.

Fuller, V.L., Lilley, C.J., Urwin, P.E., 2008. Nematode resistance. New Phytologist 180, 27–44. Available from: https://doi.org/10.1111/j.1469-8137.2008.02508.x.

Gheysen, G., Vanholme, B., 2007. RNAi from plants to nematodes. Trends in Biotechnology 25, 89–92. Available from: https://doi.org/10.1016/j.tibtech.2007.01.007.

Guan, W., Zhao, X., Dickson, D.W., Mendes, M.L., Thies, J., 2014. Root-knot nematode resistance, yield, and fruit quality of specialty melons grafted onto *Cucumis metulifer*. HortScience: a Publication of the American Society for

Horticultural Science 49, 1046–1051. Available from: https://doi.org/10.21273/HORTSCI.49.8.1046.

Guan, W., Haseman, D., Nowaskie, D., 2020. Rootstock evaluation for grafted cucumbers grown in high tunnels: yield and plant growth. HortScience: A Publication of the American Society for Horticultural Science 55, 914–919. Available from: https://doi.org/10.21273/HORTSCI14867-20.

Jesse, T., Wijbrandi, J., Heinen, L., Hogers, R., Frijters, A., Groenendijk, J., et al., 1998. The tomato Mi-1 gene confers resistance to both root-knot nematodes and potato aphids. Nature Biotechnology 16, 1365–1369. Available from: https://doi.org/10.1038/4350.

Jones, J.T., Haegeman, A., Danchin, E.G.J., Gaur, H.S., Helder, J., Jones, M.G.K., et al., 2013. Top 10 plant-parasitic nematodes in molecular plant pathology. Molecular Plant Pathology 14, 946–961. Available from: https://doi.org/10.1111/mpp.12057.

Karaağaç, O., Balkaya, A., 2013. Interspecific hybridization and hybrid seed yield of winter squash (*Cucurbita maxima* Duch.) and pumpkin (*Cucurbita moschata* Duch.) lines for rootstock breeding. Scientia Horticulturae 149, 9–12. Available from: https://doi.org/10.1016/j.scienta.2012.10.021.

López-Pérez, J.-A., Le Strange, M., Kaloshian, I., Ploeg, A.T., 2006. Differential response of Mi gene-resistant tomato rootstocks to root-knot nematodes (*Meloidogyne incognita*). Crop Protection 25, 382–388. Available from: https://doi.org/10.1016/j.cropro.2005.07.001.

Marques de Carvalho, L., Benda, N.D., Vaughan, M.M., Cabrera, A.R., Hung, K., Cox, T., et al., 2015. Mi-1-mediated nematode resistance in tomatoes is broken by short-term heat stress but recovers over time. Journal of Nematology 47, 133–140.

Ohkawa, K., Saigusa, T., 1981. Resistance of rose rootstocks to *Meloidogyne hapla*, *Pratylenchus penetrans*, and *Pratylenchus vulnus*. HortScience: A Publication of the American Society for Horticultural Science 16, 559–560. Available from: https://doi.org/10.21273/HORTSCI.16.4.559.

Omwega, C.O., Thomason, I.J., Roberts, P.A., 1988. A nondestructive technique for screening bean germplasm for resistance to *Meloidogyne incognita*. Plant Disease 72, 970–972.

Pofu, K.M., Mashela, P.W., Mphosi, M.S., 2011. Management of *Meloidogyne incognita* in nematode-susceptible watermelon cultivars using nematode-resistant *Cucumis africanus* and *Cucumis myriocarpus* rootstocks. African Journal of Biotechnology 10, 8790–8793. Available from: https://doi.org/10.5897/AJB10.1252.

Rick, C.M., Fobes, J., 1974. Association of an allozyme with nematode resistance. Report of the Tomato Genetics Cooperative 24, 25.

Roberts, P.A., 1990. Resistance to nematodes: definitions, concepts, and consequences. In: Starr, J.L. (Ed.), Methods for Evaluating Plant Species for Resistance to Plant-Parasitic Nematodes. Society of Nematologists.

Roberts, P.A., Matthews, W.C., Veremis, J.C., 1998. Genetic mechanisms of host-plant resistance to nematodes. In: Barker, K.R., Pederson, G.A., Windham, G.L., Bartels, J.M. (Eds.), Plant and Nematode Interactions. Agronomy Monographs. American Society of Agronomy, Madison, WI, USA. https://doi.org/10.2134/agronmonogr36.c11.

Sidhu, G.S., Webster, J.M., 1981. The genetics of plant-nematode parasitic systems. The Botanical Review 47, 387–419. Available from: https://doi.org/10.1007/BF02860579.

Smith, P.G., 1944. Embryo culture of a tomato species hybrid. Proceedings of the American Society of Horticultural Science 44, 413–416.

Starr, J.L.R.J., Cook, Bridge, J., 2002. Plant Resistance to Parasitic Nematodes. CABI, Wallingford, Oxon, UK, ISBN-13: 978-0851994666.

Tan, J.-A.C.H., Jones, M.G.K., Fosu-Nyarko, J., 2013. Gene silencing in root lesion nematodes (*Pratylenchus* spp.) significantly reduce reproduction in a plant host. Experimental Parasitology 133, 166–178. Available from: https://doi.org/10.1016/j.exppara.2012.11.011.

Tatu Nyaku, S., Amissah, N., 2018. Grafting: an effective strategy for nematode management in tomato genotypes. In: Recent Advances in Tomato Breeding and Production. IntechOpen Limited, London, UK. https://doi.org/10.5772/intechopen.82774.

Thies, J.A., Fery, R.L., 1998. Modified expression of the N gene for southern root-knot nematode resistance in pepper at high soil temperatures. Journal of the American Society for Horticultural Science 123, 1012–1015. Available from: https://doi.org/10.21273/JASHS.123.6.1012.

Thies, J.A., Ariss, J.J., Hassell, R.L., Buckner, S., Levi, A., 2015. Accessions of *Citrullus lanatus* var. citroides are valuable rootstocks for grafted watermelon in fields infested with root-knot nematodes. HortScience 50, 4–8. Available from: https://doi.org/10.21273/HORTSCI.50.1.4.

Walters, S.A., Wehner, T.C., Barker, K.R., 1997. A single recessive gene for resistance to the root-knot nematode (*Meloidogyne javanica*) in *Cucumis sativus* var. *hardwickii*. Journal of Heredity 88, 66–69. Available from: https://doi.org/10.1093/oxfordjournals.jhered.a023060.

Wang, L.H., Gu, X.H., Hua, M.Y., Mao, S.L., Zhang, Z.H., Peng, D.L., et al., 2009. A SCAR marker linked to the N gene for resistance to root knot nematodes (*Meloidogyne* spp.) in pepper (*Capsicum annuum* L.). Scientia Horticulturae 122, 318–322. Available from: https://doi.org/10.1016/j.scienta.2009.04.011.

Wesemael, W., 2021. Screening plants for resistance/susceptibility to plant-parasitic nematodes. In: Perry, R.N., Hunt, D., Subbotin, S.A. (Eds.), Techniques for work with plant and soil nematodes. CABI, Wallingford, UK, 2021. ISBN-13: 9781786391759.

Williamson, V.M., 1999. Plant nematode resistance genes. Current Opinion in Plant Biology 2 (4), 327–331.

Williamson, V.M., Kumar, A., 2006. Nematode resistance in plants: the battle underground. Trends in Genetics 22, 396–403. Available from: https://doi.org/10.1016/j.tig.2006.05.003.

Wright, J.C., Lacy, M.L., 1988. Increase of disease resistance in celery cultivars by regeneration of whole plants from cell suspension cultures. Plant Disease 72, 256–259.

Index

Note: Page numbers followed by "*f*" and "*t*" refer to figures and tables, respectively.

A

Abelmoschus enbeepeegeearnse, 176–177
Acid phosphatase-1 (*Aps-l*), 271–272
Acidovorax anthurii, 53
Activated disease resistance 1 (ADR1), 70–71
Adenosine 5′-diphosphate (ADP), 76–77
Adenosine triphosphate (ATP), 76–77
Adult plant resistance, 51–52
African cassava mosaic virus (ACMV), 252
African nightshade (*Solanum scabrum*), 183
Agaricus bisporus, 12–13
Age–related resistance, 51–57
  seedpods or silicles of money plant infected with white rust pathogen, 54*f*
Aggressiveness, 103, 268–269
Agricultural Research Service (ARS), 184
Agrobacterium, 232–233
Agrobacterium tumefaciens, 35–36, 233
Agromycin, 234
Agronomic crops, 227
Air circulation, 133
Air filters, 132–133
Airborne platforms, 161
Airlock-based systems, 132–133
Ají, 179
Albersheim, Peter, 86–87
Albugo candida, 53, 248
Alleles, 249–250
Alliance, 181
Allium roylei, 178–179
Almond (*Prunus amygdalus*), 273–274
α-tomatine, 26
Alternaria, 116, 146–147
  alternata, 229
  alternata f. sp. cucurbitae, 1–2, 205
  blight, 2, 229
  cucumerina, 177
  mali, 162–163
  solani, 189
American chestnut (*Castanea dentata*), 162–163
American Type Culture Collection (ATCC), 100–101
Ampicillin, 113
Amplified fragment length polymorphisms (AFLP), 211
Analysis of variance (ANOVA), 218–219
Aneuploidy, 189
Anguina, 267
Anthracnose, 146, 155
  Colletotrichum lindemuthianum, 255–256
  Colletotrichum phomoides, 1–2
  Glomerella cingulata, 146
Antibiosis, 14, 30
Antibiotic resistance genes, 108–109
Anticipatory breeding, 257
Antimicrobial agents, 22–23
Aphanomyces, 137, 146–147
Aphelenchoides, 267
Apodanthera sagittifolia, 162
Apple (*Malus domestica*), 28, 162–163, 235
Apple scab (*Venturia inaequalis*), 137
Arabidopsis thaliana, 11–12, 32–33, 69
Arachis hypogaea, 45
Area under disease progress curve (AUDPC), 75, 161–162
Arms race, 246
Asparagus (*Asparagus acutifolius*), 273–274
Asparagus officinalis, 47–48
Assessment of disease, 145
Autoimmune responses, 87–88
Avirulence genes (*Avr* genes), 68, 103–104, 247–248, 266
Avocado (*Persea americana*), 104
Avoidance, 46–47, 56, 255
AvrBs2 gene, 40, 104

B

Baby leaf lettuce, 127–128
Bacillus amyloliquefaciens, 274
Bacillus thuringiensis (Bt), 227–228
Bacillus thuringiensis eggplant, 227–228, 231–232
Backcross method, 197–199, 198*f*
Backcrossing, 198
Bacteria, 67, 107, 257–258, 265–266
  genetic variation of, 107–113
  transformation, transduction, and conjugation, 110–113

283

Bacterial angular leaf spot (*Pseudomonas syringae* pv. *lachrymans*), 83
Bacterial blight, 8
Bacterial cells, 107–108
Bacterial chromosome, 110
Bacterial leaf spot (*Xanthomonas campestris* pv. *vesicatoria*), 250
Bacterial leaf streak (*Xanthomonas oryzae* pv. *oryzicola*), 35
Bacterial spot resistance (*Bs*), 40
Bacterial variation, 109
Bacterial wilt (*Ralstonia solanacearum*), 216–217
Bacteriophages, 111
Banana (*Musa acuminata*), 1, 103–104, 183, 252
Banana streak virus (BSV), 12
Banana wilt (*Xanthomonas campestris* pv. *musacearum*), 252
Barley (*Hordeum vulgare*), 72, 186
Barley stem rust (*Puccinia graminis*), 72
Barratt, R. W., 153–154
Barriers, 32
Barrus, Mortier F., 9–10
Basic leucine zipper (bZIP), 237
Bean (*Phaseolus vulgaris*), 46–47, 195, 230, 236, 248, 269
Bean common mosaic virus (BCMV), 230
Bean leafroll virus (BLRV), 1–2, 205
Bean yellow mosaic virus (BYMV), 135–136
Beet curly top virus (BCTV), 185–186
Benton citrange, 200
Benzothiadiazole (BTH), 45
Bergelson, Joy, 246
Biffen, Rowland, 9–10, 67, 83–84
Biosynthetic gene clusters (BGCs), 237–238, 246

Biotechnology, 227
 approaches to plant-parasitic nematode control, 271–272
 cisgenesis, 234–235
 CRISPR-Cas 9 system, 235–236
 direct gene transfer/transformation, 232–234
 fungus-resistant GMO plants, 236
 future of GMO and disease resistance, 238–239
 metabolic engineering, 237–238
 pan-genomics, 231–232
 pyramiding resistance genes, 229–230
 resistance gene analogs/comparative genetics/synteny, 230–231
 tissue culture, 228–229
 viral cross-protection, 236–237
Biotypes, 14
Bioversity International, 182
Black pod (*Phytophthora palmivora*), 12, 162
Black pod rot (*Phytophthora tropicalis*), 12
Black stem rust fungus (*Puccinia graminis*), 37–38, 72
Blumeria graminis f. sp. *hordei*, 72
Botryosphaeria dothidea, 128
Botrytis (*Botrytis cinerea*), 2, 23–24, 146–147, 199
 plant defense to, 25–30
 resistance, 162–163
BOTRYTIS-INDUCED KINASE 1 gene (*BIK1* gene), 27
Bottle gourd (*Lagenaria siceraria*), 277–278
Brassica napus, 254
Brassica oleracea, 246–247
Brassica/Raphanus (BR), 107
Brassinosteroids, 46

Breeding. *See also* Classical breeding methods
 disease-resistant horticultural plants
  bountiful plates and plants of healthy peppers, 6f
  historical perspective, 7–8
  Koch's postulates, 8–13
  principal terms, 13–17
  terminology, 13
 host–pathogen, 157–158
 method, 67, 246–247, 263
 for multiple disease resistance, 205
 disease-resistant rootstock, 214–223
 F_1 hybrids, 208f
 GWAS, 211–214
 interactions, 206–210
 marker serendipity, 214
 MAS, 210–211
 seed packet of Celebrity tomato, 206f
 strategies, 43
 symbols, 201–203
Bremia lactucae, 53–54, 132–133, 248
Bridge crosses, 179
Bridging-host hypothesis, 9
Broad bean (*Vicia faba*), 33–34, 140
Broad spectrum resistance, 14
Broccoli (*Brassica oleracea* var. *italica*), 199–200
Bromegrass (*Bromus* sp.), 9
Brown canker (*Coniothyrium*), 146
Brown rots (*Monilinia fructicola*), 46, 49
Brussels sprouts (*Brassica oleracea* var. *gemmifer*), 199–200
Bulked-segregate analysis (BSA), 212–213
Burkholder, Paul R., 10
Burkholderia andropogonis, 35
Burrill, Thomas, 8
Bursaphelenchus, 267

C

Cabbage (*Brassica oleracea* var. *capitata*), 33–34, 146, 199–200, 231–232
Cabbage black rot (*Xanthomonas campestris* pv. *campestris*), 78
Cabbage yellows (*Fusarium oxysporum* f. sp. *conglutinans*), 135–136
Cacao (*Theobroma cacao*), 12
Callus cultures, 228–229
Camelina sativa, 12–13
Campbell, C. Lee, 161–162
Campbell, Laurence V., 161–162
Candytuft (*Iberis sempervirens*), 147
Cane spot (*Elsinoe veneta*), 49–50
Canola (*Brassica napus*), 236
Cantaloupe, 267
Capsicum baccatum, 179
Capsicum breeding programs, 164
Carbohydrate-active enzymes (CAZymes), 27
Carboxyl-terminal LRRs, 88–89
Carica papaya, 11
Carnation (*Dianthus caryophyllus*), 105–106, 147, 275
Carroll, Lewis, 245–246
Carrot (*Daucus carota*), 47, 270, 273–274
Cartographer, 213
Cassava (*Manihot esculenta*), 183, 252
Cassava mosaic virus disease (CMD), 252
Cauliflower (*Brassica oleracea* var. *botrytis*), 78, 199–200
Celery (*Apium graveolens* var. *dulce*), 147, 273–274
Cell-death–inducing proteins (CDIPs), 26, 28
Cells, 152
centiMorgan (cM), 211
Centraalbureau voor Schimmelcultures (CBS), 101
Cercospora, 149–150
Cervantes, Diana, 53
Chamber effect, 130–131
Changsha mandarin (*Citrus reticulata*), 200
Chenopodium album, 246
Chestnut blight (*Cryphonectria parasitica*), 162–163
Chile wilt (*Phytophthora capsici*), 5–6
Chinese cabbage (*Brassica rapa*), 147, 199–200
Chitinases, 236
Chloramphenicol, 113
Chlorophyll fluorescence, 148
Chr02–1126 marker, 211–212
Chromosomal breakage, 189
Chromosome, 86, 108
Chrysanthemum (*Chrysanthemum indicum*), 104
Cisgenes, 234–235
Cisgenesis, 234–235
Citrulus lanatus, 278
Citrus, 187
Citrus canker (*Xanthomonas axonopodis*), 146
Citrus tristeza virus (CTV), 200, 236–237
Cladosporium leaf mold (*Cladosporium fulvum*), 30, 205
Classical breeding methods, 195
 backcross method, 197–199
 breeding symbols, 201–203
 doubled haploids, 201
 hybridization, 196–197
 mass selection, 196
 pedigree method, 199
 pure line selection, 195
 recurrent selection, 199
 single plant selection, 196
 somatic hybridization, 199–200
Cleaved amplified polymorphic sequences (CAPS), 211
Clubroot disease (*Plasmodiophora brassicae*), 199–200
Clubroot-resistant cabbage (*Brassica oleracea* var. *capitata*), 199–200
Clustered regularly interspaced short palindromic repeats (CRISPR), 12, 187
Clustered regularly interspaced short palindromic repeats-associated protein 9 system (CRISPR-Cas9 system), 84–85, 235–236
Coccinia grandis, 162
Cochliobolus victoriae, 39
Cocoa (*Theobroma cacao*), 162
Coconut palm (*Cocos nucifera*), 104
Coffee (*Coffea arabica*), 128–129, 228–229, 275–276
Coffee berry disease (*Colletotrichum kahawae*), 128–129, 228–229
Coiled-coil sequence (CC sequence), 72
Cole crops (*Brassica* species), 273–274
Collections, 101–102
 culture collections, 100–101
Colletotrichum, 146
Colletotrichum lindemuthianum, 9–10, 45, 146, 255–256
Colletotrichum orbiculare, 1–2, 83
Colorado potato beetle (*Leptinotarsa decemlineata*), 227–228
Colorimetric sensor, 159–160
Commercial plant breeders, 175–176
Common scab (*Streptomyces scabies*), 149–150
Comparative genetics, 230–231
Conjugation, 110–113

Constitutive resistance, 14
Consultative Group for International Agricultural Research (CGIAR), 182
Controlled environment, 130–131, 133
Coprinus psychrombidus, 129
Core collections, 184–186
Corky root (*Pyrenochaeta lycopersici*), 166–167, 217
Corn (*Zea mays*), 149–150
Corn leaf blight (*Exserohilum turcicum*), 149–150
Cotton (*Gossypium hirsutum*), 205–206, 227, 266
Cotyledons, 152
Cowpea (*Vigna unguiculata*), 33–34, 205–206
Cowpea rust (*Uromyces phaseoli* var. *vignae*), 33–34
Criollos de Morelos 334, 215
CRISPR-associated protein 9 (Cas9), 12, 187
Crop management, 22
Crop production systems, 2
Crop yields, 1
Cropping systems, 127–128
Cross-pollinated crop, 196
Cross–protection, 14, 44–46, 236–237
  zucchini crop in greenhouse conditions, 44f
Cruikshank, Ian Alfred Murray, 41–42
Cryptic disease, 6–7
Cryptic resistance, 175
CsLOB1 gene, 187–188
Cucumber (*Cucumis sativus*), 1–2, 41–42, 76, 104, 135–136, 164, 201, 231–232, 267
Cucumber green mottle mosaic virus (CGMMV), 222
Cucumber mosaic virus (CMV), 1–2, 177, 201, 205, 233
Cucumber scab (*Cladosporium cucumerinum*), 1–2, 205

Cucumber target spot (*Corynespora cassiicola*), 1–2, 205
Cucumber vein yellowing virus (CVYV), 12, 235–236
Cucumis amarus, 278
Cucumis pustulatus, 278
Cucurbit aphid-borne yellows virus (CABYV), 177
Cucurbit leaf crumple virus (CuLCrV), 177
Cucurbita argyrosperma, 179
Cucurbits, 179
Curly top virus, 185–186
Cylindrocladium, 146–147
Cyst nematode, 266
Cytoplasmic inheritance, 85–86
Cytoplasmic male sterility (CMS), 86, 199–200

D

Dahlias (*Dahlia pinnata*), 146
Daily light integral (DLI), 140–141
Damage-associated molecular patterns (DAMPs), 70
Davis, Bernard, 157–158
de Bary, Heinrich Anton, 8
Decoy model, 87
Defense-related enzymes, 220–221
Dehybridizing seeds, 175–176
Deletion, 189
Derived cleaved amplified polymorphic sequences (dCAPS), 211
Developmental resistance. *See* Age–related resistance
2,6 dichloroisonicotinic acid (INA), 45
2,4-dichlorophenoxyacetic acid, 112–113
Diplodia, 146–147
Direct gene transfer, 232–234
Disease index, 148–149, 149f
Disease rating, 218–219
Disease resistance, 148–149
  evaluation of, 149–153

genes, 215
Disease screen, 148–149, 149f
Disease severity, 30, 149–150, 155, 159, 219
Disease Severity Index (DSI), 218–219
Disease triangle, 14
Disease-resistant horticultural plants, 156–157
Disease-resistant plants, 189
Disease-resistant rootstock, 214–223
Ditylenchus, 267
Ditylenchus dipsaci, 265–266
"Divide and Conquer" approach, 207
DNA, 233–234
  fragments, 109–110
  markers, 230
  molecules, 110
  plant virus, 106
  sequences, 12, 78
Domesticated tomato (*Solanum lycopersicum*), 168, 214, 247
Dominant resistance genes (*Dm* genes), 53–54
Double-stranded RNA (dsRNA), 272–273
Doubled haploids, 201
Downy Mildew, 163–164, 199, 238
  Bremia lactucae, 248
  Hyaloperonospora parasitica, 52–53, 78, 248
  Peronospora belbahrii, 184–185
  Peronospora destructor, 178–179
  Pseudoperonospora cubensis, 153, 177–181, 184–185, 205
Drosophila, 72
Duncan type grapefruit (*Citrus paradisi*), 200
Duncan's multiple comparison test, 218–219
Durability, 14
Durable resistance, 246–247

anticipatory breeding/
preemptive breeding,
257
emerging disease, 251–252
evolutionary forces, 257–259
Fusarium yellows symptoms
on susceptible cabbage
plant, 247*f*
multilines, 255–257
principles of disease control,
255
systems approach, 252–254
wise resistance management,
254
Dutch hyacinth (*Hyacinthus orientalis*), 56–57

E

Early blight (*Alternaria solani*),
189
Earworm resistant sweet corn,
227
East African cassava mosaic
virus (EACMV), 252
Ecballium elaterium, 162
Ectoparasitic *Xiphinema*
species, 275
Effector binding elements
(EBEs), 110–111
Effector function resistance
(EFR), 35–36
Effector triggered immunity
(ETI), 26, 70–71, 97
Eggplant (*Solanum melongena*),
185, 271
eIFiso4E, 187
Electrical resistance blocks, 139
Electromagnetic spectrum, 159
Electronic noses (e-nose),
159–160
Electroporation, 233–234
Elicitor, 33
Elicitor-Receptor Model,
86–87
Elongation factor Tu (Ef-Tu),
35–36
Elsinoe veneta, 49
Embryo culture, 180
Embryo rescue, 180–181

Emerging disease, 251–252
Endogenous apple scab
(*Venturia inaequalis*),
235
Endoparasites, 267
Endoparasitic plant-parasitic
nematode, 265
Endophytic bacteria, 31–32
English pea, 147
Enhanced disease
susceptibility-1 (EDS1),
238
Environmental interaction, 127
environmental variables,
135–137
growth chamber, 130–131
light, 140–141
monitoring equipment,
137–138
phytotron, 131–132
protected cultivation,
129–130
relative humidity, 138–139
soil moisture, 139
vertical farms, 132–135
Environmental variables,
135–137
Enzymes, 112
5-epi-aristolochene 1,3-
dihydroxylase (EAH),
36
5-epi-aristolochene synthase
(EAS), 36
Eradication, 255
Eriksson, Jakob, 9
Erysiphe cichoracearum, 1–2,
23, 74
Erysiphe necator, 12, 156
Erysiphe pisi, 1–2
Escapes, 269
Ethylene, 46
Ethylene-responsive factor
(ERF), 237
Ethylmethane sulphonate
(EMS), 186
Eukaryotic translation initiation
factor 4E proteins
(eIF4Es), 187, 235–236
Exclusion, 255

F

False flax (*Camelina sativa*),
12–13
Fava/broad bean (*Vicia faba*),
33–34
Fen gene, 214
Field resistance, 53–54
Filamentous fungi, 117
Fire blight (*Erwinia amylovora*),
8, 46, 146
Flax (*Linum usitatissimum*), 38
Flax rust (*Melampsora lini*), 38
Food and Agriculture
Organization (FAO), 1
Food and Drug Administration
(FDA), 12–13
Food chain, 264–265
Food Security, 25–26
Formae speciales (f. sp.), 9
Founder effect, 14
Fruits, 152
Fungal spores, 132–133
Fungi, 67, 114–115, 265–266
Fungicides, 81
Fungus, 25
fungus-resistant GMO plants,
236
genetic variation of, 114–119
horizontal chromosome
transfer, 117–118
host jump, 118–119
parasexual cycle, 115–116
sexual incompatibility, 117
sexual reproduction,
116–117
Fusarium, 146–147
Fusarium circinatum, 118–119
Fusarium crown and root rot
(*Fusarium oxysporum* f.
sp. *radicis-lycopersici*),
217
Fusarium head blight
(*Gibberella zeae*), 117
Fusarium oxysporum, 246–247,
275
Fusarium wilt
*Fusarium oxysporum f. sp.
conglutinans*, 135–136,
246–247

Fusarium wilt (*Continued*)
  Fusarium oxysporum f. sp. *cubensis*, 1
  Fusarium oxysporum f. sp. *lycopersici*, 1–2, 24, 99, 205, 208, 217
  Fusarium oxysporum f. sp. *melonis*, 177
  Fusarium oxysporum f. sp. *pisi*, 1–2
  Fusarium oxysporum f. sp. *radicis-lycopersici*, 207–208
  Fusarium oxysporum f. sp. *tracheiphilum*, 56–57
Fusarium xylarioides, 275–276
Fusarium yellows symptoms on susceptible cabbage plant, 247*f*

G

Gametangia, 116–117
Gametoclonal variations, 188
Garden pea, 1–2, 135–136, 205
Gas chromatography–flame ionization detection system (GC-FID system), 160–161
Gas chromatography–mass spectrometry (GC–MS), 159–160
Gene amplifications, 189
Gene pyramiding, 230
Gene-for-gene hypothesis, 67
Gene-for-gene system, 249–250
Gene-for-gene theory, 67–68
Genebanks, 183–184
Genepools, 178–179
General resistance, 13
Genetic composition, 10–11
Genetic engineering, 236
Genetic exchange, 106–107
Genetic linkage, 175
Genetic modified organism (GMO), 187
Genetic systems, 267
Genetic transformation, 190
Genetic variation, 103–104
  of bacteria, 107–113

of fungus, 114–119
of oomycetes, 113–114
of pathogens, 103–104
of viroids and viruses, 104–107
Genetically modified organisms (GMOs), 227
  crops, 11
  future of GMO and disease resistance, 238–239
Genome, 108
Genome sequencing, 30
Genome-wide association studies (GWAS), 98, 211–214
Genomic resources, 79
Genomic segments, 73–74
Genotype, 264–265, 268
  classes of disease resistance proteins, 71–72
  cytoplasmic inheritance, 85–86
  gene-for-gene theory, 67–68
  genotype-based selection methods, 79
  helper nucleotide-binding leucine-rich repeats, 70–71
  inhibitor genes, 84–85
  lock and key concept, 68
    interactions among genotypes of host and pathogen, 69*t*
  loss-of-susceptibility concept, 80–84
  marker-assisted selection, 78–80
  molecular analysis, 88–89
  nucleotide-binding and leucine-rich repeat receptors, 69–70
  quantitative disease resistance, 73–77
  resistance models, 86–88
    model of integrated decoys in NLR Protein Pairs, 88*f*
  six characteristics of quantitative disease resistance, 77–78

Genotype-by-sequencing method (GBS method), 74–75, 211–212
Gentamicin, 113
Gerbera hybrida, 23, 74
Germplasm, 258–259, 263
Germplasm repositories, 181–184
Germplasm Resources Information Network (GRIN), 182–183
Global Plan of Action (GPA), 182
Globe artichoke (*Cynara cardunculus*), 273–274
Globodera pallida, 265–266
Globodera rostochiensis, 265–266
Globodera species, 275
Glucanase, 236
Glycine max, 12–13
Glycosylinositol phosphorylceramide (GIPC), 26
Golovinomyces cichoracearum, 23, 74
Golovinomyces orontii, 72
Grafted tomato, 216–217
Grafting, 215–216, 222–223
Granular matrix sensors, 139
Grape (*Vitis vinifera*), 12, 23, 105–106, 156, 238
Grapevine Algerian latent virus (GALV), 105–106
Gray leaf spot (*Cercospora zeae-maydis*), 149–150
Gray leafspot (*Stemphylium solani*), 205, 247
Gray mold (*Botrytis cinerea*), 133, 147
Green beans (*Phaseolus vulgaris*), 146, 164, 230
Greenhouses, 75, 129–130
  greenhouse-grown tomato plants, 3
  tests, 268
Growth chamber, 130–131
Guard model hypothesis, 87

Gummy stem blight (*Stagonosporopsis citrulli*), 162
Gypsophila paniculata, 105–106
Gypsum blocks. *See* Electrical resistance blocks

H
Haploid organisms, 106
Haploid sporophyte, 201
HcrVf2 (resistance gene), 235
Heart rot (*Rhizoctonia solani*), 147
Heath, Michelle C., 33
Heirloom varieties, 176
Helper nucleotide-binding leucine-rich repeats (hNLRs), 70–71
Heterodera, 275
Heterodera avenae, 272
Heterodera glycines, 272
Heterodera schachtii, 272
Heterokaryon, 15
High resolution melting (HRM), 211
Historical perspective of breeding disease-resistant horticultural plants, 7–8
Hollyhock (*Alcea rosea*), 147
Holub, Eric, 248
Honesty or Money Plant (*Lunaria annua*), 53
Horizontal resistance, 73–74
Horsfall, James G., 153–154
Horsfall–Barratt Scale, 153–154, 165*t*
Horticultural crops, 231–232
Horticultural traits, 175
Host differential, 99–100
Host jump, 118–119
Host-pathogen evolution, 102
Host resistance
  quantifying, 153–156
  standard area diagrams for early blight severity on potato leaves, 154*f*
Hybridization, 195–197, 263
of *Capsicum chinense* in Thailand, 197*f*
Hybrids, 257
Hypersensitive resistance, 40
Hypersensitive response (HR), 14, 37–40, 98
  flax leaves displaying resistance and susceptibility to rust, 39*f*

I
Immune-suppressing molecules, 29–30
Immunity, 14
Inclusionary resistance, 25
Incubation period, 14
Induced mutation, 186
Induced resistance, 209, 235–236
Induced systemic resistance (ISR), 41–44
Infection efficiency, 14
Infection frequency, 15
Infection type, 15
Infectious period, 15
Inheritance of plant-parasitic nematode resistance, 266
Inheritance of resistance, 263
Inhibitor genes, 84–85
Inhibitor of Phytophthora capsici resistance gene (Ipcr gene), 84
Innate immune system, 22
Innate resistance, 15, 22–25
Institut National de la Recherche Agronomique (INRA), 229
Institut national de recherche pour l'agriculture, l'alimentation et l'environnement (INRAE), 254
Inter-simple sequence repeat (ISSR), 211
Interaction phenotype, 15, 145–148
  area under disease progress curve, 161–162
  automated data collection, 157–161
  detached leaf screening, 162–164
  disease screen/index, 148–149
  evaluation of disease resistance, 149–153
  quantifying host resistance, 153–156
  rating scales, 164–167
  scoring fatigue, 156–157
  statistics for assessing disease resistance, 167–169
Interactions, 206–210. *See also* Environmental interaction
International Board for Plant Genetic Resources (IBPGR), 182
International Center for Tropical Agriculture (CIAT), 182
International genebanks, 183
International Institute on Tropical Agriculture (IITA), 183
International Network for the Improvement of Banana and Plantain (INIBAP), 182
International Plant Genetic Resources Institute (IPGRI), 182
International Potato Center (CIP), 183
International Treaty on Plant Genetic Resources for Food and Agriculture, 182
Interspecific hybridization, 178
Isozyme, 211

J
Japanese pear (*Pyrus pyrifolia*), 116
Jasmonate, 46
Jefferson, Thomas, 1

JoinMap, 213
Jones, Jonathan, 87

K
Kamoun, Sophien, 87
Kanamycin, 113
Kedrostis leloja, 162
Koch, Robert Hermann, 8
Koch postulates, 8–13
Kompetitive allele-specific PCR (KASP), 211, 213
Kyuri green mottle mosaic virus (KGMMV), 177

L
Landraces, 176
Larkin, Philip J., 188
Late blight (*Phytophthora infestans*), 159–160, 189, 205
Latent period, 15
Leaf blight, 149–150, 229
Leaf mold of tomato (*Cladosporium fulvum*), 30
Leonards-Schippers, Christiane, 73–74
Leptosphaeria maculans, 254
Lettuce (*Lactuca sativa*), 53–54, 127–128, 166, 248
Lettuce corky root (*Rhizomonas suberifaciens*), 166–167
Lettuce infectious yellows virus (LIYV), 177
Leucine-rich repeat (LRR), 11, 32–33, 230–231
Leucine-rich repeat receptor-kinase (LRR-kinase), 35–36
Leucine-zipper (LZ), 72
Li, Zhi-Kang, 77
Light, 140–141
Light detection and ranging sensors (LiDAR sensors), 159
Light-emitting diode (LED), 134
Lily (*Lilium longiflorum*), 233
Lima bean (*Phaseolus lunatus*), 33–34

Limonium sinuatum, 105–106
Linde, Celeste, 257–258
Linkage, 213
  maps, 213
Linkage drag, 99
Litylenchus, 267
Longidorus, 275
Loss-of-susceptibility concept, 80–84, 187

M
Madeira vine (*Anredera cordifolia*), 183
Maize (*Zea mays*), 72, 117, 186, 227, 231–232
Maize bacterial leaf stripe (*Burkholderia andropogonis*), 35
Maize dwarf mosaic (MDM), 149–150
Maize leaf spot (*Cochliobolus carbonum*), 72
Male sterile cytoplasm, 199–200
Mandryk, M., 41–42
Mapmaker, 213
Mapmanager, 213
Marker genes, 234
Marker serendipity, 214
Marker-assisted gene pyramiding, 229–230
Marker-assisted selection (MAS), 78–80, 210–211, 271–272
Mass selection, 196
Mating types, 2
Mature seedling resistance. *See* Age-related resistance
McDonald, Bruce A., 257–258
McGee, Rebecca J., 213
McIntosh, Robert A., 257
McRostie, Gordon P., 10
Melampsora lini, 38
Meloidogyne arabicida, 275–276
Meloidogyne arenaria, 270–271
Meloidogyne enterolobii, 271
Meloidogyne haplanaria, 271

Meloidogyne incognita, 56–57, 147, 265–266
Meloidogyne javanica, 56–57, 270–271
Melon (*Cucumis melo*), 81–82, 177
Mendel, Gregor, 9
Mendel's laws, 85
Meristem, 152
Metabolic engineering, 237–238
Michelmore, Richard C., 53–54
Microbe-Associated Molecular Pattern (MAMP), 15, 21, 97
Microbes, 103
Mildew locus O gene (*Mlo* gene), 80–81
Mitochondria, 105
Moisture, 137
Molecular markers, 210–211
Molecular patterns-triggered immunity (MTI), 32
Monitoring equipment, 137–138
Monosporascus root rot (*Monosporascus cannonballus*), 177
Morgan, Thomas Hunt, 211
Moroccan watermelon mosaic virus (MWMV), 177
Multiline varieties, 255–257
Multiple disease resistance, 153
Multiple pest resistance, breeding for, 275–276
Mushroom (*Agaricus bisporus*), 12–13
Mutation, 186–188, 257–258
Mutation breeding, 186
Mycelia, 29
Myeloblastosis (MYB), 237
Myelocytomatosis (MYC), 237
Myriosclerotinia borealis, 129

N
N required gene 1 (NRG1), 70–71
National Science Foundation (NSF), 100–101
National seed banks, 182–183

Natural epiphytotic diseases, 145
Natural sources of resistance, 175–179
Navel orange (*Citrus sinensis*), 200
Nearest percent estimates (NPEs), 165–166
Necrotroph, 15
Nematodes (*Meloidogyne incognita*), 1–2
  management, 264–265
  nematode-resistant rootstocks, 276–278
  root galls, 147
  species, 263
Nep1-like proteins (NLPs), 26
NewLeaf, 227–228
Nicotiana benthamiana, 35–36
Nicotiana tabacum, 97
Nitrogen deficiency, 220
Non-Mendelian inheritance. *See* Cytoplasmic inheritance
Nonexpressor of PR gene (NPR), 238
Nongrafted tomato, 218f
Nonhost resistance, 15, 22–25, 34–35
Nonhosts green bean (*Phaseolus vulgarus*), 33–34
Nonrace-specific disease resistance (NDR1), 238
Nucleic acid, 104–105
Nucleotide binding and leucine-rich repeat receptors (NLR), 21, 67
Nucleotide sequence, 106
Nucleotide-binding site (NBS), 11, 32–33, 72, 230–231
Nucleotide-binding site leucine-rich repeat (NBS-LRR), 87, 104
Nucleotide–binding and leucine–rich repeat proteins (NB–LRR proteins), 5, 15, 34–35, 69–70, 76–77

O
Ocimum americanum, basilicum, campechianum, gratissimum, kilimanadascharicum, tenuiflorum, 184–185
Okra (*Abelmoschus esculentus*), 176–177, 267
Okra enation leaf curl virus (OELCuV), 176–177
Okra yellow vein mosaic virus (OYVMV), 176–177
Oligogenic, 266–267
Olive (*Olea europaea*), 217–218
Onion (*Allium cepa*), 48, 48f, 178–179, 273–274
Onion white rot (*Sclerotium cepivorum*), 137
Ontogenic resistance. *See* Age–related resistance
Oomycetes, 67
  genetic variation of, 113–114
Ophiostoma novo-ulmiin, 251
Orange bell pepper, 221
Oriental pear species (*Pyrus calleryana*), 46
Orthologs, 230–231
Orton, William Allen, 205–206

P
Pan-genomics, 231–232, 232f
Panama disease (*Fusarium oxysporum* f. sp. *cubensis*), 1
Panstruga, Ralph, 83
Papaya (*Carica papaya*), 70, 236–237, 273–274
Papaya ring spot mosaic virus-W (PRSV-W), 235–236
Papaya ring spot virus (PRSV), 1–2, 11, 177, 205
Parasexual cycle, 115–116
Parasexuality, 115
Particle bombardment, 232–233

Pathogen-associated molecular patterns (PAMPs), 15, 26–27, 70
Pathogen-triggered immunity (PTI), 15
Pathogenesis related gene (PR), 238
Pathogenic variants, 153
Pathogenicity, 15, 97–98, 102–103, 117–118
Pathogens, 21–22, 34, 97, 128, 246
  acquisition and maintenance, 98–99
  culture collections, 100–101
  genetic variation of bacteria, 107–113
  transformation, transduction, and conjugation, 110–113
  genetic variation of fungus, 114–119
  horizontal chromosome transfer, 117–118
  host jump, 118–119
  parasexual cycle, 115–116
  sexual incompatibility, 117
  sexual reproduction, 116–117
  genetic variation of oomycetes, 113–114
  genetic variation of pathogens, 103–104
  genetic variation of viroids and viruses, 104–107
  genotypes, 249–250
  host differential, 99–100
  pathogenicity/virulence, 102–103
  specialized and working collections, 101–102
Pathotypes, 15, 153
Pathovar (pv.), 16
Pattern recognition receptors (PRRs), 15–16, 21, 67
Pattern-triggered immunity (PTI), 35–36, 97
Pea (*Pisum sativum*), 33–34, 275–276

Pea enation mosaic virus (PEMV), 1–2, 205
Pea seedborne mosaic virus (PSbMV), 1–2, 205
Pea wilt (*Fusarium oxysporum* f. sp. *pisi*), 275–276
Peaches (*Prunus persica*), 5, 276
Peanut (*Arachis hypogaea*), 266
Peanut late leaf spot (*Phaeoisariopsis personata*), 45
Pear (*Pyrus communis*), 8, 146
Pecan (*Carya illinoinensis*), 166
Pecan scab (*Fusicladium effusum*), 166
Pedigree method, 199
Pepper (*Capsicum annuum*), 5–6, 32–33, 70, 99, 127, 152, 154–155, 203*f*, 209–212, 230, 253–254, 266
  screened for resistance to Phytophthora root rot, tray of, 149*f*
Pepper mild mottle virus (PMMoV), 230
Pepper veinal mottle virus (PVMV), 82
Peppermint (*Mentha* X *piperita*), 186
Perfect marker, 211
Peronospora tabacina, 41–42
Pesticides, 45–46, 255
Phaeoisariopsis personata, 45
Phaseolus vulgaris (bean), 230
Phenotype
  age-related resistance, 51–57
    seedpods or silicles of money plant infected with white rust pathogen, 54*f*
  cross-protection, 44–46
    cross-protected zucchini crop in greenhouse conditions, 44*f*
  effectors, 30–37
  hypersensitive response, 37–40

Flax leaves displaying resistance and susceptibility to rust, 39*f*
induced systemic resistance, 42–44
manipulation of plant architecture, 46–51
  onions with various levels of wax on leaves, 48*f*
nonhost (innate) resistance, 22–25
plant defense to *Botrytis cinerea*, 25–30
systemic acquired resistance, 40–42
  normal VF36 tomato plants, 41*f*
Phenylpropanoid biosynthesis, 42–43
Phoma, 146–147
Photocell, 153–154
Photosynthetic photon flux (PPF), 140–141
Photosynthetic photon flux density (PPFD), 140–141
Photosynthetic active radiation (PAR), 140–141
Physiological races, 209–210
Phytoalexin-deficient 4 (PAD4), 238
Phytoalexins, 16, 24
Phytoanticipins, 22–23
Phytohormones, 228–229
Phytophthora, 136–137, 146–147, 155
Phytophthora austrocedri, 137
Phytophthora blight, 211–212
Phytophthora capsici, 5–6, 98, 152, 209–210, 237–238, 253–254
  phenotypic response of New Mexico Recombinant Inbred Line-S plant 3 days after inoculation, 210*f*
Phytophthora colocasiae, 113–114
Phytophthora cryptogea, 39

Phytophthora infestans, 24, 73–74, 97–98, 251
Phytophthora palmivora, 12, 162
Phytophthora parasitica var. *nicotianae*, 97
Phytophthora ramorum, 252
Phytophthora tropicalis, 12
Phytoplasmas, 147
Phytotron, 131–132
Pineapple (*Ananas comosus*), 267
Pinus radiata, 118–119
Pitch canker disease (*Fusarium circinatum*), 118–119
Plant architecture
  manipulation of, 46–51
  onions with various levels of wax on leaves, 48*f*
Plant breeders, 127, 129–130, 175, 227
Plant defense system, 28
Plant disease management, 253
Plant germplasm, 184
Plant immune sensory system, 21
Plant immune system, 38
Plant immunity, 69
Plant protoplasts, 233
Plant resistance, 264–265
Plant tissue culture, 228
Plant-cell-wall degrading enzymes (PCWD enzymes), 27
Plant-parasitic nematodes, 263
  biotechnology approaches to plant-parasitic nematode control, 271–272
  breeding for multiple pest resistance, 275–276
  evaluating interaction phenotype, 268–270
  genetic variation for resistance, 266–268
  nematode-resistant rootstocks, 276–278
  RNAi-based nematode resistance, 272–275

sources of resistance, 270–271
Plantain (*Plantago*), 183
Plant–pathogen systems, 32–33
Plasmids, 108, 112–113
Plasmogamy, 115
Plasmonic nanocolorants, 159–160
Plum (*Prunus domestica*), 276
pmr6 resistance, 80–81
Poland, Jesse A., 73
Polyethylene glycol (PEG), 233
Polygalacturonase genes (PG genes), 27
Polyhouses, 129–130
Polymorphism, 248
Polyploidy, 189
Potato (*Solanum tuberosum*), 1–2, 24, 70, 97–98, 149–150, 183, 227–228, 254, 266
Potato aphid (*Macrosiphum euphorbiae*), 270–271
Potato early blight (*Alternaria grandis*), 154
Potato spindle tuber disease (PSTVd), 105
Potato virus X (PVX), 189
Potato virus Y (PVY), 4, 189, 230
Potyvirus, 78–79
Powdery mildew, 12, 156, 199, 205, 238
  Erysiphe pisi, 205
  Podosphaera aphanis, 52
  Podosphaera xanthii, 153, 177, 180–181, 185–186, 205
Pratylenchus, 275
Pratylenchus thornei, 273–274
Pre-formed resistance, 67
Presence/absence variations (PAV), 231–232
Prevost, Isaac Benedict, 8
Programmed cell death (PCD), 39
Promoter, 234
Protected cultivation, 129–130
Protection, 30–31, 255

Protoplast fusion, 271
Protoplasts, 233–234
Prunus domestica, 49
Pseudomonas syringae, 108–109
Pseudomonas syringae pv. *glycinea*, 11
Pseudomonas syringae pv. *lachrymans*, 1–2
Pseudoperonospora cubensis, 1–2, 83
Pto locus, 214
Puccinia chrysanthemi, 37–38
Puccinia dispersa, 37–38
Puccinia helianthin, 99
Puccinia psidii, 118–119
Puccinia tritcina, 7, 9, 37–38, 99, 257
Pumpkin (*Cucurbita maxima*), 215–216, 277–278
Pumpkin (*Cucurbita pepo*), 237
Pure line selection, 195
Pyramiding resistance genes, 229–230
Pyrus pyrifolia, 116
Pythium, 134, 137, 146–147

Q
Qualitative resistance, 254
Quantitative disease resistance (QDR), 16, 73–77
  six characteristics of, 77–78
Quantitative resistance, 254
Quantitative resistance loci (QRL), 16
Quantitative resistance traits (QRT), 73–74
Quantitative trait loci (QTL), 16, 53–54, 73–74, 98, 128, 211–212
Quantitative trait nucleotide (QTN), 16, 78

R
R-genes, 269
Race-specific resistance, 212–213
Races, 16
Radish (*Raphanus sativus*), 199–200

Radopholus similis, 265
Ralstonia, 101
Ralstonia pseudosolanacearum, 108–109
Ralstonia solanacearum, 1, 35–36, 72, 108–109, 213–214
Ralstonia solanacearum species complex (RSSC), 108–109
Random amplification of polymorphic DNA (RAPD), 211
Rating scales, 164–167
  Horsfall–Barratt Scale, 165*t*
Reactive oxygen species (ROS), 21
Receptor like proteins (RLPs), 26–27
Receptor-like cytoplasmic protein kinases gene (*RLCK* gene), 27
Receptor-like kinases (RLKs), 26–27
Recombinant inbred lines (RILs), 210*f*
Recurrent parent, 149–150
Recurrent selection, 199
Red bell pepper, 221
Red queen, 245–246
Red–green–blue (RGB), 159
ReFen 1, 186
Relative humidity (RH), 135, 137–139
Reproduction rate, 16
Required for Mla specified resistance (RAR), 238
Resistance, 16, 255
Resistance genes, 266–267
  protein, 87–88
  pyramids, 258
Resistance interaction phenotypes, 35, 145
Resistance models, 86–88
  model of integrated decoys in NLR Protein Pairs, 88*f*
Resistance phenotype, 148
Resistant accessions, 185
Resistant genes, 11

Resistant germplasm, 270
Resistant rootstock, 214–215
Restriction fragment length polymorphism (RFLP), 211, 272
Rhizoctonia, 146–147
Ribosomes, 105
Rice (*Oryza sativa*), 11–12, 31–32, 69
  defensive system, 77
Rice black spot (*Xanthomonas oryzae* pv. *oryzae*), 35
Ripe rot (*Gloeosporium fructigenum*), 180–181
Ripening-inhibitor tomatoes, 227
RNA interference (RNAi), 82, 272–273
  RNAi–based nematode resistance, 272–275
  technique, 85
RNA plant virus, 106
RNA-containing sequences, 272–273
Robigus, 7
Root rot (*Aphanomyces euteiches*), 147, 152
  diseases, 159
Root-knot nematode (*Meloidogyne incognita*), 208, 264–265, 269, 277
Root-lesion nematode (*Pratylenchus brachyurus*), 267
Rootstocks, 215–216, 222–223, 272
Rose (*Rosa* sp.), 99, 185, 199
Rose black spot (*Diplocarpon rosae*), 99, 185, 199
Rose rosette disease (RRD), 199
Rose-scented geranium (*Pelargonium graveolens*), 229
Ross, A. Frank, 45
Rotylenchulus, 275
Rotylenchulus reniformis, 275–276
Row spacing, 127–128
Rubus idaeus, 49

Rust
  Puccinia antirrhini, 147
  Puccinia malvacearum, 147
  Puccinia sorghi, 149–150
  Uromyces caryophyllinus, 147
Rust (*Puccinia graminis* f. sp. *tritici*), 10

S

Saha, Partha, 78
Salicylic acid, 40
Sansome, Eva, 113–114
Scab (*Streptomyces scabie*), 189
Scarlet runner bean (*Phaseolus coccineus*), 230
Scarlet wisteria (*Sesbania grandiflora*), 183
Scion, 215–216
Scoring fatigue, 156–157
Scowcraft, William R., 188
Screening
  methods, 251
  protocol, 268
Seedless grape cultivars, 180
Seeds, 152
Selection, 195
Semiochemicals, 160–161
Sensor nucleotide-binding leucine-rich repeat receptors (sNLRs), 70–71
Sequence-related amplified polymorphism (SRAP), 211
Sequenced Characterized Amplified Regions (SCAR), 272
Sequential inoculations, 153
Serine kinase catalytic region, 71
Sexual incompatibility, 117
Sexual recombination, 103–104
Sexual reproduction, 116–117
Shapiro-Wilk test, 218–219
Shotgun method, 232–233
Sicana odorifera, 162
Sigatoka leaf spot disease (*Mycosphaerella fijiensis*), 186

Single nucleotide polymorphisms (SNPs), 74–75
Single plant selection, 196
Single-celled organisms, 115–116
Single-nucleotide polymorphism (SNP), 211
Small interfering RNAs (siRNAs), 272–273
Smith, Erwin Frink, 8
Snapdragon (*Antirrhinum majus*), 147
Snf1 kinase, 27–28
Snow mold pathogens (*Microdochium nivale*), 129
Soil moisture, 139
Soil temperature, 135–136
Soilborne disease, 160–161
Soilborne pathogens, 219–220
Soilborne plant pathogens, 159
Solanum acanthodes, 271
Solanum bulbocastanum, 36
Solanum lycocarpum, 271
Solanum mammosum, 105–106
Solanum peruvianum, 270–271
Solanum scuticum, 271
Solanum sisymbriifolium, 271
Solanum subinerme, 271
Somaclonal mutation, 189*f*
Somaclonal resistance, 189
Somaclonal variation, 188–189
Somatic hybridization, 103–104, 199–200
Somatic hybrids, 199–200
Sour orange (*Citrus aurantium*), 200
Sources of resistance
  core collections, 184–186
  embryo rescue, 180–181
  genetic transformation, 190
  germplasm repositories, 181–184
  mutation, 186–188
  natural sources of resistance, 175–179

somaclonal variation, 188–189
species bridge, 179
South African cassava mosaic virus (SACMV), 252
Southern blight (*Athelia rolfsii* = *Sclerotium rolfsii*), 217
Southern corn leaf blight (*Bipolaris maydis*), 149–150
Soybean (*Glycine soja*), 227
Species bridge, 179
Species jump, 118–119
Spectinomycin, 113
Sphaerotheca fuliginea. *See* *Podosphaera xanthii*
Spinach (*Spinacia oleracea*), 163–164
Spinacia oleracea, 246
Split-root technique, 276
Spontaneous haploids, 201
Spore production, 16
Sporulation capacity, 16
Spring mix, 127–128
Spur blight (*Didymella applanata*), 49
Squash (*Cucumis maxima*), 277–278
Squash mosaic virus (SqMV), 177
Stacking resistance genes. *See* Pyramiding resistance genes
Stakman, Elvin C., 10
Staskawicz, Brian J., 11
Stemphylium lycopersici, 247
Stemphylium vesicarium, 47–48
Stems, 152
Stewart's wilt (*Pantoea stewartia*), 149–150
Strain-specific resistance, 212–213
Strains, 16, 153
Strawberry (*Fragaria* × *ananassa*), 231–232, 273–274
Streptomycin, 113

Sudden oak death (*Phytophthora ramorum*), 252
Sulfonamides, 113
Sunflower (*Helianthus annuus*), 99, 231–232
Susceptibility, 17
Susceptibility genes (S-genes), 82
Sustainable agriculture, 43–44
Sweet basil (*Ocimum*), 184–185
Sweet corn (*Zea mays*), 5, 35, 149–150
Sweet corn smut (*Ustilago maydis*), 147
Sweet leaf bush (*Sauropus androgynus*), 183
Sweet pea (*Lathyrus odoratus*), 273–274
Sweet potato (*Ipomoea batatas*), 183
Synteny, 230–231
Synthetic cultivars, 201–203
Systemic acquired resistance (SAR), 27, 40–42, 45
normal VF36 tomato plants, 41f
Systems approach, 252–254

T
T-cytoplasm, 86
Temperature, 135
Tempered glass, 129–130
Tensiometers, 139
Terminology, 13
Tetracycline, 113
Theophrastus, 7
Therapy, 255
Threonine kinase catalytic region, 71
Threonine-protein kinase receptor (RPK2), 76
Thrips (*Thrips tabaci*; *Frankliniella schultzei*), 48
Tilletia tritici, 8
Time domain reflectometry (TDR), 139
Tissue culture, 228–229
Tm-1 allele, 222

Tm-2 allele, 222
Tm-22 gene, 3–4
Tobacco (*Nicotiana tabacum*), 33–34, 236, 266
Tobacco etch virus (TEV), 4, 72
Tobacco mosaic virus (TMV), 45, 135–136, 207–208, 236–237
Tobamovirus, 213–214, 222
Tolerance, 17
Toll-interleukin-1 receptor (TIR), 69
Toll-like receptors (TLRs), 32
Tomato (*Solanum lycopersicum*), 1–2, 24, 33–34, 70, 99, 159–160, 177, 205, 213–214, 231–232, 247, 266–267
high tunnel, 216f
somaclonal mutation, 189f
sources of resistance to, 178f
Tomato brown rugose fruit virus (ToBRFV), 2–3
Tomato canker (*Clavibacter michiganensis*), 146
Tomato mosaic virus (ToMV), 1–3, 178, 205
Tomato mottle mosaic virus (ToMMV), 3–4
Tomato spotted wilt virus (TSWV), 230
Tomato yellow leaf curl virus (TYLCV), 213–214
Transcription-activator-like effector (TALE), 110–111
Transduction, 110–113
Transformation, 232–234
Translocation, 189
Trifoliate orange (*Poncirus trifoliata*), 200
Trimethoprim, 113
Tuber scabs, 152
Tumor-inducing genes (T-DNA), 234
Turnip mosaic virus (TuMV), 107
Type A resistance, 135–136
Type B resistance, 135–136

Typhula incarnata, 129
Typhula ishikariensis, 129

U

U.S. Agency for International Development (USAID), 227–228
U.S. Department of Agriculture, 8, 97, 105, 117–118, 153, 165–166, 184, 205–206, 213, 250
U.S. National Plant Germplasm System (NPGS), 182–183
Ulocladium leaf spot (*Ulocladium cucurbitae*), 1–2, 205
UN Food and Agriculture Organization (FAO), 1, 182
Universidade Federal de Lavras (UFLA), 255–256
US Agency for International Development (USAID), 227–228

V

Van der Biezen, Erik, 87
van der Hoorn, Renier A. L., 87
Vanderplank, James Edward, 103
Vertical farming, 132
Vertical farms, 132–135
Verticillium wilt
  resistance gene orthologs, 230–231
  Verticillium albo-atrum, 1–2, 24, 205
  Verticillium dahliae, 114–115, 186, 207–208, 217
Vertifolia effect, 17
Viral cross-protection, 236–237
Viral-infected phenotypes, 105
Viroids, 104
  genetic variation of, 104–107
Virulence, 102–103
Virulence profile, 17
Virulence source population, 17
Virulent nematodes, 265–266

Virus-resistant papaya, 227
Virus-resistant summer squash (*Cucurbit pepo*), 227
Viruses, 2, 67, 104, 257–258
  genetic variation of, 104–107
Visual fatigue, 156
Vitis cinerea, 23
Vitis davidii, 23
Vitis doaniana, 23
Vitis labrusca, 23
Volatile organic compounds (VOCs), 159–160

W

Ward, Harry Marshall, 9
Watermelon (*Citrullus lanatus*), 215–216, 237, 275–276
Watermelon chlorotic stunt virus (WmCSV), 177
Watermelon mosaic virus (WMV), 1–2, 177, 205, 237
Wax gourd (*Benincasa hispida*), 277–278
Weber–Fechner law, 153–154
Western flower thrips (*Frankliniella occidentalis*), 132–133
Wheat (*Triticum aestivum*), 7, 37–38, 67, 99, 257
Wheat bunt (*Tilletia tritici*), 8
Wheat leaf rust (*Puccinia triticina*), 152
Wheat–leaf yellow rust (*Puccinia glumarum*), 37–38
White mold disease (*Sclerotinia sclerotiorum*), 2, 29, 47, 164, 184, 230
White pine blister rust (*Cronartium ribicola*), 118–119
White rot (*Coniothyrium diplodiella*), 180–181
Wide hybridization, 17
Wild radish (*Raphanus raphanistrum*), 43

Wild watermelon (*Cucumis africanus*), 278
Wild woodland strawberries (*Fragaria vesca*), 23–24
Winter squash fruit (*Cucurbita moschata*), 55
Wise gene management, 254
Wise resistance management, 254
World Federation of Culture Collections (WFCC), 101
World *Phytophthora* Genetic Resource Collection (WPC), 101
World Vegetable Center (WorldVeg), 183
Wound-induced resistance, 30
WRKY, 237

X

Xanthomonas spp., 101, 110–111
Xanthomonas campestris, 16, 104, 248
Xanthomonas euvesicatoria, 111
Xanthomonas hyacinthi, 56–57
Xanthomonas oryzae pv. *oryzae*, 77
Xanthomonas oryzae pv. *oryzicola*, 35
Xylella fastidiosa, 11

Y

Yam (*Dioscorea alata*), 183, 229
Yellow bell pepper, 221
Yellow leaf blight of maize (*Didymella zeaemaydis*), 86
Yellow rust (*Phragmidium rubi-idaei*), 49, 67

Z

Zehneria pallidinervia, 162
Zoospores, 113–114, 209–210
Zucchini yellow mosaic virus (ZYMV), 1–2, 12, 44, 177, 205, 235–236
Zygote, 116–117

Printed in the United States
by Baker & Taylor Publisher Services